Occupational Asthma

EMIL J. BARDANA, JR., MD
Professor & Vice Chairman, Department
of Medicine
Head, Division of Allergy and Clinical
Immunology
Oregon Health Sciences University
Portland, Oregon

ANTHONY MONTANARO, MD
Associate Professor of Medicine, Divisions
of Allergy and Clinical Immunology,
and Arthritis and Rheumatic Diseases,
Department of Medicine
Director, Occupational and Environmental
Allergy Laboratory
Oregon Health Sciences University
Portland, Oregon

MARK T. O'HOLLAREN, MD
Assistant Professor of Medicine, Division
of Allergy and Clinical Immunology,
Department of Medicine
Director, Allergy and Asthma Clinic
Oregon Health Sciences University
Portland, Oregon

HANLEY & BELFUS, INC./Philadelphia
MOSBY — YEAR BOOK, INC./St. Louis • Baltimore • Boston • Chicago • London
Philadelphia • Sydney • Toronto

Publisher: HANLEY & BELFUS, INC.
                  210 S. 13th Street
                  Philadelphia, PA 19107
                  (215) 546-7293

North American and worldwide sales and distribution:

                  MOSBY–YEAR BOOK, INC.
                  11830 Westline Industrial Drive
                  St. Louis, MO 63146

In Canada: THE C.V. MOSBY COMPANY, LTD.
                  5240 Finch Avenue East
                  Unit 1
                  Scarborough, Ontario M1S 5A2
                  Canada

Occupational Asthma   ISBN 1-56053-017-0

Library of Congress Catalog Card Number 91-58457

Last digit is the print number: 9 8 7 6 5 4 3 2 1

CONTRIBUTORS

DONALD W. AARONSON, MD, JD
Clinical Assistant Professor
University of Illinois Medical School
Chicago, Illinois

EMIL J. BARDANA, JR., MD
Professor & Vice Chairman, Department
  of Medicine
Head, Division of Allergy and Clinical
  Immunology
Oregon Health Sciences University
Portland, Oregon

DAVID E. GRIFFITH, MD
Associate Professor of Medicine
Department of Medicine
University of Texas Health Center
Tyler, Texas

RICHARD S. KRONENBERG, MD
Professor and Chairman
Department of Medicine
University of Texas Health Center
Tyler, Texas

JEFFREY L. LEVIN, MD, MSPH
Assistant Professor of Medicine
Department of Medicine
University of Texas Health Center
Tyler, Texas

JERRY WAYNE McLARTY, PhD
Chairman and Professor of Epidemiology
Department of Epidemiology
University of Texas Health Center
Tyler, Texas

ANTHONY MONTANARO, MD
Associate Professor of Medicine, Divisions of
  Allergy and Clinical Immunology, and
  Arthritis and Rheumatic Diseases,
  Department of Medicine
Director, Occupational and Environmental
  Allergy Laboratory
Oregon Health Sciences University
Portland, Oregon

MARK T. O'HOLLAREN, MD
Assistant Professor of Medicine, Division of
  Allergy and Clinical Immunology,
  Department of Medicine
Director, Allergy and Asthma Clinic
Oregon Health Sciences University
Portland, Oregon

SHELDON SPECTOR, MD
Clinical Professor of Medicine, Department
  of Medicine, UCLA Medical Center
Director, Allergy Research Foundation
Los Angeles, California

Acknowledgment

The Editors wish to acknowledge the many tireless hours devoted to
the typing of the manuscript by Ms. Edie Kacalek. As well, credit goes to
Mr. Robert Hare as the photographer for the majority of illustrations.

PREFACE

The major impetus that drove us to write and edit a book on occupational asthma originated both from an intense clinical interest in the area and from the lack of an available, up-to-date, comprehensive reference source. This lack became more apparent in the face of an impressive array of new chemicals and resin systems, which continued to be introduced into the work environment on almost a daily basis. The number of agents implicated in the causation of occupational asthma has grown steadily over the past several decades. For these reasons we decided the clinician was in need of a compendium that would provide a classification of the agents involved, their similarities and differences, and their clinical effects, and it should also offer a practical approach to the patient with suspected work-related asthma.

The basis of this text rests on our collective clinical experience with occupational asthma. We have attempted to provide the reader with a critical perspective of the available data, augmented by our own evolutionary learning process. We have taken a great deal of effort to ensure that the presentation is not a series of disjointed and sometimes contradictory chapters (as many multi-authored texts are inclined to be). Chapters are arranged in a sequential fashion, tending to build on each other and carefully interwoven to complement each other. We feel the book should be useful to any individual who evaluates patients with possible work-related asthma.

As we review the completed work, one recurring theme has been stressed throughout. When evaluating patients for occupational asthma, it is critical that the evaluator have a comprehensive and accurate account of the *medical history*. Without this essential foundation, the accuracy of the diagnosis suffers greatly. This is reminiscent of the anonymous admonition quoted by Paul Dudley White in the introduction of the second edition of *Clues to the Diagnosis and Treatment of Heart Disease*:

> . . . . A doctor who cannot take a good history and a patient who cannot give one are in danger of giving and receiving bad treatment . . . .

Emil J. Bardana, Jr., MD
Anthony Montanaro, MD
Mark T. O'Hollaren, MD

Chapter 1

BRIEF HISTORY OF OCCUPATIONAL MEDICINE

Emil J. Bardana, Jr., MD

I for one have done all that lay in my power, and have not thought it beneath me to step into workshops of the meaner sort now and again and study the obscure operations of the mechanical arts; all the more that nowadays medicine has been almost entirely converted into a mechanical art, and in the schools they chatter continually about automatism.

Bernardo Ramazzini
De Morbis Artificum, 1713

The inherent dangers of the workplace have been widely appreciated for many decades. The list of physical hazards has run very long, and has included everything from the unpredictability of inclement weather at sea to the overwhelming levels of irritating dusts and vapors regularly encountered by the ancient stone cutters, builders, and miners. The concept of occupational medicine began with the ancient physicians and scholars who took note of work-related problems. The *Sallier papyri* relate some of the unsalutory effects of certain occupations upon the Egyptians of that time. Hippocrates (460–377 B.C.) taught his pupils the cardinal feature of work-related disease by admonishing them to observe the environment of their patients.[1] He also provided the earliest descriptions of lead colic as well as many other toxic properties of this metal as a work-related disorder. Lead was one of the first metals man learned to produce. It was used extensively by the Egyptians and Romans for piping, cooking utensils, and pottery glazes. Some lead water pipes made by the ancient Romans are still in use today.

Part of the Greek philosophy of the ruling classes that prevailed into the early and middle ages was disdain for manual labor. Despite the admonitions of Hippocrates, very little attention was paid to the working classes and their occupational hardships.[2] Aside from these attitudes, many of the early physicians and scholars discussed the adversities of the work environment. Aulus Cornelius Celsus (25 B.C.–50 A.D.) was an ancient scholar who spent his life in the pursuit of broad learning. He authored eight books on medicine that made up his *De Re Medicina*, the only surviving portion of his writings. Though never given appropriate recognition during his life, the eight books were rediscovered by Renaissance scholars and were among the first medical texts to be published by order of the Pope.[3] It was Celsus who provided us with one of the earliest descriptions of bronchial asthma, in the eighth chapter of Book 4. He classified asthma into acute and chronic forms, and described its severity with respect to the presence of increasing dyspnea and orthopnea. He provided extensive directions as to its treatment.

The formal concept of allergy or sensitivity to work-related antigens does not appear until the middle ages, but the first mention of a severe allergic reaction "on-the-job" extends back to the death of King Menes of Memphis. Though controversial, it is said that he met his death as a result of an anaphylactic reaction to a hornet sting.[3] At the time, he was commanding an Egyptian boat under sail and heading back to his home port.

1

The second instance of recorded allergy could very well be construed to be of an occupational origin. It relates to Britannicus (Tiberius Claudius Germanicus) born in 41 A.D., the son of Emperor Claudius and his third wife, Messalina. Claudius gave his son the surname Britannicus in honor of his successful campaign in Britain, 43 A.D. However, Britannicus was maneuvered out of the line of succession by his father's fourth wife, Agrippina, who wanted the job for her own son, Nero. Britannicus' allergy to horse dander played a pivotal role in this political event. He as unable to ride at the head of the young patricians during ceremonies, because as soon as he mounted a horse, his face swelled, his eyes teared, and he developed a terrible rash. Therefore, the honor of leading the patricians fell by default to Nero, as the Emperor's adopted son,[3] who eventually poisoned Britannicus.

Perhaps one of the earliest forms of industrial hygiene was described by Pliny the Elder (A.D. 23–79) in his *Natural History*, who noted that stone carvers and miners covered themselves in sacks and used animal bladders as masks to protect themselves against heavy dust. Many of the earliest physicians and scholars such as Martial, Herodicus, and Pedanius Dioscorides discussed the influence of occupation on the health of workers. Dioscorides gathered a great deal of information traveling the known world as one of the surgeons serving in Nero's armies (54–68 A.D.). His *De Materia Medica*, in which are described over 600 plants and plant derivatives, became the leading treatise on pharmacotherapy *for 16 centuries*. It was Dioscorides who first recommended sulfur for its rapid and loosening action on the catarrh of asthma.

At about the same time, another notable Greek physician named Galen (130–201 A.D.) practiced medicine in Rome and wrote voluminously. Galen is often described as the greatest Greek physician after Hippocrates. He was among the earliest physicians to discuss afflictions peculiar to miners, tanners, fullers, chemists, and other craftsmen. Galen was one of the principal innovators of purging to expel the causative agent of illnesses. However, for asthma he believed, along with Dioscorides, in the efficacy of smoke from burning sulfur. He dispatched many affluent asthmatics of his time to the slopes of Mt. Etna to inhale its fumes.[3]

Georgius Agricola (1494–1555), a physician-scholar who lived in the mountains of Silesia and Bohemia on the German-Czechoslovakian border, observed workers in the process of mining and smelting of gold and silver. In his treatise on mining (*De Re Metallica*) he described the consumptive lung disease that prematurely took the lives of many miners.[2,3] Subsequently other observers recorded the relationship between occupations such as mining and quarrying and cough, dyspnea, and wasting disorders. In particular, Paracelsus (1493–1541), a Tyrolean physician, authored the first monograph on occupational diseases of mining and smelting operations (*Von der Bergsucht und anderen Bergkrankheiten* [On miners' sickness and other miners' diseases]).[4] This seminal work is in three books, the first concerned mainly with pulmonary diseases of miners, the second covering diseases of smelter workers and metallurgists, and the third addressing diseases caused by mercury.[31]

However, in connection with the subject of this chapter, one name among the notable early physicians stands out over all the others. In a century that produced Newton, Galileo, Boyle, Harvey, Malpighi, and Ivan Leeuwenhock, there was born in Capri in 1633 the father of occupational medicine, Bernardino Ramazzini (1633–1714). After graduating from the University of Parma in 1659, he continued his studies at Rome under Professor Antonio Maria Rossi. In 1670, he moved to Modena where he assumed the chair in medicine. During his life, his ability to observe, investigate, and then to describe illness has rarely been matched since his death. His pursuits marked him as a truly accomplished historian, poet, philosopher, clinician, epidemiologist, and sanitarian.[5] In addition to his classic descriptions of the occupational diseases of his day, Ramazzini left two statements that bear repeating as dictums for contemporary clinicians evaluating workers for possible work-related disease. The first was his warning to all physicians to ask of their patients not only the usual questions regarding their health, but also to inquire "of what trade you are." He also urged physicians to learn more about the nature of occupational disease by actually visiting the shops, sawmills, mines, and endless other work sites. Whereas Osler believed that clinical medicine was best learned on the wards, Ramazzini professed that occupational disorders were most effectively studied in the actual work environment.

Ramazzini's treatise on occupational illness, *De Morbis Artificum*, is considered a compendium of health hazards of the medieval crafts.[5] This celebrated monograph contains

41 chapters dealing with diseases in all types of trades, including silk workers, painters, dyers, glass makers, tanners, bakers, stone workers, metal workers, chemists, and others. A supplement to the work included 12 additional chapters on occupations such as printers, confectioners, grinders, and soap-makers. Ramazzini is credited with the earliest descriptions of "bakers' asthma." His clinical description of the disorder is classic, but his explanation for the mechanism is unusual and dated. He assumed that the inhaled flour-dust formed wads of dough in the baker's respiratory passages and thus obstructed breathing. Of those working with mercury, he observed that they became asthmatic, paralytic, and liable to vertigo. He noted that few persisted in that work, for if they did, they succumbed or became miserable with tremors, loss of dentition, and weakened limbs. He noted that ill health among workers not only stemmed from noxious dusts and fumes, but also from accidental falls, strains, and poor postures.

Although Ramazzini devoted most of his treatise to the manual trades, he also noted that the professionals had their vocational diseases. He observed that their knees would stiffen with too much sitting, and they would get constipated for lack of exercise. He also wrote about their eye strain from working far into the night over fine work by candlelight. Unlike the manual tradesman who would retire to bed tired and sleepy, scholars would frequently suffer from insomnia. He recommended a cup of warm chocolate, which had recently been introduced to Europe by the Portuguese.

Ramazzini was truly a patron to all laborers, who continue to benefit from his observations. While others may have championed the cause for better wages, shorter working hours, and better industrial relations, Ramazzini dedicated his life's work to improvement of the conditions under which men have to toil. He condemned the lack of ventilation and unsuitable temperatures, and urged that laborers in dusty trades should work in spacious, ventilated rooms. He recommended rest intervals in work of prolonged duration as well as exercise and correct posture. He established the foundations of industrial medicine and sanitation of contemporary times.

One of the earliest forms of occupational allergies among the professions was the result of ipecacuanha root (*Cephaelis ipecacuanha*) introduced from Brazil to European pharmacies as an emetic. This dried root has expectorant, anti-dysenteric, and emetic properties.

Its chief alkaloid was subsequently named emetine. Thomas Dover of Bristol had the unusual distinction of being both a physician and sea captain. He developed so-called "Dover's Powder," which contained both emetine and opium and which is still used for coryza and cough. Its great popularity meant that apothecaries were often called upon to grind the ipecacuanha root for prescriptions. Reports of adverse effects of inhaling the powder soon made their appearance. In 1776, Murray reported cases of breathing difficulty, nosebleeds, and eye irritation among pharmacists.[3] There is even a report of a pharmacist's wife experiencing asthma while her husband was preparing the root for use in prescriptions. A century or so later Armand Trousseau noted that some pharmacists had to turn over all such prescriptions to "non-allergic" colleagues and to leave the premises while the work was being done. Oddly enough, ipecacuanha became a major treatment for asthma right up to the turn of this century. A remedy that was favored as effective and without danger included two ounces each of tincture of lobelia and wine of ipecac to be taken every half hour until expectoration or nausea was induced. Subsequently, reports of asthma in pharmacists were also noted in the preparation of pumpkin seed and sulfur ointments.[3]

BIRTH OF EPIDEMIOLOGY

The earliest epidemiologic thinking dates to John Graunt (1620–1674), a member of the Privie Council in London in the mid-16th century. In 1532 a weekly tally was begun in London parishes on the number of persons who died from various causes.[6] This enabled the community leaders to keep track of the number of plague deaths and other deaths in the community. Graunt realized this wealth of data should be reviewed and synthesized to a few critical tables accompanied by a brief description and conservative interpretation.[6] He was moved to write his Natural and Political Observations Made Upon the Bills of Mortality, which went through four editions. However, his most important contribution may have been the devising of the life table based on survival, the predecessor of modern actuarial tables used in the insurance industry. Graunt used only two rates of survival, at ages 6 and 76.

For some 200 years after Graunt there was very little progress in the ideas he had put forth. It was not until William Farr (1807–1883) became the Superintendent of the Statistical Department of the General Register Office in 19th century Great Britain that some of these early epidemiologic concepts were expanded.[7] Farr instituted the first systematic evaluation of the relationship between occupation and the cause of death. He noted that grinders inhaled sharp particles of stone and steel and suffered excessive mortality after the age of 45. He also noted that earthenware manufacture was one of the unhealthiest trades in the country, with a mortality after age 35 that almost doubled the average.[7] Farr's law concerns the curve followed by the incidence of an epidemic disease, rising steeply at first, leveling near its peak, then falling more steeply than it rose.

Later, John Snow (1813–1858) was able to build on these initial observations and lay down the principles of modern epidemiology. Working on the problem of cholera deaths, he was able to recognize the association between exposure and disease and deduced the hypothesis that sewage in the water caused the cholera. He then collected evidence substantiating his theory and was able to minimize the collection of false information. Ultimately it was Snow's work that led to the prevention of cholera.[8]

In recent times epidemiologists have endeavored to study exposed persons rather than diseased individuals. Persons working in industry have daily contact with large numbers of exposures, including chemicals, noise, dust, heat, trauma, exertion, radiation, etc. Some of these exposures have ultimately been related to disease. This has led to the modern concept of the case controlled study and to conducting cohort studies in industrial populations (see Chapter 5).

Between the middle of the 19th century and the middle of the 20th century, epidemiology progressed quite slowly. Much emphasis was placed on the theory of how epidemics begin. Before 1940, cancer of the lung was essentially a medical curiosity, but as World War II ended, it became apparent that more males were dying of lung cancer. Around 1950 a number of studies were carried out to determine the reason for this increased rate of lung cancer. Among the many possible causes, tobacco abuse was a prime suspect. In 1947 Doll and Hill carried out an early example of a case-controlled study to determine whether patients with carcinoma of the lung differed from other persons in respect to their smoking habits.[9] The results of this study showed that 97% of persons with lung cancer were cigarette smokers and only 92% of individuals with other diseases were smokers. Conversely, only 3% of persons with lung cancer were nonsmokers in contrast to 8% of persons with other diseases. There was still a great deal of skepticism about the interpretation of these data, and in 1951 Doll and Hill undertook a large cohort study, sending a questionnaire to all British physicians and reviewing the death certificates of any physician who died in the next 25 years.[10,11] In reviewing those data, there appeared to be a significant relationship between cigarette smoking and lung cancer, with a death rate ten times the rate for nonsmokers.

DIFFICULTIES POSED BY DOSE-RESPONSE

The first man-made chemical was synthesized in 1856 in England. William Henry Perkin, a student of von Hofmann, produced an aniline dye called mauveine. Mauveine (mauve, chrome violet) was a dye prepared by the oxidation of a mixture of aniline and toluidine by potassium chromate. Its chemical name was phenyl-phenosafranine. It was extensively employed to dye silk reddish-violet in the textile industry. It also was used in the printing trades, and especially in the printing of postage stamps. In 1895, Ludwig Rehn (1849–1930), a German surgeon, reported the first three cases of bladder cancer in exposed workers. World War I interrupted importation of the dye, and in 1916 the Chamber Works were built in southern New Jersey to supply mauveine and other chemicals in the U.S. In 1931 the first cases of bladder cancer were diagnosed in workers from that plant, which eventually led to very strict production controls and finally its closure.[12] Unfortunately, it took many decades to recognize the fact that the disease would follow exposure only after a long latency period.

The issue of disease latency has and will remain a difficult concept to appreciate. This phenomenon has resulted in an understandable delay in accepting the potential health repercussions of asbestos exposure. Asbestos is a material that has been employed for many centuries. The Romans mined it from the Italian alps and the Ural mountains. Herodotus (circa 450 B.C.) described a cremation cloth made from asbestos, and Plutarch (circa 70 A.D.) described the perpetual lamps made of wicks of asbestos, which could not be consumed by fire.[13] In the late 19th and early 20th centuries asbestos was processed in the textile industry in a manner similar to that employed with cotton. Later its fire-resistant properties allowed its adaptation to a variety of building and insulating requirements.

One of the major oversights in early epidemiologic investigations of asbestos health effects was in a report by Walter E. Fleischer and his associates as part of a U.S. Navy study.[14] These investigators found no significant hazards resulting from insulation work in U.S. Navy shipyards. Unfortunately, the vast majority of the workers examined had begun work less than 3 years previously. The general assurances provided by this study, i.e., the very low incidence of asbestosis among pipe coverers in the shipyards (0.29% or 3 cases in 1074), influenced regulators for years to come in concluding that this material was not that dangerous in insulators. It was not recognized by these investigators that asbestos-induced malignancy and asbestosis required a latent period of between 10 and 20 years.

INDUSTRIAL REVOLUTION
AND WORKER SAFETY

The industrial revolution moved workers from the safety of their homes—so-called cottage industries—into large, poorly illuminated, and ill-ventilated factories. Typically during this era, wives and children as well as family heads had to work if the family unit was to survive. Within several decades following the signing of the Declaration of Independence, hundreds of spinning mills sprang up in New England. An experiment in progressive working conditions that attracted attention both in the U.S. and Europe was conducted in Lowell, Massachusetts in 1836. Young girls came in increasing numbers to work in its mills and were promised many benefits in their new work setting. Charles Dickens was very laudatory in describing his inspections of the Lowell factories.[15] Although touted as a showplace, the work day duplicated the sunup to sundown span on the farm, with 14-hour days required. After deduction of lodging and meals, the take home pay was $2.00.[16]

By 1836, the first child-labor law was enacted in Massachusetts, which required that every child under 15 years of age be given 3 months of schooling during the work year.[17] A year before that saw the appearance of the first American treatise on the influence of work on health.[18] In 1842 the Massachusetts

child labor law was amended to forbid children less than 12 from working more than 10 hours a day in factories. In 1847, New Hampshire established the first 10-hour work day, and in 1848, Pennsylvania banned children under 12 from working in textile plants. The age limit was raised to 14 in 1849. In 1868, the first federal law was enacted, limiting the work day to 8 hours per day for any employment on behalf of the U.S. Government.[17]

In 1884 Bismark initiated reforms in Germany to safeguard workers. In 1897, Great Britain developed a system of workers' compensation, under which the employer was financially responsible for injury or death regardless of fault. The amount of compensation was limited by statute and did not fully compensate for the injury.

The United States lagged behind Europe in protecting its workers. In 1877, Massachusetts passed the first occupational safety law, and in 1893 legislation was passed by the U.S. Congress regulating railroad safety.[19] It was not until 1911 that various states in the U.S. began to develop workers' compensation systems, the first of which were modeled on the British system. By 1920, 40 states had workers' compensation laws. Mississippi was the last state to pass such a law, in 1948. Most of these laws emphasized safety at the workplace.[20] The implications of these statutes are discussed by Dr. Aaronson in Chapter 3.

DEVELOPMENT OF
OCCUPATIONAL MEDICINE

Perhaps the earliest application of industrial medicine occurred on the southern plantations, where occasionally physicians were put on retainer to treat slaves.[17] In 1868 the first hospital devoted to the care of a company's employees was opened in Sacramento, CA. This enterprise was also the first to employ an industrial nurse.[21] In the following years, many eminent retail stores and related businesses instituted programs staffed by nurses, e.g., National Cash Register (1901), Gimbel Brothers (1902), and Filene's (1904).[17]

Industrial medicine was very slow to develop in the United States. Corporations were very strong and confronted the American workforce with a variety of new dangers by introducing new and complex machinery, toxic materials, and the use of lifting tackle and conveyors. In general these early work conditions were deplorable and represented an industrial ethic that placed property rights above human rights, i.e., industrial accidents were inevitable and simply represented the price of progress. Consider the following description of the work of enameling tubs in 1912 from Alice Hamilton's *Exploring the Dangerous Trades*[32]:

> In front of the great furnaces stood the enameler and his helper. The door swung open and, with the aid of a mechanism which required strength to operate, a red-hot bathtub was lifted out. The enameler then dredged as quickly as possible powdered enamel over the hot surface, where it melted and flowed to form an even coating. His helper stood beside him working the turntable on which the tub stood so as to present all its inner surface to the enameler. The dredge was big and so heavy that part of its weight had to be taken by a chain from the roof. The men during this procedure were in a thick cloud of enamel dust, and were breathing rapidly and deeply because of the exertion and the extreme heat. I found that I could not stand the heat any nearer than twelve feet but the workmen had to come much closer. They protected their faces and eyes by various devices, a light tin pan with eyeholes and a hoop to go around the head, or a piece of wood with eyeholes and a stick nailed at a right angle so that it could be held between the teeth.

In the early 1900s Dr. Alice Hamilton (1869–1970) was living among the immigrant working class of Chicago. She began her long career of studying toxic exposures in American workers, and her work on lead toxicity received national attention. In 1919 she was made an assistant professor of industrial medicine and became the first female faculty member at Harvard Medical School. She has been appropriately termed the matriarch of American Occupational Medicine.[22,23]

REGULATORY AGENCIES AND LEGISLATION

State workers' compensation laws came into being around 1910. New York State was the first to formulate such a law. It was initially very controversial and was declared unconstitutional. Subsequently new laws were upheld and by 1948 all states had such legislation. In 1914, the United States Public Health Service established an office of Industrial Hygiene and Sanitation. This entity was created to stimulate and carry out research in the field of industrial health. Subsequently this office became the Bureau of Safety and Health Services in the Health Services and Mental Health Administration. Under the Occupational Safety and Health Act of 1970, the latter was restructured to become the National Institute for Occupational Safety and Health (NIOSH). One of the primary functions of NIOSH is to provide recommended standards to the U.S. Occupational Safety and Health Administration (OSHA) in the form of criteria documents. Criteria documents for particular hazards are prepared from critical evaluations of all available relevant information from scientific, medical, and engineering research. The criteria document has become a widely accepted method of recommending standards. The method allows for the wide distribution of criteria to industry, academia, unions, etc. as a basis of controlling hazards. After due circulation the document is passed to OSHA where the data are synthesized and official standards are published in the Federal Register.

A very significant law affecting workplace safety in the U.S. was the National Labor Relations Act of 1935. This law legitimized unionization and collective bargaining. The Public Contracts Act (Walsh-Healey) of 1936 developed labor standards in government contracts, but it never proved to be forceful legislation.[24] The Fair Labor Standards Acts of 1938 defined the principles of maximum hours and minimum wages as applied to all workers of industries engaged in interstate commerce. Another landmark piece of legislation was the 1941 Federal Mine Inspection Act and the Federal Employees Health Service Act, which authorized federal agencies to institute limited occupational health programs. The Labor Management Relations Act of 1947 subsequently provided that an employee might quit work in good faith because of abnormally dangerous conditions.

The first air-quality standards were published in 1912 by Kobert and included 20 compounds.[25] In 1921 the Bureau of Mines published the first federal compendium.[26] Henderson and Haggard were the first to publish a list of substances that considered both acute adverse health effects and potential chronic effects.[27] In 1946 the American Conference of Governmental Industrial Hygienists (ACGIH) published its initial list of 140 substances.[28] This trend has expanded to include many other lists, and the number of compounds has grown considerably.

The Federal Coal Mine and Safety Act of 1969 established the start of the government's effort to provide a safe workplace through specific and detailed regulations. Finally, the Occupational Safety and Health Act of 1970 was passed, the product of many years of human experience with industrial environments.[29] The drafters of the Act realized that before the Occupational Safety and Health Administration (OSHA) could implement rule-making procedures outlined in the Act, there must be a set of standards in place. At the time the largest collection of such standards was the list of threshold limit values published by ACGIH. Additional standards were produced by the American National Standards Institute (ANSI). These were consolidated and published as a list of about 400 substances in a document called the Z-Tables of the current Code of Federal Regulations.[30]

SUMMARY

Work-related injuries have been an issue since the beginning of recorded history. Mankind had to endure a long series of work-related epidemics before the progress of the 19th and 20th centuries was made. If we are to improve our capacity to develop standards in a more timely fashion, consideration should be given to a more generic approach. That is, rather than attempting to develop industry criteria for specific chemicals on an individual basis, an effort should be made to develop standards covering groups of agents with the capaciity to cause injury in certain ways. This appears indicated in the case of neurotoxic agents, cholinesterase-inhibiting substances, and perhaps asthmogenic agents. Safety and health regulations are essential, and they must be designed, promulgated, and then enforced so that a reckless society is at least subject to some control, with a riskless society being the ultimate and probably idealized goal.[19]

REFERENCES

1. Chadwick MA, Mann WN: The Medical Works of Hippocrates. Oxford, Blackwell Scientific Publications, 1978, pp 90–111.
2. Morgan WKC: Historical and legal aspects of industrial disease. In Morgan WKC, Seaton A (eds): Occupational Lung Diseases, 2nd ed. Philadelphia, W.B. Saunders, 1984, pp 1–8.
3. Hunter D: The Diseases of Occupations. London, Hodder & Stoughton, 1975.
4. Ramazzini B: *De Morbis Artificium Diatriba,* 1713 (Diseases of Workers, tr. by WC Wright). Chicago, Universiity of Chicago Press, 1940.
5. Harper DS: Footnots on Allergy. Uppsala, Sweden, Pharmacia AB, p 54.
6. Graunt J: Natural and political observations made upon the bills of mortality. In Wilcox WF (ed): Baltimore, Johns Hopkins Press, 1939.
7. Farr W: Vital statistics. In Humphreys NA (ed): A Memorial Volume of Selections from the Reports and Writings of William Farr. London, Office of the Sanitary Institute, 1885.
8. Snow J: Snow on Cholera. New York, Hafner, 1965.
9. Doll R, Hill AB: Smoking and carcinoma of the lung. Br Med J 2:739, 1950.
10. Doll R, Hill AB: Mortality of doctors in relation to their smoking habits. A preliminary report. Br Med J 1:1451, 1954.
11. Doll R, Peto R: Mortality in relation to smoking: 20 years' observation on male British doctors. Br Med J 2:1525, 1976.
12. Selikoff IJ: Keynote address. In Landrigan PJ, Selikoff IJ (eds): Occupational Health in the 1990s. Ann NY Acad Sci 572(4):1989.
13. Cooke WE: Pulmonary asbestosis. Br Med J 2:1024, 1927.
14. Fleischer WE, Viles FJ, Gade RL, et al: A health survey of pipe covering operations in constructing naval vessels. J Ind Med Toxicol 28:9, 1946.
15. Dickens C: American Notes for General Circulation and Pictures from Italy. London, Chapman and Hall, 1914, pp 56–58.
16. Miles HA: Lowell, As It Was and As It Is. Nathaniel L. Dayton and Merriel and Heywood, 1846, p 129.
17. Felton JS: 200 years of occupational medicine in the U.S. J Occup Med 18:809, 1976.
18. McCready BW: On the influence of trades, professions and occupations in the United States in the production of disease. Trans Med Soc State NY 3:91, 1935 (reprinted by the Johns Hopkins Press, 1943, with introduction by GW Miller).
19. Lemen RA, Mazzuckelli LF, Niemeier RW, et al: Occupational safety and health standards. In Landigan PJ, Selikoff IJ (eds): Occupational Health in the 1990s. Ann NY Acad Sci 572:100, 1989.
20. Gersuny C: Work Hazards and Industrial Conflict. Hanover, NH, University Press of New England, 1981.
21. Watson EM: Cited in Hazlett TL, Hummel WW: Industrial Medicine in Western Pennsylvania 1850–1950. Pittsburgh, University of Pittsburgh Press, 1957, p 43.
22. Hamilton A: Exploring the Dangerous Trades. Boston, Little, Brown, 1943.
23. Hamilton A, Hardy H: Industrial Toxicology, 3rd ed. Acton, MA, Publishing Sciences Group, 1974.
24. Rady RB: Walsh-Healey Public Contracts Act. Arch Environ Health 10:576, 1965.
25. Schrenk HH: Interpretation of permissible limits. Am Indust Hyg Assoc 8:55, 1947.
26. Fieldner AC, Katz SH, Kinney SP: Gas masks for gases met in fighting fires. Bureau of Mines and Tech. Paper. 248:56, 1921.
27. Henderson Y, Haggard H: Noxious gases and the principles influencing their action. New York, 1927 (cited by Shrenk in Ref. 25).
28. ACGIH Threshold Limit Values for 1946. Cincinnati, OH, American Conference of Governmental Industrial Hygienists, 1946.
29. Occupational Safety and Health Act of 1970, Public Law 91-596.
30. Code of Federal Regulations, 1987, 29 CFR 1910.1000, Air Contaminants.
31. Rosen G: The History of Miners' Diseases. New York, Schuman's, 1943, pp 64–87.
32. Hamilton A: Exploring the Dangerous Trades. Boston, Little, Brown, 1943.

Chapter 2

WORKERS' COMPENSATION AND OCCUPATIONAL ASTHMA

Donald W. Aaronson, MD, JD

Workers' Compensation laws in each of the states of the United States hold that if there is a work-connected injury, the injured worker is entitled to compensation regardless of who was at fault. The right to receive benefits is a statutory, societal decision based upon the concept that society has an obligation to support (and prevent destitution of) workers injured because of a work-connected injury. The ultimate payer for work-related injury is the consumer, because workers' compensation is funded by insurance whose premiums are paid by employers and subsequently passed on in the cost of the product or service. In a typical approach, the Supreme Court of Illinois said:

> The primary purpose of the Workmans' Compensation Act is to provide employees a prompt, sure and definite compensation together with a quick and efficient remedy for injuries or deaths suffered by such employees in the course of their employment . . . and to require the cost of such injuries to be borne by the industry itself and not by its individual members.[1]

A typical workman's compensation act has the following features:

1. An employee is automatically entitled to certain benefits whenever he suffers personal injury arising "out of and in the course of his employment."

2. There is no need to prove negligence or fault by the employer, because the injured worker gets paid whether or not the employer was negligent—it is the mere fact of being injured that triggers the payment. Indeed the worker could have contributed to his own injury

injury by his own negligence, and he would still be paid.

3. The only persons eligible to collect are employees—not independent contractors. Each state will specifically define in its statute which persons (employees) are covered by the act.

4. Benefits to be paid to the injured person: These usually cover a percentage of wages (one-half to two-thirds), hospital and medical expenses, and death benefits for dependents when such occurs. Arbitrary limits are usually imposed upon these award amounts.

5. The employee, in exchange for guaranteed benefits, gives up his right to sue his employer for damages for any injury covered by the act. Indeed, an employee who is covered under the act does not have the option to proceed either with a workers' compensation claim or a negligence suit against his employer—he must proceed with a workers' compensation claim.

6. If there was a third party whose negligence caused the injury, the worker may sue that third party. However, generally any recovery must first reimburse the employer or the Workers' Compensation Commission for payments that have already been made. The balance will go (after expenses) to the injured worker.

7. The administration of the act is usually left to an administrative commission appointed by the state. Rules of procedure and evidence are usually quite relaxed, so that most types of evidence can be introduced in order to bring about a fair result.

8. Employers are required by statute to purchase workers' compensation insurance (in some instances, self-insurance may be allowed).

9

In 1972, a national commission was appointed to study enlarging the scope of and possibly making more uniform the 50 state workers' compensation laws. The ultimate recommendations adopted by the United States Department of Labor were as follows:

1. Compulsory law.
2. No numerical exemption.
3. Farm employment coverage.
4. Full coverage of occupational diseases.
5. Rehabilitation division in Workers' Compensation agency.
6. Maintenance of benefits during rehabilitation.
7. Full medical care for accidental injuries.
8. Full medical care for occupational diseases.
9. Authority for Workers' Compensation agency to supervise medical aid.
10. Worker's initial choice of physician.
11. Broad second injury fund.
12. Adequate time to file occupational disease claims.
13. Waiting period for benefits of not more than 3 days and retroactive benefits after 2 weeks.
14. Death benefits during widowhood.
15. Permanent total disability benefits for period of disability.
16. Temporary total disability benefits equal to two-thirds of the state's average wage.[2]

Most state statutes do not comply with the above recommendations. States were given until 1975 to come into compliance, yet as of 1990 more than 40% of the states are not in substantial compliance.

OCCUPATIONAL DISEASE COVERAGE

General compensation coverage for occupational diseases also exists now in all of the 50 states. The expansion of workers' compensation to include occupational diseases has occurred through methods varying from enactment of a specific occupational disease act in some states to an increasingly broad definition of the term "injury," and occasionally to a list of covered diseases and a catch-all provision after the list so as to include all diseases that were not named. In most states, the benefits for occupational diseases are the same as for other workers' compensation-covered injuries, but there are still a number of states that significantly limit patient recovery for diseases due to dusts (silicoses, asbestoses, and other forms of pneumoconiosis). The original reason for this limitation was the fear that the system would be unable to fund full liability for dust-caused diseases because they were so widespread. Although this is no longer the case, compensation acts have not been rewritten to address this inequality.

DEFINITION OF OCCUPATIONAL DISEASE

A singular problem in the occupational disease area is the definition of the term "occupational disease." The question of how much of a disease can be considered to have a significant relationship in some way to an occupational exposure and therefore be compensable is raised, versus those conditions that are common to mankind and may not be distinctly associated with employment and therefore are not compensable. Indeed, the general tendency during much of this century, when the general coverage of workers' compensation law was expanding, was to limit coverage for occupational disorders to those that clearly were a result of an occupational exposure and were not usual diseases of mankind. A not uncommon scenario is demonstrated by examining the following occupational disease statute and interpretive case law. The law in Illinois, until amended in 1975 (as we shall see below), provided no coverage for ordinary diseases of life. The statute read:

> Ordinary diseases of life to which the general public is exposed outside of employment shall not be compensable, except where diseases follow as an incident of an occupational disease . . . .[3]

In an Illinois case, decided in 1979 but still governed by the old statute, a 42-year-old laborer had had a variety of jobs working in and around grain elevators for 20 years. His work involved frequent exposure to grain dusts. He was to have worn a small mask but often chose not to wear one (either because it was not available or he thought it unnecessary). He passed out one day at work, and subsequent examinations revealed emphysema with large bullous cysts and blebs of the left lung requiring surgery. He had a history of smoking from 1-2 packs per day. He was disabled. His doctor testified that he believed the patient had had a pre-existing condition of emphysema that was aggravated by his exposure to grain dusts. The Illinois Court held that, since emphysema is an ordinary disease of life, the mere showing that the condition of one's employment aggravated the pre-existing emphysematous condition was not sufficient to support an award for compensation.[4] This case is illustrative of the general holdings in many states until very recent years and clearly poses the problem of how we should deal with the combined situation of diseases of ordinary life and their exacerbation by occupational exposures.

The current Illinois Statute on occupational diseases is much more expansive in its definition, stating that:

> In this act, the term 'occupational disease' means a disease arising out of and in the course of the employment or which has become aggravated and rendered disabling as a result of the exposure of the employment. Such aggravation shall arise out of a risk peculiar to or increased by the employment and not common to the general public. A disease shall be deemed to arise out of the employment if there is apparent, to the rational mind upon consideration of all circumstances, a causal connection between the conditions under which the work is performed and the occupational disease. The disease need not to have been foreseen or expected, but after its contraction it must appear to have had its origin or aggravation in a risk connected with the employment and to have flowed from that source as a rational consequence.[5]

This definition is particularly important in providing for compensation for an ordinary disease of life, such as bronchitis or asthma, that is aggravated by an occupational exposure. Indeed, according to an Illinois writer, ". . . it is conceivable that a hazard of the employment sufficient to cause an aggravation of pre-existing conditions could be found in a drafty window, the blast of an air conditioner or a furnace, an overheated or underheated work room, a dusty occupation (and which one is not) [or] a work environment in which noxious fumes were inhaled."[6] In 1990, however, we begin to see a turning back of the pendulum, which had swung to broader and broader coverage of occupational and workers' injuries. In both Texas and Oregon there has been a definite narrowing of the definitions of compensable injury and occupational disease.[7] Oregon, in particular, now requires that the worker's employment be the

major contributing cause of an occupational disease. In addition, in both states a number of restrictions have been placed on compensation in amount and duration. All of this adds up toward a movement to the center in the way we deal with balancing the rights of workers with the interests of business when it comes to injuries that were somehow related to the workplace. It is clear that in coming years there will be further revisions of these statutes.

ALLERGY AND EMPLOYMENT EXPOSURES

There is still a good deal of disagreement as to whether a disability caused by an individual's own allergic nature is an occupational disease under the general definition of the term. In one case, an employee was assigned work in a milling company, which exposed him to intense concentrations of wheat dust from handling the wheat that came into the plant (he was exposed to grain dust and not to milled flour). He was entirely free from respiratory disease when he began working, but within 2 years he began to notice some respiratory symptoms. Over the next 22 years his mild cough had progressed to symptoms of chest pain, shortness of breath, and inability to walk more than a block without stopping 2–3 times to rest. A claim was filed for workers' compensation due to occupational lung disease. The court, in that case, defined occupational disease as a "disease which is the natural incident or result of a particular employment and is peculiar to it, usually developing gradually from the effects of long-continued work at the employment and serving because of its known relation to the employment to attach to the employment a risk or hazard which distinguished it from the ordinary run of occupations and is in excess of that attending employment in general." The court then went on to deny benefits to the claimant "for the reason that the asthma or emphysema from which he suffered, even though brought on by prolonged inhalation of wheat dust and even though not uncommon among people engaged in the milling industry, was nevertheless not a natural result or incident of the employment itself but instead . . . was attributable to the employee's own individual innate sensitivity or allergy to the properties of the wheat dust . . . . It was him and not his occupation that was primarily responsible for his condition."[8]

In another case decided at the same time, a 60-year-old man went to work in a logging company plant where exposure to smoke and fumes caused him to develop symptoms of sneezing, sore throat, burning eyes, and a progressively more severe problem of shortness of breath. His doctor diagnosed asthma, which he attributed to the workplace exposure. The man had never been ill with respiratory disease before he started working at the plant. He worked there for a total of 4 years and was considered disabled when he stopped working. The court, in that case, was charged with interpreting a statute that defined an occupational disease as "those diseases or infections as arise naturally and proximately out of an extra hazardous employment." In holding for the claimant, the court said that a disease is an occupational disease "where it has been proved that the conditions of the extra hazardous employment in which the claimant was employed, naturally and proximately produced the disease and that *but for* the exposure to such conditions, the disease would not have been contracted."[9]

A man who had worked as a baker from 1936 to 1947 and again briefly in 1951 and 1952, before he died as a result of his disease, was awarded compensation by a workers' compensation board. In upholding the award, the New York Court stated that the disease (baker's asthma) "was a natural hazard of his employment as a baker and was due to exposure to flour dust . . . . It is clear from the medical evidence that baker's asthma is an occupational hazard of the work."[10]

Another issue that has been raised is whether an already existing state of asthma which is merely exacerbated is compensable as an occupational disease. In a seminal opinion, a court in Pennsylvania examined a case of a claimant who worked for many years in the manufacturing of beer. He had a variety of jobs, but for most of his more than 20-year employment he was exposed to chlorine and its fumes, as well as to the fumes of other chemical agents such as caustic soda and sulfuric acid. He had also been a heavy smoker. A diagnosis of asthma as well as chronic obstructive lung disease was made. The employee filed a claim for compensation under both the Workers' Compensation and Occupational Disease Acts. The Pennsylvania statute had been amended in 1972 and now covered "injury to an employee regardless of his previous physical condition arising in the course of his employment and related thereto and such disease . . . as is

aggravated, reactivated or accelerated by the injury." The court went on to state that "in determining whether an employee has suffered a compensable injury, his previous condition is of no consequence . . . . The job-related aggravation of a disease is a category of 'injury' for compensation purposes." In other words, it can be said that "an employer takes an employee as he comes."[11] In agreement is another case in which an employee who had a history of chronic obstructive lung disease was the victim of a single, fairly intense exposure to acrylic auto body paint fumes and then was found to be totally disabled. In this case the employee claimed that his pre-existing, non-occupational disease was aggravated by an occupational exposure. He was awarded compensation under the workmans' compensation statute.[12] In Michigan, where the statute requires "causes and conditions which are characteristic of and peculiar to the business of the employer,"[13] and in Wisconsin, whose statutes contain no definition, the courts have held that unusual susceptibility and individual allergy do not defeat claims for occupational disease.[14]

As one examines the legal literature relative to occupational lung disease (lung cancer, emphysema, bronchitis, and asthma) occurring in workers with a heavy smoking history and with occupational exposures (such as the inhalation of asbestos or textile fibers, noxious fumes, acrid smoke, or irritating dusts), one can find states that award compensation (California to a fireman for lung cancer related to smoke inhalation from fire-fighting and a pack-a-day smoking habit;[15] New Jersey to a roofer who smoked two packs a day; Oregon to a heavy smoker who was exposed to dust from sanding and grinding operations and to paint fumes, and who developed chronic bronchitis[16]), and states where compensation has been denied (Michigan for a smoker's lung condition allegedly due to dust from grinding up tree limbs;[17] North Carolina for alleged byssinosis in a cotton mill worker who had smoked for 3 years[18]).

Most state courts have held that pre-existing disease—allergy or other predisposition—does not prevent a worker from being compensated for aggravation of a pre-existing condition. The employer takes a worker as he finds him. In the cases where the claimants were not awarded compensation, the general conclusion was that there was failure to prove that the employment might or could have caused or contributed to the disease as a factual matter.

THE ROLE OF THE PHYSICIAN IN ASSESSING A PATIENT WHO CLAIMS TO HAVE AN OCCUPATIONAL LUNG DISEASE

We physicians are increasingly called upon to participate in evaluations of workers who claim disability due to an occupational exposure. Our knowledgeable participation is necessary to effect a fair result both to the claimant and to the involved employer. We must, in an impartial way, present the facts and whatever reasonable conclusions can be drawn from the facts. We must accept the actuality that there are no absolute proofs in the area of workers' compensation related to occupational disease. We must present our opinions as a reasonable medical certainty that an exposure (or series of exposures) did or did not cause the condition we are evaluating.

In our American system, the determination of disability usually follows and adversarial hearing in which expert opinions, which usually conflict with each other, are presented by each side, either to a workers' compensation panel or to an administrative law judge, or ultimately to a trial court. These panels must choose between the battling experts. In the U.S., 90% of respiratory disease claims are litigated, and in 75% the issue is causation, whether the claimant's condition might or could be connected to the occupational exposure. The issue usually involves "very complex scientific testimony and a costly battle of experts."[19] This is in contrast to the system in Europe and Canada where difficult questions are referred to experts who are regular consultants to the compensation agency, rather than being witnesses for the employer or claimant.

Disability Versus Impairment

It is the responsibility of the physician to determine the degree of impairment of the respiratory system. Most physicians confuse this with an assumed responsibility to determine the amount of disability. Impairment, however, cannot be equated with disability. Disability is generally defined as an inability to carry out a specific job or task. "Respiratory impairment is best defined as an abnormality of physiologic function that persists after treatment; in short, an inability of the organs of respiration to carry out one or more of the three components of respiration: ventilation, diffusion or perfusion."[20] In order for a physician to give an opinion as to whether an employee is disabled, he must be fully aware of all of the requirements of the employee's job. The court or the party for whom the physician is carrying out the evaluation may ask the physician to give an opinion as to disability, but this would require a great deal more investigation and knowledge on the doctor's part.

Disability determinations are usually made by the workers' compensation panel or an administrative law judge—normally nonphysicians—who must evaluate not only the amount of respiratory impairment, the causes of the impairment, and the likelihood of further injury from continued workplace exposure, but also the age, educational level, intelligence, motivation of the employee, and the energy requirements of the job. All of these latter facts are usually not in the area of expertise of the examining physician. We physicians generally do best with scientific investigations and reports rather than with socioeconomic evaluations for which we are not trained.

The ultimate conclusion of the physician relative to impairment or disability should be expressed in terms of a reasonable medical certainty and must be based upon the kinds of data and information usually considered by physicians in making these determinations. The physician should use both accepted literature and accepted tests and test methods in order to ensure that the opinion will be accepted and relied upon by the ultimate decider of the questions of disability and compensation. If the physician cannot substantiate the methods or opinions as ones that would be generally accepted in the field, he or she will not be properly advising and representing either the employer or the employee. Let us now look at the processes that the examining physician should follow in undertaking an evaluation of impairment and possible disability.

Diagnosis

The most important tool available for the diagnosis of occupational asthma is a careful and extremely thorough history. A recounting of asthma symptoms related to work is essential. Occupational asthma should be suspected in a patient who reports the sudden onset of asthma with no previous history of allergy symptoms. Presenting symptoms of asthma late in the work day or only at night are a helpful clue. Be alert for the patient who works shifts other than 9 to 5 and has a diagnostically suggestive but unrecognized history of asthma during the day when he or she is asleep. Some patients will also give a history of asthma that clears on nonwork days or over vacations.

Because some symptoms may last for long periods of time after the exposure is ended, the history must also include a careful evaluation of previous work exposures. While this pattern is fairly typical for exposure to western red cedar or toluene di-isocyanate, many other occupational exposures can also result in asthma, which can be present for years after the exposure has ended. It is important to determine whether other workers have similar symptoms. This history, while certainly not diagnostic, may suggest that the symptoms are due to a direct irritant effect rather than being the result of allergy.

It is important to delve as deeply as possible into the specifics of the workplace exposure, because some manufacturing processes may generate many unsuspected potential allergens or irritants. Another item of historical importance is to determine when the symptoms became referrable to the work situation. If environmental exposure results in an allergic reaction, the history will usually reveal a fairly prolonged period of exposure prior to the onset of asthma. On the other hand, irritants may cause respiratory symptoms quite early in the exposure period. It is important historically to determine whether there was a history of nonoccupational asthma present at an earlier time in life, and whether that disease is now aggravated by an irritant nonallergic exposure. It is also very important in the history to determine whether or not there is a smoking history, either in the past or at the time of examination. Ultimate determinations of whether or not a worker will receive compensation will, as we have seen above, frequently be affected by a smoking history. It is important for the examining physician to be prepared to deal with questions involving the impact of smoking in a prospective manner. As part of the history, there should be a chronologic list of jobs, beginning with the patient's first job and leading up to the time of evaluation. This should include evaluating all of the exposures involved in each of these jobs. The history should also include pet exposures as well as a thorough evaluation of the patient's hobbies, both now and in the past.

Physical Examination

This may be the least important portion of the evaluation. It is not uncommon to have a normal chest examination if the worker is examined in your office and not in the work environment or if the primary symptom is cough. The presence of wheezing in and of itself does not establish either a diagnosis or a degree of impairment. It is only suggestive. Persistent crackles that are present through mid- or late inspiration suggest the possible presence of fibrosis.

Radiographic Examination

In the great majority of patients with occupational ashtma chest x-rays are most often normal and provide no helpful information. A finding of hyperinflation has no bearing in making an assessment of the degree of respiratory impairment.

Laboratory Tests

There are few helpful laboratory tests. The presence of elevated numbers of eosinophils in the blood or sputum—eosinophilia—may suggest that an allergic process is present. It is not a confirmatory finding and normal levels of eosinophils do not rule out the presence of allergic disease. Immunologic studies to demonstrate antibodies to potential sensitizers in the patient's environment merely demonstrate exposure and do not establish a causative relationship relative to the degree of impairment.

Pulmonary Function Testing

Pulmonary function testing is required and, along with the history, forms the basis for concluding whether or not occupational asthma is present. Pulmonary function tests can be useful in demonstrating the degree of bronchial hyperreactivity, the amount of respiratory impairment, and in estimating the amount of dyspnea. Measurements of diffusing capacity (except if fibrosis is suspected) or arterial blood gases do not seem helpful in making determinations of impairment. Some governmental agents still require arterial blood gas measurements even though wide variations from normal may not correlate with the presence or absence of respiratory impairment. Descriptions of methods of lung function measurements, as well as demonstration of airway reactivity, are discussed elsewhere in this text and will not be covered here.

A number of measurements are important in coming to conclusions about impairment and disability and in establishing their relationship to occupational exposures. The most useful and best understood measures are the FVC, FEV_1 and FEV_1/FVC ratio. These tests are easily performed and are considered reliable. Lack of patient effort or attempts to produce falsely low values can usually be identified. Measurements of airflow should be done when the patient is relatively asymptomatic as well as during and after exposure to the suspected causative workplace agent(s).

Spirometry before and after an inhaled bronchodilator is useful in confirming the presence of reversible airway obstruction, although methacholine challenge, as noted below, may be necessary. It is usually helpful once you have a baseline of nonwork day peak flows (done at least every 3–4 hours) to measure the patient's peak flows at work. While this is subject to patient cooperation and honesty, it does give a fairly good picture of the patient's sensitivity to the workplace exposure.

It would be most helpful if we could achieve a level of sophistication and trust whereby employers would allow measurements of airflow by a respiratory technician during suspected or claimed occupational exposures. This would eliminate the need for laboratory challenges, which are difficult to do and require special facilities and equipment. It is very useful to assess bronchial reactivity at a number of times. Methacholine or histamine challenge to determine the amount of airway reactivity can be a very useful tool in determining not only the degree of occupational asthma but also how severe is the respiratory impairment. If possible, methacholine (or histamine) challenge should be done after a period away from the occupation, then shortly after an occupational exposure, and then serial follow-up challenges once the exposure has been discontinued. These can be very persuasive in demonstrating that the suspect occupational exposure did or did not result in an increase in airway reactivity. Reports that show significant changes (or no change) due to a suspect exposure, and then a loss of airway hyperreactivity with elimination of the exposure, can be very useful to a workers'

TABLE 1. *Degree of Shortness of Breath Graded from 0–4*

Grade	Description
0	No shortness of breath with normal activity. Shortness of breath with exertion comparable to a well person of the same age, height, and sex.
I	More shortness of breath than a person of the same age while walking quietly on a level surface or on climbing an incline or two flights of stairs.
II	More short of breath and unable to keep up with persons of the same age and sex while walking on a level surface.
III	Short of breath while walking on a level surface and while performing everyday tasks at work.
IV	Shortness of breath while carrying out personal activities, e.g., dressing, talking, walking from one room to another.

compensation panel reviewing a claim. In assessing respiratory impairment, some measures of "dyspnea" are most helpful to a panel that must decide whether or not disability is present and, if so, how much disability indeed exists. There are no good measures of dyspnea, which is a very subjective complaint. Exercise testing has not been proven to be useful and is easily manipulated. A rough guide to assessing dyspnea can be found in Table 1.[21]

This can be roughly correlated with Table 2.[22] Using these two tables together may help you to determine the degree of dyspnea in a given patient. Lastly, in attempting to quantify the pulmonary function testing in relationship to respiratory impairment, you are referred to Table 3.[23]

Physician's Report

The physician who is assessing a patient for occupational asthma should be aware of the myriad of occupational exposures that can cause asthma. These are fully discussed in other chapters of this book. In preparing a

TABLE 2. *Relationship Between Grade of Dyspnea and FEV_1 in Subjects Not Seeking Disability Awards*

Grade of Dyspnea	Mean FEV_1 (liters)
0	3.2
I	2.4
II	1.8
III	1.2
IV	0.75

TABLE 3. *Criteria for Grading Impairment of Pulmonary Function**

Test	Mild	Moderate	Severe
Obstructive Impairment			
MVV (% predicted)	65–80	45–60	Less than 45
VC (% predicted)	Normal	Usually normal	Slight to moderate reduction
FEV$_1$ (% predicted)	65–80	45–60	Less than 45
FEV$_1$/FVC%†	55–75	45–55	Less than 45
Blood gases‡ (% sat)	Normal	Usually normal	Hypoxemia
DL$_{CO}$ (% predicted)	Normal	Normal or slight reduction	Slight to moderate reduction
Restrictive Impairment			
MVV (% predicted)	Normal	Normal	50–80
VC (% predicted)	60–80	50–60	Less than 50
FEV$_1$ (% predicted)	60–80	50–60	Less than 50
FEV$_1$/FVC%†	Normal	Normal	Normal
Blood gases % sat	Normal	Normal	Usually normal
DL$_{CO}$ (% predicted)	Normal	50–75	Below 50
Interstitial Lung Disease			
MVV (% predicted)	Normal	Normal	60 or above
VC (% predicted)	70 or greater	50–70	Less than 50
FEV$_1$ (% predicted)	70 or greater	50–70	Less than 50
FEV$_1$/FVC%†	Normal	Normal	Normal
Blood gases % sat	94–96	90–94	90 or less
(A-a)O$_2$ mm†	15–30	30–40	Above 40
DL$_{CO}$ (% predicted)	Normal	40–75	Less than 40

* Reproduced from Morgan WKD, Seaton A: Occupational Lung Diseases, 2nd ed. Philadelphia, W.B. Saunders, 1985, p 74, with permission.
† Age-related.
‡ Unreliable in obstructive impairment.
MVV = maximum voluntary ventilation; VC = vital capacity; FEV$_1$ = forced expiratory volume in 1 second; FVC = forced vital capacity; DL$_{CO}$ = diffusing capacity for carbon monoxide.

report for the patient's employer, the following should be included:

1. Complete and detailed history, as noted above.

2. Physical findings including documentation of wheezing, if present.

3. Specific identification of the causative agent and documentation with references that this agent can cause asthma (it is very helpful to all concerned if you can supply copies of some relevant articles along with the report).

4. Results of all pulmonary function testing, documenting airway obstruction and the presence of reversibility. Documentation of airway reactivity and changes on exposure to the occupational allergen or irritant. Results of all challenges, including the conditions under which the challenges were done and the conclusion from the pulmonary function test and challenge assessments.

5. Discussion of the amount of respiratory impairment and level of dyspnea. This should include estimates of permanence of pulmonary function changes if possible. It should address whether there is risk in returning to the former workplace and what kinds of exposure should be avoided in the future.

6. Discussion of disability should be avoided unless specifically requested. If this is requested, you must be certain that you are fully aware of all of the factors listed above relative to determining disability. You will also need to be aware of which occupations are possible for the patient and which exposures will occur from participation in a new occupation.

7. Lastly, a statement that with a reasonable medical certainty (51 to 49%) you believe, or do not believe, that the workplace exposure was, or was not, the cause of the claimant's lung disease.

REFERENCES

1. O'Brien v. Rautenbush, 139 NE 2nd 222, 226 (1956).
2. U.S. Department of Labor. Reprinted in Roddy JP: Basic Aspects of the Workers' Compensation Act in Workers' Compensation. Springfield, IL, Illinois Institute of Continuing Legal Education, 1990, pp 1-6, 1-7.
3. 48 IL Rev Stat 172.36 (d).
4. Bunney v. Industrial Commission (appeal of Long) 389 NE 2nd 536.
5. 48 IL Rev Stat Supra.
6. Kane AO: Occupational Diseases in Workmen's Compensation, Springfield IL, Illinois Institute of Continuing Legal Education, 1990, pp 9-5.

7. SB 1 Texas (Workers' Compensation Act) 1990. Oregon Rev Stat 656.802 (2).
8. Sanford v. Valier-Spies Milling Company, 235 SW 2nd 92 (1950).
9. Simpson Logging Co. v. Dept of Labor and Industry, 202 P 2nd 448 (1949).
10. Morrocco v. Mohican Stores Inc. 230 NYS 2nd 526 (1962).
11. Pawlowsky v. WCAB 525 A 2nd 1204 (1987).
12. Arlington Auto Body Serv v. WCAB (Bosack) 492 A 2nd 496 (1985).
13. Bird v. Pennfield Agric School Dist 83 NW 2nd 595 (1957).
14. Kroger Grocery and Baking Co. v. Industrial Comm. 1 NW 2nd 802 (1942). Consolidated Papers Inc. v. Dept. of Industry, Labor and Human Relations 251 NW 2nd 69 (1977).
15. McAllister v. WCAB 445 P 2nd 313 (1968).
16. Bolger v. Chris Anderson Roofing 285 A 2nd 228.
17. Foster v. City of Detroit 224 NW 2nd 714 (1974).
18. Nardella v. Campbell Machine Inc. 525 F 2nd 46 (1975).
19. Richman SI: Why change? A look at the current system of disability determination and workers' compensation for occupational lung disease. Arch Intern Med 97:908, 1982.
20. Morgan WKC: Pulmonary disability and impairment. Can't work? Won't work? In American Thoracic Society: Basics of Respiratory Disability. New York, American Thoracic Society, 1982.
21. Id.
22. Morgan WKC, Seaton D: Pulmonary physiology: Its application to the determination of respiratory impairment and disability in industrial disease. In Morgan WKC, Seaton D (eds): Occupational Lung Diseases, 2nd ed. Philadelphia, W.B. Saunders, 1984, p 66.
23. Id., p 74.

Chapter 3

PULMONARY FUNCTION TESTING AND DISABILITY EVALUATION

David E. Griffith, MD
Richard S. Kronenberg, MD

PULMONARY FUNCTION TESTING

Pulmonary function testing is a widely used technique that offers a broad range of information to practicing physicians. The utility of pulmonary function testing has continued to expand to the extent that some authors believe it should be part of the routine examination of subjects at risk for pulmonary disease. This discussion will focus on **spirometry** because, of the many tests of pulmonary function, spirometry is best suited for medical surveillance. Spirometry, defined as the measurement of inhaled or exhaled gas, is simple to administer, rapid, inexpensive, safe, and both sensitive and specific when properly applied and interpreted. Spirometry is particularly suited for evaluation of occupational exposures where the principal adverse respiratory effect is a pattern of obstructive lung disease such as occurs with occupational asthma.

Extensive guidelines are available for the standardized performance of spirometry. These guidelines include standardization of equipment and performance of tests,[1] qualifications of personnel administering the tests,[2] recommendations for computer assistance,[3] quality assurance,[4] and infection control.[5] By using accurate and validated spirometers and performance techniques, information from different types of spirometers, from different labs, and from one time period to the next can be appropriately compared.

Certainly pulmonary function tests also have limitations. Specifically, they are tests of physiologic function and must be interpreted both with caution and in the context of other clinical information when evaluating diseases defined anatomically, such as emphysema, or diseases defined symptomatically, such as chronic bronchitis. Because they are tests of physiologic function, however, they are well suited for evaluation of functional abnormalities such as asthma.

In the occupational setting, screening or pre-employment pulmonary function testing allows identification of pre-existing pulmonary disorders for proper job placement. In addition, spirometry may detect early changes in pulmonary function in individual workers while intervention might still be effective, and allows accumulation of data to evaluate how well exposure controls are working. Additional benefits to the occupational epidemiologist include providing exclusionary criteria to identify subjects without lung disease, inclusionary criteria for subjects with specific diseases or degrees of dysfunction, identification of the prevalence of adverse responses to environmental exposures, and definition of differences in lung function attributable to other causes.

Spirometry

Spirometry involves the forced expiratory maneuver that is the most widely used in standardized testing of lung function. During this maneuver the subject inhales maximally to total lung capacity and exhales as rapidly and forcefully as possible. Expired volume can be plotted against time to generate a spirogram

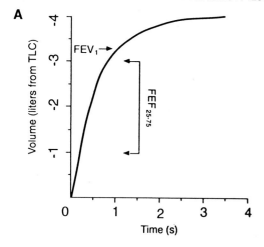

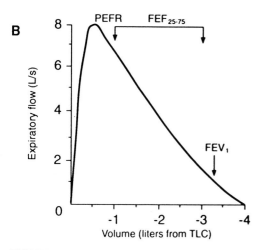

FIGURE 1. The forced expiratory maneuver. **A,** Expired volume plotted against time to generate a spirogram. **B,** Expired volume plotted against expiratory flow rates to generate a flow volume curve.

regardless of which section of the flow volume curve is used. Some typical spirograms and flow volume curves are illustrated in Figure 2.

Several useful variables may be derived from the forced expiratory maneuver. The maximal effort **forced vital capacity** (FVC) is the volume of air exhaled with a maximally forced effort from total inspiration (expressed in liters). Analysis of this curve permits computation of the volume exhaled over time (FEV_T), the ratio of FEV_T to FVC, and average flow rates during different portions of the curve.

The **time-forced expiratory volume** (FEV_T) is the volume of air exhaled in a specific time during the performance of FVC. For example, FEV_1 is the **volume of air exhaled during the first second of FVC** (expressed in liters). The FEV_1 incorporates the early effort-dependent portion of the flow volume curve, but also enough of the midportion to make it reproducible and sensitive for clinical purposes.

The forced expiratory volume over time can also be expressed as a percentage of FVC. The ratio of FEV_1 to FVC has been defined precisely in healthy subjects. This ratio declines with age, but abnormally decreased ratios indicate airway obstruction. Normal or increased ratios do not exclude airway obstruction, particularly in the presence of decreased FVC due to an interstitial pulmonary process, a chest wall restriction, or in subjects who fail to make a maximal effort throughout the expiratory maneuver.

Average forced expiratory flow can be calculated over different portions of the expiratory curve. The most widely used measurement is the FEF_{25-75}, which is **the mean expiratory flow during the middle half of FVC.** This test was previously called the maximal midexpiratory flow rate. This measurement was intended to reflect the most effort-independent portion of the curve and may be more sensitive to airflow obstruction in small airways. The FEF_{25-75}, however, shows marked variability in studies of large samples of healthy subjects, so that the 95% confidence limits for normal values are so large as to limit their sensitivity in detecting disease in an individual subject.[6,7]

Coefficients of Variation

Changes in FVC, FEV_1 or FEF_{25-75} may be found in the same subjects studied repeatedly on the same day or on consecutive days.[8] This issue is important in the setting of occupational asthma surveillance where repeated spirometry

or plotted against instantaneous expiratory flow rates to yield a flow-volume curve (Fig. 1).

The flow-volume curve during forced exhalation demonstrates a characteristic appearance, with a rapid ascent to peak flow followed by a slow linear descent proportional to volume. The initial 25 to 33% of the curve is effort-dependent. As a subject exerts increasing effort during exhalation, associated with increasing intrathoracic pressure, increasing flow is generated. Following the development of peak flow, flow subsequently diminishes in proportion to volume until residual volume is reached. This portion of the curve is relatively effort-independent, in that for each point on the volume axis, a maximal flow exists that cannot be exceeded regardless of the pressure generated by the respiratory muscles. An inadequate effort, however, can invalidate spirometric tests,

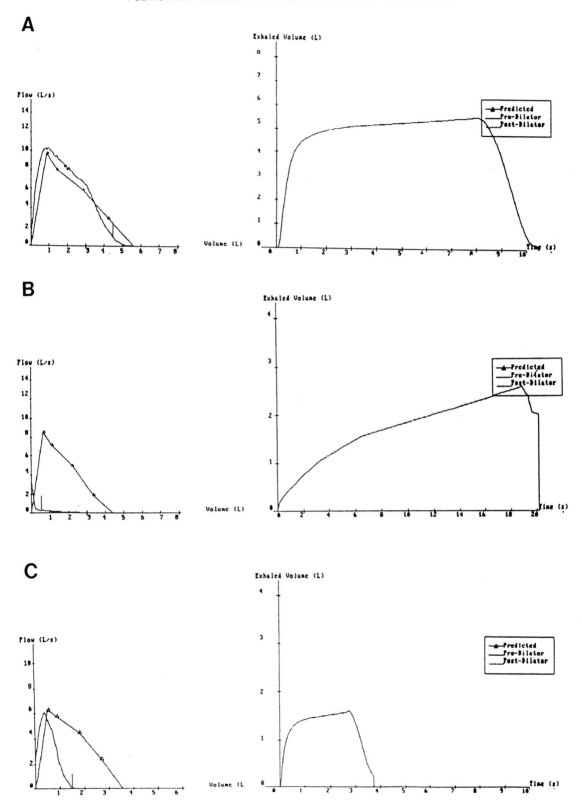

FIGURE 2. Typical spirograms and flow volume curves for **A**, normal subject, **B**, airflow obstruction, and **C**, restrictive pattern.

is an essential aspect of subject evaluation. When multiple measurements are made, the variability of the data can be expressed as the coefficient of variation for a specific test. It is impossible to determine if a specific environment has had a significant effect on pulmonary function without taking into account the coefficient of variation for each variable measured. Therefore, to establish the limits for a significant change over a work shift, the day-to-day variability of spirometric parameters must be considered. A reasonable figure for the day-to-day within-subject coefficient of variation for the FVC and the FEV_1 in normal subjects is 3%.[8] For the FEF_{25-75} the coefficient of variation is between 8 and 21%.[8,9] The coefficient of variation is significantly higher for each of these parameters in patients with airflow obstruction and increases with the degree of pulmonary dysfunction.[8,10,11] For instance, in patients with asthma, coefficients of variation from week to week for FVC, FEV_1 and FEF_{25-75} are 11%, 13%, and 23%, respectively.[8] In general, the coefficient of variation also increases with longer time periods between measurements.

Decrements in FEV_1 over a work shift of more than 5%, provided this decrement is repeated on more than one occasion, should induce follow-up clinical evaluation in consideration of limiting further exposure.[8,12] If only one shift examination is available, then a greater than 10% decrement is necessary to prevent false-positive results in the absence of repeat examinations.[12] For subjects with an FEV_1 less than 3 liters, a fall in FEV_1 greater than 150 milliliters should be considered significant, because the absolute change in milliliters associated with a 5% decrement in FEV_1 can become extremely small or fall within the background noise for the measurement.

Concepts of Normality

There are several thorough discussions of normality in pulmonary function testing that are strongly recommended to the reader.[13-15] Expected normal values for spirometric tests are based on regression equations derived from studies of large numbers of (usually) normal subjects to yield an expected mean value. This mean value is the expected result if a sizable number of normal subjects of the same height, weight, age, sex, and race as the patient were studied. "Normality" then depends on the variability in a normal population of

the parameter measured and the variability of the test itself. The regression equations account for 60 to 70% of the variability in the specific test within a population. The remaining variability is probably related to genetic and environmental factors. A number of good regression equations are available for use, each derived from a population with unique characteristics.[16-19] No single regression equation is ideal, and the appropriate regression equation for the population being studied should be matched as carefully as possible to populations from which the regression equations were derived. Some prediction equations, for instance, have been based on studies of unique religious and ethnic groups that may not be representative of a particular occupational cohort.[19] For example, it is inappropriate to use reference values derived from an all-white community to evaluate an ethnically mixed occupational population. Studies of black populations show that the various measurements of lung functions appear to be approximately 13% larger for a given height in whites compared with blacks.[20]

Determination of normality or the degree of abnormality in a pulmonary function test is based on the degree of deviation from predicted normal values calculated from the regression equations. There are several approaches to define the limits, usually the lower limits, of normality. A commonly used "traditional" approach has been to label a value abnormal if it deviates by 20% or more from the mean normal value. This approach is simplistic, inaccurate, and misleading, particularly for tests with wide intersubject variability, such as FEF_{25-75}. This approach also assumes that the test variation increases as the test value increases, thereby overestimating the actual variations between subjects with large lung volumes or flows and underestimating the variations in subjects with small volumes or flows.

A better method for determining the lower limits of normal is to define the 95% confidence interval for a given test. Ninety-five percent confidence intervals are available for most spirometric parameters, and with the aid of computer-assisted reports, individualized normal ranges are possible. The 95% confidence limits can be calculated using the predicted value ± 1.96 times the **standard error of the estimate** (SEE) around the regression line for the two-tailed t-test approach, and the predicted value ± 1.65 times time the SEE for the more commonly recommended one-tailed t-test.[16,21] The interindividual variation of lung function differs greatly between tests. In a normal population, the FVC and FEV_1 have relatively narrow 95% confidence limits of approximately 21%, whereas in order for the FEF_{25-75} to be judged abnormal a change of greater than 40% below predicted is frequently necessary.[8,16] It is clear that the "20%" method is probably functionally adequate for the FVC and FEV_1, but not for tests with wide interindividual variability, such as the FEF_{25-75}. Two assumptions yet to be validated for the 95% confidence interval method are that the confidence interval for all ages and heights is a constant and that the distribution about the predicted value is Gaussian. Critera for grading the severity of airflow obstruction using 95% confidence intervals are listed in Table 1.

The 95% confidence interval must be used with caution to determine the clinical significance of any pulmonary function test. By itself the lower limit of normal cannot be used to predict the probability of lung disease in a given patient. This is a particular problem for occupational screening if there is only a cursory or even no attempt to obtain a detailed history or physical examination from an individual patient. For example, a subject with an FEV_1 of 85% of predicted, who is an asymptomatic with no history of pulmonary dysfunction, may indeed be normal; whereas, an individual with an FEV_1 of 85% of predicted, with cough, dyspnea, and wheezing, who normally has an FEV_1 of 110% of predicted, is clearly abnormal. In this scenario the patient's history and physical examination are crucial elements in the decision about whether the subject is indeed normal. In the evaluation of occupational asthma the ability to test and retest individuals does, to some degree, eliminate this problem. Using the patient's own values as controls permits greater accuracy in detecting significant changes in lung function and in defining normality or abnormality for a given patient.

Acceptability, Reproducibility and Test Failure

The subject should be instructed in the FVC maneuver, and the appropriate technique should be demonstrated. The technician should make sure the patient understands the instructions and performs the maneuver with a good start, a maximum inspiration, and a smooth continuous exhalation with maximal effort.

TABLE 1. *Criteria for Mild, Moderate and Severe Airflow Obstruction Using 95% Confidence Intervals (CI)**

Level of Obstruction	FEV_1/FVC %
Normal	< 1 CI
Mild	≥ 1 to 2 CI
Moderate	≥ 2 to 4 CI
Severe	≥ 4 CI

* Adapted from Ref. 21.

Criteria for unacceptibility of the FVC maneuver due to poor performance are outlined in Table 2.

Ambient temperature is an important variable to recognize for field testing and for repetitive tests. A significant temperature change between two measurements can introduce potentially significant error in FEV_1 measurements.[22] Spirometry should be performed at relatively constant, moderate temperatures. Ambient temperature should also always be recorded.

A minimum of three acceptable FVC maneuvers should be performed. Generation of fewer than two acceptable curves is the only criterion for unacceptable subject performance that necessitates elimination of the results from further consideration.[1] Subjects should not be asked to perform more than seven or eight FVC maneuvers because fatigue will affect results.

A goal of test performance is that the largest FVC and second largest FVC from acceptable curves should not vary by more than 5%, expressed as a percentage of the largest observed FVC or 0.10 liters, whichever is greatest.[1] In addition the largest FEV_1 and second largest FEV_1 should not vary by more than 5% of the reading of the largest FEV_1 or 0.10 liters, whichever is greater.[1]

The reproducibility criteria are used as a guide to whether more than three FVC

TABLE 2. *Criteria for Unacceptable Performance of the FVC Maneuver*

1. An unsatisfactory start of expiration characterized by excessive hesitation or false start.
2. Coughing during the first second of the maneuver or any cough interfering with accurate measurement.
3. Valsalva maneuver (glottis closure).
4. Early termination of expiration (less than a 6-second maneuver).
5. A leak in the system.
6. An obstructed mouth piece.

maneuvers are needed. These criteria are not intended to exclude results for reports or subjects from a study. The criteria for acceptance for spirometric maneuvers discussed above should be followed and unacceptable studies discarded before applying reproducibility criteria.

The lack of reproducible lung function tests does not necessarily imply poor measurement techniques or poor subject effort. In longitudinal evaluations of several occupational-based cohorts, Eisen et al. found that nonreproducibility of spirograms is not random (i.e., some individuals have a tendency to "fail"), subjects with persistent nonreproducibility have an annual rate of decline in FEV_1 greater than subjects with more reproducible spirograms, and as the measurement of FEV_1 becomes more variable (less reproducible), the annual FEV_1 decline gets steeper.[23-26] An individual's inability to perform an adequate spirogram on a single occasion was indicative of decreased ventilatory capacity, and the persistent inability to perform successfully over time indicated an even greater cross-sectional decrease in capacity. It is clear from these observations that exclusion of individuals based on reproducibility criteria can lead to estimates of FEV_1 for a study population that are biased upward and estimates of dose response relationships that are biased towards no effect. In the study of occupationally related bronchospasm, it is also noteworthy that asthmatics may have an FEV_1 that varies during the repetitive performance of pulmonary function testing, which adversely impacts reproducibility.[27] Reproducibility of spirometry results is certainly desirable, but a lack of reproducibility alone (i.e., with otherwise technically acceptable spirograms) is not sufficient to discard or disallow the information obtained from these spirograms.

Poor reproducibility is still one consequence of poor effort or cooperation and may be the first evidence of poor effort by a subject[28] (Table 3). By itself, however, poor reproducibility is not adequate to determine poor effort with certainty. Other features of poor

cooperation include decreased vital capacity; relatively normal expiratory airflows; increased FEV_1 to FVC ratio; decreased **maximal voluntary ventilation** (MVV); uneven, slurred, or irregularly recorded spirograms; decreased TLC; and decreased pleural pressure. In the context of screening for occupational asthma, submaximal efforts may paradoxically mask an obstructive defect. In some cases poor effort may be very difficult to document with certainty. If poor effort or cooperation is suspected and is deemed important to prove, then lung volumes and MVV or transdiaphragmatic pressures can be measured to better document effort.

Peak Flow Measurements

Respiratory flow reaches a transient peak early in the forced expiratory maneuver. Peak flow occurs during a very effort-dependent portion of the respiratory maneuver, so low values can result from even slightly submaximal effort rather than from airway obstruction. When a maximal effort is made, peak flow is largely a function of the caliber of large airways; it is also influenced by the transient flow caused by expulsion of air from compressed central airways. Inexpensive plastic peak-flow meters are readily available for distribution to working populations. Their use involves minimal instruction to the worker and does not require technical supervision or equipment requiring calibration or standardization. All of these features ultimately conserve working time. The proper performance and interpretation of **peak expiratory flow rates** (PEFRs) does, however, require subject effort and cooperation.

Where cross-sectional spirometry may miss delayed asthmatic reactions, serial recording of PEFR in a timed log, along with symptoms, may provide better assessment of diurnal respiratory variation. For late asthmatic responses occurring many hours after exposure to a chemical sensitizer, PEFR done in the evening or on awakening may be more sensitive than measurement of spirometry before and after work shifts. Peak expiratory flow rate also allows assessment of function for other periods when spirometry is impractical, such as on weekends or during periods of temporary disability. Serial measurement of PEFR has been used successfully to identify workers who have developed asthma among cohorts at high risks.[29-30]

TABLE 3. *Poor Effort or Cooperation with the FVC Maneuver*

1. Poor reproducibility of FVC maneuvers
2. Uneven, slurred or irregular spirograms
3. Decreased vital capacity
4. Increased FEV_1/FVC ratio
5. Decreased maximal voluntary ventilation (MVV)

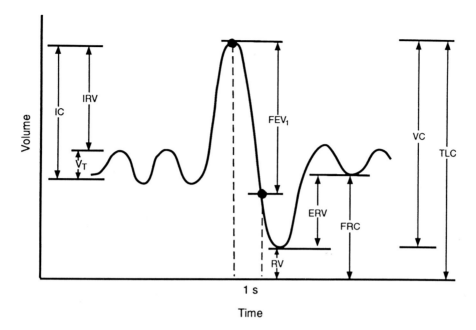

FIGURE 3. Lung volumes and capacities:

Lung Volumes
a. Tidal volume (V_T) is the volume of gas inhaled or exhaled during each respiratory cycle.
b. Inspiratory reserve volume (IRV) is the maximal volume of gas inspired from end-inspiration.
c. Expiratory reserve volume (ERV) is the maximal volume of gas exhaled from end-expiration.
d. Residual volume (RV) is the volume of gas remaining in the lungs following a maximal exhalation.

Lung Capacities
a. Total lung capacity (TLC) is the amount of gas contained in the lung at maximal expiration.
b. Vital capacity (VC) is the maximal volume of gas that can be expelled from the lungs by a forceful effort following maximal inspiration.
c. Inspiratory capacity (IC) is the maximal volume of gas that can be inspired from the resting expiratory level.
d. Functional residual capacity (FRC) is the volume of gas in the lungs at resting respiration.

Some of the factors that make PEFR recording easy and convenient contribute to its limitations. Peak flow is highly effort-dependent, and there is no mechanism for determining if low values for peak flow are effort-related or due to airflow obstruction. The measurements are self-administered and cannot be observed; therefore, there can be no checks of adequacy of effort as can be made with spirometry. Also sufficient data from large populations are not yet available for standardizing normal and abnormal diurnal variation of PEFR. Lastly, its utility for identifying preclinical and subclinical cases of asthma among asymptomatic employee populations has not yet been demonstrated. A combination of respiratory studies might improve the utility of PEFR. For instance, the demonstration of compatible changes in PEFR with an increase in airway reactivity during periods when the subject is working, and improvement in PEFR and airway reactivity when the patient is away from work suggest an occupational relationship.

Lung Volumes and Diffusing Capacity

Lung volumes and capacities are graphically illustrated in Figure 3. Determination of lung volumes is important, primarily for evaluating restrictive pulmonary processes, but it can also be used as an adjunct to spirometry for evaluating adequacy of subject cooperation (Table 4). The "gold standard" for lung volume measurement is body plethysmography, which is too bulky, delicate, and time-consuming for use in medical surveillance. Inert gas techniques utilizing helium, nitrogen, and carbon monoxide are also available and potentially useful for population screening. These techniques, however, are subject to errors because they do not detect trapped gas that does not communicate with the tracheobronchial tree. Therefore, they can seriously underestimate functional residual capacity (FRC) in patients with obstructive lung diseases. Lung volume determinations in this manner may be useful for screening purposes

TABLE 4. *Spirometric and Lung Volume Characteristics of Airflow Obstruction and Interstitial Lung Disease*

Airflow Obstruction	Interstitial (Restrictive) Disease
FVC normal or reduced	FVC reduced
FEV_1 reduced	FEV_1 reduced
FEF_{25-75} reduced	FEF_{25-75} normal or reduced
FEV_1/FVC reduced	FEV_1/FVC normal or increased
TLC normal or increased	TLC reduced
RV increased	RV reduced
DLCO normal or reduced	DLCO reduced

in normal subjects, but they are not adequate for evaluation of populations with airflow obstruction.

The **diffusing capacity of the lung to carbon monoxide** (DLCO) is also a useful test evaluating pulmonary disorders of multiple etiologies (Table 5). Its sensitivity to diverse pathophysiologic processes significantly complicates DLCO interpretation. It is, therefore, very difficult to adequately interpret an abnormal DLCO without concomitant spirometry, lung volumes, and, frequently, patient history. These considerations complicate its use as a screening or surveillance tool. The diffusion capacity for carbon monoxide can be measured several ways, but the single-breath technique is particularly amenable to field studies. The duration of testing is short and

TABLE 5. *Some Conditions Altering the Diffusing Capacity for Carbon Monoxide (DLCO)*

Decreases in DLCO
  Obstructive lung diseases
    Emphysema, cystic fibrosis
  Interstitial lung diseases
    Idiopathic pulmonary fibrosis, sarcoidosis, asbestosis, hypersensitivity pneumonitis
  Pulmonary involvement in systemic diseases
    Rheumatoid arthritis, systemic lupus erythematosus
  Cardiac diseases
    Cardiogenic pulmonary edema
  Pulmonary vascular diseases
    Primary pulmonary hypertension, pulmonary embolism
  Anemia
  Cigarette smoking
  Infections
    Pneumocystis carinii pneumonia

Increases in DLCO
  Polycythemia
  Pulmonary hemorrhage
  Asthma

the equipment required is relatively simple. This technique assumes that all carbon monoxide uptake occurs during breath-holding, but uptake of carbon monoxide actually occurs during inspiration and expiration as well. Significant error can, therefore, occur with prolonged expiration in patients with airflow obstruction. Asthmatic subjects frequently have an increased single-breath DLCO, possibly as a result of recruitment of capillary blood volume secondary to their more negative pleural pressure swings.[31] The DLCO is a better screening technique for interstitial lung diseases and as an adjunct to spirometry and lung volumes for evaluating differential diagnosis for a particular subject. Lower limits of normal for DLCO should also be calculated by 95% confidence intervals due to the wide interindividual variability of this test.[32]

Nonspecific Bronchial Hyperreactivity

Asthma is a disease characterized both by episodic airflow obstruction and bronchial hyperresponsiveness, a term used to characterize the extreme sensitivity of asthmatic airways to bronchial constricting effects of a variety of physical, chemical, or pharmacologic stimuli. All techniques employed to measure **nonspecific bronchial reactivity** (NSBR) pharmacologically involve inhalation of an aerosol containing a known bronchial-constricting agent. Inhalation is begun with a low concentration or dose of agonist, and as the dose is progressively increased, an index of airway narrowing is measured at each step so that the dose-response relationship can be constructed. A variety of techniques of delivering agonists and of measuring the response and expressing the results have been developed. Because of the reliability and simplicity of the equipment needed to measure the FEV_1, this parameter is used most frequently. Changes in other parameters such as the FVC, FEF_{25-75}, or specific airway conductance have also been utilized but do not offer a significant advantage over the FEV_1.[33,34]

Methacholine is probably the best nonspecific bronchial-constricting agent available for testing of NSBR. Histamine responses correlate well with methacholine, but histamine causes more side-effects such as cough and flushing, prostaglandin F_2 leads to cough and retrosternal irritation, and carbachol is a long-acting bronchial constricting agent.[35-37] Cold-air challenge is also safe, specific for asthma, and easy to perform.[38-40] However, it requires expensive, sophisticated equipment and so far has not been as readily adapted for widespread occupational surveillance.

The results of bronchial provocation tests are expressed by a dose-response curve plotted on semi-log paper. The doses expressed on the log abscissa are the cumulated dose units (1 dose unit equals one inhalation of a 1 mg per ml concentration of bronchial-constricting substance). The response on the ordinate is a linear percent change from control value (baseline FEV_1). The **provocative dose or provocative concentration to decrease the FEV_1 by 20%** (PD_{20} or PC_{20}) is then calculated from the curve and is expressed as dose units of inhaled substance.

There are two major published protocols for methacholine challenge that differ in inhalation technique and aerosol generation methods.[41,42] These two protocols do, however, correlate well when expressed as PD_{20}.[43] In general, a baseline FEV_1 is established. The patient then inhales several breaths of diluent and a repeat FEV_1 is done to establish a control value. Starting with a methacholine concentration of 0.075 mg/ml, the subject inhales several breaths. A repeat FEV_1 is measured within 1 to 2 minutes. If the FEV_1 is not decreased by 20%, several breaths of the next concentration are inhaled and a repeat FEV_1 is measured. The subject then continues to inhale several breaths of increasing concentration of methacholine until the test is completed or until the FEV_1 is decreased by 20%. The concentrations of methacholine commonly used are 0.075, 0.15, 0.31, 0.62, 1.25, 2.5, 5.0, 10.0, and 25.0 mg/ml.

Field use of methacholine challenge may require shortening the usual laboratory protocol, which can take an hour or more to perform for nonasthmatic subjects.[44-48] Abbreviated protocols involve: (a) using only three concentrations of methacholine (0.5, 2.0, and 8.0 mg/ml) and using fourfold rather than twofold dose increments,[46] (b) varying the initial concentration of aerosolized solution depending on symptoms and FEV_1,[45] and (c) decreasing the time of dose inhalation and the time between successive doses.[47-48] The choice of field method for methacholine challenge should be guided by the purpose of screening.

Bronchial challenge testing with nonspecific pharmacologic agents has been found to have a high degree of sensitivity but only a moderate degree of specificity in identifying subjects with asthma (Table 6). In general the PC_{20} of methacholine is lower than 8 mg/ml

TABLE 6. *Some Conditions Associated with Nonspecific Bronchial Hyperreactivity*

1. Asthma
2. Atopy (hay fever)
3. Bronchiolitis
4. Chronic obstructive pulmonary disease (COPD)
5. Cystic fibrosis
6. Foreign body aspiration
7. Near drowning
8. Occupational chemical irritant exposures
9. Post-adult respiratory distress syndrome
10. Sarcoidosis
11. Smoke inhalation
12. Viral upper respiratory infection

in asthmatics subjects, whereas in subjects with normal pulmonary function and negative histories it is usually greater than 16 mg/ml.[41,49] The frequency distribution of methacholine response is unimodal, however, so that overlap exists. Nonasthmatic subjects with conditions such as atopy and disorders such as chronic bronchitis may demonstrate NSBR in the range of the asthmatic response (Table 6.).[51,51] Severity of response can be graded on the basis of methacholine or histamine dosage associated with PC_{20}; severe, <0.25 mg/ml; moderate, <2 mg/ml; mild, <8 mg/ml; and slight, <16 mg/ml.[41]

Asthma affects up to 6% of the adult U.S. population. Therefore, it is reasonable to assume that every common occupation involves a significant number of workers with asthma and preexisting NSBR. In a workplace with the potential for development of occupational asthma, the number of workers with preexisting NSBR or asthma may, in fact, be less than that found in the general population. Subjects with preexisting asthma or NSBR who experience exacerbations of their symptoms in the workplace are probably less likely to join or stay in such an environment. It is important to identify bronchial hyperreactivity both in those who developed NSBR in the workplace and in those with preexisting NSBR who may be at risk for exacerbation of symptoms as a result of workplace exposures. Many agents encountered in the workplace may have little or no effect on nonasthmatic workers but can cause profound symptomatic bronchial constriction in workers with asthma. Unfortunately, testing for NSBR cannot discriminate between those with preexisting NSBR and those who develop NSBR as a result of their workplace exposure. The identification of NSBR in the workplace does not necessarily identify a cause-and-effect relationship between the occupation and the NSBR, but may still identify subjects at risk for exacerbation of lung disease. Time studies, specific exposures studies, and correlation with functional studies may be required to identify with certainty the association of NSBR with a specific occupational exposure.

EVALUATION AND GRADING OF PULMONARY DISABILITY

Most clinicians who see patients with respiratory problems make an assessment of disability during the patient's initial visit and at regular intervals thereafter. These patients complain primarily of dyspnea on exertion that can be quantitated in terms of some standard or familiar activity. The patient's ability to hold a job, walk some distance without stopping for breath, climb stairs, mow his or her lawn, or do housework are common examples that appear in the respiratory patient's history. This type of historical assessment should allow a reasonably accurate categorization of the patient's impairment or disability (Table 7). Thus, a patient with significant respiratory symptoms and even moderately abnormal pulmonary function, but who is still able to work full time, might be considered mildly or moderately impaired, whereas a patient no longer able to work because of respiratory symptoms would be categorized as totally disabled. Unfortunately, there may be little or nothing in the way of objective findings that differentiates these two patients. This difficulty in objectively determining the degree of disability in individual patients—a problem greatly compounded by our legal, insurance, and social security system—has led to a number of formal schemes for determining respiratory disability. This section will review the methods proposed for determining and grading respiratory disability and discuss the problems with the concept of disability assessment.

TABLE 7. *Clinical Criteria for Grading Disability*

None	Able to work full time. No impairment of life style.
Mild	Able to work with minimal restrictions. Loss of ability to do vigorous activity.
Moderate	Can work to a limited extent. Can keep up with most people of same age on level but not on stairs.
Severe	Cannot work. Some restriction of activities of daily living.

TABLE 8. *Definition of Terms Relating to Disability*

Source	Term	Definition
ATS[52,53]	Impairment	A medical condition resulting from a functional abnormality
	Disability	The effect of impairment on a patient's life
WHO[55]	Impairment	Loss of function
	Disablement	Loss of exercise capacity
	Handicap	Total effect of impairment on patient's life

Definitions

Before proceeding further, it is necessary to deal with some definitions. Although many clinicians use the words "impairment," "disability," and "handicap" interchangeably, these terms have been given precise definitions by various organizations interested in the evaluation and grading of disability. Unfortunately these definitions vary somewhat in different countries. The United States and Canada have generally adopted the definitions proposed by the American Thoracic Society (ATS).[52,53] The ATS has defined an **impairment** as a purely medical condition resulting from a functional abnormality (Table 8). This medical condition may or may not be stable at the time the evaluation is made and may be temporary or permanent. Impairments may be of varying degrees of severity up to and including those that would preclude any gainful employment. Impairments are not exclusively dependent on the patient's lung function. They may be environmentally related, such as a patient with occupational asthma who is impaired when exposed to inciting agents, or a patient with tuberculosis who is impaired in terms of contact with others for public health reasons.

In contrast to "impairment," the ATS defines **disability** as the total effect of an impairment on a patient's life. Thus, disability is not just related to a purely medical condition (impairment) but involves complex psychosocial factors. A farmer and an accountant may both be equally impaired in terms of their ability to operate heavy machinery, but only the farmer would be disabled. Some people feel the assessment of an impairment is totally within the capability of a physician, whereas the determination of disability requires input from other professionals such as psychologists and social workers.[54]

European countries tend to use the definitions of these terms proposed by the World Health Organization (WHO) instead of the ATS definitions. The WHO definitions attempt to take into account the lack of correlation between individual organ function and the overall function of the individual.[55] The WHO defines "impairment" as loss of function, "disablement" (in terms of the respiratory system) as loss of exercise capacity, and "handicap" as the total effect of impairment on a patient's life. Unless specifically noted, the ATS definitions will be used here.

Methods for Assessing Pulmonary Disability

Virtually every scheme for the objective assessment of respiratory disability starts with pulmonary function testing. Pulmonary function laboratories are now standardized in terms of equipment and testing techniques.[1,16] The main issue in terms of disability assessment is what tests to perform. Patients referred for disability assessment are assumed to have disease. The issue for the laboratory is not the early detection of subtle obstruction in the small airways but the correlation of significant pulmonary function abnormalities with work capacity. Therefore, the pulmonary function tests used for disability evaluation are simple spirometry with emphasis on the forced vital capacity (FVC) and forced expiratory volume in one second (FEV_1). Since these tests are designed to measure primarily airways disease, the single-breath DLCO is also used to assess the magnitude of interstitial disease. The FEV_1 and FVC are simple to perform and require relatively inexpensive equipment.[56] Most laboratories now use electronic, computerized equipment. In addition, the FVC and FEV_1 are quite reproducible when compared to other tests of pulmonary function with a coefficient of variation of about 5%.[56] The DLCO is fairly easy for the patient to perform but requires more complex and expensive equipment than spirometry. It also has considerably more variability (about 15 to 20%).[32,56]

The results of these pulmonary function tests in an individual patient are compared against normal values to determine a percent of predicted value. The published algorithms for grading disability usually specify which set of normal values to use. The validity of pulmonary function testing is critically dependent on obtaining a maximum effort from the patient. Repeated forced exhalations done at maximum effort by the same individual will produce nearly identical flow rates at any given lung volume.[57] This effect can be most easily seen by viewing superimposed maximum expiratory flow versus volume curves done in succession by the patient. Valid curves will be virtually superimposable.[58] Computerized spirometry that allows the pulmonary function technician to view several flow versus volume curves simultaneously has greatly improved the speed and accuracy of disability assessment using pulmonary function tests.[56]

To reiterate, impairment is the loss of function of a particular organ or organ system, whereas disability is the effect of this impairment on the life of the individual.[52] Thus, pulmonary function testing really is a measure of organ impairment and not disability. Translating an abnormal pulmonary function test into a degree of disability requires a number of assumptions about the relationship between abnormal lung function and work capacity. In order to assess that relationship more directly, a number of schemes for assessing respiratory disability advocate exercise testing in addition to resting pulmonary function testing, at least for certain groups of patients.[59-61] Exercise testing has the advantage of integrating the function of a number of organ systems into a single testing session. It is theoretically possible by using exercise testing to attribute the loss of exercise capacity to respiratory, cardiac, or muscular (lack of conditioning) causes.[62] Since actual work load is one of the variables measured during exercise testing, it is also possible to determine the work capacity of the patient, or at least the work level at which the patient became symptom-limited. There are also some diseases such as subtle pulmonary vascular disease that may only show up on exercise testing.[63] Of course these measurements are somewhat invasive and require sophisticated and expensive equipment. Therefore, exercise testing should only be performed when the resting pulmonary function tests are not clearcut. There is no point in doing exercise testing of someone with an FEV_1 of less than a liter. In many individuals, however, exercise testing remains the best means of integrating the multiple factors that produce disability.

Grading the Degree of Disability

There are several published schemes for grading the degree of disability in an individual patient. In most instances the choice of which criteria to use will not be left to the doctor's discretion. If the disability is acquired as a result of an individual's occupation, workers' compensation rules apply. The definition of disability under workers' compensation varies from state to state. In addition there are some federal programs specific to certain occupations or classes of workers, such as the Federal Employees' Compensation Program and the Black Lung Program.[64] Each of these programs has its unique rules and application process. Payments under workers' compensation are designed to replace lost wages, cover medical costs, and provide for the expense of rehabilitation. Workers' compensation cases not infrequently seek final adjudication in the courts where the degree of disability is generally defined by the case law of the state where the court is located.

People who become disabled from illness or injury that is not related to their employment may apply for assistance under Social Security Disability Insurance (SSDI).[65] The philosophy governing payments under SSDI is all together different from payments under workers' compensation. SSDI benefits are designed to prevent people who are unable to earn over $300 per month from becoming totally impoverished.[66] Individuals must have been unemployed for at least 6 months and must be expected to remain disabled for at least 12 months. Two-thirds of SSDI applicants are initially disapproved, but a number of the initial disapprovals are reversed on appeal, with a post-appeal approval rate of 47%.[66]

The most widely used current schemes for disability grading for respiratory diseases are those of the American Thoracic Society (ATS),[52,53] the Canadian Thoracic Society (CTS),[67] the American Medical Association (AMA),[59] and the Social Security Administration (SSDI).[65] Some of the features of these various schemes are outlined in Table 9. The

ATS and AMA criteria for disability from respiratory problems are quite similar, the only difference being the inclusion of maximum volume of oxygen utilization ($\dot{V}_2MAX$) measurements obtained from exercise testing in the AMA criteria. Both the ATS and AMA schemes emphasize pulmonary function testing as the main determinant of the degree of disability. The FEV_1 and the FVC are the primary pulmonary function tests used. Diffusion (DLCO) is added in the presence of restrictive disease. Measurement of maximum voluntary ventilation (MVV) is specifically not recommended, and exercise testing is deemphasized, with the recommendation it be used in only exceptional cases where an individual's work requires sustained heavy exertion. In such a circumstance routine pulmonary function testing might underestimate the degree of disability.

The CTS criteria use more classes of impairment than the ATS and AMA criteria. The CTS criteria also incorporate symptoms, $\dot{V}_2MAX$, and arterial blood gases in their grading scheme. Obstructive and restrictive disease are treated separately by the CTS criteria. SSDI criteria for disability are extremely stringent. The SSDI plan makes no provision for partial disability. For an average size man, SSDI accepts the presence of disability only if the FEV_1 is equal to or less than 1.4 liters.[65] This is close to the severest impairment class according to ATS and AMA criteria. Individuals with this level of pulmonary function abnormality would not be able to perform most jobs that require a moderate degree of exertion and would be limited to clerical and other similar occupations. SSDI also has stringent criteria for disability measured by arterial blood gases (PO_2 less than 55 mmHg) or diffusion (DLCO less than 9 ml/mmHg × min).

Another technique for grading the degree of disability is to determine the energy expenditure required for a given occupation or task and to then compare this requirement against the amount of energy the patient can generate. The energy requirements of a number of occupations and tasks have been determined with reasonable precision (Table 10). In several occupations these requirements have been refined to precisely specify the task involved.[68] This type of comparison requires exercise testing in order to make a precise measurement of the patient's $\dot{V}O_2MAX$. Attempts have been made to estimate

TABLE 9. *Schemes for Grading Respiratory Disability*

Source	Features
ATS[53]	Four classes of disability based almost entirely on pulmonary function tests. Exercise not recommended.
AMA[59]	Virtually same four classes as ATS but exercise criteria based on $\dot{V}_2MAX$ included.
CTS[67]	Five classes of impairment. Symptoms, $\dot{V}_2MAX$, and blood gases are part of criteria. Obstructive and restrictive diseases are given separate criteria.
Social Security[65]	Very stringent criteria approaching the severe class of ATS. No partial disability.

TABLE 10.   *Relationship Between AMA Disability Classes and Work Requirements**

Class	1	2	3	4
$\dot{V}_{2MAX}$ ml/(kg-min)	>25	20–25	15–20	>15
Occupation or activity	Mailman	Heavy labor	Sweeping	Walking 3 mph on level
	Climbing stairs	Using heavy tools	Paper hanging	Bedmaking
	Lift and carry 80 lb			Clerical work
	Shoveling heavy load			Truck driving

Adapted from refs. 68, 77, and 78.

$\dot{V}O_2MAX$ from pulmonary function tests, but the correlation has been relatively poor.[69] Other less invasive measures of $\dot{V}O_2MAX$ such as heart rate[68] and the 12-minute walk[70] have also been introduced, but these will require more study to determine their validity. A major conceptual problem with the concept of comparing the patient's $\dot{V}O_2MAX$ with the energy requirements for a given job lies in the failure of this technique to account for short, intense energy requirements. Most people can sustain activity of 40% of their $\dot{V}O_2MAX$ for an indefinite period. Thus, if an individual has a value for 40% of his $\dot{V}O_2MAX$ testing that is greater than the energy requirements for his occupation, he should not be disabled for that particular job. This analysis, however, usually only considers the average energy requirements for a particular job, when, in fact, the job might regularly require short periods of intense energy that are beyond the patient's capability.

Special Problems in Disability Evaluation

Dyspnea.   A major problem with any disability evaluation is that a patient's ability to function is usually limited by symptoms that are difficult to quantify or measure objectively. This is a difficult problem with any type of disability, but it is especially difficult when the limiting symptom is shortness of breath. With some symptoms such as musculoskeletal pain there is a reasonable correlation between the symptom and a measurable loss of function, such as limitation in range of motion. Dyspnea, however, is related to a complex interaction of neurological, chemical, and behavioral factors that are quite poorly correlated with pulmonary function tests.[71] Exercise testing might have some advantage in that it can sometimes identify at least the major organ system that limits the patient's ability to perform.[62] It is possible to quantitate dyspnea using analog scales,[72] and this technique appears to be valid when used to assess

the effect of treatment in the same individual.[73] Thus far it has not been used for disability evaluation.

Patient Motivation.   While it is generally true that the symptom of dyspnea does not correlate with pulmonary function abnormalities, it is also true that there ought to be at least some correlation. A patient claiming total disability on the basis of being too short of breath to work should in most instances have at least some measurable abnormality on routine pulmonary function testing.[74] This raises the entire question of patient motivation in disability assessment. At least one study suggests patients claiming disability tend to exaggerate their symptoms. Cotes compared FEV_1 values in 150 coal miners claiming disability and seeking compensation with FEV_1 values in 60 consecutive hospitalized patients.[75] At the same degree of breathlessness, the disability claimants had an appreciably better FEV_1 (% predicated) than the hospitalized patients. Interestingly, one could also conclude from this study that the disability claimants as a group did not deliberately try to underperform during the pulmonary function testing. This may still be a problem, however, with individual patients. Using flow versus volume loops helps to identify patients who are intentionally or inadvertently underperforming. It is essentially impossible for a patient to achieve the reproducibility and characteristic appearance of a well-performed flow versus volume loop without a maximum effort.[58] Patients who do not perform well on pulmonary function testing will sometimes respond if told their tests are not interpretable and cannot be graded without a better effort on their part.

Reversible or Intermittent Disease.   Another special problem concerns the assessment of disability in patients with reversible or intermittent disease. This is particularly true in the patient with occupational asthma who may be entirely asymptomatic away from the inciting agent. These individuals are only disabled for a particular job or environment and may have perfectly normal pulmonary and exercise function at other times. The ATS recognizes the difficulty of evaluating the asthmatic patient by recommending periodic evaluation.[53] In patients with exercise-induced bronchospasm not preventable by bronchodilators, the ATS recommends assessing impairment after exercise. Chan-Yeung has suggested a more elaborate protocol which includes: (1) periodic evaluation with changing clinical status; (2) measurement of bronchial hyperresponsiveness with methacholine or exercise; (3) if bronchial hyperresponsiveness cannot be measured, asthma severity should be documented by the minimal amount of medication necessary to control symptoms; and (4) consideration of the degree of bronchial hyperresponsiveness in the assessment of disability.[76]

CONCLUSION

In the final analysis disability can only be considered in the context of the individual and his or her life situation. Thus the distinction between "impairment" and "disability" or "handicap" is not a trivial one. Obviously the same impairment might be disabling in one type of job and not in another. A patient may be too short of breath to work as a laborer but not as an accountant. Unfortunately, it is not always realistic for a patient to be retained for a job within his or her work capacity. Can a laborer who develops chronic obstructive lung disease in his mid-50s learn how to be an accountant? Would someone hire him even if he did? The answer to both these questions is almost certainly "no," and this individual should be considered totally disabled even though it is theoretically possible for him to perform less strenuous jobs. Motivation is another major factor in whether or not an impairment becomes a disability. There is some evidence that motivation may be linked to education. Only about 20% of laborers return to work after a pneumonectomy as opposed to 70–80% of those in the professions.[74] All of these factors must be considered and integrated into a final decision regarding whether or not an individual is disabled. Although this is a decision the physician is often asked to make, he or she may not be the best qualified person to make it. As more progress is made in this field we may learn how to develop a more comprehensive approach to the problem.

REFERENCES

1. Gardner RM (chairman): Standardization of spirometry—1987 update. Am Rev Respir Dis 136:1285–1298, 1987.
2. Gardner RM (chairman): Pulmonary function laboratory personnel qualifications. Am Rev Respir Dis 134: 623–624, 1987.
3. Gardner RM (chairman): Computer guidelines for pulmonary laboratories. Am Rev Respir Dis 134:628–629, 1986.
4. Gardner RM (chairman): Quality assurance in pulmonary function laboratories. Am Rev Respir Dis 134: 625–627, 1986.
5. Tablan OC, Williams WW, Martone WJ: Infection control in pulmonary function laboratories. Infect Control 6:442–444, 1985.
6. McCarthy DS, Craig DB, Cherniak RM: Intraindividual variability in maximal expiratory flow-volume and closing volume in asymptomatic subjects. Am Rev Respir Dis 112:406–411, 1975.
7. Cochrane GM, Prieto F, Clark TJ: Intrasubject variability of maximal expiratory flow volume curve. Thorax 32:171–176, 1977.
8. Pennock BE, Rogers RM, McCaffree DR: Changes in measured spirometric indices. Chest 80:1, 97–99, 1981.
9. Lam S, Abboud R, Chan-Yeung M: Use of maximal expiratory flow-volume curve with air and helium-oxygen in the detection of ventilatory abnormalities in population surveys. Am Rev Respir Dis 123:234–237, 1981.
10. Rossoff L, Csima A, Zamel N: Reproducibility of maximum expiratory flow in severe chronic obstructive pulmonary disease. Bull Eur Physiopathol Respir 15:1129–1136, 1979.
11. Rozas CJ, Goldman AL: Daily spirometric variability: Normal subjects and subjects with chronic bronchitis with and without airflow obstruction. Arch Intern Med 124:1287–1291, 1982.
12. Hankinson JL: Pulmonary function testing in the screening of workers: Guidelines for instrumentation, performance, and interpretation. J Occup Med 28:10, 1081–1091, 1986.
13. Buist AS: Evaluation of lung function: Concepts of normality. Current Pulmonology 4:141–165, 1982.
14. Becklake MR: Concepts of normality applied to the measurement of lung function. Am J Med 80:1158–1164, 1986.
15. Glindmeyer HW: Predictable confusion. J Occup Med 23:12, 845–846, 1981.
16. Crapo RO, Morris AH, Gardner RM: Reference spirometer values using techniques and equipment that meets ATS recommendations. Am Rev Respir Dis 123:659–664, 1981.
17. Knudson RJ, Lebowitz MD, Holberg CJ, et al: Changes in the normal maximal expiratory flow-volume curve with growth and aging. Am Rev Respir Dis 127:725–734, 1983.
18. Knudson RJ, Slatin RC, Lebowitz MD, et al: The maximal expiratory flow volume curve. Am Rev Respir Dis 113:587–600, 1976.
19. Morris JF, Koski A, Johnson LC: Spirometric standards for healthy nonsmoking adults. Am Rev Respir Dis 3:55–61, 1971.
20. Rossiter CE, Weill H: Ethnic differences in lung function: Evidence for proportional differences. Int J Epidemiol 3:56–61, 1974.
21. Morris AH, Kanner RE, Crapo RO, Gardner RM: Clincial Pulmonary Function Testing: A Manual of Uniform Laboratory Procedure, 2nd ed. Salt Lake City, Intermountain Thoracic Society, 1984.

22. Hankinson JL, Villa JO: Dynamic BTPS correction factors for spirometric data. J Appl Physiol 55:1354–1360, 1983.
23. Eisen EA, Robins JM, Greaves IA, Wegman DH: Selection effects of repeatability criteria applied to lung spirometry. Am J Epidemiol 120:5, 734–742, 1984.
24. Eisen EA, Oliver LC, Christiani DC, et al: Effects of spirometry standards in two occupational cohorts. Am Rev Respir Dis 132:120–124, 1985.
25. Eisen EA, Robins JM: Estimation of ventilatory capacity in subjects with unacceptable lung function tests. Int J Epidemiol 15:3, 337–342, 1986.
26. Eisen EA, Dockery DW, Speizer FE, et al: The association between health status and the performance of excessively variable spirometry tests in a population-based study in six U.S. cities. Am Rev Respir Dis 136:1371–1376, 1987.
27. Fayrard P, Orehek J, Grimaud C, et al: Bronchoconstrictor effects of a deep inspiration in patients with asthma. Am Rev Respir Dis 3:433–439, 1975.
28. Krowka MJ, Enright PL, Rodarte JR, Hyatt RE: Effect of effort on measurement of forced expiratory volume in one second. Am Rev Respir Dis 136:829–833, 1987.
29. Burge PS, O'Brien IM, Harries MG: Peak flow rate records in the diagnosis of occupational asthma due to colophony. Thorax 34:308–316, 1979.
30. Burge PS, O'Brien IM, Harries MG: Peak flow rate records in the diagnosis of occupational asthma due to isocyanates. Thorax 34:317–323, 1979.
31. Cotton D, Mink J, Graham B: Effect of high negative inspiratory pressure on single-breath CO diffusing capacity. Respir Physiol 54:19–29, 1983.
32. Crapo RO, Morris AH: Standardized single breath normal values for carbon monoxide diffusing capacity. Am Rev Respir Dis 123:185–189, 1981.
33. Michoud MC, Ghezzo H, Amyot R: A comparison of pulmonary function tests used for bronchial challenges. Bull Eur Physiopathol Respir 18:609–621, 1982.
34. Dehaut P, Rachiele A, Martin R, et al: Histamine dose-response curves in asthma: Reproducibility and sensitivity of different indices to assess response. Thorax 38:516–522, 1983.
35. Juniper EF, Frith PA, Dunnett C, et al: Reproducibility and comparison of response to inhaled histamine and methacholine. Thorax 33:705–710, 1978.
36. Salome C, Schoeffel R, Woolcock A: Comparison of bronchial reactivity to histamine and methacholine in asthmatics. Clin Allergy 10:541–546, 1980.
37. Thomson N, Roberts R, Bandouvakis J, et al: Comparison of bronchial responses to prostaglandin F2-alpha and methacholine. Allergy Clin Immunol 68:392–398, 1981.
38. Assoufi BK, Dally MB, Newman-Taylor AJ, et al: Cold air test: A simplified standard method for airway reactivity. Bull Eur Physiopathol Respir 22:349–357, 1986.
39. Weiss ST, Tager IB, Weiss JW, et al: Airways responsiveness in a population sample of adults and children. Am Rev Respir Dis 129:898–902, 1984.
40. O'Byrne PM, Ryan G, Morris M, et al: Asthma induced by cold air and its relation to nonspecific bronchial responsiveness to methacholine. Am Rev Respir Dis 125:281–285, 1982.
41. Cockcroft DW, Killian DN, Mellon JJA, et al: Bronchial reactivity to inhaled histamine: A method and clinical survey. Clin Allergy 7:235–243, 1977.
42. Chai H, Farr RS, Froehlich LA, et al: Standardization of bronchial inhalation challenge procedures. J Allergy Clin Immunol 56:323–327, 1975.
43. Ryan G, Dolovich MB, Roberts RS, et al: Standardization of inhalation provocation tests: Two techniques of aerosol generation and inhalation compared. Am Rev Respir Dis 123:195–199, 1981.
44. Enarson DA, Chan-Yeung M, Lam S, et al: Does determination of bronchial reactivity add anything to prevalence studies of respiratory disease in the occupational setting? Am Rev Respir Dis 129(suppl):A160, 1984.
45. Hendrick DJ, Hughes J, Fabbri LM, et al: Epidemiologic measurement of bronchial reactivity in polyurethane workers. Am Rev Respir Dis 127(suppl):154, 1983.
46. Enarson DA, Tabona MZ, Dorken E, et al: Bronchial reactivity to methacholine in nonatopic grainhandlers: Relation to age, smoking, and initial lung function. Am Rev Respir Dis 127(suppl):154, 1983.
47. Ryan G, Cookson WOC, Musk AW: Allergy and non-allergic bronchial reactivity as determinants of work-related respiratory symptoms in seasonal grain handlers. Chest 87(suppl):215S, 1986.
48. Chatham M, Bleeker ER, Norman P, et al: A screening test for airways reactivity. An abbreviated methacholine inhalation challenge. Chest 82:15–18, 1982.
49. Malo JL, Pineau L, Carter A, et al: Reference values of the provocative concentrations of methacholine that cause 6% and 20% changes in forced expiratory volume in one second in a normal population. Am Rev Respir Dis 128:8–11, 1983.
50. Braman SS, Barrows AA, DeCotiis BA, et al: Airway hyperresponsiveness in allergic rhinitis. Chest 91:671–674, 1987.
51. Bahous J, Cartier A, Ouimet G, et al: Nonallergic bronchial hyperexcitability in chronic bronchitis. Am Rev Respir Dis 129:829–832, 1982.
52. American Thoracic Society: Evaluation of impairment/disability secondary to respiratory disease. Am Rev Respir Dis 126:945–951, 1982.
53. American Thoracic Society: Evaluation of impairment/disability secondary to respiratory disorders. Am Rev Respir Dis 134:1205–1209, 1986.
54. Becklake MR, Rodarte JR, Kalica AR: NHLBI workshop summary: Scientific issues in the assessment of respiratory impairment. Am Rev Respir Dis 137:1505–1510, 1988.
55. World Health Organization: International classification of impairments, disabilities, and handicaps. Geneva, World Health Organization, 1980.
56. Clausen JL (ed): Pulmonary Function Testing Guidelines and Controversies: Equipment, Methods and Normal Values. A project of the California Thoracic Society. Orlando, FL, Academic Press, 1982.
57. Mead J, Turner JM, Macklem PT, Little JB: Significance of the relationship between lung recoil and maximum expiratory flow. J Appl Physiol 22:95–108, 1967.
58. Wilson AF (ed): Pulmonary Function Testing Indications and Interpretations. A project of the California Thoracic Society. Orlando, FL, Grune & Stratton, 1985.
59. American Medical Association Guide to the Evaluation of Permanent Impairment. Chicago, American Medical Association, 1984.
60. Bates DV: Disability and compensation. Chest 78:361–362, 1980.
61. Veterans Administration: Schedule for rating disability. Section 6600 for bronchitis, 6603 for emphysema, and 6802 for pneumoconiosis. September, 1975.
62. Jones NL: Clinical Exercise Testing, 3rd ed. Philadelphia, W.B. Saunders, 1988.

63. Loke J: Distinguishing cardiac versus pulmonary limitation in exercise performance. Chest 83:441–442, 1983.

64. Richman S: Why change: A look at the current system of disability determination and workers' compensation for occupational lung disease. Ann Intern Med 97:908–914, 1982.

65. U.S. Department of Health and Human Services: Social Security Administration disability evaluation under Social Security. SSA Publication No. 05-10089, 1986.

66. Carey T, Hadler N: The role of the primary physician in disability determination for social security insurance and workers' compensation. Ann Intern Med 104:706–710, 1986.

67. Ostiguy GL: Summary of the task force report on occupational respiratory disease (pneumoconiosis). CMA Journal 121:414–421, 1979.

68. Harber P, Tamimie J, Emory J: Estimation of the exertion requirements of coal mining work. Chest 85:226–231, 1984.

69. Cotes JE, Zejda J, King B: Lung function impairment as a guide to exercise limitation in work-related lung disorders. Am Rev Respir Dis 137:1089–1093, 1988.

70. McGavin CR, Gupta SP, McHardy GJR: Twelve-minute walking test for assessing disability in chronic bronchitis. Br Med J 1:822–823, 1976.

71. Tobin MJ: Dyspnea. Pathologic basis, clinical presentation, and management. Arch Intern Med 150:1604–1613, 1990.

72. Altose M, Cherniack N: Respiratory sensations and dyspnea. J Appl Physiol 58:1051–1054, 1985.

73. Man GCW, Hsu K, Sproule BJ: Effect of aprazolam on exercise and dyspnea in patients with chronic obstructive pulmonary disease. Chest 90:832–836, 1986.

74. Morgan WKC: Clinical significance of pulmonary function tests. Disability or disinclination? Impairment or importuning? Chest 75:712–715, 1979.

75. Cotes JE: Assessment of disablement due to impaired respiratory function. Bull Physiopathol Respir 11:210–217, 1975.

76. Chan-Yeung M: Pulmonary perspective. Evaluation of impairment/disability in patients with occupational asthma. Am Rev Respir Dis 135:950–951, 1987.

77. Barnhart S: Evaluation fo impairment and disability in occupational lung disease. In Rosenstock L (ed): Occupational Pulmonary Disease. Occup Med State Art Rev 2:227–241, 1987.

78. Becklake MR: Organic or functional impairment. Overall perspective. Am Rev Respir Dis 129(suppl):S96–S100, 1984.

Chapter 4

DETERMINATION OF AIRWAY HYPERREACTIVITY TO ALLERGENS AND OTHER BRONCHOCONSTRICTIVE SUBSTANCES

Sheldon L. Spector, MD

Various inhaled substances can be administered that produce bronchial obstruction. Such inhaled substances have the ability to help clarify the role of mediators and other factors that determine airway hyperreactivity. The most widely employed bronchial provocation tests measure "nonspecific airway reactivity," which reflects the extent to which the airways are generally irritable or reactive to nonallergic agents.[1] Bronchial provocation tests can also be employed to measure the effects of specific allergenic substances found in the environment or in occupational settings.[2] Even though the distinctions are not always clear, it is convenient to talk about them by subcategorizing challenges into nonspecific and specific challenges. In general, asthmatic subjects are considerably more reactive to the so-called nonspecific stimuli than are the normal nonasthmatic controls. Patients with bronchitis and hay fever tend to fall in between the normals and the asthmatics. Reactivity tends to be increased in patients with allergies as well as those who are longtime smokers. Hyperreactivity is generally measured by a PC_{20} or PD_{20}, which stand for provocative concentration or provocative dose, where there is a 20% fall in a pulmonary function parameter, usually FEV_1. Individual patients that fall out of an accepted range are thought to have hyperreactive airways, but the break-off point where hyperreactivity begins has not been clearly defined.

INHALATION CHALLENGES WITH AGENTS OTHER THAN ANTIGENS

Acetylcholine (ACh). Acetylcholine was one of the first agents to be used clinically. It was first popularized by Tiffeneau[3,4] and is still occasionally used by investigators in Europe[5] and in the Far East.[6] Its main disadvantages are its rapid inactivation in the body by cholinesterases and its short half-life, with the associated difficulty in obtaining serial measurements.

Carbamylcholine (Carbaminocholine Chloride). This derivative of acetylcholine is not metabolized by acetylcholinesterase and therefore has a longer duration of action. It has the advantage of being stable in solution. Although certain European investigators still describe its use,[7] it has never gained in popularity among American investigators. Moreover, Cropp noted adverse reactions of an unknown mechanism, which further dampened enthusiasm for its use in the United States.[8]

Methacholine (Acetyl-β-methylcholine [Mecolyl]). Methacholine is also an analogue of acetylcholine but lacks the nicotine action of acetylcholine. It is not as stable in solution as carbamylcholine but has become one of the most widely used bronchoconstrictors to assess nonspecific reactivity. Spector and Farr popularized the concept of keeping the number of breaths constant and increasing the concentration, a method later accepted by

35

an NIH panel to standardize bronchial inhalation challenges.[9,10]

Histamine Phosphate (β-Imidazolyethylamine Phosphate). Histamine is similar in popularity to methacholine and probably constricts airway-smooth muscle both directly[11] and reflexly.[12] Although methacholine and histamine have been compared and often show similar reactivity in a given individual,[13] certain subjects have a disparity between the two responses[14] that implies a different mechanism behind its mode of action in these individuals.

Hypertonic Saline. Hypertonic saline may cause bronchoconstriction in asthmatic subjects,[15] and its action is probably mediated predominantly through the release of histamine from mast cells, with a minor contribution being made by prostanoids.[16]

Prostaglandins. Asthmatic subjects are nearly 8,000 times more sensitive to prostaglandin $F_2\alpha(PGF_2\alpha)$ than healthy controls. This compares to an increased sensitivity to histamine of 10- to 100-fold. Although the F series of prostaglandins produce bronchoconstriction, many of the E family of prostaglandins produce bronchodilatation.[17,18] On the other hand, both $PGF_2\alpha$ and PGE have proven irritating to many individuals and commonly cause cough in an asthmatic subject. Theories put forth to explain idiosyncrasy associated with the use of aspirin and other nonsteroidal anti-inflammatory agents in asthmatic subjects often involve prostaglandins and other products of arachidonic acid metabolism.[19,20] One explanation suggests the enhancement of the metabolism of the lipoxygenase pathway, leading to increased leukotriene formation.[21,22] Aspirin-sensitive asthmatics are reported to be more sensitive to histamine than $PGF_2\alpha$.[23] They also show a selective and marked increase in airway responsiveness to leukotriene E4 (LtE4) compared to histamine. After desensitization with aspirin, an average 33-fold reduction in LtE4 responsiveness can be found.[24] Anticholinergic agents such as atropine and β_2 stimulants can significantly inhibit the bronchoconstrictive response to $PGF_2\alpha$, whereas cromolyn sodium, thymoxamine, and ipratropium bromide have no blocking effect.[25]

Leukotrienes. Inhaled LtC4 produces a prominent central and slight peripheral airway response. By contrast, inhaled histamine results in a predominantly peripheral airway constriction.[26] LtD4 may mediate cold air isocapnic bronchoconstriction.[27] LtB4 probably does not have an important role in bronchial hyperresponsiveness.[28]

Serotonin. Although the exact role of serotonin in human bronchial constriction is not known, serotonin may potentiate vagal effects on airway smooth muscle in dogs.[29] Certain solutions of serotonin appear to rapidly decompose. It is not found in the mast cells of man per se but is released from human platelets.[30]

Adenosine. Adenosine and its metabolite, adenosine 5' monophosphate (AMP), may produce bronchoconstriction partially through the release of histamine. Selective H_1-antihistamines like terfenadine and astemizole inhibit AMP-induced bronchoconstriction by more than 80% and displace the concentration response curve to the right.[31]

Other Bronchoconstrictive Substances. It would be impractical to give detailed descriptions of all possible agents that have been employed to induce bronchoconstriction in normals or asthmatic subjects. Almost any agent given in large enough quantities or with unusual physical characteristics (e.g., too low or too high a pH) can serve as a potent irritant to an asthmatic or even a healthy subject. Obstruction can be produced with cold air, hypotonic saline, and a magnitude of drugs such as propranolol.[32-35]

Bradykinin is thought to act directly on smooth muscle. However, given as an aerosol, its primary action may involve vagal reflexes in man.[36] Exercise can also produce nonspecific bronchial provocation. It can be performed in an office setting by running a patient up and down the stairs or on a treadmill, controlling for temperature and humidity. Cold air is though to be the initial stimulus for this bronchoconstriction. Possible drawbacks of exercise provocation is the rendered refractory period induced after the initial stimulus and the standardization in humidity and temperature ideally required.[37]

COMPARISON OF DIFFERENT BRONCHOCONSTRICTIVE CHALLENGES

Although good correlation might be present between two tests of bronchial obstruction, the dissimilarities between certain responses are often more interesting than the similarities, because different mechanisms exist between the two challenges studied. For example, some asthmatic subjects have a negative exercise challenge yet will have a significant fall in FEV_1 after a methacholine or histamine challenge.[38-41] During an upper respiratory infection, normal individuals develop a transient hyperreactivity of their airways in response to exercise with cold air as well as to histamine.[42] Although both of these tests of hyperreactivity are well correlated and can be blocked by atropine, in certain individuals a disparity exists in the recovery from the two stimuli. After 6 weeks, exercise with cold air no longer produces a decrease in (SG_{aw}; $p < 0.05$), yet by 6 weeks airway reactivity to histamine remained decreased in 9 of 13 subjects.[42] Certain individuals are more responsive to methacholine than to respiratory heat loss and vice versa.[43] Hajos studied 158 asthmatic subjects and found 18% reacted only to 0.2% serotonin and not histamine or acetylcholine (ACh).[44] Most investigators, however, feel that histamine and ACh given by inhalation produce similar bronchial reactivity, especially if used in relatively equal doses.[45,46]

Although the similarities between responsiveness to methacholine and histamine have been mentioned, Spector and Farr found a small group of asthmatic subjects that could tolerate increasing doses of histamine without a corresponding fall in FEV_1 and who became unresponsive to the highest test dose.[14] Similar observations were observed by Itkin in a few subjects[47] and Schoeffel and co-workers.[48] Spector and Farr also reported on one patient who was highly reactive to histamine inhalation (i.e., who had a fall in FEV_1 after a very low concentration) who subsequently showed marked improvement after ingestion of an antihistamine.[14]

Histamine and methacholine reactivity can also be distinguished by the ability of hexamethonium (a ganglionic blocking agent) to block the former but not the latter.[49]

In general, anticholinergics such as ipratropium bromide prevent methacholine and not histamine bronchoconstriction, and antihistamines such as chlorpheniramine prevent histamine- but not methacholine-induced bronchoconstriction. It is therefore presumed that receptor sites involved in bronchial provocation by these two agents are different.[50] It has also been observed that there is a significant cumulative dose effect with methacholine and not with histamine.

STORAGE OF BRONCHOCONSTRICTIVE AGENTS

A discussion of the details involved in the storage of these bronchoconstrictive agents or techniques to appropriately deliver these challenges is beyond the scope of this article, but references are provided for those interested in these specific details of the above.[1,51]

INDICATIONS FOR PERFORMING BRONCHIAL CHALLENGE WITH BRONCHOCONSTRICTIVE SUBSTANCES (OTHER THAN ANTIGENS)

To Define the Hyperreactive State or Atypical Asthma

Virtually all individuals with asthma, with rare exceptions, have hyperreactive airways.[1] Even though this finding is characteristic of asthma, it is not unique to this diagnosis. For example, a small number of healthy subjects and up to 50% of patients with hay fever have an abnormally exaggerated response.[1] It may be that humans are born with bronchial hyperresponsiveness and genetic or environmental factors influence its loss thereafter.[52] Hyperreactivity might also be acquired, because it is found with conditions such as bronchitis, sacroidosis, tuberculosis, silicosis, and cystic fibrosis.[1] The acute respiratory distress syndrome (ARDS) is often associated with hyperreactive airways.[53] Interestingly, those patients who experience cough while on angiotensin-converting enzyme (ACE) inhibitors appear to be those with underlying bronchial hyperreactivity. Often the bronchial hyperreactivity persists despite cessation of the ACE-inhibitors.[54] Lindgren and co-workers reported that after 1–2 weeks of enalapril, the PC_{20} value for histamine challenge was reduced along with an increased dermal response to anti-human IgE.[55]

To Correlate Hyperreactivity with Other Factors

Histamine Inhalation Challenge.   Various investigators have related histamine reactivity to other factors such as the severity and duration of asthma.[56,57] Townley et al. did not find a relationship between the level of reactivity and the duration of symptoms, but they did find the reactivity was less in patients free of symptoms for more than 2 years.[58] On the other hand, Spector and co-workers noted that the greatest reactivity to histamine or methacholine was found in those admitted for intensive inpatient care at a younger age who had an earlier age of onset and had asthma longer than patients with less airway reactivity.[59] Townley and co-workers reported that hay fever sufferers had intermediate methacholine reactivity compared to normals who could tolerate high concentrations and asthmatics who could only tolerate low concentrations.[60]

Spector and Farr reported that patients who were not very methacholine reactive were statistically the least severe patients as measured by their discharge doses of corticosteroids.[14] Cockcroft and co-workers also related heightened reactivity to the more severe asthmatic.[61]

A correlation has also been noted with the degree of hyperresponsiveness and the amount of treatment needed to control symptoms.[61a] Staudenmayer et al. found that asthmatic patients who were highly reactive to histamine and who had a low panic-fear profile were those who were hospitalized at exceptionally high rates relative to others.[62] There is still debate regarding the relationship between reactivity to methacholine or histamine and severity of asthma. In fact, Josephs and co-workers assessed the relationship between nonspecific reactivity and the day-to-day clinical expression of asthma by measuring methacholine reactivity every 2 to 3 weeks over a period of 12–18 months.[63] They concluded that the association of nonspecific reactivity and exacerbations of bronchial asthma was not sufficiently close to be of practical use.

Antigen Inhalation Challenge. The greater the nonspecific reactivity of an asthmatic subject, the more likely a reactivity will occur to an aerosolized allergen mixture. For example, the mean bronchial threshold dose to the mite antigen is significantly higher in the asymptomatic individual than in as asthmatic subject who is highly reactive to histamine. There is also a relationship between histamine responsiveness and bronchial responsiveness to other allergens. Investigators must be cautious in giving too high a concentration of antigen to produce a decrease in pulmonary function, i.e., a positive response. Even asymptomatic or hay fever patients can be induced to wheeze for the first time when the concentration of antigen is pushed high enough. Additionally, this can prove potentially dangerous.[64] At least two factors have been related to a positive bronchial inhalation challenge: nonspecific airway hyperreactivity and a positive skin test.[65] One must always keep in mind the clinical meaning of the challenge result as it relates to the history and the nature of the patient's illness.

The pulmonary function tests employed can influence the results. For instance, a differential response had been noted between patients with allergic rhinitis (hay fever) and asthma.[66] Fish et al. speculated that there might be hyperreactivity of both central and peripheral airways in asthmatic subjects, but only hyperreactivity of central airways in nonasthmatic subjects.[67] However, there also might be a difference in physiologic response to the test itself.[68-70]

Other Tests of Bronchial Lability. Reactivity to nonspecific substances and exercise can be compared to other tests as a means of better understanding mechanisms that have been previously discussed.[1]

Response to Medications. Various investigators have tried to demonstrate a relationship between nonspecific reactivity and response to certain medications, such as prednisone. Oppenheimer was unsuccessful in doing so, but he only studied a small number of subjects.[71] Hargreave and co-workers reported that the lower the peak flow values were in the morning (along with high histamine hyperreactivity), the greater the response to albuterol. This Canadian group has noted the relationship between bronchial responsiveness and the level of treatment required to control symptoms, with the amount and strength of medication increasing for those who are the most reactive.[61a]

To Assess Effectiveness of Treatment Modalities by Their Ability to Block the Hyperreactive Airway Disease

It would be logical to assume that if a new agent can block or normalize hyperreactivity to, for example, methacholine or histamine, this agent might have potential usefulness in the treatment of asthma. The agents that seems to block hyperreactivity best over the long term are the corticosteroid aerosols,[61a,72,73] even though some investigators feel that the reduction of bronchial responsiveness may be minimal or of questionable clinical relevance.[22,188] Cromolyn sodium also can block hyperreactivity especially if treatment is given for greater than 12 weeks.[73a,74] Surprisingly, the antibiotic troleandomycin raises the threshold of an asthmatic subject to methacholine and can sometimes dramatically improve asthmatic symptoms.[75,76] Prolonged treatment is associated with the best effect on hyperreactivity. It is not clear whether improvements in airway responsiveness and clinical asthma are maintained with prolonged use. Juniper and co-workers reduced or discontinued budesonide after 1 year of vigorous therapy. They found that even though improvements in airway responsiveness can be maintained for at least 3 months, deterioration in spirometry and symptoms may occur as a forerunner of increased responsiveness.[76a] Immunotherapy can also affect not only late-phase reactions but bronchial hyperresponsiveness as well.[77] In pollen-sensitive individuals given birch pollen immunotherapy, bronchial responsiveness to histamine became less in the immunotherapy-treated group but not in the control group.[78]

To Place Occupational Asthma in Perspective

Contact with certain occupational agents has been associated with a subsequent increased reactivity to methacholine or histamine.[79] In fact, a continued reactivity implies continued exposure to the presumed offender.[80,81] Unfortunately, almost any noxious stimulus such as a pollutant or virus can cause the same increased nonspecific responsiveness. Thus any assumptions about cause-and-effect relationships must be made cautiously.

The initial exposure to an agent can cause either a temporary or more sustained change in nonspecific reactivity, depending on the strength and chronicity of the initial exposure. Histamine inhalations before and after exposure to dimethyl ethanolamine, Western red cedar sawdust, and pyrolysis products of polyvinyl chloride have been associated with an increased reactivity.[82-85] In many circumstances, several months after removal from exposure to such agents as California redwood, grain dust, and isocyanates, reactivity decreases only to increase again with re-exposure. In certain individuals increased reactivity remains even when the initial exposure or continued exposure is not obvious.[85]

Brooks and co-workers have described an asthma-like illness called "reactive airways dysfunction syndrome" (RADS).[86] Presumed normal individuals developed symptoms of shortness of breath, cough, wheezing, and chest tightness within 24 hours after exposure to high levels of noxious irritants such as vapors, fumes and smoke.[87] Despite this brief exposure, symptoms and increased airways responsiveness continued for more than 1 year. Tarlo et al. suggested an expanded definition

to include exposure not limited to a single accident or incident at work.[88] However, the distinction made between RADS and other types of occupational exposures needs to be further clarified and better understood.

ALLERGEN INHALATION CHALLENGES

Provocation challenges with allergens are less widely employed than challenges with other bronchoconstrictive substances. They are conducted in a similar manner to a histamine or methacholine challenge but with increasing concentrations of antigens, using dilutions of allergens predicted from the skin-prick method as a built-in safety feature. In contrast to the "nonspecific" provocations, airway response to allergen occurs more slowly. Immediate reactions typically occur after 15 or 20 minutes, followed in many circumstances by a late-phase reaction (which will be discussed subsequently). The following are indications for allergen challenges:

A Means to Understand the Role of Allergy in Asthma.   Perhaps the most common use nowadays of allergen challenge is to better understand allergic mechanisms as they relate to early- and late-phase reactions in asthma. The potential benefit of a new agent for the treatment of asthma might also be based on its ability to block these early- and late-phase reactions. Standardized allergen extracts have made these challenges more reproducible and lipophilized extracts have solved a storage problem that often had been associated with loss of stability.

If allergen inhalation challenge (AIC) provides different information than a skin test or in vitro test, then there is rationale for its use.[89,90] This is of particular interest in occupational asthma if a new agent is suspected, because skin testing to that agent may not have been standardized. Mast cells themselves have different sensitivities in different parts of the body, i.e., there is mast cell heterogeneity.[91] There is also a difference in basophil response compared to the tissue mast cell response.[92] It is still not clear if there is local production of IgE in the tracheobronchial tree so that a skin test per se would not provide the same information as an IgE challenge to the organ of interest.

Huggins and Brostoff concluded that there is a local production of IgE in nasal secretions.[93] They found patients with a positive clinical history and positive nasal provocation despite negative skin tests and negative RAST to dust mite. In looking at a possible causal relationship between an allergen and clinical symptoms, an important decision must be made regarding the maximum dose of antigen that should be employed to clarify this relationship. This point is illustrated by studies of Townley and co-workers, who performed AIC in normals and patients with hay fever and asthma.[60] When they used an antigen concentration of 10,000 PNUs, 11 of 14 patients with hay fever had a positive bronchial inhalation challenge response even though they had never wheezed before. This implies that too high a concentration was used to differentiate hay fever patients from asthmatics, even though the latter was the condition sought for clarification.[60]

Cavanaugh and colleagues reported similar results, concluding that patients who by inhalation challenge responded only to high concentration of antigens, behave as a separate population, i.e., with a higher incidence of negative skin test reactions compared with other subjects tested.[94] When we first performed antigen challenges we also noticed severe reactions if the allergen extract concentration given was too high so as to get a positive AIC with no clinical meaning. In fact, it led us to recommend bronchial challenges with concentrations of antigens greater than 10^{-2} or 10,000 PNUs (protein nitrogen units).[9] As mentioned previously, there is a relationship between responses to histamine or methacholine and the allergic responses.[65] When there is increased reactivity, a more severe allergic reaction would be anticipated. If too high a concentration of antigen leads to a late asthmatic response, there is potential to perpetuate and accentuate hyperreactivity.

Comparison of Skin Tests, In Vitro Tests, and Others. Allergen provocation tests have been touted by some as an absolute standard to which other tests should be compared, because they measure the locally secreted IgE in the organ of involvement, e.g., the lung in an asthmatic subject. Occasionally an in vitro test may be negative despite a positive antigen inhalation test and/or a positive skin test.

Aas and co-workers compared pollen and house dust reactivity by skin tests and AIC.[89] They found that the type of antigen and the degree of skin test reactivity both influence the results of an AIC response. There was a greater likelihood for a positive bronchial challenge response in patients with pollen reactivity compared to house dust reactivity.

Interestingly, patients with positive skin test results and negative bronchial challenge responses had nasal allergies to the pollens. The implication of this is that skin tests reveal IgE reactivity but not which organ is susceptible to this IgE effect. Aas et al. also studied the relationship between skin test reactivity and AIC. The greater the skin test reactivity, the greater the chance for subsequent positive AIC. We often find historical data are not very helpful because many of our patients have perennial symptoms. On the other hand, if a patient has a positive skin test with an accompanying strong history of a reaction to that antigen, the AIC will give a predictably positive response in more than 90% of the circumstances.[90,95] A level of skin test reactivity will often allow one to predict a subsequent allergen inhalation challenge, especially if the nonspecific reactivity is known.

Replacement for Skin Tests If They Cannot Be Performed. Skin disorders such as severe eczema might disallow skin testing. In vitro testing, which is a more expensive and less sensitive alternative to skin testing, may have to be employed under such circumstances. It also may have to be employed if a patient is on one of the long-acting antihistamines that will suppress skin test reactivity for weeks or months.

Clarification of Mediators and Mechanisms. Antigen inhalation challenges have been associated with elevated histamine levels and a sustained or biphasic release of neutrophil chemotactic factor.[96] Investigators have also found liberation of what was formerly called slow-reacting substance of anaphylaxis (SRS-A)[97] and the purified equivalents, the leukotrienes, especially C4 and D4.[98] Schwartz and co-workers described a method to assess mast cell activation in vivo as contrasted with the activation of basophils.[99] They found that an elevated plasma or serum tryptase level had diagnostic value for indicating mast cell-related events such as would occur with anaphylactic reactions. Serum complement falls during bronchospasm induced by antigen and not by methacholine. However, Arroyave and associates also found a decrease in complement in some of their controls, making interpretation of these data difficult.[100] Other investigators have also reported a drop in hemolytic complement level after AIC, which cromolyn could prevent in a small number of patients.[101] Although platelets are activated after allergen challenge, the platelet-derived thromboxene A2 does not appear to be important in the early bronchoconstrictor response.[102]

Deal and co-workers have contrasted AIC with hyperventilation after cold air. The former challenge produced a prolonged release of neutrophil chemotactic factor; the latter did not.[103]

LOCATION OF RESPONSE AS A CLARIFICATION OF THE MECHANISM

The pattern of change in mechanics of gas exchange in the lung during AIC has been investigated by various researchers. Olive and Hyatt noted the first effect of inhaled antigen was to cause a parallel shift in the maximum expiratory flow volume (MEFV) curve with no change in slope.[104] Not all patients showed the same pattern. One-third of the 15 subjects had closure of the units with no change in MEFV slope; another third initially produced the same pattern but at the height of the response showed a MEFV slope change, which suggested that other airways increased their resistance. The final one-third had an immediate change of slope with all but one showing an increase in residual volume. Thus, the site of airway obstruction may be different among some asthmatic subjects. Some investigators have suggested that an indicator of small airway response such as the flow iso-volume (Viro V) would be a better indicator of airway response to AIC than a measurement of large airways such as SG_{aw}.[105]

Oligati and co-workers found a greater involvement of peripheral airways in the seven patients they studied.[106] There was a decrease in mean arterial oxygen saturation after ragweed challenge, but not methacholine challenge, for comparable severity of bronchospasm as measured by SG_{aw}.

IMMEDIATE VERSUS LATE ASTHMATIC RESPONSE: IMPLICATIONS FOR MECHANISMS

Following exposure to allergens, an immediate- and/or late-phase reaction may develop. Typically the immediate component occurs within minutes, followed thereafter by a late phase that is thought to be inflammatory in nature and is often associated with a hyperreactive state. The late-phase reaction (LAR) has been defined as occurring from 4–12 hours after the immediate reaction and can occur in organs other than the lungs, such as the skin and nose. Most investigators feel that the late reaction is IgE-mediated, involving mast cells and other inflammatory cells such as eosinophils and polymorphonuclear cells. The prevalence of these late-phase responses usually ranges from 40 to 60%.[107-110] Some of the variables that determine the differences in prevalence involve: (1) the parameter used to determine a positive response, such as FEV_1 vs. another pulmonary function; (2) what percent fall is considered positive; (3) the IgE reactivity of the patient; and (4) the quantity of antigen administered.

Bundagaard and Boudet did not find the LAR to be very reproducible, because only one of the five subjects studied had similar positive allergen challenge when done on a second occasion.[111] Ihre et al. could change isolated late reactions following allergen challenge to dual reactions by increasing the allergen dose.[112] Thus, late asthmatic responses are more likely with certain antigens compared to others, high concentrations of allergens, and high levels of circulating IgE in the early response as measured by skin tests or mediator release. There is not necessarily a correlation between the late-onset skin reaction compared to the bronchial reaction.[113]

Other investigators have suggested that there is no need to perform allergen inhalation challenge if the skin test reactivity and nonspecific reactivity are known.[114] However, such predictability would not carry over to late asthmatic responses after occupational exposure or a new substance in the environment. This has important implications, because LAR might help explain the perpetuation of asthma in an individual. The inhalation of allergens, either experimentally or through natural exposure, can increase nonspecific bronchial responsiveness to substances such as histamine and methacholine.[115,116] This increasing reactivity can be demonstrated shortly after the immediate airway response or during the interval following LAR. The increased responsiveness may then persist for days or even weeks after the initial exposure.

Durham et al. found that in subjects who developed LAR after exposure to occupational agents there was an increase in nonspecific bronchial responsiveness to methacholine at 2–3 hours after the challenge.[117] Clinically there is an increase in nonspecific bronchial responsiveness during seasonal pollen exposure,[118] and reduction in reactivity can occur after prolonged allergen avoidance[119] or after immunotherapy.[120,121]

Although mediator release has been described during the discussion of early phase reactions, certain mediators are also released during late-phase responses. Neutrophil chemotactic factor activity (NCF-A) has been consistently found with late-phase responses.[122,123] Histamine has only been found sporadically.[122]

Metabolites of arachidonic acid have been noted.[124,125] The leukotriene LTB4, which is a potent neutrophil chemotactic factor in humans, has been found in plasma specimens obtained during the development of both an early and a late asthmatic response following AIC.[122,125] Using a sheep model, Abraham found that dual-responders produced more leukotrienes and were more sensitive to leukotrienes than the early responders.[126]

Those patients with an LAR had a significantly increased concentration of lyso form of platelet activating factor (PAF) compared with patients having a single immediate response 6 hours after the antigen challenge.[127] There were no differences in PAF level at 20 minutes, however.

Immunoglobulin levels have also been measured, and in 6 or 7 patients with dual reactions to dust mite there was higher IgG$_1$ antibody level compared to the 5 patients with isolated immediate reactions.[128] Also in the presence of high IgG$_1$ antibodies there was a propensity to develop LAR.

Gonzales and co-workers measured the number of helper (OKT$_4$) and suppressor (OKT$_8$) T-cells in blood and lavage fluid in patients with immediate or dual reactions.[129] There was a significant increase in the percentage of OKT$_4$ cells in the blood with the single early responders. The perecentage OKT$_4$ was much lower ($p < 0.005$) on the antigen day in the early responders than on the antigen day in the late-phase responders. This suggests the possibility that suppressor T-cells are mobilized into the lung after antigen-induced single early reactions, and that this might be associated with the presence of subsequent late-phase response.

Diaz and co-workers found a significant increase in lymphocytes, neutrophils, and eosinophils ($p < 0.05$)) in late-phase responders compared to the isolated early responders, also supporting the role of eosinophils and their products in late-phase injury responses.[130] Frick and Busse reported an increase in the proportion of peripheral blood eosinophils that are hypodense, only in those patients with both IAR and LAR. They concluded that the percent of hypodense eosinophils better reflects the severity of asthma than the concentration of total peripheral blood eosinophils.[131]

Various medications can affect both immediate and late challenge to allergen. The pharmaceutical industry has utilized blocking properties to predict possible effectiveness in various allergic diseases, especially asthma. Corticosteroids taken orally classically block a late response very well but do not block the immediate response in most systems. On the other hand, oral steroids given 3 hours before an AIC in sheep blocked both.[132] Martin and co-workers found that prednisone blocked both the immediate antigen response to pollens when given at 40 mg daily for 7 days before and on the day of the challenge.[133]

In an Italian study, prednisone not only inhibited the LAR and the increased airway responsiveness after TDI exposure, but also normalized the number of leukocytes and the concentration of albumin found in the bronchial-alveolar lavage fluid.[134] Unlike oral steroids, corticosteroid aerosols inhibit both the immediate and late response. Cromolyn also inhibits both according to most investigators.[135-137] Theophylline can block the late response, and only slightly alter the early one.[138] Pauwels suggests that theophylline affects airway inflammation.[139] Nedocromil, not yet released in the U.S., blocks both early- and late-phase reactivity to antigen.[140] Classically beta agonists only block the early response; however, many long-acting beta agonists have not been adequately studied using this model.[141] Ipratropium bromide has little if any effect on immediate response to antigen challenge.[141]

Specific PAF antagonists block early bronchoconstriction, with a tendency towards blockage of residual bronchial hyperreactivity for 6 hours after an AIC.[142] Guinot et al. considered a specific PAF inhibitor a potentially useful medication in the treatment of asthma.[142] Interestingly, indomethacin is reported by some to inhibit the LAR but not the early response.[143,144]

Although the late-phase response model has served as a possible explanation for persistence of hyperreactivity, future studies and further clarifications are necessary to put immediate and late responses in proper perspective for the following reasons: (1) The concentration of antigen itself may be responsible for the production of certain late-phase reactions.[145] This has been demonstrated by various investigators who could convert early allergen response to dual response just by administering a large dose of allergen, e.g, with a short-acting β_2 agonist. Interestingly, when a beta agonist accompanied the allergen challenge, there was no accompanying increase in nonspecific hyperresponsiveness.[146] (2) Nonasthmatic, allergic subjects (e.g., hay fever patients) can show hyperreactivity after an allergen challenge, and many nonallergic asthmatics have hyperresponsiveness, so it is unclear which environmental factor is perpetuating the symptoms of these two groups.[147] (3) In some studies of occupational exposure, increased airway responsiveness may occur after an early response alone, and the late phase response is not necessary.[148] Exercise and possibly distilled water have been associated with increased LAR without increased nonspecific responsiveness. (5) Lastly, certain medications, such as indomethacin, inhibit the late responses yet are not a useful treatment for asthma.[143,144]

In summary, the late-phase model has proved interesting and provocative. It possibly may explain perpetuation of hyperreactivity in certain individuals, yet there are certain questions with respect to its usefulness as a model that have not yet been clarified.

ADDITIONAL INDICATIONS FOR ALLERGEN CHALLENGES

Evaluation of New Allergens in Pulmonary Disease. The literature swells with papers on new allergens that may produce pulmonary disease. Although many are organic substances, some are not. Some of these agents are discussed in Chapters 7 to 20.

Evaluation of New Treatments in Blocking Agents. Pharmaceutical manufacturers typically test new medications for their ability to block an early or a late (or both) antigen inhalation challenge. Such studies should take into account the peak action and duration of action of the blocking agent that is to be examined. If too high a concentration of antigen is used, erroneous conclusions might be drawn regarding the ability of a blocking agent to accomplish its goal, especially if the challenge itself has no clinical meaning for the patient.

Evaluation of the Therapeutic Effect of Immunotherapy. As discussed briefly before, allergen challenges have been used to evaluate the benefit of hyposensitization, as reflected by a decrease in bronchial reactivity after treatment. In many instances improvement is associated with the loss of the late reaction. Immunotherapy to dust mite and cat dander in particular has been shown to cause a change in late-phase reactivity and clinical improvement.

Recently Van Bever and Stevens reported the complete resolution of the LAR in 5 of 15 children after 1 year of house dust immunotherapy.[149] Furthermore, as a group the subjects showed a less severe LAR after 1 year of house dust. Although the PD_{20} of the IAR was not changed, the severity of the IAR was also reduced after 1 year of house dust immunotherapy.

Convincing the Patient of Cause-and-effect Relationships. Occasionally a double-blind challenge is used by a physician to convince a patient that he or she is symptomatic after exposure to that allergen.

Guidelines for a Safe Inhalation Challenge Procedure

A person having asthmatic symptoms should not be given a potential bronchoconstrictor, which can further compromise pulmonary function. Persons with moderate-to-severe impairment of lung function, e.g., an FEV_1 of 1 liter or less, should only be tested if the necessary precautions are taken. The biggest potential decrement of function occurs within minutes after a histamine challenge or methacholine challenge. There are a few individuals with prolonged reaction (lasting 1–2 hours) to the latter for reasons that are not clear. Their reaction is readily reversed by an aerosolized beta-agonist bronchodilator. Such individuals may have a defect in acetylcholinesterase metabolism. A beta blocker may also prolong the action of methacholine.

Antigen inhalation challenges can provoke prolonged or late reactions that require more precautions. They should not be done routinely in an office setting, especially with inexperienced personnel. The guideline for an antigen challenge is an initial antigen concentration that produces a 2+ reaction on intracutaneous injection. A 2+ equals a wheal greater than 5 mm in diameter minus the diameter of the wheal produced by the diluent control. Using the puncture technique, a 5% solution of 1:20 W/V diluent of aqueous solutions of antigen is usually applied to the skin. A wheal greater than 2 mm in diameter is considered equivalent to a positive intradermal test, with the solution having a concentration of antigen of 1:10,000 +/– one dilution.

When allergen skin tests are performed, a "negative" diluent control and a positive histamine control should accompany the skin test with antigens. With intradermal tests, the injected histamine solution consists of 0.02 mm of 0.1% base solution. For prick tests, a 1% solution of histamine base is recommended. Ideally, no medications should be withheld, but since this is impractical, guidelines for withholding medications are listed in Table 1.

Discussion of Preparation of Patient for Challenge

It should be remembered that smoking, cola drinks, coffee, and chocolate should be treated in a similar way to medication and stopped at least 6 hours before testing. Exercise and exposure to irritants should also be avoided 2 hours before the bronchial challenge, so that the patient can remain in a relatively asymptomatic state. Ideally patients should not be told they will receive a bronchodilator or a bronchoconstrictor. The suggestion itself could influence the result.[150,151] Challenges should be performed at a consistent time of the day if possible, because circadian rhythms can also influence challenge results.[152] Human susceptibility to antigens may be greater during menstruation.[153]

Deciding on the Proper Pulmonary Function Tests

In deciding on the proper pulmonary function tests, certain substances primarily affect small airways, whereas others primarily influence large airways.[154,155] If such information is known, it might determine which pulmonary function test might be ideal for a given challenge. If this information is not known, parameters that describe both small and large airways should be included in the testing. An adequate baseline pulmonary function must be obtained, recording the nature and time of the last bronchodilator usage. Even if a bronchodilator cannot be completely discontinued, it can be given in a similar manner to subsequent challenges. The timing of the measurement may be important, because pulmonary function tests of both spirometry and body plethysmography may be technically difficult to perform if data must be collected quickly.

A pulmonary function test should be relatively sensitive and specific. A change in SG_{aw} during a methacholine challenge, for example,

TABLE 1. Suggestions for Withholding Medications Prior to Inhalation Challenge

Medication*	Time of Avoidance
β-adrenergic-stimulating agents (aerosols)	At least 8 hours
Sustained-release β-agonists[†]	At least 24 hours
Short-acting theophylline derivatives[†]	At least 8 hours
Sustained-release theophylline derivatives[†]	At least 24 hours
α-Adrenergic blocking agents	At least 8 hours
Anticholinergic agents	At least 8 hours
Cromolyn sodium	At least 24 hours
Common antihistamines	At least 48 hours
Hydroxyzine or long-acting antihistamines[†]	At least 96 hours

* In general, patients on beta-adrenergic blocking agents should not be challenged due to a prolonged or exaggerated effect or altered response to treatment.
[†] Medications presumably will still be present in the bloodstream.

may be five times greater than the change in FEV_1. The SG_{aw} need not be more sensitive. Any relatively large change must be considered in relation to the wide variability of the test and its standard error. Although the SG_{aw} may appear to be more sensitive, it is also quite variable and cumbersome. One cigarette can decrease SG_{aw} more than 35% in normal subjects, and certain asthmatic patients may have a 35% or greater fall with just the suggestion that they may experience bronchial obstruction. Various standardization panels have advocated a minimal acceptable change in FEV_1 of 20% and SG_{aw} of 35%; however, these are somewhat arbitrary. FEV_1 has less variability from day to day compared to SG_{aw}. A significant difference from normal is usually defined as the value that would be expected in less than 5% of normal subjects. Changes observed should exceed 2 SD for repeated measures before statistical significance is reached. Ideally, coefficients of variation should be done for measurements within a given day, as well as from week to week.

Pennock and co-workers suggested that significant change in expiratory volumes or flow after a bronchodilator is 1 SD outside the limits of normal intertrial variability.[156] Thus, a significant change would be greater than 5% for FEV_1 and FVC, and greater than 13% for FEF_{25-75} during the middle half of the FVC in normal persons, and greater than 13% for FEV_1, greater than 11% for FVC, and greater than 23% for FEF_{25-75} in obstructed persons.

I would suggest that the FEV_1, even with its limitations, should be included as one of the measurements of a bronchoconstrictor response after occupational agents, methacholine, or histamine. Pulmonary function measurements can be added, depending on their availability and the need for other information about the bronchoconstrictive response. Factors affecting response include environmental influences as well as viruses, vaccines, and recent exposures to allergens.

Herxheimer and Tiffeneau postulated that hyposensitization by the inhalation route can occur if very dilute antigens are given initially and progression with more concentrated antigen follows.[157,158] In other words, less antigen would be required to produce a positive response due to previous exposure to the antigen. A contrasting phenomenon is the priming effect characterized by a heightened reactivity to an allergen due to previous exposure— which is usually in a high concentration of antigen. Both of these phenomena have not been well studied but are not thought to be a problem during a routine antigen challenge.

Various investigators have suggested that baseline airway caliber has the potential of modifying bronchial hyperreactivity during the pollen season, although present data are not very convincing. Vedal et al. also postulated that airway caliber and possibly immunologic sensitivity to plicatic acid are associated with the occurrence of bronchial hyperresponsiveness in Western red cedar workers.[159] Hume and Gandevia reported that as the FEV_1 and forced vital capacity improves, so does the absolute response until it reaches a maximum.[160] Absolute response is poor if the initial value is low. Goldberg and Cherniack described the greatest changes after therapy as taking place when airway resistance is highest.[161]

Influence of the Pulmonary Function Measurement Itself

Different methods used to measure airway response, such as maximal expiratory flow maneuvers and submaximal flow maneuvers for airway resistance are often included. The disadvantage of a forced expiratory maneuver as measured by spirometry is a reduction of normal tone that occurs after inspiration to total lung capacity[154,162] or after induced bronchoconstriction in normals[163] and asthmatic subjects.[164] In contrast, a deep inspiration or expiration causes bronchoconstriction in asthmatic patients, which is prevented by anticholinergics such as atropine.[155,165,166] Body plethysmography is expensive and therefore not widely available. The panting maneuver itself may be affected by laryngeal narrowing induced by a particular drug administered during bronchial provocation. Measurements of airways resistance and maximum flow should be made at the same lung volume.[167-169] Although the FEV_1 maneuver can be effort-dependent, it has survived the test of time in minimally variable test of pulmonary function.

Influence of Medications

Theophylline Derivatives. According to Cockcroft and co-workers, theophylline blocks a nonspecific challenge with blood levels of greater than 10 mg/L. No blocking effect occurs with less than 10 mg/L.[170] Both enprophylline and theophylline given intravenously cause a small dose-related increase in methacholine PC_{20} threshold.[171] Theophylline reduces antigen-induced bronchospasm, as well as the rise in plasma histamine and in the serum neutrophil chemotactic activity.[172] The protective effect is also related to the serum theophylline level.[138,173]

Beta Agonists and Antagonists. Inhaled albuterol or ingested albuterol can protect against an aerosolized histamine provocation challenge or shift histamine reactivity.[170,174] Propranolol given systemically or by inhalation produces little if any bronchoconstriction in healthy subjects.[175,176] Yet, certain investigators have reported a mild bronchoconstriction even in normals.[177] There is general agreement that asthmatic subjects may develop severe bronchial obstruction after propranolol.[178] Beta-adrenergic agonists such as inhaled fenoterol (800 μg) are reported to be more effective than cholinergic antagonists such as ipratropium bromide (80 μg) in preventing early allergen-induced bronchospasm.[179] Martin and associates reported that terbutaline sulfate (2.5 mg every 6 hours for 36 hours) significantly blocked AIC.[172]

Cromolyn Sodium. Cromolyn has partially or completely blocked methacholine or histamine challenge with short-term administration.[180] After long-term treatment with cromolyn, there is a report of reduced bronchial hyperresponsiveness as measured by histamine challenge in patients with perennial asthma.[181] Although most studies indicate that cromolyn blocks immediate bronchial challenge response to allergens, not all patients demonstrate such an inhibition.[182-184] Cromolyn sodium usually blocks late reactions.

Corticosteroids. Many investigators have not found that oral corticosteroids change airway reactivity to inhaled parasympathetic drugs in asthmatic patients.[185,186] Inhaled steroids have a significant blocking effect with time according to most investigators, although one group found that methacholine was unaffected by beclomethasone.[187,188] In many studies oral corticosteroids do not block bronchoconstriction produced by high concentrations of house dust and wheat flour antigens.[189,190] Martin and co-workers reported that oral prednisone 40 mg for 7 days inhibited their immediate bronchial challenge with pollen antigens.[172] Aerosol beclomethasone dipropionate given 30 minutes before allergen challenge inhibits the late, but not the immediate, allergen-induced reaction, as has been mentioned.[191]

Anticholinergic Agents. As reviewed elsewhere,[1] anticholinergic agents abolish bronchial constriction induced by aerosols of methacholine, citric acid, and carbon dust. It also completely or partially blocks inhalation of cold air, exercise, antigen challenges, and the effect of suggestion. When various doses of atropine are used, it minimally or completely blocks histamine and antagonizes the effect of propranolol. It partially blocks the bronchoconstrictor response to $PGF_2\alpha$ in asthmatic subjects but not in normals. Ipratropium bromide (SCH 1000), an analogue of atropine, can block methacholine-induced asthma better than histamine-induced asthma in aerosol doses of 40 and 80 μg. On the other hand, the protective effect of ipratropium against histamine is less than the protective effect of a beta agonist such as fenoterol, even though they both have the ability to partially block histamine challenges.

Atropine blockade of AIC is a more controversial topic, especially since there is an implication regarding the role of reflexes in airway constriction of asthmatic subjects. Most investigators do not find significant block of atropine in antigen-induced bronchoconstriction, although Yu and associates reported that 1.5–2.5 mg of atropine could block antigen reactions when given by IV route.[192] There may also be patient variability, because some investigators have found complete blockage while others have only found partial blockage.[193-195] The dose of antigen may also influence results. The cholinergic effect may be more obvious at a lower antigen dose.[193,196] At least two factors of nonspecific airway reactivity and skin test positivity influence an antigen challenge. These variables may also play a role as to the degree of blockage.[65,197] They correspond to a similar observation that certain patients show a greater blocking effect to histamine inhalation with aerosolized atropine than do others.[198]

Alpha-adrenergic Blocking Agents. Although alpha-adrenergic receptors in human airway smooth muscle are present sparsely, there may be an increase in the presence of lung disease.[199,200] In any case, their role is presumed to be minimal in asthma. Nevertheless, alpha receptor antagonists such as phentolamine or thymoxamine can block exercise or histamine challenge in asthmatic subjects.[201-203] Thymoxamine can inhibit AIC when given intravenously and even to a small degree when given by inhalation.[204]

Other Medications. Inhibitors of prostaglandin synthesis do not block immediate decrements in pulmonary function after AIC in asthmatic patients.[205]

Nifedipine, a potent inhibitor of transmembrane calcium ion flux, can inhibit histamine provocative challenges and exercise-induced asthma.[206,207]

Pretreatment with aerosolized lidocaine will block methacholine-induced bronchoconstriction.[208] The response to inhaled histamine is correlated with the 24-hour urinary excretion of sodium, a high rate of sodium excretion being associated with increased airways reactivity. It may even explain increased infant mortality related to increased table salt purchases.[209]

Treatment with ascorbic acid can block a methacholine-induced bronchoconstriction. The ameliorative action of ascorbic acid can be blocked by the ingestion of indomethacin, implicating prostaglandin pathways.[210] Ascorbic acid can protect histamine-induced airway constriction according to some investigators but not others.[211]

Influence of Emotional Factors

Emotional factors in asthma are thought to be experienced mainly through the parasympathetic nervous system. A significant number of asthmatic subjects respond to psychological stimuli with bronchoconstriction.[150,151] Those asthmatic patients with the most hyperreactive airways are the ones most likely to respond to bronchoconstrictive suggestion.[150,151] Cholinergic antagonists such as atropine can block this bronchoconstriction implicating the parasympathetic nervous system.

Menstrual Cycle

Premenstrual exacerbation of asthma has been noted by various investigators.[153] Pauli and co-workers did not find a change in methacholine reactivity throughout the menstrual cycle to explain the deterioration in asthma.[212]

Circadian and Other Body Rhythms

An increase in histamine hyperreactivity has been found in asthmatic and bronchitic subjects during nighttime hours.[213] Bronchial reactivity to histamine and acetylcholine follows a circadian pattern.[214,215]

Other Disease States

Congestive heart failure is also associated with hyperresponsiveness.[216,217] Yet, Seibert and co-workers found normal airway responsiveness to methacholine in cardiac asthma.[218]

Pregnancy

Juniper and co-workers found a twofold improvement in airway responsiveness during pregnancy in 16 females they studied, which corresponded to an associated improvement in clinical asthma as measured by medication reduction. Symptoms and spirometry remained unchanged during pregnancy. There also was no correlation with progesterone or estrogen levels.[219]

AEROSOL GENERATION, DELIVERY, AND PENETRANCE

Large particles tend to sediment in proximal airways and smaller particles tend to penetrate into the peripheral airways. Particles of < 0.4 μm in diameter and $> 5\mu m$ have decreased deposition. Ideally inhaled particles should range between 0.3 and 0.4 μm. Individual nebulizers may vary considerably in the median aerodynamic diameter of particles produced.

Two popular aerosol delivery systems are the dosimeter method and continuous flow method. Details regarding their use and comparison studies have been described.[2,220] The use of spacer devices or cones favors a more peripheral alveolar distribution and also has certain disadvantages. Particle size and distribution of the dose may not be as critical as was once thought; however, there are variables that should be considered for their potential influence on response, especially during disease states.

A standard way of expressing data on bronchoconstrictive substances including allergens is by calculations of cumulative doses. This is based on the assumption that the dose of the substance generated is retained and cumulated, which in reality is not always correct. An antigen typically is accumulated and, to a small degree, methacholine might also be accumulated in the body.

Histamine and other substances may have relatively short-lived effects that are completely dissipated in the body. Much of the generated dose is not only inhaled and exhaled, but lost in equipment, metabolized, or removed from the sites of distribution. Ideally the baseline FEV_1 prior to starting a challenge should be 80% or greater of a previously-observed highest value, and not so low as to compromise a minimal reserve in pulmonary function.

According to standardization protocols, five successive breaths of a bronchoconstrictive substance such as methacholine or antigen are given (Tables 2 and 3). A positive result for a methacholine challenge is a 3-minute sustained fall in FEV_1 of 20% or more from the control FEV_1 value. If the test result is negative, five breaths of the next dilution are given. If the result is borderline, then fewer than five breaths of the next dilution may be given. A positive result for an antigen challenge is a 10-minute fall, sustained for at least 10 minutes. Results are expressed by a dose-response curve using a semilogarithmic plot, and on the logarithmic abscissa the cumulated dose is plotted. On the linearly expressed ordinate, the response is measured by percent of the diluent control aerosol. The plot shows a best-lined fit curve, and the cumulative dose at which lung function has deteriorated by at least 2 standard deviations below control values is considered the PD. The antigen or other provocative substance is multiplied by the number of breaths (usually 5) to get the cumulated dose for each exposure. Sensitivity is determined by the PD itself, whereas reactivity

TABLE 2. *Cumulative Doses for Bronchial Inhalation Challenge Using Bronchoconstrictive Agents* at Five Breaths Per Dilution*

Concentration (mg/ml)	Inhalation Units[†] (per 5 breaths)	Cumulative Dose (inhalation units)
Lengthy Protocol		
0.03	0.15	0.15
0.06	0.30	0.45
0.12	0.60	1.05
0.25	1.25	2.30
0.50	2.50	4.80
1.0	5.00	9.80
2.0	10.00	19.80
5.0	25.00	44.80
10.0	50.00	94.80
25.0	125.00	219.00
Shortened Protocol (For Methacholine)		
0.025	0.125	0.125
0.25	1.25	1.375
2.5	12.5	13.88
10.0	50.0	63.88
25.0	125.0	188.88

* At concentrations of antigens of 1:100 and above, the clinical meaning is unclear.
[†] One inhalation unit = one breath of solution with 1 mg of drug/ml.

is determined by the slope. Abbreviated protocols have been suggested by some but have the disadvantage of less safety and less standardization. A way of expressing data other than the dose-response plot would be the area under the curve, which has the advantage of defining the degree of sensitivity. After certain occupational exposures, such as Western red cedar, patients may continue to demonstrate increased bronchial responsiveness to inhaled methacholine or histamine, even years after exposure to red cedar.

TABLE 3. *Cumulative Doses for Bronchial Inhalation Challenge Using Allergen at Five Breaths per Dilution*

Allergen* Concentration (W/V)	Inhalation Units[†] (per 5 breaths)	Cumulative Units (per 5 breaths)
1:1,000,000	0.025	0.025
1:500,000	0.05	0.075
1:100,000	0.25	0.325
1:50,000	0.5	0.825
1:10,000	2.5	3.32
1:5,000	5.0	8.32
1:1,000	25.0	33.3
1:500	50.0	83.3
1:100	250.0	300.3

W/V = weight per volume
* At concentrations of allergens of 1:100 and above, the clinical meaning is unclear.
[†] One inhalation unit = one breath of 1:500 W/V dilution.

Safety Considerations

It is rare that a positive bronchial challenge will provoke a permanent decrement in lung function, especially by using the standardization techniques with step-wise increases in antigen concentration. Antigen challenges should require constant observation, especially in view of the late-phase reactions. Safety considerations require the presence of resuscitation equipment, oxygen, and appropriate medication including aerosolized bronchodilators. A physician or nurse familiar with challenges should be directly available. Ideally, technicians who administer antigen bronchial challenges should not have an allergic background or have a history or family history of asthma. A well-ventilated room helps to prevent excessive antigen exposure from the air.

REFERENCES

1. Spector SL: Bronchial inhalation challenges with aerosolized bronchoconstrictive substances. In Spector SL (ed): Provocative Challenge Procedures: Bronchial, Oral, Nasal and Exercise: Vol. I. Boca Raton, FL, CRC Press, 1983, pp 137–176.
2. Spector SL: Allergen inhalation challenge procedures. In Spector SL (ed): Provocative Challenge Procedures: Background and Methodology. Mount Kisco, NY, Futura Publishing, 1989, pp 293–340.
3. Tiffeneau R: Hypersensibilite pulmonaire de l'asthmatique a l'acetylcholine et a l'histamine. Similitude, differentiation pharmacodynamique. Therapie 11:715, 1956.
4. Tiffeneau R: Hyperexcitabilite bronchomotrice de l'asthmatique, sequelle des agressions bronchoconstrictive allergiques. Acta Allergol 14:416, 1959.
5. Chapman TT: Hypersensitivity to inhalation of acetylcholine related to asthma. Irish J Med Sci 443:507, 1962.
6. Muranaka M, Nakajima K, Suzuki S: Bronchial responsiveness to acetylcholine in patients with bronchial asthma after long-term treatment with gold salt. J Allergy Clin Immunol 67:350, 1981.
7. Orehek J, Gayrard P, Smith AP, et al: Airway response to carbachol in normal and asthmatic subjects. Am Rev Respir Dis 115:937, 1977.
8. Cropp G: Personal communication.
9. Spector SL, Farr RS: Bronchial provocation tests. In Weiss EB, Segal MS (eds): Bronchial Asthma Mechanisms and Therapeutics. Boston, Little Brown, 1976, pp 639–647.
10. Chai H, Farr RS, Froelich LA, et al: Standardization of bronchial inhalation challenge procedures. J Allergy Clin Immunol 56:323–327, 1975.
11. Dale HH, Laidlaw PP: The physiological action of beta-iminoazolyethylamine. J Physiol (Lond) 41:318, 1910.
12. DeKock MA, Nadel JA, Zwi S, et al: New method for perfusing bronchial arteries: Histamine bronchoconstriction and apnea. J Appl Physiol 21:185, 1966.

13. Juniper EF, Frith PA, Dunnett C, et al: Reproducibility and comparison of responses to inhaled histamine and methacholine. Thorax 33:705-710, 1978.

14. Spector SL, Farr RS: A comparison of methacholine and histamine inhalations in asthmatics. J Allergy Clin Immunol 56:308-316, 1975.

15. Anderson SD, Schoeffel RE, Finney M: Evaluation of ultrasonically nebulized solutions as a provocation in patients with asthma. Thorax 38:284-291, 1983.

16. Finnerty JP, Wilmot C, Holgate ST: Inhibition of hypertonic saline-induced bronchoconstriction by terfenadine and flurbiprofen. Am Rev Respir Dis 140:593-597, 1989.

17. Cuthbert MF: Bronchodilator activity of aerosols of prostaglandin E_1 and E_2 in asthmatic subjects. Proc R Soc Med 64:15, 1971.

18. Mathe AA, Hedqvist P: Effects of prostaglandin F_2 alpha and E_2 on airway conductance in healthy subjects and asthmatic patients. Am Rev Respir Dis 111:313, 1975.

19. Harnett JC, Spector SL, Farr RS: Aspirin idiosyncrasy, asthma and urticaria. In Middleton E Jr, Reed CE, Ellis EF (eds): Allergy: Principles and Practice. St. Louis, C.V. Mosby, 1978, pp 1002-1021.

20. Szczeklik A, Gryglewski RJ, Czerniawska-Mysik G, Zmuda A: Aspirin-induced asthma and urticaria. J Allergy Clin Immunol 58:10, 1976.

21. Spector SL, Wangaard CH, Farr RS: Aspirin and concomitant idiosyncrasies in adult asthmatic patients. J Allergy Clin Immunol 64:500-506, 1979.

22. Goetzl EJ: Mediators of immediate hypersensitivity derived from arachidonic acid. N Engl J Med 303:822, 1980.

23. Mathe AA, Hedqvist P, Holmgren A, Svanbord M: Bronchial hyperreactivity to prostaglandin F_2 alpha and histamine in patients with asthma. Br Med J 1:193, 1973.

24. Arm JP, O'Hickey SP, Spur BW, Lee TH: Airway responsiveness to histamine and leukotriene E_4 in subjects with aspirin-induced asthma. Am Rev Respir Dis 140:148-153, 1989.

25. Georgopoulos D, Giulekas D, Ilonidis G, Sichletidis L: Effect of salbutamol, ipratropium bromide and cromolyn sodium on prostaglandin F_2a-induced bronchospasm. Chest 96:809-814, 1989.

26. Pichurko BM, Ingram RH Jr, Sperling RI, et al: Localization of the site of the bronchoconstrictor effects of leukotriene C_4 compared with that of histamine in asthmatic subjects. Am Rev Respir Dis 140:334-339, 1989.

27. Israel E, Juniper EF, Callaghan JT, et al: Effect of leukotriene antagonist, LY171883, on cold air-induced bronchoconstriction in asthmatics. Am Rev Respir Dis 140:1348-1353, 1989.

28. Black PN, Fuller RW, Barnes PJ, Collery CT: Effect of inhaled leukotriene B_4 alone and in combination with prostaglandin D_2 on bronchial responsiveness to histamine in normal subjects. Thorax 44:491-495, 1989.

29. Hahn HL, Wilson AG, Graf PD, et al: Interaction between serotonin and efferent vagus nerves in dog lungs. J Appl Physiol 44:144, 1978.

30. Halpern BN, Neveu T, Spector SL: On the nature of the chemical mediators involved in anaphylactic reactions in mice. Br J Pharmacol 20:389, 1963.

31. Phillips GD, Polosa R, Holgate ST: The effect of histamine-H_1 receptor antagonism with terfenadine on concentration-related AMP-induced bronchoconstriction in asthma. Clin Exper Allergy 19:405-409, 1989.

32. Wells RE, Walker JEC, Hickler RB: Effects of cold air on respiratory air flow resistance in patients with respiratory tract disease. N Engl J Med 303:822, 1980.

33. Varonier HS, Panzani R: The effect of inhalations of bradykinin on healthy and atopic (asthmatic) children. Int Arch Allergy Appl Immunol 34:293, 1968.

34. Newball HH, Keiser HR: Relative effects of bradykinin and histamine on the respiratory system of man. J Appl Physiol 35:552, 1973.

35. Gerritsen J, Koeter GH, Vander-Weele LT, Knol K: Propranolol inhalation challenge in relation to "histamine" response in children with asthma. Thorax 43:451-455, 1988.

36. Simonsson BG, Skoogh BE, Bergh NP, et al: In vivo and in vitro effect of bradykinin on bronchial motor tone in normal subjects. Respiration 30:378, 1973.

37. Godfrey S: Bronchial challenge by exercise or hyperventilation. In Spector SL (ed): Provocative Challenge Procedures: Background and Methodology. Mount Kisco, NY, Futura Publishing, 1989, pp 365-394.

38. Kiviloog J: Bronchial reactivity to exercise and methacholine in bronchial asthma. Scand J Respir Dis 54:347, 1973.

39. Eggleston PA: A comparison of asthmatic response to methacholine and exercise. J Allergy Clin Immunol 63:104, 1979.

40. Anderton RC, Cuff MT, Frith PA, et al: Bronchial responsiveness to inhaled histamine and exercise. 63:315, 1979.

41. Mellis CM, Kattan M, Keens TG, Levison H: Comparative study of histamine and exercise challenges in asthmatic children. Am Rev Respir Dis 117:911, 1978.

42. Aquilina AT, Hall WJ, Douglas RG Jr, Utell MJ: Airway reactivity in subjects with viral upper respiratory tract infections: The effects of exercise and cold air. Am Rev Respir Dis 122:3, 1980.

43. Hargreave FE, Ryan G, Thomson NC, et al: Bronchial responsiveness to histamine or methacholine in asthma: Measurement and clinical significance. J Allergy Clin Immunol 68:347, 1981.

44. Hajos M-K: Clinical studies on the role of serotonin in bronchial asthma. Acta Allergol 17:358, 1962.

45. Popa V, Douglas JS, Bouhuys A: Airway responses to histamine acetylcholine and antigen in sensitized guinea pigs. J Lab Clin Med 84:226, 1974.

46. Makino S: Clinical significance of bronchial sensitivity to acetylcholine and histamine in bronchial asthma. J Allergy 38:127, 1966.

47. Itkin IH: Bronchial hypersensitivity to mecholyl and histamine in asthma subjects. J Allergy 40:245, 1967.

48. Schoeffel RE, Anderson SD, Gillam I, Lindsay DA: Multiple exercise and histamine challenge in asthmatic patient. Thorax 35:164, 1980.

49. Holtzman MJ, Sheller JR, Dimeo M, et al: Effect of ganglionic blockade on bronchial reactivity in atopic subjects. Fed Proc 38:1110, 1979.

50. Woenne R, Kattan M, Orange RP, Levison H: Bronchial hyperreactivity to histamine and methacholine in asthmatic children after inhalation of SCH1000 and chlorpheniramine maleate. J Allergy Clin Immunol 62:119, 1978.

51. Merck & Co: The Merck Index, 11th ed. Rahway, NJ, Merck & Co, 1989.

52. Lesouef PN, Geelhoed GC, Turner DJ, et al: Response of normal infants to inhaled histamine. Am Rev Respir Dis 139:62-66, 1989.

53. Simpson DL, Goodman M, Spector SL, Petty TT: Long-term follow-up and bronchial reactivity testing in survivors of the adult respiratory distress syndrome. Am Rev Respir Dis 117:449–454, 1978.

54. Kaufman J, Casanova JEE, Riendl P, Schlueter DP: Bronchial hyperreactivity and cough due to angiotensin-converting enzyme inhibitors. Chest 95:544–548, 1989.

55. Lindgren BR, Rosenqvist U, Ekstrom T, et al: Increased bronchial reactivity and potentiated skin responses in hypertensive subjects suffering from cough during ACE-inhibitor therapy. Chest 95:1225–1230, 1989.

56. Curry JJ: Comparative action of acetyl-beta-methylcholine and histamine on the respiratory tract in normals, patients with hay fever, and subjects with bronchial asthma. J Clin Invest 26:430, 1947.

57. Curry JJ, Lowell FC: Measurement of vital capacity in asthmatic subjects receiving histamine and acetyl-beta-methylcholine: A clinical study. J Allergy 19:9, 1948.

58. Townley RG, Ryo UY, Kolotkin BM, Kang B: Bronchial sensitivity to methacholine in current and former asthmatic and allergic rhinitis patients and control subjects. J Allergy Clin Immunol 56:429, 1975.

59. Spector SL, Staudenmayer H, Kinsman RA, et al: Methacholine and histamine inhalation challenges in asthma: Relationship to age of onset, length of illness, and pulmonary function. Allergy 34:167–173, 1979.

60. Townley RG, Dennis M, Itkin IH: Comparative action of acetyl-beta-methylcholine, histamine and pollen antigens in subjects with hay fever and patients with bronchial asthma. J Allergy 36:121, 1965.

61. Cockcroft DW, Killian DN, Mellon JJA, Hargreave FE: Bronchial reactivity to inhaled histamine: A clinical survey. Clin Allergy 7:235, 1977.

61a. Juniper EF, Frith PA, Hargreave FE: Airway responsiveness to histamine and methacholine relationship to minimum treatment to control symptoms of asthma. Thorax 36:575–579, 1981.

62. Staudenmayer H, Kinsman RA, Dirks JF, et al: Medical outcome in asthmatic patients: Effects of airway hyperreactivity and symptom-focused anxiety. Psychosom Med 41:109–118, 1979.

63. Josephs LK, Gregg I, Mullee MA, Holgate ST: Nonspecific bronchial reactivity and its relationship to the clinical expression of asthma. Am Rev Respir Dis 140:350–357, 1989.

64. Spector SL, Farr RS: Bronchial inhalation challenge with antigen. J Allergy Clin Immunol 64:580–586, 1979.

65. Nathan RA, Kinsman RA, Spector SL, Horton DJ: Relationship between airways response to allergens and nonspecific bronchial reactivity. J Allergy Clin Immunol 64:491–499, 1979.

66. Bruce CA, Rosenthal RR, Lichtenstein LM, Norman PS: Quantitative inhalation bronchial challenge in ragweed hay fever patients: A comparison with ragweed-allergic asthmatics. J Allergy Clin Immunol 56:331, 1975.

67. Fish JE, Rosenthal RR, Batra G, et al: Airway responses to methacholine ion allergic and non-allergic subjects. Am Rev Respir Dis 113:579, 1976.

68. Fish JE, Peterman VI, Cugell DW: Effect of deep inspiration on airway conductance in subjects with allergic rhinitis and allergic asthma. J Allergy Clin Immunol 60:41, 1977.

69. Ankin MG, Peterman VI, Fish JE: Effects of lung inflation on maximum flow responses to methacholine and antigen in hay fever and asthma subjects. Am Rev Respir Dis 119(Supp 2):55, 1979.

70. Fish JE, Kelly JF: Measurements of responsiveness in bronchoprovocation testing. J Allergy Clin Immunol 64:592, 1979.

71. Oppenheimer EA, Rigatto M, Fletcher CM: Airways obstruction before and after isoprenaline, histamine, and prednisolone in patients with chronic obstructive bronchitis. Lancet i:552, 1968.

72. Kerrebijn JF, van Essen-Zandvliet EEM, Neijens HJ: Effect of long-term treatment with inhaled corticosteroids and beta agonists on the bronchial responsiveness in children with asthma. J Allergy Clin Immunol 79:653–659, 1987.

73. Dutoit JI, Salome CM, Woolcock AJ: Inhaled corticosteroids reduce the severity of bronchial hyperresponsiveness in asthma, but oral theophylline does not. Am Rev Respir Dis 136:1174–1178, 1987.

73a. Hoag JE, McFadden ER: Long-term effect of cromolyn sodium on nonspecific bronchial hyperresponsiveness: A review. Ann Allergy 66:53–63, 1991.

74. Cockcroft DW, Murdock KY: Comparative effects of inhaled salbutamol, sodium cromoglycate, and beclomethasone dipropionate on allergen-induced early asthmatic responses, late asthmatic responses, and increased bronchial responsiveness to histamine. J Allergy Clin Immunol 79:734–740, 1987.

75. Spector SL: Use of provocation techniques for the evaluation of drug efficacy. J Allergy Clin Immunol 64:677–684, 1979.

76. Spector SL, Katz FH, Farr RS: Troleandomycin: Effectiveness in steroid dependent asthma and bronchitis. J Allergy Clin Immunol 54:367–369, 1974.

76a. Juniper EF, Kline PA, Vanzieleghem MA, Hargreave FE: Reduction of budesonide after a year of increased use. J Allergy Clin Immunol 87:483–489, 1991.

77. Assen ESK, McAllen MD: Changes in challenge tests following hyposensitization with mite extract. Clin Allergy 3:161, 1973.

78. Rak S, Lowhagen O, Venge P: The effect of immunotherapy on bronchial hyperresponsiveness and eosinophil cationic protein in pollen-allergic patients. J Allergy Clin Immunol 82:470–480, 1988.

79. Salvaggio JE, Hendrick DJ: The use of bronchial inhalation challenge in the investigation of occupational asthma. In Spector SL (ed): Provocative Challenge Procedures: Background and Methodology. Mount Kisco, NY, Futura Publishing, 1989, pp 417–450.

80. Lam S, Wong R, Yeung M: Nonspecific bronchial reactivity in occupational asthma. J Allergy Clin Immunol 63:28, 1979.

81. Cockcroft DW, Cartier A, Jones G, et al: Asthma caused by occupational exposure to a furan-based binder system. J Allergy Clin Immunol 66:458, 1980.

82. Valliers M, Cockcroft DW, Taylor DM, et al: Dimethyl ethanolamine-induced asthma. Am Rev Respir Dis 115:867, 1977.

83. Cockcroft DW, Cotton DJ, Mink JT: Nonspecific bronchial hyperreactivity after exposure to Western Red Cedar. Am Rev Respir Dis 119:505, 1979.

84. Boushey HA, Empey DW, Laitinen LA: Meat wrapper's asthma: Effect of fumes of polyvinyl chloride on airways function. Physiologist 18:148, 1975.

85. Boushey HA, Holtzman MJ, Sheller JR, Nadel JA: Bronchial reactivity: State of the art. Am Rev Respir Dis 121:389, 1980.

86. Brooks SM, Weiss MA, Bernstein IL: Reactive airways dysfunction syndrome (RADS). Chest 88:376, 1985.

87. Braman SS, Corrao WM: Bronchoprovocation testing. Clin Chest Med 10:165–176, 1989.

88. Tarlo SM, Broder I: Irritant-induced occupational asthma. Chest 96:297–300, 1989.
89. Aas K: The Bronchial Provocation Test. Springfield, IL, Charles C Thomas, 1975.
90. Spector SL: Bronchial provocation tests. In Weiss EB, Segal MS, Stein M (eds): Bronchial Asthma: Mechanisms and Therapeutics, 2nd ed. Boston, Little, Brown, 1985, pp 360–379.
91. Patterson R, Suszko IM, Zeiss CR Jr: Reactions of primate respiratory mast cells. J Allergy Clin Immunol 50:7, 1972.
92. May CD, Williams CS: Further studies concerning the fluctuating insensitivity of peripheral leukocytes to unrelated allergens and the meaning of nonspecific "desensitization": Clin Allergy 3:319, 1973.
93. Huggins KG, Brostoff J: Local production of specific IgE antibodies in allergic rhinitis patients with negative skin tests. Lancet ii:148, 1975.
94. Cavanaugh MJ, Bronsky EA, Buckley JM: Clinical value of bronchial provocation testing in childhood asthma. J Allergy Clin Immunol 59:41, 1977.
95. Spector SL, Farr RS: Bronchial Inhalation procedures in asthmatics. Med Clin North Am 58:71–84, 1974.
96. Bhat KN, Arroyave CCM, Manney SM Jr, et al: Plasma histamine changes during provoked bronchospasm in asthmatic patients. J Allergy Clin Immunol 58:647, 1976.
97. Ahmet T, et al: Abnormal mucociliary transport in allergic patients with antigen-induced bronchospasm: Role of slow reacting substance of anaphylaxis. Am Rev Respir Dis 124:110, 1981.
98. Marom Z, et al: Slow-reacting substances, leukotrienes C_4 and D_4 increase the release of mucus from human airways in vitro. Am Rev Respir Dis 126:449, 1982.
99. Schwartz LB, Metcalfe DD, Miller JS, et al: Tryptase levels as an indicator of mast-cell activation in systemic anaphylaxis and mastocytosis. N Engl J Med 316:1622, 1987.
100. Arroyave CCM, Stevenson DD, Vaughan JH, et al: Plasma complement changes during bronchospasm provoked in asthmatic patients. Clin Allergy 7:173, 1977.
101. Pyrjma J, et al: Decrease of complement hemolytic activity after an allergen-house dust-bronchial provocation test. J Allergy Clin Immunol 70:306, 1982.
102. Lupinetti MD, Sheller JR, Catella F, Fitzgerald GA: Thromboxane biosynthesis in allergen-induced bronchospasm. Am Rev Respir Dis 140:932–935, 1989.
103. Deal EC Jr, Wasserman SM Jr, Soter NA, et al: Evaluation of role played by mediators of immediate hypersensitivity in exercise-induced asthma. J Clin Invest 65:659, 1980.
104. Olive JR Jr, Hyatt RE: Maximal expiratory flow and total respiratory resistance during induced bronchoconstriction in asthmatic subjects. Am Rev Respir Dis 106:366, 1972.
105. Ahmed T, Fernandez RJ, Wanner A: Airway responses to antigen challenge in allergic rhinitis and allergic asthma. J Allergy Clin Immunol 67:135–145, 1981.
106. Olgiati R, Birch S, Rao A, et al: Differential effects of methacholine and antigen challenge on gas exchange in allergic subjects. J Allergy Clin Immunol 67:325–329, 1981.
107. Price JF, Warner JO, Hey EN, et al: Controlled trial of hyposensitization to Dermatophagoides pteronyssinus in children with asthma. Lancet ii:912–915, 1978.
108. Robertson D, Kerigan AT, Hargreave FE, et al: Late asthmatic responses induced by ragweed pollen. J Allergy Clin Immunol 54:244, 1974.
109. Paggiaro PL, Chan Yeung M: Pattern of specific airway responses in asthma due to Western red Cedar (Thurja plicata): Relationship with length of exposure and lung function measurement. Clin Allergy 17:333–339, 1987.
110. Booij-Noord H, DeVries K, Sluiter HJ, et al: Late bronchial obstruction reaction to experimental inhalation of house dust extract. Clin Allergy 2:43–61, 1972.
111. Bundgaard A, Boudet L: Reproducibility of the late asthmatic response (abstract). Eur J Respir Dis 137:284, 1988.
112. Ihre E, Axelsson IGK, Zetterstrom O: Late asthmatic reactions and bronchial variability after challenge with low doses of allergen. Clin Allergy 18:557–567, 1988.
113. Atkins PC, Martin GL, Yost R, et al: Late onset reactions in humans: Correlation between skin and bronchial reactivity. Ann Allergy 60:27–30, 1988.
114. Cockcroft DW, Murdock KY, Kirby J, et al: Prediction of airway responsiveness to allergen from skin sensitivity to allergen and airway responsiveness to histamine. Am Rev Respir Dis 135:264–267, 1987.
115. Tiffeneau R: Hypersensibilite cholinergo-histaminique pulmonaire de l'asthmatique. Acta Allergol 13:187, 1958.
116. Rosenthal RR, Norman PS, Summer WR: Bronchoprovocation: Effect on priming and desensitization phenomena in the lung. J Allergy Clin Immunol 56:338, 1975.
117. Durham SR, Carroll M, Lee TH, et al: Mechanisms of early and late asthmatic reactions. In Reed CE (ed): Proceedings XII International Congress of Allergology and Clinical Immunology. St. Louis, C.V. Mosby Co, 1987, pp 229–236.
118. Boulet LP, Cartier A, Thomson NC, et al: Asthma and increases in nonallergic bronchial responsiveness from seasonal pollen exposure. J Allergy Clin Immunol 71:339–406, 1983.
119. Platts-Mills TA, Mitchell EB, Nock P, et al: Reduction of bronchial hyperreactivity during prolonged allergen avoidance. Lancet ii:675–678, 1982.
120. Metzger WJ, Donnelly A, Richerson HB: Modification of late asthmatic responses during immunotherapy for Alternaria-induced asthma. J Allergy Clin Immunol 75:121A, 1983.
121. Warner JO, Price JF, Soothill JF, et al: Controlled trial of hyposensitisation to Dermatophagoides pteronyssinus in children with asthma. Lancet ii:912–915, 1978.
122. Lemanske RF Jr, Kaliner M: Late-phase IgE-mediated reactions. J Clin Immunol 8:1–13, 1988.
123. Nagy L, Lee TH, Kay AB: Neutrophil chemotactic factor activity in antigen-induced late asthmatic reactions. N Engl J Med 306:497–501, 1982.
124. Murray JJ, Tonnel AB, Brash AR, et al: Release of prostaglandin D_2 into human airways during acute antigen challenge. N Engl J Med 315:800–804, 1986.
125. Goetzl EJ, Pickett WC: Novel structural determinants of the human neutrophil chemotactic activity of leukotriene. Br J Exp Med 153:482–487, 1981.
126. Abraham W: The importance of lipoxygenase products of arachidonic acid in allergen-induced late responses. Am Rev Respir Dis 135:S49–S53, 1987.

127. Nakamura T, Morita Y, Kuriyama M, et al: Platelet-activating factor in late asthmatic response. Int Arch Allergy Appl Immunol 82:57–61, 1987.
128. Ito K, Kudo K, Okudaira H, et al: IgG₁ antibodies to house dust mite *Dermatophagoides farinae* and late asthmatic response. Int Arch Allergy Appl Immunol 81:69–74, 1986.
129. Gonzalez MZ, Diaz P, Galleguillos FR, et al: Allergen-induced recruitment of bronchoalveolar helper (OKT₄) and suppressor (OKT₈) T-cells in asthma. Am Rev Respir Dis 136:600–604, 1987.
130. Diaz P, Gonzalez MC, Galleguillos FR, et al: Leukocytes and mediators in bronchoalveolar lavage during allergen-induced late-phase asthmatic reactions. Am Rev Respir Dis 139:1383–1389, 1989.
131. Frick WE, Sedgwick JB, Busse WW: The appearance of hypodense eosinophils in antigen-dependent late phase asthma. Am Rev Respir Dis 139:1401–1406, 1989.
132. Delehunt JC, Yerger L, Ahmed T, et al: Inhibition of antigen-induced bronchoconstriction by methylprednisolone succinate. J Allergy Clin Immunol 73:479–483, 1984.
133. Martin GL, Atkins PC, Dunsky EH, et al: Effects of theophylline, terbutaline, and prednisone on antigen-induced bronchospasm and mediator release. J Allergy Clin Immunol 66:204–212, 1980.
134. Boschetto P, Fabbri LM, Zocca E, et al: Prednisone inhibits late asthmatic reactions and airway inflammation induced by toluene diisocyanate in sensitized subjects. J Allergy Clin Immunol 80:261–267, 1987.
135. Burge PS, Efthimou J, Turner-Warwick M, et al: Double blind trials of inhaled beclomethasone dipropionate and fluocortin butyl ester in allergen-induced immediate and late asthmatic reactions. Clin Allergy 12:523–531, 1982.
136. Mattoli S, Foresi A, Corbo GM, et al: Effects of two doses of cromolyn on allergen-induced late asthmatic response and increased responsiveness. J Allergy Clin Immunol 79:747–754, 1987.
137. Pelikan Z, Pelikan-Filipek M, Schoemaker MC, et al: Effects of disodium cromoglycate and beclomethasone dipropionate on the asthma response to allergen challenge. I. Immediate response (IAR). Ann Allergy 60:211–216, 1988.
138. Pauwels R, Van Renterghem D, Van Der Straeten M, et al: The effect of theophylline and enprofylline on allergen-induced bronchoconstriction. J Allergy Clin Immunol 76:583–590, 1985.
139. Pauwels R: The effects of theophylline on airway inflammation. Chest 92:32A–37S, 1987.
140. Bonifazi F, Antonicelli L, Pieretti C, et al: Double-blind crossover trial to compare the activity of nedocromil sodium and placebo in antigen challenge. Allergol Immunopathol 15:151–153, 1987.
141. Howard PH, Durham SR, Lee TH, et al: Influence of albuterol, cromolyn sodium and ipratropium bromide on the airway and circulating mediator responses to allergen bronchial provocation in asthma. Am Rev Respir Dis 132:986–992, 1985.
142. Guinot P, Brambilla C, Duchier J, et al: Effect of BN 52063, a specific PAF-acether antagonist, on bronchial provocation test to allergens in asthmatic patients: A preliminary study. Prostaglandins 34:723–731, 1987.
143. Fairfax AJ: Inhibition of the late asthmatic response to house dust mite by non-steroidal anti-inflammatory drugs. Prostaglandins Leukotrienes Med 8:239–248, 1982.
144. Joubert JR, Shephard E, Mouton W, et al: Non-steroidal anti-inflammatory drugs in asthma: Dangerous or useful therapy? Allergy 40:202–207, 1985.
145. Hargreave FE, Dolovich J, Robertson DG, Kerigan AT: The late asthmatic responses. Can Med Assoc J 110:415–424, 1974.
146. Lai CKW, Twentyman OP, Holgate ST: The effect of an increase in inhaled allergen dose after rimiterol hydrobromide on the occurrence and magnitude of the late asthmatic response and the associated change in nonspecific bronchial responsiveness. Am Rev Respir Dis 140:917–923, 1989.
147. Smith RM, Richerson HB: A longitudinal study of airway responsiveness to methacholine in ragweed hay fever patients (abstract). Am Rev Respir Dis 137:284, 1988.
148. Machado L: Increased bronchial hypersensitivity after early and late bronchial reactions provoked by allergen inhalation. Allergy 40:580–585, 1985.
149. Van Bever HP, Stevens WJ: Suppression of the late asthmatic reaction by hyposensitization in asthmatic children allergic to house dust mite (*Dermatophagoides pteronyssinus*). Clin Experimental Allergy 19:399–404, 1988.
150. Spector SL, Luparello TJ, Kopetzky MT, et al: Response of asthmatics to methacholine challenge and suggestion. Am Rev Respir Dis 113:43–50, 1976.
151. Horton DG, et al: Bronchoconstrictive suggestion in asthma: A role for airways hyperreactivity and emotions. Am Rev Respir Dis 117:1029, 1978.
152. Gervais P, Reinberg A, Gervais C, et al: Twenty-four-hour rhythm in the bronchial hyperreactivity to house dust in asthmatics. J Allergy Clin Immunol 59:207, 1977.
153. Smolensky M, Reinberg A, Quent JT: The chronobiology and chronopharmacology of allergy. Ann Allergy 47:234, 1981.
154. Vincent NJ, et al: Factors influencing pulmonary resistance. J Appl Physiol 29:236, 1970.
155. Orehek J, et al: Bronchomotor effect of bronchoconstriction-induced deep aspirations in asthmatics. Am Rev Respir Dis 121:297, 1980.
156. Pennock BE, Rogers RM, McCaffree DDR: Changes in measured spirometric indices. What is significant? Chest 80:97, 1980.
157. Tiffeneau R: Amples variations due degre de l'allergie pulmonaire produites par administration d'allergenes par voie respiratoire. Int Arch Allergy 17:193, 1960.
158. Herxheimer H: Bronchial hypersensitization and hyposensitization in man. Int Arch Allergy 2:40, 1951.
159. Vedal SS, Enarson DA, Chan H, et al: A longitudinal study of the occurrence of bronchial hyperresponsiveness in Western red cedar workers. Am Rev Respir Dis 27:651–655, 1988.
160. Hume KM, Gandevia B: Forced expiratory volume before and after isprenaline. Thorax 12:276, 1957.
161. Goldberg I, Cherniack RM: The effect of nebulized bronchodilator delivered with and without IPPB on ventilatory function in chronic obstructive emphysema. Am Rev Respir Dis 91:13, 1965.
162. Green M, Mead J: Time dependence of flow volume curves. J Appl Physiol 37:793, 1974.
163. Nadel JA, Tierney DF: Effect of a previous deep inspiration on airway resistance in man. J Appl Physiol 16:717, 1961.
164. Orehek J, et al: Influence of the previous deep inspiration on the spirometric measurement of provoked bronchoconstriction in asthma. Am Rev Respir Dis 123:269, 1981.

165. Gimeno F, et al: Spirometry-induced bronchial obstruction. Am Rev Respir Dis 105:66, 1972.

166. Gayrard P, et al: Bronchoconstrictor effects of a deep inspiration in patients with asthma. Am Rev Respir Dis 111:433, 1975.

167. Ingram RH Jr, McFadden ER Jr: Localization and mechanisms of airway responses. N Engl J Med 297:596, 1977.

168. Ingram RH Jr, et al: Relative contributions of large and small airways to flow limitation in normal subjects before and after atropine and isoproterenol. J Clin Invest 49:696, 1977.

169. Spector SL, Souhrada JF: Maximal midexpiratory flow as an index of acute airway changes. Chest 68:851–852, 1975.

170. Cockcroft DW, Killian DN, Mellon JJA, Hargreave FE: Protective effect of drugs on histamine-induced asthma. Thorax 32:429, 1979.

171. Koeter GH, Kraan J, Boorsma M, et al: Effect of theophylline and enprofylline on bronchial hyperresponsiveness. Thorax 44:1022–1026, 1989.

172. Martin GL, Atkins PC, Dunsky EH, et al: Effects of theophylline, terbutaline, and prednisone on antigen-induced bronchospasm and mediator release. J Allergy Clin Immunol 66:204, 1980.

173. Falliers C: Assessment of oral antiasthmatic drugs by inhalation challenge. J Allergy Clin Immunol 64:685, 1979.

174. Casterline CL, Evans R III, Ward GW Jr: The effect of atropine and albuterol aerosols on the human bronchial response to histamine. J Allergy Clin Immunol 58:607, 1976.

175. Townley RG, McGeady S, Bewtra A: The effect of beta-adrenergic blockade on bronchial sensitivity to acetyl-beta-methacholine in normal and allergic rhinitis subjects. J Allergy Clin Immunol 57:358, 1976.

176. Zaid G, Beall GN: Bronchial response to beta-adrenergic blockade. N Engl J Med 275:580, 1966.

177. Orehek J, Gayrard P, Grimaud CH, Charpin J: Effect of beta-adrenergic blockade on bronchial sensitivity to inhaled acetylcholine in normal subjects. J Allergy Clin Immunol 55:164, 1975.

178. Ryo UY, Townley RG: Comparison of respiratory and cardiovascular effects of isoproterenol, propranolol, and practolol in asthmatic and normal subjects. J Allergy Clin Immunol 57:12, 1976.

179. Booij-Noord H, Quanjer PH, DeVries K: Protektive wirkung von berotec bei provokation-stetsen mit spezfisher allergen inhalation und histamin. Int J Clin Pharmacol 6(Suppl 4)69, 1972.

180. Woenne R, Kattan M, Levison H: Sodium cromoglycate-induced changes in the dose-response curve of inhaled methacholine and histamine in asthmatic children. Am Rev Respir Dis 119:927, 1979.

181. Chhabra SK, Guar SN: Effect of long-term treatment with sodium cromoglycate on nonspecific bronchial hyperresponsiveness in asthma. Chest 95:1235–1238, 1989.

182. Engstrom I, Vejinolovna J: The effect of disodium cromoglycate on allergen challenge in children with bronchial asthma. Acta Allergol 25:382, 1970.

183. Herxheimer HGJ, Brewersdorff H: Disodium cromoglycate in the prevention of induced asthma. Br Med J 2:220, 1969.

184. Frith PA, Ruffin RE, Juniper EF, et al: Inhibition of allergen-induced asthma by three forms of sodium cromoglycate. Clin Allergy 11:67, 1981.

185. Tiffeneau R, Dunoyer P: Action de la cortisone sur l'hypersensibilite cholinergique pulmonaire de l'asthmatique. Presse Med 64:719, 1956.

186. Arkins JA, Schleuter DP, Fink JN: The effect of corticosteroids on methacholine inhalation in symptomatic bronchial asthma. J Allergy 41:209, 1968.

187. Easton JG: Effect of an inhaled corticosteroid on methacholine airway reactivity. J Allergy Clin Immunol 67:388, 1981.

188. Ryan G, Latimer KM, Juniper EF, et al: Effect of beclomethasone dipropionate on bronchial responsiveness to histamine in controlled nonsteroid-dependent asthma. J Allergy Clin Immunol 75:25–30, 1985.

189. Nakazawa T, Toyada T, Furukawa M, et al: Inhibitory effects of various drugs on dual asthmatic responses in wheat flour-sensitive subjects. J Allergy Clin Immunol 58:1, 1976.

190. Booij-Noord H, Orle NGM, DeVries K: Immediate and late bronchial obstructive reactions to inhalation of house dust and protective effects of disodium cromoglycate and prednisone. J Allergy Clin Immunol 48:344, 1971.

191. Pepys J, et al: The effects of inhaled beclomethasone dipropionate (Becotide) and sodium cromoglycate on asthmatic reactions to provocation tests. Clin Allergy 4:12, 1974.

192. Yu DTC, Galant SP, Gold WM: Inhibition of antigen-induced bronchoconstriction by atropine in asthmatic patients. J Appl Physiol 32:823, 1972.

193. Rosenthal RR, Norman PS, Summer WR, et al: Role of the parasympathetic system in antigen-induced bronchospasm. J Appl Physiol 42:600, 1977.

194. Fish JE, Rosenthal RR, Summer WR, et al: The effect of atropine on acute antigen-mediated airway constriction in subjects with allergic asthma. Am Rev Respir Dis 115:371, 1977.

195. Itkin IH, Anand SC: The role of atropine as a mediator blocker of induced bronchial obstruction. J Allergy 45:178, 1970.

196. Drazen JM, Austen KF: Atropine modification of the pulmonary effects of chemical mediators in the guinea pig. J Appl Physiol 38:834, 1975.

197. Bryant DH, Burns MWS: Bronchial histamine reactivity: Its relationship to the reactivity of the bronchi to allergens. Clin Allergy 6:523, 1976.

198. Casterline CL, Evans R, Ward GW: The effect of atropine and albuterol aerosols on the human bronchial response to histamine. J Allergy Clin Immunol 58:607, 1976.

199. Guirgis HM, McNeill RS: The nature of adrenergic receptors in isolated human bronchi. Thorax 24:613, 1969.

200. Anthracite RF, Vachon L, Knapp PH: Alpha-adrenergic receptors in the human lung. Psychosomat Med 33:481, 1971.

201. Bianco S, Griffin JP, Kamburoff PL, et al: The effect of histamine-induced bronchospasm in man. Br J Dis Chest 66:27, 1972.

202. Beil M, DeKock A: Role of alpha-adrenergic receptors in exercise-induced bronchoconstriction. Respiration 35:78, 1978.

203. Kerr JW, Govindaraj M, Patel KR: Effect of alpha-receptor blocking drugs and disodium cromoglycate on histamine hypersensitivity in bronchial asthma. Br Med J 2:139, 1970.

204. Patel KR, et al: The effect of thymoxamine and cromolyn sodium on post-exercise bronchoconstriction in asthma. J Allergy Clin Immunol 57:285, 1976.

205. Fish JE, et al: Indomethacin modification of immediate-type immunologic airway responses in allergic asthmatic and non-asthmatic subjects. Am Rev Respir Dis 123:609, 1981.

206. Cerrina J, Denjean A, Alexandre G, et al: Inhibition of exercise-induced asthma by a calcium antagonist, nifedipine. Am Rev Respir Dis 123:156, 1981.

207. Williams DO, Barnes PJ, Vickers HP, Rudolf M: Effect of nifedipine on bronchomotor tone on histamine reactivity in asthma. Br Med J 283:348, 1981.

208. Weiss EB, Patwardhan AV: The response to lidocaine in bronchial asthma. Chest 72:429, 1977.

209. Burney PGJ, Neild JE, Twort CHC, et al: Effect of changing dietary sodium on airway response to histamine. Thorax 44:36–41, 1989.

210. Ogilvy CS, DuBois AB, Douglas JS: Effects of ascorbic acid and indomethacin on the airways of healthy male subjects with and without induced bronchoconstriction. J Allergy Clin Immunol 67:363, 1981.

211. Zuskin E, Lewis AJ, Bouhuys A: Inhibition of histamine-induced airway constriction by ascorbic acid. J Allergy Clin Immunol 51:218, 1973.

212. Pauli BD, Reid RL, Munt PW, et al: Influence of the menstrual cycle on airway function in asthmatic and normal subjects. Am Rev Respir Dis 140:358–362, 1989.

213. DeVries K, Goei JT, Booij-Noord M, Orie NGM: Changes during 24 hours in the lung function and histamine hyperreactivity of the bronchial tree in asthmatic and bronchitic patients. Int Arch Allergy 20:93, 1962.

214. Tammeling GJ, DeVries K, Kruyt EW: The circadian pattern of the bronchial reactivity to histamine in healthy subjects and in patients with obstructive lung disease. In McGovern JP, Smolensky M, Reinberg A (eds): Chronobiology in Allergy and Immunology. Springfield, IL, Charles C Thomas, 1976.

215. Reinberg A, Gervais P, Morin M, Abulker C: Circadian rhythms in the threshold of bronchial response to acetylcholine in healthy and asthmatic subjects. Scheving L, Halberg F, Pauly J (eds): Tokyo, Igaku Sjoin, 1974, p 174.

216. Sasaki F, Ishizaki T, Mifune J, et al: Bronchial hyperresponsiveness in patients with chronic congestive heart failure. Chest 97:534–538, 1990.

217. Pison C, Malo J-L, Rouleau J-L, et al: Bronchial hyperresponsiveness to inhaled methacholine in subjects with chronic left heart failure at a time of exacerbation and after increasing diuretic therapy. Chest 96:230–235, 1989.

218. Seibert AE, Allison RC, Bryars CH, Kirkpatrick MB: Normal airway hyperresponsiveness to methacholine in cardiac asthma. Am Rev Respir Dis 140:1805–1806, 1989.

219. Juniper EF, Daniel EE, Roberts RS, et al: Improvement in airway responsiveness and asthma severity during pregnancy. Am Rev Respir Dis 140:924–931, 1989.

220. Ryan G, Dolovich MB, Roberts RS, et al: Standardization of inhalation provocation tests: Two techniques of aerosol generation sand inhalation compared. Am Rev Respir Dis 123:195, 1981.

Chapter 5

EPIDEMIOLOGY AND OCCUPATIONAL ASTHMA

Jerry McLarty, PhD

Epidemiology is the study of disease in populations. This includes the study of the presence and occurrence of disease and the causes and control of disease in defined populations.[1] Although the impetus for epidemiologic studies in occupational diseases may often be clinical observations of single individuals, the ultimate result is a study of well-defined and often large populations of individuals. Such large studies require a number of methods unique to epidemiology. These methodologies include special study designs and special analytical techniques. Epidemiology can be roughly categorized into three specific kinds of methodology: descriptive, analytic, and experimental.

Descriptive epidemiology is concerned with the occurrence of disease and the relationship of disease to basic characteristics such as age, race, sex, and occupation. Descriptive epidemiology is usually based on surveys, public records and other information collected routinely, sometimes for other purposes. The technique is often "hypothesis-generating," that is, clues to the occurrence of disease or its link to possible causative factors are discovered in the data analysis.

Analytic epidemiology involves studies specifically designed to examine associations—to identify or measure the effects of risk factors or the health effects of specific exposures. Analytic studies are more often than not "hypothesis-testing" studies. The three most common analytic studies are case-control, cross-sectional, and cohort studies.

Experimental epidemiology also involves hypothesis testing, but the key feature is the control of the exposure and response situation, rather than simple observation and measurement. Experimental epidemiology is most closely linked with randomized, controlled trials.

There are at least six uses for epidemiologic methods in the identification and control of occupational pulmonary disease:[2]

1. to identify disease in an occupational setting;
2. to measure the incidence, prevalence, and severity of disease;
3. to identify the cause of disease;
4. to help limit, prevent, or control the disease;
5. to establish industrial hygiene standards; and
6. to establish baseline data, population norms, and procedures for the measurement of occupational disease.

Other applications, perhaps overlapping with the ones listed above, include establishing a dose-response relationship between identified causative agents and disease; designing preventive measures and evaluating their efficacy; convincing responsible parties that an occupationally related health problem exists; and better defining the definitions of normal and diseased so that the two can be discriminated.

In this chapter, some fundamental concepts and the common types of epidemiologic studies are described, and their strengths and weaknesses are presented with respect to the study of occupational asthma. Some of the common problems associated with epidemiologic studies and the methods used in occupational asthma are discussed.

55

EPIDEMIOLOGIC CONCEPTS

Several terms and concepts are fundamental to the understanding of epidemiology. The measurement of the presence and occurrence of diseases, the rates at which they occur, the comparison of risk between exposed and non-exposed populations, and the evaluation of screening tests all have specific terminology and situations to which they best apply.

Two of the most commonly misused terms are prevalence and incidence. **Prevalence** measures the amount of disease (percentage or number of persons with disease) present at a particular time or over a period of time, and **incidence** measures the occurrence of new cases over a period of time. When used without qualification, the term prevalence usually refers to the situation at a particular time (**point prevalence**) and **period prevalence** refers to the number of persons with the disease at any time during a specified period.[1] Lifetime prevalence, for example, means the number of persons known to have had the disease at some time during their lifetime. The prevalence of asthma (point prevalence) is estimated to be 4.3% of the U.S. population, or approximately 9.5 million persons.[3] Occupational asthma is estimated to represent about 15% of the total asthma prevalence.[4]

Incidence is usually expressed as number of new cases per person-years. For example, the incidence of mesothelioma is less than 1 case per 100,000 person-years. An early estimate (underestimate, as it turned out) of the frequency of byssinosis in British cotton workers was 6 cases per year in 58,000 workers.[2] This can be expressed as approximately 10.3 cases per 100,000 person-years.

It is common in epidemiologic studies to adjust incidence or prevalence rates for age, sex, race, smoking, or other common factors. This is done so that comparisons between groups are more meaningful. A number of different methods have been developed for adjustment. Comparison of disease rates in different populations leads to different measures of risk, including relative risks and risk factors. A **relative risk** can be defined as the risk of disease (or death) among exposed persons divided by the risk of disease in non-exposed persons. For example, a study of occupational exposures to fiberglass yielded a 1.8 relative risk of asthma by dividing the age- and smoking-adjusted asthma prevalence rates of fiberglass-exposed workers by the same prevalence rate of nonexposed persons.[5] This would generally be interpreted to mean that persons occupationally exposed to fiberglass are almost twice as likely to develop asthma as persons not so exposed.

A term often used interchangeably with relative risk is **"odds ratio."** For rare diseases, the two can be virtually equivalent, but for common diseases this is not the case. The following matrix illustrates this point:

	Exposed	Unexposed
Disease	a	b
No disease	c	d

Where a, b, c, and d are the numbers of persons in the four categories.

The odds ratio is defined to be ad/bc. The disease rate in exposed persons is $a/(a + c)$; in unexposed persons it is $b/(b + d)$. The relative risk of disease in the exposed (as compared to unexposed) is then:

$$\frac{a/(a + c)}{b/(b + d)} = \frac{a}{b} \times \frac{(b + d)}{(a + c)} \cong \frac{ad}{bc}$$

If the disease is rare, i.e., a and b are small compared to c and d, then relative risk is approximately equal to the odds ratio. The major point is that odds ratios are not necessarily the same as relative risks, even though the two terms are often used interchangeably.

Odds ratios are also commonly estimated by a special regression technique called **logistic regression,** which uses the logarithm of the odds ratio as the dependent variable with multiple independent variables (covariates).

Another term used to quantify risk is the SMR, the **standardized mortality** (or morbidity) **ratio,** which is the ratio of the number of events (deaths to cause, or incidence of disease) in an occupationally exposed study population to the number of events that would be expected if the study population had the same rates as a standard population. The ratio is multiplied by 100. So an SMR of 100 indicates no excess risk, and an SMR greater than 100 indicates excess risk in the study population. Because of the "healthy worker" effect, SMRs of less than 100 are common in occupational studies.

Risk factors are things that are associated with increased risk but may or may not be causal. For example, smoking is known to be associated with an increased risk to asthma.[6] Smoking may play a causal role in the development of asthma, but the causal role is less clear for another risk factor—race.[7] Air pollution, infections, age, and the presence of atopy are other examples of commonly studied asthma risk factors. Logistic regression is often used to evaluate, and adjust for, the relative importance of multiple risk factors.

Another important concept in the application of epidemiology is that of the **screening test** and the terms it generates: sensitivity and specificity. The assumption of a screening test is that there is a "gold standard" of diagnosis (usually a definitive clinical diagnosis) against which a lesser standard (usually an epidemiologic test such as a questionnaire) is compared. **Sensitivity** is the proportion of truly diseased persons in the screened population identified by the screening test (often called the true positive rate). **Specificity** is the portion of truly nondiseased persons identified by the screening test (often called the true negative rate). The following table illustrates these concepts.

Screening test results	True Status		Total
	Diseased	Not Diseased	
Positive	a	b	a + b
Negative	c	d	c + d
Total	a + c	b + d	a + b + c + d
Then, sensitivity = a/(a + c) and specificity = d/(b + d)			

Realistically there is a trade-off between sensitivity and specificity. For example, a very sensitive test may detect too many false positives, and a highly specific test may not be very sensitive, i.e., would miss many true positives. The trade-off between sensitivity and specificity is illustrated by the following example: marked bronchial hyperresponsiveness is uncommon in persons without asthma, but, conversely, some persons with asthma do not have bronchial hyperresponsiveness.[8] This means that bronchial hyperresponsiveness is a sensitive test for asthma but it is not very specific. Sensitivity and specificity are usually expressed as percentages. Immunologic testing for hypersensitivity pneumonitis has been reported to have specificity from 60% to 90% and sensitivity approaching 90% to 100%.[9]

COMMON TYPES OF STUDIES

Most epidemiologic studies of occupational asthma have been etiologic studies to determine possible causative agents. Such studies include the most common study types such as descriptive studies and the analytical case-control and cohort studies. To date there have been very few experimental epidemiologic studies, but this is likely to change as the number of causative agents increases and the focus changes from identification and documentation of the problem to prevention or control of the problem. The categorization of epidemiologic studies, as discussed below, is academic and not necessarily mutually exclusive nor exhaustive; there are often indistinguishable elements of each type used in a single study. A study of the health effects of the Mount St. Helens volcanic ash is a recent example that used elements of all of the study types discussed below.[10]

Descriptive Studies

Descriptive epidemiology is usually based on information collected routinely and often for unrelated purposes. Surveys of company records, public health statistics, and insurance and workers' compensation records are examples. The characteristics often studied involve defining the person-place-time relationships between exposure and disease. Estimates of disease prevalence often are obtained from descriptive studies. The previously cited study of byssinosis in Great Britain[2] involved death records and disability pension records. In the U.S., maps of mortality by cause, county-by-county, have been the source of many hypothesis-generating studies. Often such studies are initiated in response to unusual clinical findings in a few individuals. The advantage of such studies is that they are relatively cheap, requiring only the examination of existing data and not the generation of new data. The major problem with descriptive studies, using existing records, is that undetected biases may exist in the data and that the data collected may not be appropriate to the questions being asked. Repeated analysis of nonspecific data collections can produce spurious correlations that are not upheld in subsequent hypothesis-testing studies.

The classic descriptive study, and indeed possibly the beginning of modern epidemiology, was the work of John Snow that led to the control of the 19th century cholera epidemic in London.[1] By examination of the geographic patterns of cholera cases, he identified a contaminated water source that was responsible for the epidemic. The relevance to occupational asthma is that the problem was identified and eliminated without any knowledge of the actual etiologic agent; the cholera vibrio was discovered 30 years later by Koch. Effective control measures may be instituted in occupational settings long before definitive analytic studies can be done.

Case-control Studies

Case-control studies and cohort studies are usually hypothesis-testing or hypothesis-confirming studies rather than hypothesis-generating. Relative risks and odds ratios are common products of case-control studies. Case-control studies compare persons with a specific disease (cases) to persons thought to be similar in important aspects but who do not have the disease (controls). More than one control group may be used. The groups are compared with respect to exposure, suspected risk factors, and perhaps factors that may be protective. A key element in case-control studies is comparability of the cases and controls in all factors except disease. Such comparability is necessary to eliminate bias, such as selection bias or recall bias. Case-control studies, when first initiated early in this century,[11] represented a major departure from the random sample designs commonly used in statistics at that time. The cases and controls are not necessarily random nor representative samples at all.

The purpose of case-control studies is to confirm the relationships of putative etiologic agents and disease, or to estimate the strength of the relationships, and to investigate possible interactions between various risk factors. Examples of pure case-control studies are not as numerous in occupational asthma as in other fields, such as cancer research. A good recent example is a study in an electronics factory to evaluate etiologic factors for work-related asthma.[12]

One major advantage of case-control studies is that they are relatively cheap and efficient. A single study can evaluate many causal hypotheses simultaneously. The entire exposed cohort need not be studied, just the identified cases and an appropriate number of similar controls. The major limitation is the susceptibility to bias, especially selection bias, that may cause cases to be fundamentally different from controls. Other forms of bias include the possibility that cases may answer questions concerning exposure differently than persons without disease. An inherent problem

in case-control studies of occupational asthma is the definition of a case (or the definition and measurement of disease). An excellent reference text on the design and analysis of case-control studies was written by Breslow and Day.[11]

Cohort Studies

Cohort studies are also used for hypothesis testing. Commonly, estimates of incidence are obtained from cohort studies. A cohort is an identified group of persons, usually with one or more unique features in common, such as occupation. Cohort studies can be characterized as prospective or retrospective, depending upon whether the group has been followed (studied) subsequent to or prior to identification. The unique feature of cohort studies is that the persons will be studied with respect to disease occurrence over a number of years; they can be observed before the occurrence of disease. Rates of disease occurrence can then be compared between exposed and nonexposed, or between varying degrees of exposure. The effects of multiple risk factors and confounding variables can also be considered.

A major advantage of cohort studies is that recall and selection bias can be eliminated. Because persons are identified for study by their presence in the cohort and not by their disease, selection bias is not the problem it is for case-control studies. Recall of important covariates such as smoking behavior is much less likely to be biased, especially in prospective cohort studies. Another advantage of cohort studies is that predisease biologic parameters can be recorded. This is particularly relevant to occupational asthma studies, because the presence or absence of atopy is of special interest in the etiology of disease and may change dramatically in the time before and after onset of the disease. Repeated measures of exposure and confounding variables can help minimize measurement and misclassification errors. The obvious disadvantage to cohort studies is their expense; usually large groups of persons and several years of observation are required.

If the occurrence of asthma is rare in a particular occupation, then the required numbers of person-years can be especially large. Retrospective cohort studies can be less expensive but may suffer from the same recall bias and lack of information as case-control studies. Selection of controls is another fundamental problem with cohort studies; often there is no naturally occurring control group, so rates from general populations are necessary for comparison. Extrapolations from unique cohorts to the general population can be difficult because of inherent differences in the populations. Breslow and Day have produced an excellent reference for the design and analysis of cohort studies.[13]

Cohort studies of occupational asthma are much more common than case-control studies. A recent example of a cohort study is the report of mortality and disability of Finnish cotton mill workers.[14] Incidence rates for respiratory and musculoskeletal diseases were obtained, in addition to mortality data. Standardized mortality ratios were also reported for respiratory, cardiovascular, and cancer deaths.

Hybrid studies are becoming common. Prentice[15] introduced a new study design called the nested case-control design that combines some of the best features of case-control and cohort studies. The idea is that cases identified from a cohort study can be used with controls selected from the same study. This is a particularly efficient study design because the entire study cohort need not get the same intensive (expensive) follow-up as the cases and selected controls.

Cross-sectional Studies

Cross-sectional studies are commonly used to document the prevalence and severity of disease by studying the characteristics of a study population at a particular point in time. The terms **field survey, frequency survey, prevalence study,** and **cross-sectional study** are used interchangeably. Etiologic relationships between exposure and other risk factors and disease can be examined by comparing subgroups with and without the disease or by documenting the presence or absence of disease in subgroups with or without the exposures. Regression analysis can accomplish the same tasks with varying levels of exposures and disease.

Cross-sectional studies are usually undertaken to study already known or suspected hazards, to investigate etiology, or to establish and monitor hygiene standards. A classic example of an occupational cross-sectional study was a survey that uncovered serious respiratory problems in Lancashire cotton mill workers in 1956.[16] These respiratory problems were associated with sudden onset at work, after a weekend off, and were characterized by increasing severity of symptoms and changes in ventilatory capacity as the week progressed. One of the first uses of cross-sectional studies to establish and monitor industrial hygiene standards was also in English cotton mills.[17-19]

Cross-sectional studies have two major disadvantages: (1) bias in study populations and (2) problems with establishing temporal relationships between exposure and dose. Both of the problems are inherent to the one-time measurement of disease and risk factors; persons measured may be self-selected survivors, i.e., they may represent a subgroup particularly immune to the problem being measured. Also, one-time measurements on many individuals may give misleading estimates of changes over time or changes with age that occur in single individuals.

Experimental Studies

Experimental studies differ from the observational and analytical studies in that the patients or their exposures or the course of their disease is deliberately altered as a part of the study. Examples in occupational asthma are rare but are becoming more frequent as attempts are made to intervene in the workplace to prevent or minimize health problems. For example, the etiology of occupational asthma has been studied in small groups of patients who have been deliberately exposed to different types of dust and monitored for symptoms and pulmonary function changes.[20] A more comprehensive workplace example is the experimental trial of cotton steaming to reduce the hazardous effects of cotton dust.[21]

Experimental studies have the advantage that they can address hypotheses directly and can eliminate the usual sources of bias and eliminate or control confounding factors. The disadvantage is that they often require large numbers of subjects and long periods of follow-up. Permanent changes in pulmonary function, for example, require many years to be detected reliably. However, acute asthmatic responses may be studied in a shorter period of time.

PROBLEMS IN EPIDEMIOLOGIC STUDIES OF OCCUPATIONAL ASTHMA

In addition to the usual epidemiologic problems of selection and recall bias, confounding factors and low power to discriminate "signal" from "noise," studies in occupational asthma have other features that make them especially difficult. The major problems include the definition and measurement of asthma, the definition and measurement of exposure, and the difficulty in establishing linkage between exposure and disease.

Definition and Measurement of Occupational Asthma

A simple definition of occupational asthma is variable airflow obstruction caused by a specific agent in the workplace.[22,23] This definition, however, does not consider the mechanisms of asthma induction, and a variety of quite different conditions could lead to the same diagnosis.[24] Clinically, asthma is characterized by intermittent respiratory symptoms, airway hyperresponsiveness, and reversible airways obstruction. For epidemiologic studies, criteria have commonly included a history of physician-diagnosed asthma or affirmative answers to questions concerning wheeze.[8] However, wheezing is not unique to asthma. Reversible airways obstruction is measured by improvement in ventilatory function after bronchodilators and challenge testing are used to demonstrate hyperresponsiveness. Not only are the pulmonary and immunologic tests for asthma nonspecific, there is considerable age-related and time-related variation in the nature of asthma.[25,26] The variety of diagnostic criteria used in occupational asthma studies can make comparisons between studies difficult, if not impossible. Obviously, incidence and prevalence rates could vary dramatically, within the same population, for different definitions of disease.

One of the most pressing needs in the epidemiology of occupational asthma is the development of easier and cheaper methods of measuring and defining asthma. Enarson and others[8] have strongly recommended that priorities be placed on the development and validation of better questionnaires for the epidemiologic assessment of asthma. Most respiratory disease questionnaires in current use are derivatives of two landmark questionnaires—the British Medical and Research Council and the American Thoracic Society standardized questionnaires.[27,28] Although these two questionnaires contain asthma-related symptoms, they are clearly not adequate for the study of occupational asthma. The documentation of questionnaire sensitivity and specificity is difficult because there is no generally accepted "gold standard" against which to compare. Symptom-related questions have been found to be neither sensitive nor specific when compared to methacholine inhalation challenge.[29] Sensitivities range from 17% (wheeze and breathlessness) to 65% (any respiratory symptom), with the corresponding specificities ranging from 95% to 58%, respectively.[26] Note the trade-off, as sensitivity improves, specificity gets worse. Physician-diagnosed asthma is more specific, (i.e., 99%) but much less sensitive (10%). Another problem with questionnaires is in associating the symptoms with the occupational exposure. The National Institute of Occupational Safety and Health has approved a set of questions suggesting work-relatedness of symptoms.[30] Much work remains to be done in the development of a standardized questionnaire and in testing its validity (sensitivity/specificity) and reliability (repeatability).

Definition and Measurement of Exposure

The strength of association between exposure and disease is highly dependent upon the effectiveness of the measurement of exposure. Historically, occupational exposures have been poorly defined.[31]

McDonald[32] has stressed that the failure to specify occupational exposure, other than in terms of total duration of exposure, is the most serious weakness in occupational health studies. For acute effects such as occupational asthma, the most important exposures may be the current exposures; for chronic disease past exposures may be more relevant. Because asthma may be caused by a variety of agents in the form of smoke, gas, fumes, and dust, quantitation of exposure is even more difficult. Measuring dust intensity levels is further complicated by the fact that the size of particle or particular components of the dust may be more important, etiologically, than total dust levels.[33,34] Simple measures such as duration of exposure are the most commonly used, because they only require an employment record for computation. Intensity categories of low, medium, and high are not ideal but are often the only practical solution. A combination of duration and intensity—a cumulative exposure index—is becoming widely used, where possible.[35]

Perhaps the ultimate measures of exposure will be tests of exposed persons for the presence or absence of agents (or the response to agents) in biologic specimens. Such measures may reflect not only exposure but perhaps retained exposure or individual susceptibility to exposure. For example, the presence of asbestos bodies in sputum has been a good index of heavy occupational exposure to asbestos.[36,37] Several studies have used hair and urine samples to estimate exposures to arsenic and other metals.[38] An interesting study (a combination of cross-sectional and historical cohort studies) of an entire community exposure to sour gas emissions used similar samples to document exposure.[39] New and powerful immunochemical methods are being developed that have great potential for documenting and quantifying occupational exposures to allergens.[26]

"Fuzzy" Linkage Between Exposure and Disease

In addition to problems in defining and measuring disease and exposure, the linkage between occupational exposure and asthma is not always clear. Asthma is not unique to the occupational setting; in fact, most asthma is not occupationally related.[40] Furthermore, occupational asthma is clinically indistinguishable from nonoccupational asthma. Not all exposed persons develop asthma; certain sensitized individuals are much more susceptible.[41] There is often a time delay between exposure and onset of disease, and symptoms may be present long after cessation of exposure. Finally, continued exposure may result in chronic airway obstruction, so that removal from exposure may not have immediate detectable effects (one of the diagnostic criteria for occupational asthma).[42]

SUMMARY AND CONCLUSIONS

It has been said that "asthma has not yet been defined with concepts that can be translated into criteria and procedures for use by epidemiologists."[25] It certainly is true that the study of occupational asthma is made difficult by some of the issues discussed above: there is no precise definition of the disease, it is hard to measure with precision, its presence is sometimes intermittent, exposure is equally hard to define and quantify, and the etiology is not unique to the occupational setting. Occupational populations are in many ways different from other clinically studied populations, with

potential selection biases inherent and many confounding variables present. Nevertheless, there is room for optimism. Many of the problems can be overcome with better questionnaires specific to the detection of occupational asthma and better techniques of documenting exposure, perhaps by immunochemical and other indirect biologic responses as indicators of exposure. There have been encouraging recent technical advances in these areas. With the development of standardized questionnaires specific to occupational asthma and standardized diagnostic criteria, the problems of case detection and between-study comparisons can be reduced.

Novel programs for registering occupationally related cancers and linking them to certain occupations have been established.[43] Similar programs could be established for respiratory disease as well. Better methods for case-finding; better work history records with special emphasis on recording duration, intensity, and type of exposure; and improved medical surveillance and recordkeeping by employers are certainly feasible and would contribute to the epidemiology of the disease.

Most of the epidemiologic studies have been cross-sectional surveys; these could be followed up with more case-control and longitudinal cohort studies. New hybrid study designs, such as nested case-control studies, are now available to improve the efficiency and power of studies. There has been very little experimental epidemiology in occupational asthma. This is a particularly rich area for study, especially in designing prevention strategies and in evaluating their efficacy. It is clear that the control and prevention of occupational asthma are a multidisciplinary problem, with an increasingly important role for epidemiology. As the precision of the measurement instruments and other technologies improve so will the power of the epidemiologic methods that can be applied to the problem.

REFERENCES

1. Last JM (ed): A Dictionary of Epidemiology, 2nd ed. Oxford, Oxford University Press, 1988.
2. Schilling RSF: Problems in the identification of occupational disease. In Occupational Pulmonary Disease, Focus on Grain Dust and Health. New York, Academic Press, 1980, pp 3–19.
3. Schacter J: Measurement of the prevalence of respiratory allergies by interview questionnaire. J Allergy Clin Immunol 55:249–255, 1975.
4. Blanc P: Occupational asthma in a national disability survey. Chest 92:613–617, 1987.

5. Lebowitz MD: Occupational exposure in relation to symptomatology and lung function in a community population. Environ Res 14:59-67, 1977.
6. Burrows B, Lebowitz MD, Barbee RA: Respiratory disorders and allergy skin test reactions. Ann Intern Med 84:134-139, 1976.
7. Mak H, Johnson P, Abbey H: Prevalence of asthma and health service utilization of asthmatic children in an inner city. J Allergy Clin Immunol 70:367-372, 1982.
8. Enarson DA, Vedal S, Schultzer M, et al: Asthma, asthmalike symptoms, chronic bronchitis, and the degree of bronchial hyperresponsiveness in epidemiologic surveys. Am Rev Respir Dis 136:613-617, 1987.
9. Grammer LC, Patterson R, Zeiss CR: Guidelines for the immunologic evaluation of occupational lung disease. J Allergy Clin Immunol 84(5, Part 2):805-814, 1989.
10. Bernstein RS, Baxter PJ, Falk H, et al: Immediate public health concerns and actions in volcanic eruptions: Lessons from the Mount St. Helens eruptions. Am J Public Health 76(suppl 3):25-37, 1986.
11. Breslow NE, Day NE: Statistical Methods in Cancer Research. Volume 1, The Analysis of Case-control Studies. IARC Scientific Publications No. 32. Lyon, International Agency for Research on Cancer, 1980.
12. Burge PS, Perks WH, O'Brien IM, et al: Occupational asthma in an electronics factory: A case-control study to evaluate aetiological factors. Thorax 34:300-307, 1979.
13. Breslow NE, Day NE: Statistical Methods in Cancer Research. Volume 2, The Design and Analysis of Cohort Studies. IARC Scientific Publications No. 82. Lyon, International Agency for Research on Cancer, 1987.
14. Koskela RS, Klockars M, Jarvinen E: Mortality and disability among cotton mill workers. Br J Ind Med 47:384-391, 1990.
15. Prentice RL, Self SG, Mason MW: Design options for sampling within a cohort. In Moolgavkar SH, Prentice RL (eds): Modern Statistical Methods in Chronic Disease Epidemiology. New York, John Wiley & Sons, 1986, pp 50-62.
16. Schilling RSF: Byssinosis in cotton and other textile workers. Lancet ii:261-265, 319-325, 1956.
17. Schilling RSF: Epidemiological studies of chronic respiratory disease among cotton operatives. Yale J Biol Med 37:55-73, 1964.
18. Roach SA, Schilling RSF: A clinical and environmental study of byssinosis in the Lancashire cotton industry. Br J Ind Med 17:1-9, 1960.
19. British Occupational Hygiene Society, Committee on Hygiene Standards: Hygiene standards for cotton dust. Ann Occup Hygiene 15:165-192, 1972.
20. McKerrow CB, Roach SA, Gilson JC, Schilling RSF: The size of cotton dust particles causing byssinosis. Br J Ind Med 19:1-8, 1962.
21. Merchant JA, Lumsden JC, Kilborn KH, et al: Intervention studies of cotton steaming to reduce biological effects of cotton dust. Br J Ind Med 31:261-274, 1974.
22. Chan-Yeung M: Occupational asthma update. Chest 93:407-411, 1988.
23. Newman-Taylor AJ: Occupational asthma. Thorax 35:241-245, 1980.
24. Balmes JR: Surveillance for occupational asthma. Occup Med State Art Rev 6(1)101-109, 1991.
25. Woolcock AJ: Epidemiologic methods for measuring prevalence of asthma. Chest 91(Suppl 96):89S-92S, 1987.
26. Smith AB, Castellan RM, Lewis D, Matte T: Guidelines for the epidemiologic assessment of occupational asthma. J Allergy Clin Immunol 84(5, Part 2):794-805, 1989.
27. Ferris BF: Epidemiology standardization project: Respiratory questionnaires. Am Rev Respir Dis 118:7-53, 1978.
28. Medical Research Council: Questionnaire on respiratory symptoms. London, Medical Research Council, 1976.
29. Klees J, Alexander M, Rempel D, et al: Evaluation of a proposed NIOSH surveillance case definition for occupational asthma. Chest 98(suppl 5):212S-215S, 1990.
30. Hoffman RE, Rosenman KD, Watt F, et al: Occupational disease surveillance: Occupational asthma. MMWR 39:119-123, 1990.
31. Baumgarten M, Oseasohn R: Studies in occupational health: A critique. J Occup Med 22:171-176, 1980.
32. McDonald JC: Epidemiology. In Weill H, Turner-Warwick M (eds): Occupational Lung Diseases: Research Approach and Methods. New York, Marcel Dekker, 1981, pp 373-404.
33. McKerrow CB, Roach SA, Gilson JC, Schilling RSF: The size of cotton dust particles causing byssinosis. Br J Ind Med 19:1-8, 1962.
34. Venables KM: Epidemiology and the prevention of occupational asthma. Br J Ind Med 44:73-75, 1987.
35. Becklake MR: Epidemiology in the workplace: Can it answer the clinician's questions? In Bernard J, Gee L, Morgan WKC, Brooks SM (eds): Occupational Lung Disease. New York, Raven Press, 1984, pp 109-118.
36. McLarty JW, Greenberg SD, Hurst GA, et al: The clinical significance of ferruginous bodies in sputa. J Occup Med 22:92-96, 1980.
37. Roggli VL, Greenberg SD, McLarty JW, et al: Comparison of sputum and lung asbestos body counts in former asbestos workers. Am Rev Respir Dis 122:941-945, 1980.
38. Agahian B, Lee JS, Nelson JH, Johns RE: Arsenic levels in fingernails as a biological indicator of exposure to arsenic. Am Ind Hyg Assoc J 51:646-651, 1990.
39. Spitzer WO, Dales RE, Schecter MT, et al: Chronic exposure to sour gas emissions: Meeting a community concern with epidemiologic evidence. Can Med Assoc J 141:685-691, 1989.
40. Bonner JR: The epidemiology and natural history of asthma. Clin Chest Med 5:557-565, 1984.
41. Becklake MR: Epidemiology and surveillance. Chest 98(Suppl 5):165S-172S, 1990.
42. Fine JM, Balmes JR: Airway inflammation and occupational asthma. Clin Chest Med 9:557-590, 1988.
43. Siemiatycki J, Day NE, Fabry J, Cooper JA: Discovering carcinogens in the occupational environment: A novel approach. J Nat Cancer Inst 66:217-225, 1981.

Chapter 6

OCCUPATIONAL BRONCHITIS

David E. Griffith, MD
Jeffrey L. Levin, MD, MSPH

As a disease entity, chronic bronchitis gets relatively little respect. This lack of serious attention stems from an inability to attribute dire pathophysiologic consequences to chronic cough with mucous hypersecretion. Interest has been restimulated in bronchitis, however, due to recent revelations about asthma as an inflammatory process and to interest in occupationally related causes of pulmonary disease in general.

Although chronic cough and mucous hypersecretion are commonly encountered, the true prevalence of these symptoms is unclear, because chronic bronchitis and emphysema are frequently lumped under the umbrella term chronic obstructive pulmonary disease (COPD). Additionally, symptoms of cough, sputum production, and wheezing are all common in populations at risk and do not, in themselves, differentiate specific respiratory syndromes.[1] Recognizing these limitations, in 1980 there were approximately 7.5 million Americans with chronic bronchitis.[2] Cigarette smoking is recognized as, by far, the most common etiologic factor in the development of chronic bronchitis, although a number of other causes including occupational exposures, air pollution,[3] viral infections,[4] and immunologic deficiencies[5] are also implicated in its development. Unfortunately, it is difficult to perform studies to assess the deleterious consequences of each of these factors due to the problem of determining relative contributions in multiple, simultaneous exposures. Even though cigarette smoking is the leading cause of chronic bronchitis, the elimination of cigarette smoking would by no means eliminate chronic bronchitis. In fact, as strategies for cigarette smoking

cessation succeed, alternative causes of bronchitis, such as occupational exposures, will only become more apparent and important.

The existence of industrial or occupational chronic bronchitis as a definable disease entity remains a controversial issue. This stems in part from a lack of standardized definitions for the obstructive lung diseases. The syndrome of **chronic bronchitis** was originally defined in symptomatic or clinical terms, as productive cough for 3 months of the year for 2 consecutive years.[6] In contrast, **asthma** is defined in functional terms as reversible airways obstruction, and **emphysema** is defined in pathologic terms as destruction of alveoli. The definition of chronic bronchitis is arbitrary (it says more about the term "chronic" than "bronchitis") and offers no clues to the pathogenesis or natural history of the disorder.

A pathologic correlate to mucous hypersecretion—mucous gland hypertrophy—was described and seemed to establish a logical series of events whereby an irritant such as cigarette smoke produced hypertrophy of bronchial mucous glands, hypersecretion of mucous, and ultimately airways obstruction. More recently, however, the pathologic processes of small-airways inflammation and emphysema have proven to be much more important in the development of airflow obstruction. As a result there is justifiable skepticism about the importance of chronic cough with mucous hypersecretion as a problem of major physiologic or functional significance. In that context, however, considerable clinical heterogeneity exists in the population of chronic bronchitics with regard to the presence or severity of concomitant pulmonary syndromes such as chronic airflow obstruction and bronchial hyperreactivity. This heterogeneity is perhaps explained by differences in individual susceptibility.

While it may be difficult to attribute specific adverse sequelae to chronic bronchitis, either mechanistically or pathophysiologically, chronic bronchitis is a sentinel symptom complex among populations at risk from inhalation of an irritant stimulus. Chronic bronchitis identifies a population at risk for more debilitating pulmonary syndromes. The majority of these subjects may not develop chronic airflow obstruction or bronchial hyperreactivity (which are due to factors difficult to define, such as individual susceptibility, host defenses, and relative degree of response). It is currently impossible, however, to determine which bronchitics will develop more serious pulmonary dysfunction.

The syndrome of chronic bronchitis is, by necessity, discussed in the context of cigarette smoke-induced bronchitis. Essentially all of the epidemiologic and pathophysiologic information about chronic bronchitis as a syndrome is derived from cigarette-smoking populations. Occupationally exposed subjects may have symptoms similar to those seen in cigarette smokers, but little is known about the pathophysiology or natural history of this disorder in the occupational setting. Most of the specific studies performed in cigarette-smoking populations have not assessed the potential contribution of occupational exposures. It is possible that conclusions based on findings in cigarette smokers are directly applicable to nonsmokers with occupational exposures. This assumption is unproven, however, and the reader should not necessarily assume that data derived in cigarette smokers are directly relevant to occupationally exposed subjects.

PATHOLOGY

Although the clinical syndrome of chronic bronchitis is defined symptomatically, it is also widely recognized to denote an inflammatory process in the bronchi. Bronchi are large airways that contain cartilage and are greater than 2 millimeters in diameter. More peripheral noncartilaginous airways less than 2 millimeters are termed bronchioles. Inflammation of the smaller airways is, therefore, more correctly termed bronchiolitis.

The development of large-airway abnormalities associated with chronic bronchitis requires a sustained and cumulative exposure to an inhaled irritant. For cigarette smokers this exposure period is several years,[7] whereas inflammatory changes in the small noncartilaginous airways may precede large-airway abnormalities.[8] It is noteworthy that in this setting large-airway inflammation may be present without significant small-airway inflammation and vice versa.

In 1954, Reid published the first comprehensive description of the disease found in the conducting airways of patients with the clinical diagnosis of chronic bronchitis.[9] Hyperplasia and hypertrophy of mucous glands in lung epithelium were associated with excess mucous within the proximal cartilaginous airways. It was assumed that inhalation of cigarette smoke and other environmental pollutants elicited hypersecretion of mucous into the airway lumens, with chronic exposure leading to mucous gland enlargement and goblet cell metaplasia. It was also presumed that chronic sputum expectoration was the clinical corollary of mucous gland hypertrophy and hypersecretion. Reid described an index of bronchial gland enlargement that presumably correlated with the amount of sputum produced.[10] The Reid index is determined by measuring the thickness of the mucous glands in a radial direction at several points around the circumference of the bronchus. This value is then normalized to the distance between the basement membrane and the inner edge of the cartilaginous plate. Subsequent studies have shown that the Reid index is normally distributed in the general population without a clear separation between bronchitics and nonbronchitics.[11,12] Therefore, somewhat surprisingly, there is not a clear correlation between the Reid index and the degree of mucous hypersecretion. More recently, however, a significant correlation has been demonstrated for absolute gland size and volume proportion of mucous glands (ratio of gland area to bronchial wall area) relative to the volume of sputum produced.[13] It took approximately 30 years to confirm that the defining symptomatology of chronic bronchitis was correlated to the characteristic morphologic change of the syndrome.

Inflammation, particularly neutrophilic inflammation, has not been a consistent or even significant pathologic feature of chronic bronchitis. This paucity of inflammatory cells in large airways raises a question of terminology. Is the term "bronchitis" really appropriate? In chronic bronchitis the inflammatory infiltrate that invades the airway mucosa, interstitium, and periglandular areas is composed predominantly of mononuclear cells.[10] The presence of inflammatory cells has had only an inconsistent association with cough and mucous hypersecretion. In a recent study, Mullen et al. confirmed not only the mononuclear nature of the inflammatory process, but also showed that the severity of this inflammatory process correlated with the size of the mucous glands.[14] Thus, mucosal inflammation in cartilaginous airways may be a factor in the production of excess mucous in chronic bronchitis.

In contrast to the paucity of inflammatory cells in pathologic specimens from chronic bronchitics, cytologic analysis of sputum from bronchitics has demonstrated a predominance of neutrophils.[15] This finding suggests differences in pathophysiology between luminal and parenchymal inflammation in chronic bronchitis. Usual methods of fixing lung tissue tend to cause the luminal contents of the airways to wash out prior to the pathologic examination, which therefore, does not necessarily reflect changes in the lumen. Bronchoalveolar lavage (BAL) studies confirm that cell recovery from the airways in chronic bronchitics demonstrates both an absolute elevation in the number of neutrophils and an increase in the percentage of neutrophils recovered.[16]

Rennard et al. have developed a bronchoalveolar lavage technique that preferentially samples central airways.[16] This specimen is termed the "bronchial sample" of the total BAL fluid recovered. The percentage of neutrophils in the bronchial sample correlates with cigarette-smoking history, sputum production, and airway obstruction. That is, subjects with more intense airway inflammation also have more severe airway obstruction and increased sputum production. It is still not clear, however, if airway neutrophilia has either etiologic or prognostic significance. Further, the mechanisms of neutrophil accumulation within the airways of chronic bronchitics have not been elucidated. A number of cell types, including alveolar macrophages, bronchial epithelial cells, eosinophils, and even neutrophils, are capable of releasing neutrophil chemoattractants.

Overall the inflammation of chronic bronchitis appears to have two distinct components, (1) mononuclear inflammation in the bronchial wall and (2) neutrophilic inflammation in the bronchial lumen. The relative importance of each type of inflammation and how they interact are unknown. The contribution of either type of inflammation to the development of chronic airflow obstruction or bronchial hyperreactivity is also unknown, although it is likely that the neutrophil has a contributing role in each of these processes.[17-19]

Potential Mechanisms of Airway Injury Secondary to Bronchial Inflammation

In airways chronically exposed to irritant substances with associated intraluminal neutrophilic inflammation, it is important to consider mechanisms of injury from both the toxic material inhaled and the secretory products of neutrophils. Because cigarette smoke contains more than 2,000 chemical components,[21] it is inappropriate to discuss direct toxic effects of cigarette smoke on the bronchial surface in the context of occupational exposures that may also be multiple and complex.

The toxicity of an inhaled occupational irritant depends on the substances inhaled, duration of inhalation, lung defense mechanisms, and nature of the subsequent inflammatory response. The ability of a variety of inhaled agents to penetrate the respiratory tract is also a function of both water solubility and particle size.[22] Those agents having high water solubility become solvated in the secretions of the upper respiratory tract. In many instances, this water solubility combined with an irritant effect may not only result in bronchoconstriction, but also serve as an early warning mechanism to alert the exposed individual to flee the area. Examples of substances causing this irritant effect include ammonia, sulphur dioxide, and hydrogen chloride.

The less soluble agents, in general, are able to penetrate the peripheral small airways and alveolar spaces. These agents, such as phosgene, oxides of nitrogen, and coal dust, are therefore more insidious in exerting their effects, typically lacking early warning characteristics and acting in a latent fashion, hours to years after exposure.

Size characteristics are equally important. Particles or fibers with diameters greater than 10 microns tend to deposit in the upper airways. Those less than 10 microns may deposit in the smaller airways, and those less than 3 microns in the alveolar spaces themselves. For substances such as coal dust, this is particularly important for air-monitoring and regulatory controls. Although controlling exposures to particles smaller than 5 microns may limit the development of pneumoconiosis, exposures to larger particles may still induce chronic bronchitis.[23] Currently, however, the specific toxic effects of most inhaled occupational substances on the bronchial mucosa are not well defined.

In contrast, the toxic effects of neutrophils have been extensively studied, and it is likely that neutrophils in the airways of chronic bronchitics are important mediators of bronchial injury. Neutrophils are also implicated in the pathogenesis of other lung disorders, including the adult respiratory distress syndrome (ARDS), idiopathic pulmonary fibrosis (IPF), emphysema, and even some occupationally related disorders such as asbestosis.[17,24-26]

Neutrophils cause bronchial injury by several mechanisms. Neutrophil-derived reactive oxidant species produce direct cell injury, oxidation of inhibitors of neutrophil proteinases, and degradation of matrix components, with alteration of connective tissue structures so that they are more susceptible to proteolysis.[27] Release of neutrophil azurophilic granule enzymes, elastase and cathepsin B, may also contribute to bronchial injury. Neutrophil elastase destroys many elements of the normal lung, including fibronectin, elastin, proteoglycans, and laminin.[28] In animal models, neutrophil elastase instilled into the tracheobronchial tree produces bronchial changes characteristic of chronic bronchitis, including mucous gland hyperplasia, reduced ciliary beat frequency, and altered ciliated epithelium.[29,30] Cathepsin B also has extensive activity against interstitial elements of the lung. Although it appears not as active as elastase, it may augment damage in association with elastase.[31] In response, the lung produces several respiratory tract antiproteinases that are found on the bronchial surface, including alpha-1-antiproteinase and bronchial proteinase inhibitor. Both of these antiproteinases are vulnerable to inactivation by oxidation.[32,33] It is possible that local inactivation of lung antiproteinases or excessive release of proteinases can produce an imbalance whereby proteolytic activity predominates. This assertion is the core of the proteinase/antiproteinase theory of emphysema development but may also be pertinent in the pathogenesis of chronic bronchitis.

Recently, two additional potential modulators of airway inflammation, lactoferrin and lysozyme, have been demonstrated in BAL fluid from chronic bronchitics.[34] Lactoferrin binds free iron, thus preventing iron-mediated catalysis of hydroxyl radical formation. Lysozyme inhibits neutrophil chemotaxis and neutrophil production of oxygen radicals. Interestingly, lactoferrin and lysozyme levels do not correlate with the number of neutrophils recovered by BAL.[34] These substances may, therefore, arise from airway epithelium in chronic bronchitics.

In chronic bronchitics airway injury is probably exacerbated during periods of acute bronchitis in which there is relatively short-lived, intense proteolytic attack on the major bronchi. The tracheobronchial tree is chronically infected with bacteria in cigarette-induced chronic bronchitis, which may play a role in these exacerbations.[35] It is also possible that colonization of airways by bacteria provides continuous stimulation of the inflammatory process with self-perpetuation of neutrophil enzyme release. The role of infection in occupationally related bronchitis is currently not known.

Beyond a cause-and-effect relationship with cough and sputum production, the significance of large-airway inflammation is unclear, primarily because it does not appear to be important pathophysiologically in the development of chronic airflow obstruction. It may, however, be more important in the development of bronchial hyperreactivity.[18,19] Bronchial injury secondary to inflammation might play an important role in exposing bronchial irritant receptors to inhaled irritants, triggering reflex or vagally mediated bronchoconstriction. The significant bronchodilating effect of anticholinergic drugs in chronic bronchitics is indirect evidence of this phenomenon.[36]

OTHER DISORDERS ASSOCIATED WITH "AIRWAY INFLAMMATION"

It is worthwhile to contrast the pathologic findings in chronic bronchitis with those found in asthma and small-airways disease with chronic airflow obstruction. Each of these disorders is characterized by "airway inflammation," which is a label that encompasses diverse findings. In this context the term "airway inflammation" is as misleading as the term "COPD." Typical pathologic and BAL findings in chronic bronchitis, small-airways disease, and asthma are summarized in Table 1. The cellular characteristics of sputum and BAL fluid recovered from asthmatics are especially different from that found in chronic bronchitics.[37,38] Asthmatics tend to

TABLE 1. *Diseases Associated with "Airway Inflammation"*

Disease	Pathologic Findings	Sputum or Bronchoalveolar Lavage Findings
Asthma[37,38,89]	Large or small airways, shedding of the epithelium, infiltration with mast cells and eosinophils, goblet cell metaplasia, basement membrane thickening, smooth muscle hypertrophy, and hyperplasia	Eosinophilia and mast cells
Chronic Bronchitis[10,14-16]	Large cartilaginous airways; hypertrophy of mucous glands, metaplasia and hyperplasia of goblet cells, excess mucous in bronchial lumen. Mononuclear infiltration of the bronchial wall	Macrophages and neutrophils
Small Airways Disease[16,42,46]	Small noncartilaginous airways; mononuclear cell infiltration in membranous bronchioles, smooth muscle hypertrophy, fibrosis primarily in membranous bronchioles, goblet cell metaplasia, pigment deposition in terminal bronchioles	Macrophages and neutrophils
Mineral Dust Airways Disease[51,52]	Similar to small-airways disease plus fibrosis (and accompanying pigment) of respiratory bronchioles and alveolar ducts	Unknown

have increased numbers of eosinophils and mast cells compared with the predominance of neutrophils found in bronchitics.

The components of airway inflammation clearly differ among subsets of patients with different pulmonary disorders, even disorders characterized by airflow obstruction. Even if the end result is similar, i.e., bronchial hyperreactivity, the specific location and cellular makeup of the inflammatory process may differ significantly between these disorders. With the present level of understanding of the pathophysiology and natural history of obstructive pulmonary diseases, it is erroneous to equate all pulmonary disorders associated with airway inflammation. Even if the various forms of airway inflammation are due to a common irritant, it is still unclear how or if they are related from an etiologic standpoint. Similarly, treatment of airway inflammation may require different approaches dependent of the specific characteristics of the inflammatory process of each disorder.

Bronchitis and Chronic Airflow Obstruction

Initially, hypertrophied mucous glands and excess mucous in bronchial lumens were thought to be the principal structural features responsible for airflow obstruction. It has since been shown that mucous hypersecretion itself has little to do with the airflow obstruction.

Epidemiologic investigations have suggested that sputum production and pulmonary impairment are related but separate phenomena. Fletcher and his colleagues longitudinally followed several hundred English postal and transport workers over an 8-year period.[39] Cigarette smoking, sputum production, and excessive decline in forced expiratory volume in 1 second (FEV_1) were strongly intercorrelated; however, the effect of cigarette smoking on lung function was much stronger than the history of sputum production. When the losses in FEV_1 were adjusted for cigarette consumption, no independent effect of sputum production upon changes in ventilatory function could be demonstrated. Peto and associates combined the results of four surveys involving more than 2,000 men from Great Britain.[40] The risk of death from COPD was strongly correlated to the degree of airflow obstruction upon admission in the study, but for men initially having a similar FEV_1, death rates were not related to the amount of mucous hypersecretion.

Structure-function analysis stands in excellent agreement with results obtained from clinical and epidemiologic studies. There is no correlation between airflow obstruction and the Reid index, volume proportion of mucous glands, or degree of mucous gland enlargement.[13,41] These data support the conclusion that airflow obstruction is a disease process largely independent of cough and mucous hypersecretion. Although interrelated, and produced by the same irritants, chronic bronchitis and limitation of airflow are separate disorders.

Small-airways Disease

Bronchiolitis is the term given to inflammation of noncartilaginous airways less than 2 millimeters in diameter. As is the case with chronic airflow obstruction, in general chronic bronchitis and small-airways disease are interrelated though separate disorders. In contrast to the relatively benign nature of mucous hypersecretion associated with large-airways inflammation, small-airways inflammation is clearly associated with airflow obstruction.[42] In fact, small airways are the principal site of airway obstruction early in chronic airflow obstruction. In severe airflow obstruction, however, small-airways inflammation is not as important a factor as anatomic emphysema.[43-45] The small airways may be affected early by inhaled irritants as reflected in studies of young, asymptomatic smokers in whom central airways are normal but small airways demonstrate bronchiolitis.[46]

The inflammation in small airways secondary to cigarette smoke appears to be dose-related and may show improvement with cessation of the irritant insult.[46-48] Tests of small-airways function, in the absence of overt airflow obstruction (i.e., diminished FEV_1), correlate, in general, with the presence of small-airways inflammation.[49] Single tests of small-airways function, however, tend to have a wide variability with poor specificity.[50] It is likely that the early preclinical stage of mild disease in distal airways might not be detected by usual tests of spirometric function.

A specific type of small-airways inflammation has been described in subjects exposed to asbestos and silica. This occupationally related small-airways inflammation has been termed mineral dust small-airways disease (MDAD) and is pathologically distinct from the airways inflammation of cigarette smokers (see Table 1).[51,52] Study of the natural history of small-airways inflammation in this occupationally exposed population has been hampered by concomitant use of cigarettes.

Small-airways inflammation is probably associated with other occupations and inhaled irritants.[53] Again, assessment is hampered by concomitant cigarette use and suboptimal tests of small-airways function. Small-airways inflammation of at least mild severity is a common finding in older nonsmoking subjects, which is additional evidence that environmental factors such as air pollution or occupational exposures inhaled over a lifetime contribute to small-airways disease.[54]

Occupational exposures will probably have to be associated with the presence of anatomic emphysema before severe chronic airflow obstruction develops. As will be discussed, there is evidence that anatomic emphysema is associated with at least some occupational exposures. The relationship between emphysema and small-airways disease, either in the occupational setting or in cigarette smokers, remains unclear.

Bronchial Hyperreactivity

Numerous studies confirm the observation that subjects with chronic bronchitis, with variable degrees of airflow obstruction, display an increase in airway responsiveness to cholinergic drugs and histamine.[55-57] Patients with chronic bronchitis tend to be less responsive to bronchoprovocating agents than asthmatic subjects, although there is considerable overlap in degree of response between the two groups of patients. In spite of these similarities there are also differences in the responses to bronchial-constricting stimuli between chronic bronchitics and asthmatics. Most bronchial provocation studies in bronchitics demonstrate a significant relationship with baseline lung function, so that the lower the initial FEV_1, the greater the increase in airway responsiveness.[56-57] It is possible that the airflow obstruction itself determines the degree of response to inhaled bronchial-constricting agents. Additionally, asthmatics show significant response to bronchial-constricting agents such as cold air and aerosolized or nebulized distilled water, which may act through mast cell mediator release.[57,58] Neither of these agents consistently causes bronchial constriction in chronic bronchitics. Airway hyperreactivity in chronic bronchitis is probably a result of epithelial injury and is not primarily immunologically mediated.

OCCUPATIONAL ETIOLOGIES

When attempting to characterize the occupational causes of chronic bronchitis, the presence of confounders such as cigarette smoking, environmental pollution, a history of multiple jobs, and the "healthy-worker effect" complicate an already difficult task. The healthy worker effect refers to the bias present in occupational cohorts due to the fact that selection for healthy workers operates both at hiring and throughout employment.[59] This bias is compounded by those workers leaving employment as a result of illness, particularly when occupationally related. Use of standardized questionnaires and the manner in which they are completed also make it problemmatic to eliminate subjectivity and consequent bias.

The prevalence of bronchitis overall is much higher in industrialized as compared with rural areas.[60] Whether this is due to the confounding variables mentioned above, as opposed to true occupational etiologies, is uncertain. Long-term exposure to respirable agents in and of itself can induce an irritant effect that precipitates the mucous hypersecretion typical of chronic bronchitis.[61] Table 2 lists many of the proposed causative agents in occupational chronic bronchitis.[62] An alternative approach is to consider inorganic substances separately from organic etiologic agents. Whichever approach is favored, it must

TABLE 2. *List of Causative Agents in Occupational Chronic Bronchitis*

Agent	Definite	Probable	Possible
Aldehydes (acrolein, formaldehyde)	+		
Ammonia	+		
Brick dust		+	
Cadmium (emphysema)			+
Chlorine	+		
Chloromethyl methyl ether	+		
Chromium	+		
Coal mine dust (bronchitis, emphysema)	+		
Cobalt		+	
Cotton dust	+		
Coke oven	+		
Diesel exhaust	+		
Endotoxin	+		
Grain dust (wheat, barley)	+		
Osmium tetroxide	+		
Oxides of nitrogen		+	
Paraquat			+
Phosgene	+		
Polychlorinated biphenyls		+	
Pottery dust	+		
Sodium hydroxide	+		
Toluene diisocyanate	+		
Tungsten carbide		+	
Vanadium		+	
Vinyl chloride monomer		+	
Western red cedar	+		
Wood dust	+		

Reprinted from Merchant JA (ed): Occupational Respiratory Diseases. DHHS (NIOSH) Publication No. 86-102. Washington, D.C., U.S. Government Printing Office, 1986, p 504.

TABLE 3. *Causative Agents in Occupational Chronic Bronchitis and Other Pulmonary Diseases with Which They Are Linked*

Agent	Disease
Oxides of nitrogen	Bronchiolitis obliterans
Toluene diisocyanate	Asthma
Chromium, coke-oven particulate	Bronchogenic carcinoma
Coal mine dust	Coal workers' pneumoconiosis
Cotton dust and related substances	Byssinosis
Western red cedar	Hypersensitivity pneumonitis

be borne in mind that many of these materials can affect lung function in ways other than causing chronic bronchitis. Table 3 provides but a few examples where this is the case. Substances listed in the tables may be encountered in multiple industrial processes.

Cigarette smoking plays a significant role in the development of chronic bronchitis in many occupational settings. Some have argued that for many individuals the occurrence of bronchitis due to tobacco products is itself an indirect result of the occupational environment. The key factor here is the occurrence of stress related to the workplace and the resultant increase in cigarette smoking that frequently accompanies this stress.[23] Whether the employer is therefore the responsible party in "causing" the illness, versus the tobacco industry or the individual smoker, is a matter of opinion and certainly beyond the scope of this discussion.

Few pathologic studies of industrial chronic bronchitis have been performed. Those studies that exist for coal miners have relied upon indices of bronchial gland enlargement (such as the Reid index) in relation to exposure. Smoking once again has represented a confounding variable. Although most of these studies have failed to demonstrate any relationship between bronchial gland size and length of employment,[63] one study of 94 autopsied miners in the United Kingdom did reveal an association between the Reid index and cumulative coal dust exposure.[64] In the same study, however, no such correlation could be shown between gland hypertrophy and degree of pneumoconiosis. The authors suggest that differences exist as a function of particle size contained within the dust. Large particle size would affect large airways but would not be respirable into the smaller airways, the target site for coal workers pneumoconiosis.

Although chronic bronchitis has a distinct clinical definition and a characteristic pathologic appearance, the most significant prognostic factor rests with the presence or absence of functional or physiologic impairment.[23] While simple bronchitis does not appear to be accompanied by shortened survival, the presence of accompanying obstruction and breathlessness worsens prognosis.[20] Some have suggested that cough and sputum production may actually be protective, with studies demonstrating a greater reduction in the FEV_1 among exposed individuals not having these symptoms.[61] Furthermore, it has also been proposed that chronic bronchitis should be defined only as a disease entity when obstruction coexists, and that compensation should be recommended only in circumstances of intense occupational exposure.[65]

In general, occupational bronchitis occurs as a result of severe prolonged exposure to a respiratory irritant. A number of agents, primarily irritant gases, can produce acute, sometimes severe, bronchitis associated with massive exposures. In this setting bronchitis is a warning symptom that can be associated with more severe pulmonary abnormalities such as ARDS or bronchiolitis obliterans. Chronic airflow obstruction is also a reported consequence of acute symptomatic exposures to ammonia, chlorine, and sulphur dioxide.[66] Why certain acute exposures result in chronic bronchitis and how this is related to disease occurrence with long-term exposure cannot currently be answered.

To complicate the picture further, the irritant effects of a variety of agents may actually decrease following repeated exposure. Response appears to be attenuated in exposed individuals through a tolerance mechanism. The phenomenon of attenuation is well described for ozone and has also been demonstrated for other agents.[67,68]

OCCUPATIONAL DISEASE PREVALENCE AND DOSE-RESPONSE RELATIONSHIPS

Although respiratory diseases do not constitute the most common occupational disorders, they are a major category and account for a significant amount of morbidity resulting in lost work time and increased health care expenditures. Whereas pneumoconiosis has been one of the most important occupational respiratory disease entities in the past, airway disease is gaining rapidly in importance. Whether this is a function of increased awareness of occupational factors in disease causation by physicians, a better informed working class, litigatory pressures, or a true increase in disease incidence and prevalence is unclear.

The prevalence data linking occupational exposure to chronic bronchitis have been substantiated only for the coal mining industry. In spite of the many etiologic factors that have been identified as potential causes of chronic bronchitis (see Table 2), these have been identified primarily in cross-sectional studies of smaller sample size, and the causal role has been less clearly supported. In addition, many of the industrial settings where a potential causative agent is used rarely result in isolated exposure to a single agent. For example, steel foundry work may result in exposures not only to coal dust, but to coke ovens, welding activities, and fibrous glass, as well as a variety of metals. Finally, individuals who have worked in the coal mine industry generally have done so to the exclusion of other types of work. This has not been the case in many of the other settings where occupational factors are at play in the development of bronchitis. Frequently, these workers have held jobs in a multitude of settings. As a result of this lack of conclusive information, only coal mine dust will be considered here to illustrate the prevalence of disease due to exposure and the dose-response relationships at play. The focus on coal dust should not diminish the importance of bronchitic symptoms with exposure to many agents and processes such as gold mining, foundry activities, and grain work.[23,53,61,62,69]

Exposure to coal dust is not limited to underground mining. Surface mining, coal preparation, and coal-use operations all represent activities where significant exposure may occur. Some estimates indicate that 200,000 workers are engaged in such activities in the United States.[70] Coal face mining, drilling, and preparation present the opportunities for greatest exposure.

The prevalence of abnormalities associated with coal dust exposure (including pneumoconiosis), the degree of clinical findings, and the level of functional impairment are related to cumulative dust exposure.[71] The latter is a function of both the number of years worked in a particular activity as well as the amount of respirable dust and free silica content. This observation explains the reason for removing an employee from further high exposure at the first evidence of disease.

The pathologic lesions of emphysema and chronic bronchitis have been known for some time to coexist with coal workers' pneumoconiosis (CWP).[72] The relative contribution of cumulative dust exposure to the development of measurable obstruction and emphysema has been demonstrated in several groups,[20,71,73-75] but cigarette smoking has not always been well controlled for in these studies.[75]

Other authors have reported a significant association between measured dust exposure and the prevalence of symptoms of chronic bronchitis in men less than 45 years of age.[76] The absence of such a relationship beyond 45 is explained by the presence of other causes of chronic bronchitis among older subjects that obscure this finding.

Rogan and colleagues have shown a clear link between cumulative coal dust exposure (in the respirable range of 1-5 microns) and degree of airways obstruction.[77] In a group of 3581 coal face workers followed prospectively, a progressive reduction in FEV_1 with increasing cumulative exposure was detected. However, increasing severity of bronchitis symptoms was associated with a loss in FEV_1 greater than that based upon dust exposure, age, and other related factors. This finding suggest that once bronchitic symptoms develop in the face of measurable obstruction, disease progression may be independent of the factors that initiate the process.

In a cross-sectional analysis of almost 9000 bituminous coal miners, Kibelstis and coworkers demonstrated that the prevalence of bronchitic symptoms and obstructive spirometric changes was greater among smokers than among nonsmokers or ex-smokers.[78] However, the prevalence of these findings was greater in coal face workers compared with surface workers, reflecting the heavier exposure among the former group. Recent data from a group of 3380 British coal miners clearly showed an additive effect of coal dust exposure and smoking on bronchitic symptoms and lung function.[79]

The presence of a dose-response relationship between degree of exposure and prevalence of findings supports a causal role between the agent and the disease. Similarly, this relationship adds support for a nonimmunologic, irritant effect of coal dust in the induction of changes leading to bronchitic complaints.

The evaluation of coal miners has been pivotal for establishing a causal role for inhaled occupational irritants in the development of chronic airflow obstruction. This relationship is, after all, the core of the concern about occupational bronchitis. Autopsy studies in coal miners with adequate allowance for confounding effects of smoking demonstrate a significant association between coal mining exposure and the presence of emphysema.[80] Similar findings have been demonstrated in South African hard rock gold miners.[81] It is unclear if these observations have relevance to all occupations associated with bronchitic symptoms, but clearly the contention that airway disease associated with occupational exposure is not a serious problem must be reconsidered.

CONTRIBUTION OF SMOKING

The presence of an interaction between occupational exposure to a respiratory toxicant and cigarette smoking in causing disease is certainly not a new concept. The synergistic relationship between occupational asbestos exposure and cigarette smoking in the development of bronchogenic carcinoma is well established.[82] Synergism implies that there is a greater rate of disease among occupationally exposed smokers than would be expected by adding the rate for occupationally exposed nonsmokers with that of nonexposed smokers.

The relationship between occupational exposure to other agents and cigarette smoking is less well established and has been reviewed elsewhere.[70] The effect of smoking is frequently difficult to isolate successfully from the effect of exposure. Many argue that while controlling occupational exposure to respiratory hazards is important, the reduction of tobacco smoking is far more critical to reducing respiratory morbidity and mortality.[83] This opinion was supported in the study by Foxman et al., who performed an analysis of mortality on a group of men from four occupational categories who had been examined 30 years earlier.[84] The report focused upon the effect of occupation, smoking, lung function, and respiratory symptoms. Overall, the all-cause mortality for the dust-exposed groups was the same or lower than for the non-dust-exposed workers. However, smokers had double the death rates of nonsmokers, consistent across all occupational groups. Although cough and sputum were associated with increased mortality regardless of smoking habits, the major determinant was poor lung function. This confirmed a previous observation by Peto et al., strongly linking the risk for subsequent death from COPD to initial airflow obstruction.[40]

EVALUATION AND TREATMENT

The evaluation of occupational bronchitis is theoretically very simple. Because bronchitis is defined symptomatically, ostensibly all that is necessary for making a diagnosis is a compatible symptom complex. A complete chronological occupational history is necessary to evaluate working environments that pose potential risks for respiratory symptoms. This line of questioning may require extensive knowledge of specific occupations on the part of the physician. Further, other potential risk factors for chronic bronchitis, outlined previously, should be explored.

Beyond recognition of the syndrome, however, is evaluation of possible associated pulmonary dysfunction. All subjects with bronchitic symptoms should have spirometry performed as a minimal requirement for assessment, if only as a basis for future comparison. Ideally, it would be desirable to have baseline spirometry done prior to occupational exposure or onset of symptoms. Follow-up spirometric examination of subjects with bronchitis is important to monitor possible development of chronic airflow obstruction. Surveillance spirometry for workers at risk should probably include asymptomatic workers as well, because not all subjects with chronic airflow obstruction have cough and sputum production.

If airflow obstruction is present on spirometry, it is clear that significant pulmonary abnormalities exist beyond inflammation of large airways. Chronic bronchitics do respond to all forms of bronchial-dilating drugs but may be particularly responsive to anticholinergic agents.[36,85] As a result of bronchial inflammation, patients may also be responsive to corticosteroids, both inhaled and intravenous. There are multiple potential mechanisms by which corticosteroids are beneficial, including inhibition of chemotactic response with diminished cell recruitment, stabilization of lysozymal membranes, and alteration of cellular protein production.

If bronchitic symptoms persist after removal from the offending environment, in the absence of frank airflow obstruction, then testing for bronchial hyperreactivity should be considered. These patients may also be at risk for development of chronic airflow obstruction and can improve with bronchial-dilating medication.

Bronchoalveolar lavage, and specifically the technique described by Rennard et al., provides the capability of evaluating endobronchial inflammation; however, its role in the evaluation and management of individual patients is not clear.[16]

RESPIRATORY IMPAIRMENT AND DISABILITY

Impairment has been defined as "an alteration of an individual's health status that is assessed by medical means."[86] Determination of **disability** includes not only assessment of medical impairment, but also is based upon socioeconomic and psychological factors. The term disability is therefore not a purely medical one. As a result, the use of objective laboratory tests in the determination of respiratory impairment represents only a single component in the evaluation of disability.

The value of a given laboratory test used for this purpose is dependent upon a number of factors.[87] The true objectivity of the test might be altered by subject effort as well as technician and observer bias. Reproducibility of any given laboratory result is also critical for the purpose of comparing these results to accepted norms. Finally, test results may not correlate well with symptoms experienced while performing a given work task. This is particularly true with regard to respiratory impairment. In healthy individuals, pulmonary functional capacity is typically much greater than the demands of most daily tasks. Therefore, a considerable reduction in measurable lung function may occur before symptoms become apparent. Furthermore, symptoms related to respiratory impairment may also be influenced by cardiac disease, as well as psychological and even socioeconomic determinants.

Many different criteria exist for measuring impairment that rely upon these testing components. Regarding chronic bronchitis, reliance on symptoms, in part, is necessary based upon the actual definition of the disease. However, spirometry is also a very useful tool, because the presence of obstruction alters prognosis. The Veterans Administration rating schedule for chronic bronchitis considers these factors.[88] In this case, a 30% or moderately severe rating of impairment is based in large part on symptoms, with only beginning evidence of chronic airway obstruction.

THE ROLE OF PREVENTION

Previous mention has been made of the prognostic value of measurable obstruction when it accompanies chronic bronchitis of industrial cause. There is considerable doubt that medical surveillance is useful for the detection of early obstructive disease. This setting would be ideal for an easily administered sensitive and specific test of small-airway dysfunction, but such a test is not yet available. Therefore, the ability to predict prospectively which individual with bronchitic symptoms is at risk for chronic airflow obstruction is also not available. If frank obstruction is already present, however, there is a more rapid rate of functional decline than expected on the basis of age alone, even where there is no significant further occupational exposure.[61] This finding suggests that medical surveillance is of little value once obstruction is already present. Furthermore, there have been no measurements made to assess the result of removal from exposure on symptoms, although discontinuation of cigarette smoking clearly reduces or eliminates bronchial symptoms. Thus, medical surveillance of symptoms may not be useful for prevention of worsened disease by guiding removal from the workplace, even though it is assumed to be the case.

Medical surveillance, although important, is no substitute for minimizing exposure where disease prevention is concerned. Clearly, cigarette smoking must be targeted as the primary culprit for chronic bronchitis in industrial settings. The question of whether cigarette smokers with bronchitic symptoms should be protected or removed from potentially offending environments is controversial. In view of the role that occupational exposures play, environmental hygiene cannot be overemphasized. Significant advances have been made in the use of personal protective devices such as respirators in recent years. Nonetheless, engineering measures for the reduction of ambient contamination continue to be the mainstay of disease prevention.

CONCLUSIONS AND FUTURE DIRECTIONS

There continues to be controversy surrounding the existence of occupational chronic bronchitis as a true disease entity. There is little doubt that continued refinement of the terminology surrounding these disease processes is critical to future study. Additional epidemiological analysis involving collaborative efforts and existent data bases is necessary to ensure adequate sample size for sound statistical conclusions. Equally important is the need for improved air-sampling strategies in order to elucidate the presence of dose-response relationships. Likewise, future analysis of data surrounding the removal of individual workers from exposure and the impact of removal on bronchitic symptoms and obstructive findings will help guide decision-making that is based upon medical surveillance. Smoking-intervention strategies and improved, but cost-effective, engineering controls are of paramount importance in the prevention of chronic bronchitis occurring in the work setting. While chronic bronchitis per se may have little functional significance, its associated symptoms supply a warning for the development or presence of more severe pulmonary abnormalities.

REFERENCES

1. Dodge R, Clinc MG, Borrows B: Comparisons of asthma, emphysema, and chronic bronchitis diagnoses in a general population sample. Am Rev Respir Dis 133:981–986, 1986.
2. Tenth Report of the Director, NHLBI. Vol 3, Lung Diseases. NIH Publication No. 84-2358, 1982.
3. Linn WS, Hackney JD, Pedersen EE, et al: Respiratory function and symptoms in urban office workers in relation to oxidant air pollution exposure. Am Rev Respir Dis 114:477–483, 1976.
4. Tager I, Speizer FE: Role of infection in chronic bronchitis. N Engl J Med 292:563–571, 1975.
5. Bjorkander J, Bake B, Oxelius V-A, Hanson LA: Impaired lung function in patients with IgA deficiency and low levels of IgG_2 or IgG_3. N Engl J Med 313:720–724, 1985.
6. Ciba Guest Symposium Report. Terminology, definitions and classification of chronic pulmonary emphysema and related conditions. Thorax 14:286–299, 1959.
7. Megahed GE, Senna GA, Eissa MH, et al: Smoking versus infection as the aetiology of bronchial mucous gland hypertrophy in chronic bronchitis. Thorax 22:271–287, 1967.
8. Sobonya RE, Kleinerman J: Morphometric studies of bronchi in young smokers. Am Rev Respir Dis 105:768–775, 1972.
9. Reid LM: Pathology of chronic bronchitis. Lancet i:275–278, 1954.
10. Reid L: Measurement of the bronchial mucous gland layer: A diagnostic yardstick in chronic bronchitis. Thorax 15:132–141, 1960.
11. Scott KWM: An autopsy study of bronchial mucous glands hypertrophy in Glasgow. Am Rev Respir Dis 107:239–245, 1973.

12. Ryder RC, Dunnill MS, Anderson JA: A quantitative study of bronchial mucous gland volume, emphysema and smoking in a necropsy population. J Pathol 104:59-71, 1971.
13. Jamal K, Conney TP, Fleetham JA, et al: Chronic bronchitis. Correlation of morphologic findings to sputum production and flow rates. Am Rev Respir Dis 129:719-722, 1984.
14. Mullen BM, Wright JL, Wiggs BR, et al: Reassessment of inflammation of airways in chronic bronchitis. Br Med J 291:1235-1239, 1985.
15. Chodosh S: Examination of sputum cells. N Engl J Med 282:854-857, 1970.
16. Thompson A, Daughton D, Robbins R, et al: Intraluminal airway inflammation in chronic bronchitis. Am Rev Respir Dis 140:1527-1537, 1989.
17. Niewoehner D: Cigarette smoking, lung inflammation, and the development of emphysema. J Lab Clin Med 111:15-27, 1988.
18. Holtman MJ, Fabbri LM, O'Byrne PM, et al: Importance of airway inflammation for hyperresponsiveness induced by ozone. Am Rev Respir Dis 127:686-690, 1983.
19. O'Byrne PM, Walters EH, Gold BD, et al: Neutrophil depletion inhibits airway hyperresponsiveness induced by ozone exposure. Am Rev Respir Dis 130:214-219, 1984.
20. Lyons JP, Ryder RC, Seal RM, Wagner JC: Emphysema in smoking and non-smoking coalworkers with pneumoconiosis. Bull Europ Physiopath Respir 17:75-85, 1981.
21. Stedman RL: The chemical composition of tobacco and tobacco smoke. Chem Rev 68:153-207, 1967.
22. Greaves IA: Occupational pulmonary disease. In McCunney RJ (ed): Handbook of Occupational Medicine. Boston, Little, Brown, and Company, 1988, pp 93-96.
23. Casey KR: Industrial bronchitis. In Rom WN (ed): Environmental and Occupational Medicine. Boston, Little, Brown, and Company, 1983, pp 267-271.
24. Weiland JE, Davis WB, Holter JF, et al: Lung neutrophils in the adult respiratory distress syndrome: Clinical and pathophysiologic significance. Am Rev Respir Dis 133:218-225, 1986.
25. Crystal RG, Bitterman PB, Rennard SI, et al: Interstitial lung diseases of unknown cause: Disorders characterized by chronic inflammation of the lower respiratory tract. N Engl J Med 310:154-166, 235-244, 1984.
26. Garcia JGN, Griffith DE, Cohen AB, Callahan KS: Alveolar macrophages from patients with asbestos exposure release increased levels of leukotriene B_4. Am Rev Respir Dis 139:1494-1501, 1989.
27. Badwey JA, Karnovsky ML: Active oxygen species and the functions of phagocytic leukocytes. Ann Rev Biochem 49:695-726, 1980.
28. Janoff A: Biochemical links between cigarette smoking and pulmonary emphysema. J Appl Physiol 55:285-293, 1983.
29. Tegner H, Ohlsson K, Roremalm NG, et al: Effect of human leukocyte enzymes on tracheal mucosa and its mucociliary activity. Rhinology 17:199-206, 1979.
30. Breurer R, Lucey EC, Stone PJ, et al: Proteolytic activity of human neutrophil elastase and porcine pancreatic trypsin causes bronchial secretory cell metaplasie in hamsters. Exp Lung Res 9:167-175, 1985.
31. Lucey EC, Stone PJ, Breurer R, et al: Effect of combined human neutrophil cathepsin G and elastase on induction of secretory cell metaplasia and emphysema in hamsters, with in vitro observations on elastolysis by these enzymes. Am Rev Respir Dis 132:362-366, 1985.
32. Carp H, Janoff A: Inactivation of bronchial mucous proteinase inhibitor by cigarette smoker and phagocyte-derived oxidants. Exp Lung Res 1:225-237, 1980.
33. Hoidal JR, Niewoehner DE: Lung phagocyte recruitment and metabolic alterations induced by cigarette smoker in humans and in hamsters. Am Rev Respir Dis 126:548-552, 1982.
34. Thompson A, Bohlin T, Payvandi F, Rennard S: Lower respiratory tract lactoferrin and lysozyme arise primarily in the airways and are elevated in association with chronic bronchitis. J Lab Clin Med 115:148-158, 1990.
35. Laes AW, McNaught W: Bacteriology of the lower-respiratory-tract secretions, sputum, and upper-respiratory-tract secretions in "normals" and chronic bronchitis. Lancet ii:1112-1115, 1959.
36. Taskin D, Ashutosh K, Bleecker E, et al: Comparison of the anticholinergic bronchodilator bromide with metaproterenol in chronic obstructive pulmonary disease. Am J Med 81(Suppl 5A):81-92, 1986.
37. Gibson PG, Girgis-Gabardo A, Morris MM, et al: Cellular characteristics of sputum from patients with asthma and chronic bronchitis. Thorax 44:693-699, 1989.
38. De Monchy JGR, Kauffman HF, Venge P, et al: Bronchoalveolar esosinophilia during allergen-induced late asthmatic reactions. Am Rev Respir Dis 131:373-376, 1985.
39. Fletcher C, Peto R, Rinker C, Speizer FE: The Natural History of Chronic Bronchitis and Emphysema: An Eight-Year Study of Early Chronic Obstructive Lung Disease in Working Men in London. Oxford, Oxford University Press, 1976.
40. Peto R, Speizer FE, Cochrane AL, et al: The relevance in adults of air-flow obstruction, but not of mucus hypersecretion, to mortality from chronic lung disease. Results from 20 years of prospective observation. Am Rev Respir Dis 128:491-500, 1983.
41. Thurlbeck WM: Chronic Airflow Obstruction in Lung Disease. Vol 5: Major Problems in Pathology. Philadelphia, W.B. Saunders, 1976.
42. Hogg JC, Macklem PT, Thurlbeck WM: Site and nature of airway obstruction in chronic obstructive lung disease. N Engl J Med 278:1355-1360, 1968.
43. Mitchell RS, Stanford RE, Johnson JM, et al: The morphologic features of the bronchi, bronchioles, and alveoli in chronic airway obstruction: A clinicopathologic study. Am Rev Respir Dis 114:137-145, 1976.
44. Hale KA, Ewing SL, Gosnell BA, Niewoehner DE: Lung disease in long-term cigarette smokers with and without chronic air-flow obstruction. Am Rev Respir Dis 130:716-721, 1984.
45. Nagai A, West WW, Thurlbeck WM: The National Institutes of Health intermittent positive-pressure breathing trial: Pathology studies II: Correlation between morphologic findings, clinical findings, and evidence of expiratory air-flow obstruction. Am Rev Respir Dis 132:946-953, 1985.
46. Niewoehner DE, Kleinerman J, Rice DB: Pathologic changes in the peripheral airways of young cigarette smokers. New Engl J Med 291:755-758, 1974.
47. Buist A, Sexton GJ, Nagy JM, Ross BB: The effect of smoking cessation and modification on lung function. Am Rev Respir Dis 114:115-162, 1976.
48. Bode FR, Dosman J, Martin RR, Macklem PT: Reversibility of pulmonary function abnormalities in smokers. A prospective study of early diagnostic tests of small airways disease. Am J Med 58:43-52, 1975.

49. Wright JL, Lawson LM, Pare PD, et al: The detection of small airways disease. Am Rev Respir Dis 129:989-994, 1984.
50. Buist SA: Current status of small airways disease. Chest 86:100-105, 1984.
51. Wright JL, Churg A: Morphology of small airway lesions in patients with asbestos exposure. Hum Pathol 15:68-74, 1984.
52. Churg A, Wright JL, Wiggs B, et al: Small airways disease and mineral dust exposure. Am Rev Respir Dis 131:139-143, 1985.
53. Cotton DJ, Graham BL, Li K-YR, et al: Effects of smoking and occupational exposure on peripheral airway function in young cereal grain workers. Am Rev Respir Dis 126:660-665, 1982.
54. Cosio MG, Hale KA, Niewoehner DE: Morphologic and morphometric effects of prolonged cigarette smoking on the small airways. Am Rev Respir Dis 122:265-271, 1980.
55. Bahous J, Cartier A, Ouimet G, et al: Nonallergic bronchial hyperexcitability in chronic bronchitis. Am Rev Respir Dis 129:829-832, 1984.
56. Yan K, Salome CM, Wookcock AJ: Prevalence and nature of bronchial hyperresponsiveness in subjects with chronic obstructive pulmonary disease. Am Rev Respir Dis 132:25-29, 1985.
57. Ramsdale EH, Morris MM, Roberts RS, et al: Bronchial responsiveness to methacholine in chronic bronchitis; relationship to airflow obstruction and cold air responsiveness. Thorax 39:912-918, 1984.
58. Ramsdale EH, Roberts RS, Morris MM, et al: Differences in responsiveness to hyperventilation and methacholine in asthma and chronic bronchitis. Thorax 40:422-426, 1985.
59. Mausner JS, Kramer S: Mausner & Bahn Epidemiology: An Introductory Text, 2nd ed. Philadelphia, W.B. Saunders, 1985, pp 319-320.
60. Anderson M: Occupational Lung Diseases: An Introduction. New York, American Lung Association, 1983, p 49.
61. Kilburn KH: Occupational chronic bronchitis. In Last JM (ed): Maxey-Rosenau Public Health and Preventive Medicine, 12th ed. Norwalk, CT, Appleton-Century-Crofts, 1986, pp 569-574.
62. Kilburn KH: Chronic bronchitis and emphysema. In Merchant JA (ed): Occupational Respiratory Diseases. DHHS (NIOSH) Publication No. 86-102. Washington, D.C., U.S. Government Printing Office, 1986, pp 503-529.
63. Churg A, Green FHY (eds): Pathology of Occupational Lung Disease. New York, Igaku-Shoin Medical Publishers, pp 144-145.
64. Douglas AN, Lamb D, Ruckley VA: Bronchial gland dimensions in coal miners: Influence of smoking and dust exposure. Thorax 37:760-764, 1982.
65. Felchsig R: Pros and cons of dust-induced bronchitis as an occupational disease. Ind Health 27:27-30, 1989.
66. Schwartz DA: Acute inhalational injury. Occup Med State Art Rev 2:297-318, 1987.
67. Horvath SM, Gliner JA, Folinsbee LJ: Adaption to ozone: Duration of effect. Am Rev Respir Dis 123:496-499, 1981.
68. Fairchild EJ: Tolerance mechanisms. Arch Environ Health 14:111-125, 1967.
69. Minette A: Is chronic bronchitis also an industrial disease? Eur J Respir Dis 146(Suppl):87-98, 1986.
70. Garcia JGN, Griffith DE, Levin JL, Idell S: Tobacco smoke exposure in occupational lung disease. Semin Respir Med 10:372-384, 1989.
71. Merchant JA: Coal workers' pneumoconiosis. In Last JM (ed): Maxcy-Rosenau Public Health and Preventive Medicine, 12th ed. Norwalk, CT, Appleton-Century-Crofts, 1986, pp 545-552.
72. Worth G: Emphysema in coal workers (editorial). Am J Ind Med 6:401-403, 1984.
73. Bates DV, Pham OT, Chau N, et al: A longitudinal study of pulmonary function in coal miners in Lorraine, France. Am J Ind Med 8:21-32, 1985.
74. Soutar CA, Hurley JF: Relation between dust exposure and lung function in miners and ex-miners. Br J Ind Med 43:307-320, 1986.
75. Ryder R, Lyons JP, Campbell H, Gough J: Emphysema in coal workers' pneumoconiosis. Br Med J 3:481-487, 1970.
76. Cotes JE, Steel JL: Work-Related Lung Disorders. Boston, Blackwell Scientific Publications, 1987, pp 373-381.
77. Rogan JM, Attfield MD, Jacobsen M, et al: Role of dust in the working environment in development of chronic bronchitis in British coal miners. Br J Ind Med 30:217-226, 1973.
78. Kibelstis JA, Morgan EJ, Reger R, et al: Prevalence of bronchitis and airway obstruction in American bituminous coal miners. Am Rev Respir Dis 108:886-893, 1973.
79. Marine WM, Gurr D, Jacobsen M: Clinically important respiratory effects of dust exposure and smoking in British coal miners. Am Rev Respir Dis 137:106-112, 1988.
80. Becklake MR: Chronic airflow limitation: Its relationship to work in dusty occupations. Chest 88:608-617, 1985.
81. Becklake MR, Irwig L, Kielkowski D, et al: The predictors of emphysema in South African gold miners. Am Rev Respir Dis 135:1234-1241, 1987.
82. Hammond EC, Selikoff IJ, Seidman H: Asbestos exposure, cigarette smoking and death rates. Ann NY Acad Sci 330:473-490, 1979.
83. Elmes PC: Relative importance of ciagrette smoking in occupational lung disease. Br J Ind Med 38:1-13, 1981.
84. Foxman B, Higgins ITT, Oh MS: The effects of occupation and smoking on respiratory disease mortality. Am Rev Respir Dis 134:649-652, 1986.
85. Griffith DE, Garcia JGN: Asthmatic bronchitis. Semin Respir Inf 3:27-39, 1988.
86. Engelberg AL (ed): Guides to the Evaluation of Permanent Impairment, 3rd ed. Chicago, American Medical Association, 1988, p 2.
87. Boehlecke B: Laboratory assessment of respiratory impairment for disability evaluation. In Merchant JA (ed): Occupational Respiratory Diseases. DHHS (NIOSH) Publication No. 86-102. Washington, D.C., U.S. Government Printing Office, 1986, pp 181-216.
88. 38 Code of Federal Regulations Pension Bonuses & Veterans' Relief, Revised as of July 1977.
89. Hogg JC: Mucosal permeability and smooth muscle function in asthma. Med Clin North Am 74:731-739, 1990.

Chapter 7

BYSSINOSIS AND TOBACCO-RELATED ASTHMA

Mark T. O'Hollaren, MD

Byssinosis is an occupational lung disorder characterized by chest tightness, wheezing, cough, and shortness of breath.[1] It may be accompanied by both variable and chronic airflow obstruction and is seen in those working with relatively high concentrations of textile dust, including cotton, flax, and soft hemp.[2,3] The respiratory symptoms seen are usually most notable after the worker returns to work following several days off (e.g., on Mondays).[1] It is a clinically distinct entity from the pneumoconioses (e.g., asbestosis and silicosis) and occupational extrinsic allergic alveolitis (e.g., farmer's lung).[4]

Although byssinosis may be characterized by cough, wheezing, and dyspnea, which may improve with bronchodilators, some investigators believe that several characteristics differentiate it from occupational asthma. Byssinosis does not require prior sensitization, and nearly all workers in an area may be affected if the concentration of cotton dust is high enough.[5] Furthermore, IgE does not appear to play a significant pathogenic role in the disease.[5]

As noted above, byssinosis is seen in those working with textile dust from cotton, flax, and soft hemp; rope workers using manila and hard hemp do not appear to contract byssinotic symptoms.[6] Although each of these materials will be discussed separately, the largest amount of research into the pathogenesis of byssinosis has been done with cotton dust.

HISTORICAL PERSPECTIVE

Manual flax processing existed in ancient Egypt.[7] Graves in Bershia (2,000 B.C.) and Luxor (1,600 B.C.) contain picture writing showing flax cultivation and processing.[7] In 1705, Ramazzini wrote " . . . those who hackle the flax and hemp to prepare it for being spun and wove, afford frequent instances of the unwholesomeness of their trades . . . ."[8] The term byssinosis (*byssos*, Greek for a fine yellow flax) was introduced by Proust in 1877 as the name for the respiratory disease characteristic of textile workers. In 1894, d'Evelyn stated "hackling is the most deadly process . . . the hacklers all die young, and all suffer from chronic diseases of the lung caused by flax dust."[9] Hackling is the combing apart of the fibers of flax or hemp.

In the early 19th century, operators of textile mills claimed that the "behavioral excesses" of the weekend were responsible for the workers' typical Monday complaints of chest tightness, cough, and dyspnea.[2] Since that time, cotton, hemp, and flax workers have been noted to develop higher frequencies of chronic cough, phlegm production, and dyspnea compared with control workers.[2,4,8,10,11]

Byssinosis has only gained widespread recognition in approximately the last 30 years, even though Ramazzini described it approximately 200 years ago.[12] The initial studies of McKerrow et al. showed that inhalation of cotton dust caused a decrease of ventilatory capacity.[13] Occupational health guidelines have been instituted limiting the amount of gravimetrically measured lint-free cotton dust in the work area of cotton mills to 0.200 mg/M^3 for yarn preparation areas, and 0.750 mg/M^3 for weaving areas of the mills.[2] The smaller, respirable dust particles are referred to as the "lint-free cotton dust."[14]

ETIOLOGIC AGENTS OF BYSSINOSIS

Cotton

Aerosols of cotton dust are composed of plant constituents including cellulose, as well as particles derived from microbial flora of the plant that include endotoxins and other proteins. It is not yet known which of these (or which combination) is the causative agent of byssinosis.[2] Through the years, investigators have implicated various chemical components of cotton plants, as well as bacteria and microfungi, as the agents responsible for byssinosis.[2]

Cotton Production. There is significant variability in the composition of raw cotton, depending on where, when, and how it is harvested.[10] After the harvested cotton is transported to a cotton gin in trailers or modules, it is thoroughly cleaned before being passed to the gin stand. At the gin stand the seed is separated from the lint.[10] The seed is processed into oil and meal, and the lint is further cleaned and packaged into bales weighing approximately 480 pounds (Fig. 1). The lint

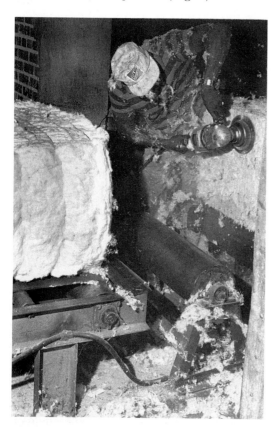

FIGURE 1. Cotton worker cleaning a 500 lb bale of compressed cotton.

bales are processed in the textile mill by first opening them, and then the cotton is carded and processed into yarn, which may be used for weaving, knitting, or further processed into other cotton products.[10] The health risks of this sequence of events have been known for many years.

Flax

It has been known for centuries that those with high flax dust exposure, such as the hacklers, are at significant risk of developing chronic lung disease. Even though flax and cotton plants are quite different botanically, those workers involved in the processing of flax may develop byssinosis similar to that seen in cotton workers.[7] The processing of flax has not changed appreciably since ancient times.[7] After the flax has been dried and deseeded in the field, it is "retted," a stage whereby a putrefactive process is used to loosen the woody parts of the plant from the fibers. The retting process is accomplished by placing the flax plants in layers in concrete containers, covering them with water, and leaving them for 1–2 weeks, depending on the ambient temperature. After drying, the retted flax is beaten with a heavy piece of wood, hackled to clean out the woody parts, combed, and then spun.

In one study of workers processing flax located in a village on the Nile Delta in Egypt, the concentration of respirable dust particles during processing was highest during hackling and combing.[7] Byssinosis was diagnosed in 22.9% of those flax workers who were examined, and 18.4% had a greater than 10% drop in their FEV_1 at the end of the first 4-hour morning work shift of the week.[7]

The severity of flax-induced byssinosis has been noted in one study to increase with longer duration of exposure to the flax dust. As with byssinosis from cotton dust exposure, cigarette smoking among flax workers increased the incidence of byssinosis in this population as well.[7] Cinkotai et al. found the incidence of byssinosis among flax scutchers to be 12.5%, despite fairly high airborne concentrations of dust, as well as high total and gram-negative bacterial concentrations in the workplace.[15]

Flaxseed and its derivatives may occur in other types of work environments besides those involved with processing the flax itself.[16,17] Flaxseed derivatives may be found in hair care products, animal feeds, insulating materials, rugs, cloth, cereals, flours, baked goods, dough, remedies, laxatives, and patent leather.[16] Jelks and Solomon note that flax is said to cross-react with mustard.[16]

Flaxseed has also been reported to cause contact dermatitis when found in paints, varnishes, furniture polish, and printer's ink.[16]

Sisal

Sisal (*Agave* sp. and *Fourcroya* sp.) is a fairly inert natural fiber used in the manufacture of sisal rope. A byssinotic condition has been reported to develop in sisal workers while processing their fiber into coarse fabrics and floor coverings.[12] There is some difference of opinion, however, on exactly what type of lung disorders may occur from sisal contact. There are conflicting reports regarding the effect of sisal dust exposure on acute changes in pulmonary function.[18] Some investigators have noted a fall in pulmonary function during a work shift in a sisal processing plant,[19-21] while others have not.[22] In one of the studies showing an acute decrease in lung function after sisal dust exposure, it appeared to be related to dust exposure levels.[19]

Baker et al. postulated that the lubricant used to soften sisal fiber may, in conjunction with the sisal, have some adverse effect on pulmonary function.[18] Overall, at present there appears to be only scant evidence that sisal dust inhalation leads to permanent lung damage, and further work in this area is clearly needed[18] (Fig. 2).

Hemp

Cannabis sativa (hemp), commonly found in central Asia and other warm regions, is a wind-pollinated plant that was planted in the American Midwest as a fiber source for making cordage.[16] Regional varieties now grow freely over great areas of the earth. Marijuana and hashish are obtained from the pistillate (female) flower clusters, and a single plant may produce 500 million pollen grains.[16] *Cannabis sativa* is known to contain over 400 compounds. As noted previously, hemp workers have been shown to develop byssinosis from the hemp dust.

Kapok

Kapok is largely imported from Indonesia.[17] The kapok tree *(Ceiba pentandra)* produces a seed hair that is used in a number of applications in connection with its relative resistance to becoming water-logged after water exposure.[16] These uses include stuffing for life jackets, boat cushions, sleeping bags, and throw pillows.[16]

Kapok has largely been replaced now by synthetic fibers and foams for these applications, but is still occasionally used. Many investigators note that kapok becomes more allergenic with age, possibly explained by oxidation of the fibers, or more likely due to contamination by mites or other microbial agents.[16,17]

Jute

Jute is obtained from two South Asian plants of the linden family *(Corchorus capsularis* and

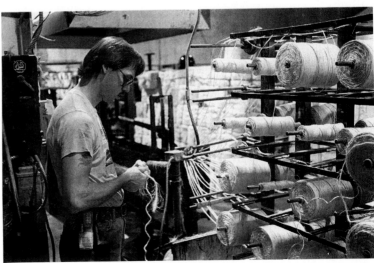

FIGURE 2. Sisal rope in a sisal processing plant.

C. olitorius). Rugs, burlap, and rope may contain jute and allergenicity has been described. However, others feel that contaminants may play a role as well.[16]

Coir

Sri Lanka produces 90–95% of the world's supply of coir.[6] Coir is the fiber obtained from the husk of the coconut and has a number of uses depending on the thickness of the fiber.[6] The long, thicker bristle is used in brushes, whereas the finer, short fibers are used as filling material for mattresses. Rope made from coir is fairly resilient and will stretch significantly without breaking. Early voyagers made cables and riggings from coir, because it was resistant to the effects of sea water.[6] It has also been used for nets, twine, brooms, and sacks.

The chemical composition of coir dust is similar to sisal dust, which, as noted above, is fairly inert.[6] In a study of 779 workers processing coir, the workers did not appear to be at any increased risk over control subjects for the development of chronic respiratory disease, including both asthma and byssinosis.[6]

EPIDEMIOLOGY OF BYSSINOSIS

Chronic airflow obstruction may result from prolonged cotton dust exposure in some workers.[12,14,23] The effects of cigarette smoking have been shown to have additive (and possibly synergistic) effects on the symptoms and pulmonary function of those workers chronically exposed to cotton dust.[4,12,14,24,25]

The prevalence of byssinosis in one large South African study of 2,411 subjects was shown to be 11.2% in spinners, 6.4% in weavers, and 6.1% in winders. The investigators in this study suspected that the actual prevalence of byssinosis was underestimated because of the high employee turnover rate compared to other countries where the cotton workers would stay longer on the job.[4]

Cinkotai et al. surveyed 4,656 textile employees in 31 textile factories engaged in spinning or weaving various cotton fibers in the United Kingdom.[25] They noted that the incidence of reported byssinotic symptoms in the 1950s was as high as 51% of exposed workers. This decreased to approximately 18% in the mid-1970s and only 3.9% by 1989.[25] They also noted a higher incidence of byssinosis in whites, compared to workers of East Indian and Pakistani descent. This difference was attributed to the relatively recent arrival (i.e., in the last 15 years) of these foreign workers into the U.K., during which time many of the workplace conditions had improved dramatically.[25]

Takam et al. compared a random sample of 125 men exposed to cotton dust in Cameroon with 68 men from nonproduction areas.[14] Workers completed a symptom-scoring questionnaire; peak expiratory flow rates (PEFRs) and airborne dust concentrations were measured in the workplace. Workers exposed to higher levels of cotton dust experienced more respiratory symptoms (particularly on Monday), and these were most prevalent in active smokers. Workers in the opening, carding, and spinning departments had the highest incidence of byssinosis, at 28%, whereas the overall prevalence in the sample was 18%. Byssinotic workers also had a higher incidence of chronic bronchitis.[14]

Although workers without prior exposure to cotton dust may exhibit the signs and symptoms of byssinosis, it is seen more often in those with a prolonged (i.e., 10 years or longer) exposure to high concentrations of cotton, flax, or soft hemp dust.[25]

Some investigators have argued that there is not excessive mortality among textile workers.[10] In Rhode Island, however, a review of the occupation and industry statements on death certificates revealed a statistically significant increase in death from nonmalignant respiratory disease among male textile workers, consistent with a pattern of mortality due to textile dust exposure. Those working with textile dyeing and finishing also had a higher incidence of cancer of the esophagus and rectum; however, smoking data, unfortunately, were not available in this study.[27]

CHEMISTRY, ANTIGEN IDENTIFICATION, AND PATHOPHYSIOLOGY OF BYSSINOSIS

The precise antigens responsible for causing byssinosis remain elusive, although considerable progress has been made in this area. It is quite likely that there are multiple substances in cotton dust that are capable of producing byssinosis.

Interestingly, in one study guinea pigs chronically exposed to cotton dust for 1 year developed hematologic changes with specific antibody formation, a fraction of which was specific for *Enterobacter agglomerans,* the most prevalent microorganism in the dust.[26]

The relevance of these findings to humans is not clear.

Allergen skin tests to cotton, hemp, flax, and jute antigens were performed in 41 patients with byssinosis.[28] Immediate skin test reactions to these antigens were rarely seen, but nearly all workers with byssinosis had delayed positive reactions. In this same study, only four patients had positive bronchial provocation with textile allergens, and these four had clinical pictures more consistent with bronchial asthma. Approximately one-half of the workers with byssinosis in this study had bronchoconstrictive responses to inhaled acetylcholine.[28]

Extracts of cotton dust have been shown to contain at least 40 distinct antigens.[29] Although IgE antibodies specific for dust have been found in some workers with byssinosis, the finding of bronchoconstriction after cotton dust challenge in a significant number of healthy volunteer subjects makes an IgE-mediated mechanism extremely unlikely.[1]

Mechanical irritation does not appear to be operative in byssinosis.[10] Extracts of cotton dust have been found to contain histamine, although Chan-Yeung et al. state that the amount of histamine is most likely not sufficient to induce acute bronchoconstriction in vivo.[1,30] Extracts of cotton dust are also capable of causing histamine release from isolated human lungs, as well as from the lung tissue of some animals.[30]

Both symptomatic cotton and flax workers were found to have significantly higher blood histamine levels on Mondays (after 2 days away from the plant) compared with asymptomatic cotton workers, suggesting a pathogenic role for the release of mediators including histamine.[1,31]

Considerable experimental and epidemiologic evidence exists to support a strong role for endotoxins from contaminating bacteria as one, if not the principal, agent of disease in acute byssinotic effects.[1,2,32-37] Laboratory animals given endotoxins by aerosol inhalation have a markedly diminished response on the second day, compared to the first, similar to the pattern seen in cotton workers on the first day of the work week.[34] Bacterial endotoxin has also been shown to activate the complement system with resultant release of allergic mediators including histamine.[36]

Rylander et al. correlated the number of gram-negative bacteria contaminating cotton bales with falls in FEV_1 on Mondays in cotton card room workers; this correlation was stronger than that with the level of dust from vertically elutriated cotton alone.[33] Others have also correlated airborne gram-negative bacteria in cotton spinning mills with the prevalence of byssinotic symptoms.[35]

Recent investigations[38] have confirmed those done earlier,[39] showing that the number of microorganisms on different parts of cotton plants still in the fields increases sharply after the first frost of the season. It is interesting that in the San Joaquin valley, cotton is rarely harvested after the first frost, and studies of cotton from this area show low levels of gram-negative bacterial contamination compared with cotton from varying regions of the cotton belt.[2,35,40,41]

Castellan et al. postulated that these lower bacterial counts may relate to the generally less notable human airway response to dust from California-grown cotton compared to other regions of the country where cotton is harvested after the first frost.[2] Castellan et al. measured acute ventilatory changes in 54 workers with acute airway responsiveness to cotton dust.[2] They monitored spirometry immediately before and 6 hours after exposure to card-generated cotton dust from seven different cottons of varying grades from several different growing regions. During the cotton-dust exposures, they sampled the air for concentrations of gravimetric dust, viable bacteria and fungi, and bacterial endotoxin. Correlation of the exposures of these components of dust with fall in FEV_1 of the study workers showed no relationship to the viable fungi. There was a statistically significant correlation between the fall in FEV_1 and the gravimetrically determined cotton dust concentration ($p < 0.05$), and there was a highly significant correlation between bacterial endotoxin concentration in the dust and fall in FEV_1 ($p < 0.00001$). The researchers concluded that bacterial endotoxin may play a major role in the acute fall in pulmonary function accompanying exposure to inhaled cotton dust.[2]

Lipopolysaccharide from *Enterobacter agglomerans*, one of the most common gram-negative bacteria found in cotton dust, has been shown to bind to pulmonary surfactant similar to that seen with *Pseudomonas aeruginosa*.[42] DeLucca et al. postulate that this may contribute to the pathogenesis of byssinosis, stating that the pulmonary tissues may become "stiffer" after interaction with this lipopolysaccharide, impairing the normal function of the lung tissue.[42]

This seemingly overwhelming evidence in favor of bacterial endotoxin as the causative agent of byssinosis is not without its flaws. Buck et al. demonstrated falls in lung function in normal volunteers exposed to extracts of cotton bract despite nearly complete removal of endotoxin, arguing for additional pathogenic mechanisms.[43]

Others have noted a heat-stable, water-soluble portion of cotton bract that is capable of inducing bronchoconstriction even after the bronchial provocation solution has been made free of endotoxin. These authors suggest another component of the cotton bract is contributing.[32,44]

One such additional contributing factor may be cotton bract tannin.[45-47] This tannin has been shown to be a polyclonal activator of human T lymphocytes in vitro, similar to the pattern seen with PHA and ConA, well-known plant lectins that also function as T-cell mitogens.[47] The response was dependent on dose of tannin and the presence of monocytes. Lipopolysaccharide from *Enterobacter agglomerans* was not a mediator of tannin mitogenicity in vitro.[47]

Lauque et al. performed bronchoalveolar lavage on anesthetized, intubated, and mechanically ventilated rabbits 4 hours after aerosol challenges with saline (control), cotton dust extracts, and tannin.[46] They found that tannin challenge did not cause as high an increase in PMNs in bronchoalveolar lavage (BAL) fluid as that seen with cotton dust extract, although BAL fluid levels of the potent bronchoconstrictor PGF_2-alpha were similar to cotton dust extract challenge. The authors concluded that the inflammatory response to cotton dust inhalation is only partially due to the tannin present in cotton dust.[46] Thus, this is probably multifactorial in origin.

SYNERGISTIC FACTORS

The effects of smoking on the clinical course of byssinosis have been studied extensively. Smoking has been shown to be additive, and perhaps synergistic, in worsening the pulmonary function tests of those suffering from byssinosis.[4,12,14,24] It is very difficult to differentiate the effects of cigarette smoking from those of cotton dust exposure in cotton workers. Schachter et al. have postulated that smoking and byssinosis damage different parts of the tracheobronchial tree and thus affect the shape of the expiratory flow volume curve differently.[23] This concept warrants further investigation.

CLINICAL PRESENTATION AND EVALUATION OF BYSSINOSIS

Clinical Syndrome

The presenting symptoms of byssinosis are most frequently chest tightness, dyspnea, and cough, which may or may not be accompanied by audible wheezing.[1] Although symptoms have been reported immediately after first contact,[10] byssinosis most frequently occurs in those workers with a significant duration of employment in the textile industry, often greater than 10 years.[25] Symptoms of byssinosis are most common in workers with a high level of exposure to cotton dust, and least common in those working in an area of the plant with less dust exposure.[1]

In contrast to most cases of occupational asthma, byssinosis is usually worse on Mondays.[3] The chest symptoms typically begin several (usually about 4) hours after the patient begins work on Monday morning.[1] If symptoms are present on Tuesday, they are usually milder, and they commonly abate by the end of the week.[1]

Although it would be unlikely to have someone with asthma working in a high dust area of a cotton mill, it is worthwhile to note that cotton dust may also exacerbate asthma.[4] However, in asthma, the patient's symptoms usually worsen within 30 minutes of exposure to the workplace, in contrast to 4–5 hours as is the case with byssinosis.[4]

A complete medical history is essential in evaluating the patient with possible byssinosis. A detailed workplace questionnaire may facilitate taking the history.

Physical Examination and Laboratory Findings

Physical findings in byssinosis are generally similar to those seen with asthma. The physician may hear wheezing and/or decreased air movement on auscultation of the lungs. Allergen skin testing is not a helpful procedure in establishing the diagnosis of byssinosis.[28] In cotton byssinosis, immediate positive skin test reactivity to cotton is usually absent.[28] In byssinosis secondary to hemp and flax (and in the byssinosis-like syndrome seen with jute), positive skin tests may be seen, but are still uncommon.[28] As mentioned previously, although delayed positive skin tests are more common in byssinosis, they are not a constant finding in byssinosis from any cause.[28]

Skin testing to cottonseed extract may be very dangerous, especially with intradermal testing, and should be done only with prick tests.[16] Cottonseed allergy may also be seen as an inhalant, and cottonseed allergens may be present in stuffing used in upholstery, mattresses, and cushions.[16] It may also be found in some animal feeds, cottonseed meal (pomace), fertilizers, and some foods.[16] The high temperatures used for the manufacture of cottonseed oil appear to denature any cottonseed protein allergen present, rendering it essentially nonallergenic.[16,17]

Pulmonary function findings noted with byssinosis include an accelerated rate of decline in FEV_1 compared to healthy controls (average loss per year in FEV_1 ranged from 48-292 ml/year compared with 30 ml/year in a healthy control group).[11,48,49] Symptoms of chest tightness, shortness of breath, and cough on Monday may be associated with a post-shift fall in FEV_1.[1]

TOBACCO

Lander and Graveson investigated clinical symptoms, spirometry (FVC and FEV_1), and serial peak expiratory flow rates (PEFRs) in 16 tobacco plant workers compared to a control group matched for sex, age, and cigarette-smoking status. Air sampling using personal breathing zone sampling pumps assayed for total dust; samplers quantifying airborne bacteria and microfungi were also used.[50] The researchers noted that 69% of tobacco workers reported symptoms compatible with asthma compared with 6% of controls. The mean diurnal change in PEFR was 14.3% for the tobacco workers compared with 9.8% for the controls, a significant difference implying increased airway caliber lability.[50]

Gleich et al. describe a 31-year-old with clear occupational asthma due to green tobacco leaf exposure (Fig. 3).[51] Cromolyn treatment did not prevent her dyspnea at work. Skin testing with green tobacco leaf and cured tobacco leaf extracts were positive, but an extract of tobacco smoke condensate was negative. RAST assay using green tobacco leaf extract as the solid phase antigen source demonstrated 15.4% binding, 150 times greater than control, nonallergic serum. Leukocytes from the patient released histamine in significant amounts compared to control cells in the presence of green tobacco extract. This patient also demonstrated positive nasal and bronchial provocation tests with green tobacco leaf extract.[51] The decrease in tobacco leaf antigenicity from green leaf stage to cured stage is probably due to protein degradation which takes place during the curing process (Fig. 4).[51]

Tobacco, because it is an organic material, may be contaminated with microfungi, which may also cause asthma and allergic extrinsic alveolitis.[52,53] As an organic dust, it is also apparent that workers with an atopic predisposition are probably at increased risk of developing occupational asthma secondary to tobacco leaf exposure.[50] Smokers in one study appeared to be at greater risk of developing obstructive lung disease than smokers not

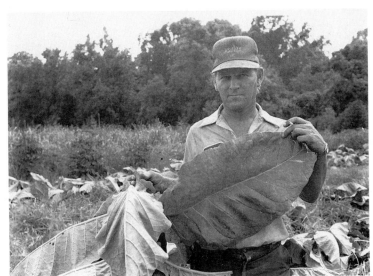

FIGURE 3. Close-up of tobacco leaf.

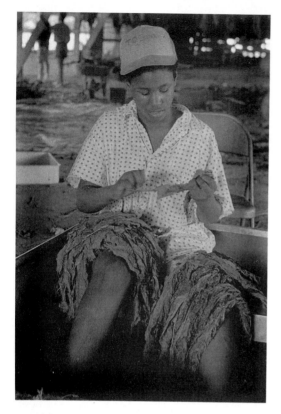

FIGURE 4.   Tobacco worker stripping tobacco leaves.

working with tobacco, but other investigators have not found this to be the case.[50]

Long-term exposure to tobacco leaf materials and dust may result in harm to the airways, even at levels as low as 0.5 mg/M^3, as evidenced by increases in bronchial hyperreactivity in some workers.[50]

TREATMENT AND WORKPLACE RECOMMENDATIONS

Byssinosis can be prevented if proper industrial hygiene measures are taken to decrease the dust burden in the air of the workplace.[3] New occupational standards should be incorporated that also take into account airborne bacterial endotoxin levels as well as the dust concentrations.[2]

Textile workers are advised to avoid smoking, as well as avoiding further exposure to the offending dust at a time when they still have adequate ventilatory reserve to prevent further functional loss.[1] Further deterioration of lung function in some hemp and cotton workers despite removal from the workplace underscores the need for prompt job change should

symptoms of byssinosis develop.[11] There is not adequate information available on the efficacy of medical therapy in byssinosis.

If occupational hygiene measures are ignored, symptoms may progress after many years of exposure to the point where chronic obstructive pulmonary disease may result.[4,5] This may be an extremely worrisome sign, because, as expected, those with an $FEV_1 < 50\%$ in the hemp industry had a higher mortality rate than those with an $FEV_1 > 50\%$ on follow-up 7 years later.[11] Prevention is clearly the preferred route, and if byssinosis is discovered, the worker needs to promptly be removed from his or her present workplace.

REFERENCES

1. Chan-Yeung M, Lam S: State of Art: Occupational asthma. Am Rev Respir Dis 133:686–703, 1986.
2. Castellan RM, Olenchock SA, Hankinson JL, et al: Acute bronchoconstriction induced by cotton dust: Dose-related responses to exdotoxin and other factors. Ann Intern Med 101:157–163, 1984.
3. Cockcroft DW: Occupational asthma. Ann Allergy 65:169, 1990.
4. White NW: Byssinosis in South Africa: A survey of 2411 textile workers. S Afr Med J 75:435–442, 1989.
5. Braman SS, Teplitz C: Occupational lung disease. Primary Care 5:425–445, 1978.
6. Uragoda CG: A clinical and radiographic study of coir workers. Br J Ind Med 32:66–71, 1975.
7. Noweir MH, El-Sadik YM, El-Dakhakhny A, et al: Dust exposure in manual flax processing in Egypt. Br J Ind Med 32:147–154, 1975.
8. Ramazzini B: A Treatise of the Diseases of Tradesmen. London, Bell, 1705.
9. d'Evelyn A: Reports by the inspector of factories upon the conditions of work in flax mills and linen factories in the United Kingdom. In Osborne EH (ed): Parliamentary Papers, 1894; Vol. VIII, C. 7287, London, HMSO.
10. Byssinosis: Clinical and Research Issues. Report of the Committee on Byssinosis, National Research Council. Washington, D.C. National Academy Press, 1982.
11. Bouhuys A, Zuskin E: Chronic respiratory disease in hemp workers: A follow-up study, 1967–1974. Ann Intern Med 84:398–405, 1976.
12. Bouhuys A, Beck GJ, Schoenberg JB: Epidemiology of environmental lung disease. The Yale Journal of Biology and Medicine 52:191–210, 1979.
13. McKerrow CB, McDermott M, Gilson JC, et al: Respiratory function during the day in cotton workers. A study in byssinosis. Br J Med 15:75, 1958.
14. Takam J, Nemery B: Byssinosis in a textile factory in Cameroon: A preliminary study. Br J Ind Med 45:803–809, 1988.
15. Cinkotai FF, Emo P, Gibbs AC, et al: Low prevalence of byssinotic symptoms in 12 flax scutching mills in Normandy, France. Br J Ind Med 45:325–328, 1988.
16. Jelks ML, Solomon WR: Airborne allergens. In Kaplan AP (ed): Allergy. New York, Churchill Livingstone, 1985, pp 255–320.

17. Solomon WR, Matthews KP: Aerobiology and inhalant allergens. In Middleton E Jr, Reed CE, Ellis EF, et al (eds): Allergy, Principles and Practice, 2nd ed. St. Louis, C.V. Mosby, 1983, pp 1143-1202.
18. Baker MD, Irwig LM, Johnson JR, et al: Lung function in sisal ropemakers. Br J Ind Med 36:216-219, 1979.
19. McKerrow CB, Gilson JC, Schilling RSF, Skidmore JW: Respiratory function and symptoms in rope makers. Br J Ind Med 22:204-209, 1965.
20. Munt DF, Gauvain S, Walford J, Schilling RSF: Study of respiratory symptoms and ventilatory capacities among rope workers. Br J Ind Med 22:196-203, 1965.
21. Valic F, Zuskin E: Effects of different vegetable dust exposures. Br J Ind Med 29:293-297, 1972.
22. Gilson JC, Stott H, Hopwood BEC, et al: Byssinosis: The acute effects on ventilatory capacity of dusts in cotton ginneries, cotton, sisal, and jute mills. Br J Ind Med 18:9-18, 1962.
23. Beck GJ, Schachter EN: The evidence for chronic lung disease in cotton textile workers. Am Statistician 37:404, 1983.
24. Schachter EN, Kapp MC, Beck GJ, et al: Smoking and cotton dust effect in cotton textile workers. Chest 95:997-1003, 1989.
25. Cinkotai FF, Rigby A, Pickering CA, et al: Recent trends in the prevalence of byssinotic symptoms in the Lancashire textile industry. Br J Ind Med 45:782-789, 1988.
26. Olanivan NS, Karol MH: Serological study of guinea pigs exposed for 12 months to cotton dust. J Toxicol Environ Health 25:185-199, 1988.
27. Dubrow R, Gute RM: Cause-specific mortality among young male textile workers in Rhode Island. Division of Surveillance, Hazard Evaluations, and Field Studies. Am J Ind Med 13:439-454, 1988.
28. Popa V, Gavrilescu N, Preda N, et al: An investigation of allergy in byssinosis: Sensitization to cotton, hemp, flax and jute antigen. Br J Ind Med 26:101, 1969.
29. Rubenstein HS: Occupational asthma: A view of synergistic causes. Occupational Health and Safety 50:32-34, 36, 38, 1981.
30. Butcher BT, O'Neil CE, Jones RN: The respiratory effects of cotton dust. In Salvaggio JE, Stankus RP (eds): Clin Chest Med 4:63-70, 1983.
31. Noweir MH: Highlights of broad spectrum industrial hygiene research activities in a developing country—Egypt. Am Ind Hyg Assoc J 40:839-859, 1979.
32. Cullen MR, Cherniack MG, Rosenstock L: Occupational medicine. N Engl J Med 322:594, 1990.
33. Rylander R, Imbus HR, Suh MW: Bacterial contamination of cotton as an indicator of respiratory effects among card room workers. Br J Ind Med 36:299-304, 1979.
34. Pernis B, Vigliani EC, Cavagna C, Finulli M: The role of bacterial endotoxins in occupational diseases caused by inhaling vegetable dusts. Br J Ind Med 18:120-129, 1961.
35. Cinkotai FF, Whitaker CJ: Airborne bacteria and the prevalence of byssinotic symptoms in 21 cotton spinning mills in Lancashire. Ann Occup Hyg 21:239-250, 1978.
36. Wilson MR, Sokol A, Ory R, Salvaggio JE, Lehrer SB: Activation of the alternative complement pathway by extracts of cotton dust. Clin Allergy 10:303-308, 1980.
37. Milton DK, Godleski JJ, Feldman HA, et al: Toxicity of intratracheally instilled cotton dusts, cellulose, and endotoxin. Am Rev Respir Dis 142:184, 1990.
38. Merchant JA, Lumsden JC, Kilburn KH, et al: Dose-response studies in cotton textile workers. J Occup Med 15:222-230, 1973.
39. Clark FE: Occurrence of cotton fiber contaminated by Aerobacter cloacae. U.S. Dept. Agriculture, Tech. Bull. 935, 1947.
40. Simpson ME, Marsh PB: Bacterial counts on commercial raw cotton from the U.S. crop of 1980. Textile Research Journal 52:1-9, 1982.
41. Simpson ME, Marsh PB: Further counts of bacteria on U.S. produced raw cotton fiber. Text Res J 54:231-237, 1984.
42. DeLucca AJ, Brogden KA, Engen R: Enterobacter agglomerans lipopolysaccharide-induced changes in pulmonary surfactant as a factor in the pathogenesis of byssinosis. J Clin Microbiol 26:778-780, 1988.
43. Buck MG, Schachter EN, Wall JH: Partial composition of a low molecular weight cotton bract extract which induces acute airway constriction in humans. In Wakekyn PE (ed): Proceedings of the Sixth Cotton Dust Research Conference. Memphis, TN, National Cotton Council, 1982, pp 19-23.
44. Douglas JS, Duncan PG, Zuskin E: Characteristics of textile dust extracts. II. Bronchoconstriction in man. Br J Ind Med 41:70-76, 1984.
45. Rohrbach MS, Kreofsky T, Rolstad RA, et al: Tannin-mediated secretion of a neutrophil chemotactic factor from alveolar macrophages. Potential contribution to the acute pulmonary inflammation reaction associated with byssinosis. Am Rev Respir Dis 139:39-45, 1989.
46. Lauque DE, Hempel SL, Schroeder MA, et al: Evaluation of the contribution of tannin to the acute pulmonary inflammatory response against inhaled cotton mill dust. Am J Pathol 133:163-172, 1988.
47. Vuk-Pavlovic Z, Russel JA, Rohrbach MS: Cotton bract tannin: A novel human T-lymphocyte mitogen and a possible causative agent of byssinosis. Int Arch Allergy Appl Immunol 87:14-18, 1988.
48. Merchant JA, Lumsden JC, Kilburn KH, et al: Intervention studies of cotton steaming to reduce biologic effects of cotton dust. Br J Ind Med 31:261-274, 1974.
49. Berry G, McKerrow CB, Molyneux MKB, et al: A study of the acute and chronic changes in ventilatory capacity of workers in Lancashire cotton mills. Br J Ind Med 30:25-36, 1973.
50. Lauder F, Gravesen S: Respiratory disorders among tobacco workers. Br J Ind Med 45:500-502, 1988.
51. Gleich GJ, Welsh PW, Yunginger JW, et al: Allergy to tobacco: An occupational allergy. N Engl J Med 302:617-619, 1980.
52. Huuskonen MS, Husman K, Jarvisalo J, et al: Extrinsic allergic alveolitis in the tobacco industry. Br J Ind Med 41:77-83, 1984.
53. Lauder F, Jepsen JR, Gravesen S: Late asthmatic reaction caused by microfungi in the tobacco industry. Ugeskr Laeger 147:2918-2919, 1985.

Chapter 8

WESTERN RED CEDAR ASTHMA AND ASTHMA SECONDARY TO OTHER WOOD DUSTS AND WOOD OR PLANT-RELATED PRODUCTS

Emil J. Bardana, Jr., MD

Since earliest times, wood dusts were felt to act as nonspecific respiratory irritants. Several pathologic lung conditions were associated with the harvesting and processing of lumber. This chapter will focus on occupational asthmatic conditions related to wood dusts as well as wood and plant-related products. The earliest descriptions of these conditions related to the exacerbation of bronchial asthma with exposure to sawdust.[1-4] Over the past three decades, a large number of studies have implicated wood dusts in the causation of adult-onset bronchial asthma, and a spectrum of wood species has been incriminated. In addition, the impressive growth and expansion of the electronics and computer industries have resulted in many workers being exposed to colophony (rosin) as an integral part of the soldering process. A variety of tree- and shrub-derived vegetable gums have also been identified as causing asthma, especially in the printing industry. Finally, occupational asthma has been described secondary to pollen and dust exposure in a variety of plant handlers. Because of the interactions that may exist, this chapter will also briefly review the major forms of allergic alveolitis directly attributed to wood dust or fungi isolated from tree bark or wood dust.

WESTERN RED CEDAR ASTHMA

The western red cedar *(Thuja plicata),* also called red cedar and giant arborvitae, is a magnificent forest evergreen and an extremely valuable timber tree, reaching up to 200 feet high. It is native from Alaska to northern California and Montana, mostly in regions of copious rainfall and fog. The use of western red cedar in the building industry increased considerably in the early part of this century. The reasons for its increased use were its beautiful natural finish, its inherent resistance to attack by insects, and its resistance to harsh weather.

Chemistry

The chemical composition of western red cedar has been extensively investigated.[5,6] It has been noted that the structural make-up of the wood (cellulose, lignin, etc.) is much the same as that found in other coniferous woods. However, cedar does differ from other woods by virtue of its characteristic extractable ingredients. It shares this property with redwood *Sequoia sempervirens)* and some *Eucalyptus* species (some Australian eucalyptus are the only trees to exceed the redwood in height).[7] These extractable ingredients have been divided into those that are volatile and those that are not. The volatile components account for about 10% of the extractable materials and include methyl thujate, thujic acid, and a variety of other tropolones. The latter have been noted to have inherent fungicidal properties. Some have also been found to manifest beta-adrenergic receptor blocking properties.[8] Several terpenoid oils have been extracted from the *Thuja* genus, and 4-isopropyltropone is considered the principal volatile oil of western red cedar.

The most important constituent in the nonvolatile class is a phenolic compound referred to as plicatic acid. This polyphenolic compound has a molecular weight of 422 daltons, is water soluble, and contains a catechol ring structure (Fig. 1). Plicatic acid is a lignin and represents main polyoxyphenol in the cedar extractives. The other principal phenolic nonvolatile component is plicathin. Other components in the nonphenolic fractions include pectic acid, starch, hemicullulose, and a variety of simple sugars.

Plicatic acid has four acidic hydroxyls, one of them a strongly acidic carboxyl group that consumes more sodium hydroxide in the cooking liquor of a pulp mill than other woods. This is associated with accelerated digester corrosion.[8] Lignans are defined as optically active plant products characterized by the beta-gamma-dibenzylbutane skeleton. Their occurrence is widespread, and they have been isolated from bark, fruit, heartwood, leaves, roots, and resinous exudates of different plants. Plicatic acid is unique among the lignans found in various species. It has a carboxylic acid group that the others do not demonstrate. A few of the other lignans, such as isotaxiresinol found in the heartwood of the yew *(Taxus baccata)* and nordihydroguiaretic acid found in the creosote bush of Mexico *(Larrea divaricata)*, have a catechol ring structure with adjacent hydroxy groups on an aromatic ring as is found in plicatic acid.

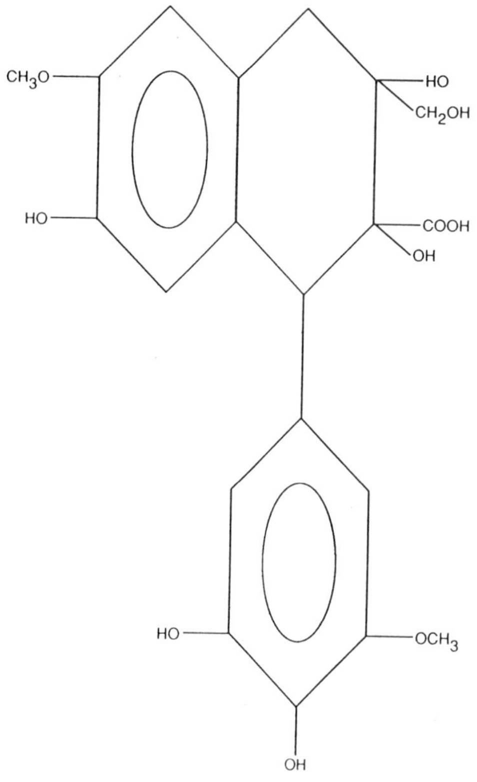

The true cedars belong to the pine family, Pinaceae. There are four basic varieties of true cedars, i.e., the deodor *(Cedrus deodara)* that grows in the Himalayas, the Atlas *(C. atlantica)* growing in the Atlas mountains of North Africa, the Cyprus cedar *(C. brevifolia)* growing on the island of Cyprus, and the cedar of Lebanon *(C. libani)*, which is mentioned in the Bible and is probably the tree originally designated cedar by the ancient Greeks. The true cedars are not related taxonomically to the thujas, but they have the same fresh, sweet odor and tough, reddish wood. There are approximately 32 genera other than the *Thuja* that are called cedar, but are not related to the *Thuja* genus. The best example is the species of red cedar, *Juniperus virginiana*, whose fragrant red heartwood is the red cedar used in chests and closets. It is also used to make oil of cedar and for lead pencils.

The *Thuja* genus is an arborvitae with five species of evergreen native to North America and Asia. Other members are not important as a source of timber with the exception of *T. occidentalis*, the white cedar that is utilized commercially for its soft, white, easily worked wood. In the past it was used in the northeastern United States as a source of telephone poles.

PLICATIC ACID

FIGURE 1. Structural formulas for plicatic acid, a polyphenolic compound with a MW 422. It is water-soluble and contains a catechol ring structure.

Clinical Features

The earliest report of western red cedar asthma was in 1926 by Seki in Japan.[1] Japanese workers were exposed to imported cedar used in building homes and furniture. A large quantity had been imported in response to an urgent need of wood following the Tokyo earthquake.[9] Doig briefly described two minor outbreaks of asthma related to cedar dust in 1949.[10] Komatsu studied a number of workers exposed to *Thuja standishei*. His observations are perhaps unique among the reports on this syndrome.[11] This investigator prepared an extract from the dust, which was interpreted as producing large (22 mm) type I wheal-and-flare reactions in workers, with smaller (12 mm) reactions in controls. Similarly, a number of additional reports from Japan emphasized the allergic nature of the clinical syndrome.[12,13]

In 1969 Sosman and his colleagues reported a spectrum of hypersensitivity lung reactions to oak, mahogany, and western red cedar. Two carpenters with cedar asthma were noted to have negative skin tests, the presence of precipitins to a crude extract of western red cedar, and a delayed response to both a fine dust and an aqueous extract of the dust.[14]

In 1969 Milne and Gandevia authored the first comprehensive description of western red cedar asthma.[15] This was followed by several reports collating their observations in six cases of asthma and four patients with rhinitis, especially as it related to bronchial provocation.[16,17] The clinical history of cedar asthma was usually characterized by a long period of exposure to cedar dust. In contrast to later studies, these initial cases did not develop work-related asthma until many years, and in some cases decades, after they entered the trade. Initially eye and nasal irritation, rhinorrhea, or nasal obstruction was noted (Table 1). Within weeks, an irritating cough developed that was characteristically worse at the end of the day or during the night. Subsequently, episodes of nocturnal cough and wheezing would begin, with production of tenacious sputum. Partial or complete relief usually occurred over weekends or in the intervals separating periods of intermittent exposure. In severe advanced cases, severe symptoms and especially nocturnal paroxysms, were noted to persist for weeks and months even after cessation of exposure.[15]

According to Gandevia and Milne, diagnosis was facilitated by a history indicating material worsening upon exposure to cedar dust. Confirmation of the diagnosis was not facilitated by skin testing. Small and inconsistent reactions were noted to cedar extract, whereas the majority of their patients showed immediate reactivity to housedust.[15] Of interest, four of the eight housedust-reactive patients failed to respond adversely to bronchial challenge. Serum precipitins were observed in most cases. These investigators confirmed the diagnosis by conducting bronchial provocation tests with an extract of western red cedar. This was

TABLE 1. *Potential Clinical Sequelae of Exposure to Western Red Cedar Dust (Thuja plicata)*

Diagnosis	Reference	Incriminated Constituent of Western Red Cedar
Allergic contact dermatitis	23	Related to tropolones and related compounds in the heartwood.
		Related to lichens (composed of fungi and algae) growing on the bark. Sensitizing compounds are usnic acid and atranorine.
		Related to liverworts (moss-like growth). Sensitizing compounds are the sesquiterpene lactones. Cross-reacts with similar chemicals in *Compositae* genus.
Contact urticaria	22	Fine western red cedar dust and possibly 4-isopropyltropone.
Rhinocon- junctivitis	17–20	Fine western red cedar dust and said to be specifically related to plicatic acid.
Chronic bronchitis	17–20	Synergy between smoking and exposure to western red cedar dust
Bronchial asthma	1–4, 9–20	Fine western red cedar dust and said to be specifically related to plicatic acid.
Allergic alveolitis	14	Fine western red cedar dust

prepared by mixing 10 grams of fine western red cedar dust and 100 ml of Coca's solution and allowing it to stand for 2 weeks. The supernatant was removed, Seitz-filtered, and tested for sterility before use. This solution was described as D strength with sequential 1:10 dilutions used to prepare C, B, and A strengths, respectively. C or D strength extract was inhaled for 90 seconds using a Wright nebulizer. Control challenges with diluent or house dust were carried out. Cedar dust challenges were not carried out. Several patients were shown to have recurrent bouts of nocturnal asthma following a single challenge, i.e., a protracted delayed reaction, and all of the asthmatic patients had a positive bronchial response.[15] The majority of cases with asthma became asymptomatic upon removal from cedar dust. During the same year, Mitchell reported a case of western red cedar asthma in which a strong immediate reaction was noted to skin tests and bronchial provocation.[18]

Chan-Yeung et al. reported their initial three cases in 1971.[19] Two patients presented with typical rhinoconjunctivitis prior to developing asthma. Crude and purified extracts of the volatile fraction of western red cedar and other wood dusts were prepared. The extract was prepared in such a way that all proteins in it were denatured. The authors do not discuss how this constituent might have related to the actual work exposures encountered by the patients.[16] A mild immediate skin test response was noted in two patients. Serum precipitins were absent in all three patients. Bronchial provocation produced an immediate reaction in one and delayed reactions (3 to 4 hours) in the remaining two patients. One of these delayed reactions persisted over 24 hours. The immediate reaction could be inhibited by cromolyn sodium. One patient developed bibasilar rales during the late reaction, suggesting the presence of an alveolitis. The pattern of the reaction suggested an "allergic" mechanism. Two normal individuals and two patients with asthma, but without exposure to cedar failed to react to a single bronchial challenge.

In 1972 Pickering et al. used the pan test that was subsequently popularized by Pepys to tip finely ground western red cedar dust as the challenge technique to reproduce bronchial symptoms. Dust was tipped from one pan to another to reproduce conditions of the work environment. Either lactose or sand could be used as a control. Using the actual western red cedar dust as a challenge seemed extremely rational and worked well to reproduce the worker's asthma.[20]

In 1973 Chan-Yeung et al. published their retrospective observations on 22 woodworkers presenting with respiratory symptoms.[21,22] This included the three patients previously reported. Most of these workers were employed by cedar sawmills. Typical symptoms arose after a latent period ranging between 4 months and 3 years of steady exposure. In a few patients, the latent period was 10 to 20 years. One patient had a history of childhood asthma, another of bronchiectasis, and four smokers had established chronic bronchitis. Family and personal history of atopic disease was usually absent. Twelve of the 22 workers developed rhinitis prior to paroxysms of cough productive of scant sputum. Symptoms were prominent nocturnally.

In arriving at a diagnosis in these 22 woodworkers, a number of studies were conducted using a dialyzed western red cedar extract prepared in such a manner as to destroy all proteins.[7] This material was then dialyzed to eliminate all high molecular weight substances. The concentration used for provocation was the same as that used in the crude extract.[19] This purified material failed to evoke a positive reaction in any patient. In addition, an extract from which all volatile components were removed was also prepared. This caused a reaction in two patients who had reacted to the crude extract.[19] Since plicatic acid was the principal constituent in the nonvolatile fraction, 16 patients and 10 control subjects (two healthy, four with chronic bronchitis, and four with bronchial asthma) were challenged once with this constituent. The inhaled dose was arbitrarily set at 50% of those used with the whole extract. No attempt was made to calibrate the nebulized dose of plicatic acid against western red cedar dust or to verify the ambient levels of plicatic acid at the workplace. An immediate asthmatic reaction was induced in four, a late asthmatic was noted in eight, and biphasic reactions were noted in six patients. Four patients failed to demonstrate any response, even with high doses. These individuals are said to have presented with a different clinical situation where their symptoms are unrelated to dust exposure and where symptoms did not improve even when they avoided further exposure. Serum precipitins to the purified extract were not observed. Positive epicutaneous tests to the extract were essentially negative except for mild immediate reactions in three patients. By virtue of these observations the authors claimed that plicatic acid was probably the compound in red cedar that caused respiratory symptoms.[21,22]

During the same year, Ishizaki et al. reported their epidemiologic survey among 1797 furniture workers in the city of Kanuma, Japan.[23] An allergic evaluation was carried out on 269 individuals. Although only a small percentage of asthmatic patients were skin tested with potent material, 85% reacted positively, and these investigators concluded that an atopic predisposition was an important factor in the development of western red cedar asthma. The latter has not been the case in almost all studies of this condition. Bronchial provocation with dust or extract was not carried out.

In 1974 Mitchell and Chan-Yeung reported the results of their research program to determine the cause of "cedar-poisoning." The term was in common use in British Columbia and was applied to skin and respiratory disorders in forest products industry workers.[24] Eighty-seven patients were evaluated and the preponderance of disease occurred on the skin (Table 1). They observed 12 workers with contact allergy to lichens and 52 with contact sensitivity to liverworts. Lichens are plants composed of a fungus and algae that contain usnic acid and atranorine as immunogens. Liverworts are related to the mosses and contain sesquiterpene lactones (Fig. 2). The latter compounds are also found in the species of the Compositae family, the largest family of plants in the world with over 30,000 species, and including such plants as chrysanthemums, ragweed, wild artichoke, and sagebrush.[24] Only a single woodworker was found to have contact sensitivity to the heartwood of western red cedar. The clinical picture was characterized by the appearance of recurrent eczema of the hands, notably affecting the finger webs. The tropolones and related compounds are felt to be responsible for this skin disease.

Mitchell and Chan-Yeung emphasized that the respiratory symptoms were due to sensitivity to the "dust itself" of western red cedar wood. Among the 35 proved cases of asthma and rhinitis due to western red cedar diagnosed to that point, there were 18 sawmill workers (Fig. 3), 12 carpenters and cabinetmakers, four construction workers, and one wood carver. There were no loggers or other forest workers.[24]

Mue et al. described 17 wood frame workers in Japan who developed western red cedar asthma. An aqueous extract was developed and fractionated. One particular fraction was reported to result in positive immediate skin test reactions and bronchial provocation.[25] Skin reactivity was demonstrated to be transferable (P-K test). Based on these observations, an antigen was felt to be present in western red cedar that was capable of inducing allergic asthma.[25] These observations have never been repeated or confirmed by other investigators.

In 1977 Chan-Yeung et al. published a series of papers reiterating and expanding some of their earlier observations.[26-28] The initial paper studied 38 patients (presumably many or all of whom were the subjects of earlier studies).[26] Fifteen of these individuals had a history of prior or current tobacco abuse. These workers underwent pulmonary function testing after they had left work 6 or more months. Twenty-seven of these workers (71%) had become totally asymptomatic with normal lung function. Three continued with symptoms of chronic bronchitis secondary to smoking, and eight continued to have recurrent episodes of bronchial asthma. All were found to have bronchial hyperreactivity on methacholine challenge. Since these patients were all studied retrospectively, it could not be determined to what

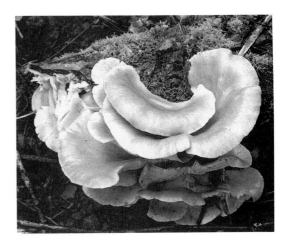

FIGURE 2.   Extensive moss and fungal growth on the bark of a tree in the Pacific Northwest.

extent the bronchial hyperreactivity preexisted western red cedar asthma and perhaps was a predisposing factor for its development. The investigators correctly indicated that preemployment physicals with performance of methacholine challenge tests would help provide answers to this question.

Chan-Yeung et al. carried out a retrospective survey of woodworkers in British Columbia to determine the prevalence of respiratory symptoms, the influence of certain job descriptions, and a variety of host factors on the expression of the disease.[27,28] The control population was not well matched to the study population. Analysis of the data suggested that workers exposed to red cedar dust had a higher prevalence of symptoms than those exposed to other wood dusts. Contrary to the

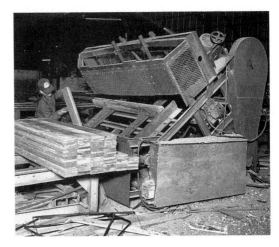

FIGURE 3.   Cedar mill worker in Oregon working proximal to a planer. Typically, no respiratory protection is being used.

observations of Gandevia in Australia,[15-17] the Canadian group reported that western red cedar asthma is likely to develop within the first 2 years of work. They presumed that the majority of affected workers left the industry early in their tenure, leaving a selected population. Although the prevalence of western red cedar asthma in this particular study was noted to be quite low, i.e., 1.1%, the authors felt that a more realistic figure was 4 or 5%.[27] There was some evidence suggesting synergy between exposure to western red cedar dust and smoking, with a greater tendency of exposed workers to develop chronic bronchitis.[27] Atopy appeared to be unrelated to the prevalence of chest symptoms or pulmonary function abnormalities, but appeared to be more common in workers with rhinoconjunctivitis.

In the late 1970s several studies considered triggers that would result in sustained bronchial hyperreactivity. Among the work-related substances, western red cedar dust was found to result frequently in either a dual or isolated late asthmatic response, which in turn was linked to a protracted state of bronchial hyperreactivity.[29,30] In addition to this observation, both these studies were important in confirming Pickering's pan test and the diagnostic applicability of fine western red cedar dust[20] as a reliable method of bronchial provocation. Other studies indicated that in addition to allergens[31,32] and occupational sensitizers,[29,30] high concentrations of gaseous irritants[33,34] and respiratory infections[35] also provoked a delayed asthmatic response with bronchial hyperresponsiveness.

By 1980, Chan-Yeung indicated that her group had diagnosed 45 patients with western red cedar asthma.[36] The typical clinical and laboratory features of western red cedar asthma were reviewed (Table 2). These investigators continued to establish the diagnosis by administering either a dialyzed western red cedar extract or a purified plicatic acid bronchial challenge. This group did not mention dust as a useful and possibly more appropriate challenge material. Carbol saline or Douglas fir dust extracts were used as controls.[36] The basic pathogenesis was not known, but based on the pattern of the reaction an allergic reaction was suspected.

In an attempt to clarify the pathogenesis of western red cedar asthma, plicatic acid was tested for its ability to activate complement and to generate chemotactic activity from pooled normal serum.[37] These studies determined that plicatic acid was capable of

TABLE 2.   *Clinical and Laboratory Features of Western Red Cedar Asthma*

Negative family and personal history of atopy or bronchial asthma.

Correlation of respiratory symptoms to significant western red cedar dust exposure (sawmill, cabinet makers, etc.)

Latent period between start of exposure and onset of symptoms.

Nonsmokers affected in higher proportion than smokers.

Only a small proportion of cedar mill workers are affected, i.e., 6-9% develop rhinoconjunctivitis and 3-5% develop asthma.

Onset of chest tightness, cough, and breathlessness, usually after work and at night.

Challenge with western red cedar dust, extract, or plicatic acid results in a dual or delayed asthmatic reaction in 90% of affected workers.

There may be prolonged persistence of bronchial hyperreactivity after any exposure to cedar dust.

Timely diagnosis and removal from work usually result in complete resolution of symptoms.

activating complement via the classical pathway independent of immunoglobulin. These observations were consistent with the probability that plicatic acid could directly induce bronchial inflammation that could precipitate in the generation of chronic bronchitis or bronchial asthma.[37]

Brooks et al. conducted an epidemiologic study of workers exposed to western red cedar and other dusts at a wood product facility in the U.S.[38] The populations studied consisted of 74 shake mill employees exposed to western red cedar, 58 planer mill workers exposed to a variety of woods (principally Douglas fir, hemlock and red alder), and 22 clerical employees. Occupational asthma was diagnosed in 10 of 73 (13.5%) workers. Workers with the highest dust exposure (sawyers, packers, splitters, and deckmen, in descending order) showed the highest prevalence of disease. Based on their observations, these investigators felt that an 8-hour time weighted average level of western red cedar dust should be below 3.5 mg/M[3] to reduce incidence of disease.[38] It is also interesting to note a high incidence of occupational asthma (5%) in workers exposed to Douglas fir, hemlock, and alder wood dusts.

Pathogenesis (Fig. 4)

Further studies relating to the pathogenesis of western red cedar asthma were reported by

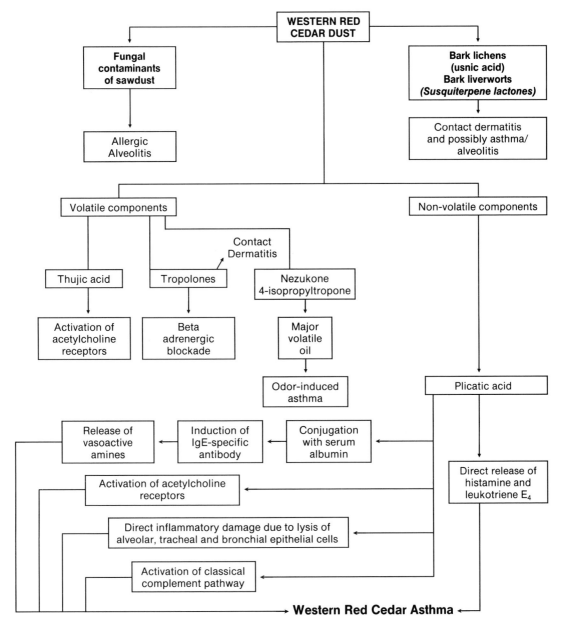

FIGURE 4.   Schematic diagram depicting possible pathogenetic mechanisms implicated in the development of western red cedar asthma.

Tse et al.[39] Because a hypersensitivity mechanism was suspected as a pathogenic explanation, specific IgE antibodies were looked for against plicatic acid-human serum albumin conjugates. There was ample precedent that such antibodies existed in the setting of low molecular weight chemical-induced occupational asthma.[40-42] Tse et al. were able to demonstrate the presence of specific IgE antibodies in about half of patients who reacted positively to plicatic acid challenge.[39] These same antibodies were not found in challenge-negative patients. Dermal testing with the same antigens was not carried out. IgE appeared to react with a crude cedar extract in which plicatic acid was said to be the major hapten. Binding to the plicatic acid conjugate was seen in only 5 of 15 challenge-positive patients. These data led the authors to believe that anti-plicatic acid IgE antibodies might be playing an important pathogenic role leading to the development of western red cedar asthma. To date this observation has not been repeated or extended, and there is no certain evidence that these antibodies play any role in the pathogenesis of this disease.

In a follow-up study designed to evaluate the prevalence of chronic western red cedar asthma, Chan-Yeung et al. investigated 125 workers who had been diagnosed with western red cedar asthma for periods ranging between 1 to 9 years.[43] Of the 125, 75 left the industry and had no subsequent exposure to cedar. Only half were said to have recovered completely. The reason why this was different from the author's earlier observation in which 71% were noted to have recovered completely was not explained.[26] However, the authors felt that the most important factor determining a favorable outcome was a timely diagnosis followed by removal from exposure (Table 2). Despite the observations that IgE-specific antibodies directed against a plicatic acid conjugate had been observed in some patients with western red cedar asthma, Chan-Yeung admitted that the pathogenic mechanism for western red cedar asthma had not yet been established.[44] Potential nonimmunological mechanisms included: (1) reflex bronchoconstriction thought to play a role in the immediate, but not the delayed asthmatic reaction; (2) direct histamine release from human basophils and mast cells[44] (additional evidence indicates that aqueous extracts of western red cedar wood are capable of releasing significant amounts of histamine directly from pig and human lung tissue in vitro[45]); (3) direct activation of the complement pathway; and (4) possible pharmacologic mediation via beta adrenergic receptor blockade by the tropolones. Immunologic mechanisms were stated to probably play a role in the pathogenesis of this disease based upon the specificity of the plicatic acid challenge test, the fact that only 3 to 5% of workers are affected, the latent period between exposure and disease, and the small amount of plicatic acid that can induce a reaction.[45]

A more recent report by Chan-Yeung's group involved a retrospective longitudinal study to determine the occurrence of bronchial hyperresponsiveness in western red cedar workers.[46] Two-hundred-twenty-seven workers employed in a Vancouver mill underwent methacholine provocation on at least two occasions during three surveys over a 2-year period. Unfortunately, many of the 652 workers evaluated initially were unable to participate through the entire study. Bronchial hyperresponsiveness was initially noted in 18% of workers. About 15% of workers without bronchial hyperresponsiveness developed it during the observation period. As well, about 15% of those who had bronchial responsiveness initially lost it during the period of follow-up. Bronchial hyperresponsiveness was associated with a decrease in the level of pulmonary function. Workers with bronchial hyperresponsiveness had a higher prevalence of plicatic acid IgE antibodies, although the percent with positive tests was never higher than 21% and in one subgroup as low a 6% positivity. These investigators felt that these results supported a contention that immunologic sensitivity to plicatic acid and change in airway caliber were associated with the occurrence of bronchial hyperresponsiveness in cedar workers. However, most observers remain skeptical that this is the case.

Additional studies by Shimoda et al. in Seattle on the contractile effects of western red cedar were directed at elucidating pathogenic mechanisms.[47] The contractile effects of thujic and plicatic acids derived from western red cedar on isolated canine tracheal smooth muscle were studied to determine if they were direct spasmogens. Both thujic acid and plicatic acids contracted the smooth-muscle preparations. Atropine and verapamil inhibited contractile responses by both thujic and plicatic acids. However, histamine (H_1,H_2)-receptor blockade as well as adrenergic and serotonin blockade failed to influence the observed contractile effect. Their observations suggested that thujic and plicatic acids contracted canine tracheal smooth muscle via activation of acetylcholine receptors. Thujic acid appeared to be more potent than plicatic acid.[47]

The effects of plicatic acid on histamine and leukotriene release in bronchoalveolar fluid was studied in six individuals with western red cedar asthma.[48] These individuals all had bronchoscopic evidence of bronchospasm within 10 minutes of challenge with plicatic acid, this despite the fact that the majority of prior bronchial challenge studies had resulted in either isolated, delayed, or dual asthmatic responses. Although six nonoccupational asthmatics were included in the study, none was challenged with plicatic acid. The latter would have proven extremely useful in determining the bronchial specificity of plicatic acid. Plicatic acid-induced bronchoconstriction was accompanied by increased levels of histamine and leukotriene E_4.

The Seattle group extended their initial observations to examine the toxicity of plicatic acid on pulmonary epithelium. Toxic effects were studied on laboratory models with monolayers of rat type II and human A549 alveolar epithelial cells, rat tracheal explants, and intact rat lungs as targets. These studies demonstrated that plicatic acid was toxic to tracheal, bronchial, and alveolar epithelial cells. The investigators hypothesized that direct toxicity of plicatic acid contributed to the acute bronchospastic syndrome and chronic bronchitis observed in some workers.[49]

Summary and Unresolved Issues

Western red cedar asthma was originally described in 1926 in Japan,[1,9,11,12] with subsequent descriptions in the United Kingdom,[10] United States,[14] and Australia.[15,16] The first comprehensive description was made by Gandevia and Milne.[17] In 1971 Chan-Yeung published the first of a large series of observations[19] on this condition and has since dominated the scientific observations in this area.[21,22,24,28-28,36,37,39,43,44,46,48] It is important to understand that all studies on this condition have been retrospective in nature. The clinical features of this condition are summarized in Tables 1 and 2.

A number of issues remain unresolved and controversial. First, the use of western red cedar extract or purified plicatic acid for the purposes of bronchial provocation has never been justified against the alternative use of freshly cut western red cedar dust. It is probable, based on data available, that plicatic acid may play a significant role in the pathogenesis of western red cedar asthma.[21,22,26] However, there is insufficient evidence at this point to exclude other constituents in western red cedar dust as also playing a role. There is ample evidence that freshly cut western red cedar dust will provoke immediate, delayed, and dual asthmatic responses.[14,20,29,30] There is no evidence that would indicate that plicatic acid is either more specific or safer as a bronchial challenge agent. In fact, there are only four nonoccupational asthmatics who are reported to have been challenged and said to have responded negatively to plicatic acid.[21] These four asthmatics were not described in terms of their status, severity, or their specific spirometric sequelae upon challenge.

An opportunity to study the bronchospastic effects of plicatic acid in some additional non-work-related asthmatic subjects was recently deferred.[48] Given the fact that plicatic acid has been shown in laboratory models or humans to: (1) directly induce bronchospasm via activation of acetylcholine receptors[47]; (2) release histamine and leukotriene E_4[48]; (3) activate the classical complement pathway independent of immunoglobulin[37]; (4) induce specific IgE antibodies to a plicatic acid-human serum albumin conjugate on selected individuals[39]; and (5) produce lytic damage to alveolar, tracheal, and bronchial epithelial cells[49] would support the view that plicatic agent induces its effects by a variety of different specific and nonspecific mechanisms (Fig. 4).

It has been maintained by many that the characteristic dual or isolated delayed asthmatic response seen with plicatic acid is more compatible with a specific immunologic response as opposed to a simple irritant effect. However, very initial observations using sophisticated spirometric measurements[22] as well as recent bronchoscopic observations demonstrated the presence of an immediate bronchospastic effect in nearly all plicatic acid challenged subjects.[48] Aside from this, it is evident that the delayed asthmatic reaction can be seen with a variety of nonimmune stimuli, such as exercise and distilled water, among others.[50,132]

Secondly, no one has ever demonstrated plicatic acid in the ambient work environment of a cedar sawmill, a cabinet shop, or similar locale. Since it is a nonvolatile constituent,[5-7] one wonders whether this agent is aerosolized in any significant amount. Finally, the dose used in bronchial provocation is totally arbitrary and has never been calibrated against the effects of western red cedar dust.[49]

The third major problem relating to the current information on western red cedar asthma relates to the retrospective nature of all the studies. Chan-Yeung has stated that the only way to determine the true prevalence of western red cedar asthma is to carry out a prospective study with a preemployment methacholine or histamine challenge test to determine initial bronchial reactivity.[26-28,51] Such a study has not been done and, as yet, it is difficult to be certain how many cases of western red cedar asthma reported in the literature represent a flare of preexisting disease or a postviral sequela.[35,52,53]

OCCUPATIONAL ASTHMA SECONDARY TO OTHER WOOD DUSTS

A variety of other wood dusts have been associated with occupational respiratory and dermatologic disease.[2-4,14,38,54,55] The woods

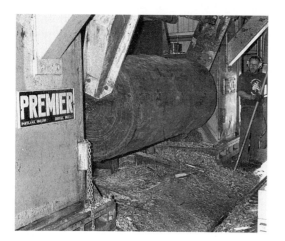

FIGURE 5. Debarking machine at a Northwest lumber mill.

causing the most significant problems are the hardwoods used for special projects, furniture, hobby needs, and so forth. Respiratory disease

has been linked to wood dust as an irritant,[2,3,45,59] as an allergen,[4,14,24] and as a cause of allergic alveolitis.[56,57] The bark of many trees or contaminants on its surface has been a source of both respiratory allergy[24,58] and a variety of contact dermatoses[24,54] (Figs. 2 and 5). The data relating to the induction of bronchial asthma de novo are quite limited and for the most part consist of anecdotal case reports. Most cases were investigated by epicutaneous skin tests, immunodiffusion for precipitins, and bronchial provocation. In the case of skin testing and examination for the presence of precipitating antibodies, aqueous or alcohol extracts of the wood dust were used. For bronchial provocation, either the dust itself was used, with a modification of the method established by Pickering et al.,[20] or an aqueous or alcohol extract was used, with modifications of previously reported techniques.[14,17,21] Table 3 summarizes the wood dusts implicated as a cause for occupational asthma.[59-74]

TABLE 3. *Wood Species Incriminated in the Induction of Occupational Asthma*

Wood Species	Patients Studied	Epicutaneous Tests	Precipitin Tests	Bronchial Provocation	Ref. No.
Kejeat wood *(Pterocorpus angolensis)*	1	Positive	ND*	ND	60
Cocabolla wood *(Dalbergia retusa)*	3	Positive†	ND	ND	4
Oak	1	Negative	Positive	Immed.	14
Mahogany	1	Negative	Positive	Dual	
Cedar *(Thuja plicata)*	2	Negative	Positive	Delayed	
Abiruana wood *(Pouteria)*	2	Positive	Negative	Dual	61
California redwood *(Sequoia sempervirens)*	2	Negative	Negative	Dual	62
Cedar of Lebanon *(Cedra libani)*	6	Negative	Negative	ND	63
Iroko or kambala *(Chlorophora excelsa)*	2	Negative	ND	Dual	74
		Positive	Negative	Delayed	20
Ramin wood *(Gonystylus bancanus)*	2	Positive‡	Negative	Immed.	64
African zebrawood *(Microberlinia)*	1	Positive‡	Negative	Dual	65
Abachi	12	Positive	Positive	NA§‡	60
Cherry	2	ND	Negative	NA	
Iroko	8	Positive	Negative	NA	
Mahogany	12	Positive(11)	Positive	NA	
Makore	18	Positive	Positive	NA	
Manzonia	24	ND	Negative	NA	
Oak	2	ND	Negative	NA	
Okume	4	Positive	Positive	NA	
Rosewood	7	ND	Negative	NA	
Soapbark dust *(Quillaja saponaria)*	1	ND‡	ND	Immed.	67
Tanganyika aningre	3	Positive	Negative	Dual	68
African maple (obeche) *(Triplochiton scleroxylon)*	11	Positive‡	Negative or ND	Immed. or dual	64,69,70 71||,75
Ebony wood *(Diospyros crassiflora)*	1	Negative	ND	Delayed	4,72
Ash wood *(Fraxinus americana)*	1	Negative‡	ND	Immed.	73
Spindle tree wood *(Euonymus europaeus)*	1	Positive	ND	Immed.	133||

* ND: not done; †: positive immediate reactions to patch testing, reverted to negative after immunotherapy; ‡: additional or solitary in vitro assays carried out confirming presence of IgE-specific antibodies, i.e., RAST or REIA; § NA: bronchial provocation done, but methodology and results not reported in detail; ||: reference 71 may include observations made in references 64 and 69; ||: RAST, RAST-inhibition and Western blot also carried out.

In addition to occupational asthma, African maple (obeche) has been implicated as a cause for contact urticaria.[70]

OCCUPATIONAL ASTHMA ASSOCIATED WITH COLOPHONY (PINE RESIN)

(Electronic Workers' Asthma)

History and Chemistry

Colophony (rosin) is a solid material left after turpentine has been distilled from the oleoresin and canal resin of pine. It has been used as a soldering flux since ancient times. It was described by Pliny in 77 A.D.[76] and is mentioned in an ancient manuscript with various recipes (*Mappa clavicula*, circa 850).[77] The recipes describe the early version of a soldering cream as containing two parts of axle grease, a third of colophony, and an equal quantity of tin filings. Since that time colophony has been the basis of soft soldering fluxes.

Gum resin is produced by collecting crude oleoresin from scarification of the pine tree. The soluble acids are removed by addition of water. The material is then distilled. The distillate is turpentine, and the residue is colophony. Colophony is a mixture of resin acids, each containing a single reactive carboxyl group. Two basic types of resins exist, i.e., the pimaric type containing a methyl or vinyl at position 7, or the abietic type with an isopropyl at position 7. There is also a neutral fraction (Fig. 6). There are 8 principal resin acids, including abietic, levopimaric, palustic, neoabietic, dehydroabietic, tetrahydroabietic, dextopimaric, and isodextropimaric. Colophonies from different species of pine differ in the ratio of abietic to pimaric type resin acids.[78,79]

Colophony can also be produced from the dead stumps of cut pines (wood rosin) or the tall oil left over after the Kraft pulp paper process (tall oil rosin). The composition and

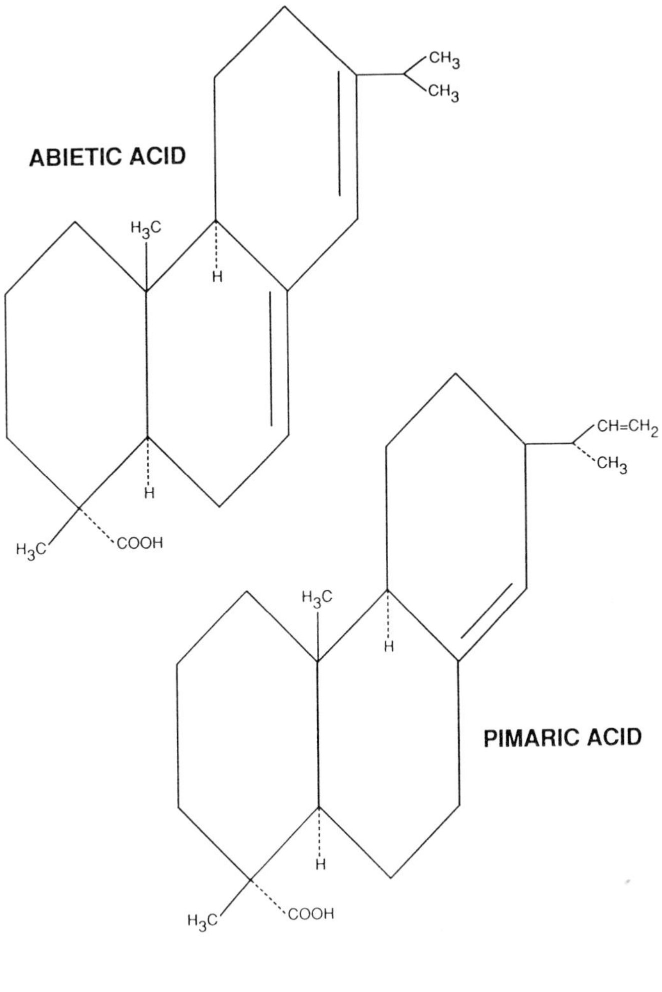

FIGURE 6. Structural formulas of the two basic types of resin acids in colophony, i.e., pimaric acid and abietic acid.

ABIETIC ACID

PIMARIC ACID

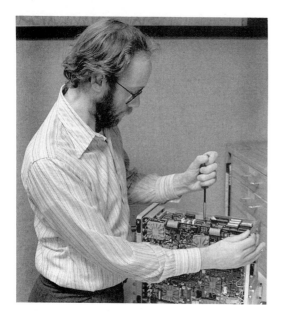

FIGURE 7.   An electronic industry worker using a soft soldering technique in the final stages of assembly.

containing particulate fluoride and a mist of unchanged ethanolamine. The latter compound belongs to the diamine class of chemicals and is used as the second major alternative to acid anhydrides as a hardener curing agent. Cable joiner workers inhaling these fumes have developed occupational asthma.[84-86]

In addition to hard soldering, soft soldering techniques have also been shown to produce occupational asthma (Fig. 7). Soft soldering employs lead/tin alloys at lower temperatures (250–450°C). In the electronics industry, non-corrosive fluxes are used that usually contain colophony. Soft corrosive fluxes are used in plumbing and in the manufacture of tin containers and radiators. Most of these fluxes contain ammonium chloride and zinc chloride. Weir et al. reported two cases of occupational asthma caused by this type of soldering flux.[87] Symptoms occurred only after a latent period of at least 12 months in both cases.

Clinical Features

The initial report of colophony-induced asthma was by Fawcett et al.[88] The flux-cored solder usually employed in electronics work is a metal alloy with a tin or lead substrate and a flux consisting of colophony with a small concentration of activator. Corrosive fluxes are used in plumbing and in the manufacture of tin containers and radiators. Subsequent expanded retrospective studies[89-94] indicated that most patients who developed colophony asthma had been exposed to solder flux fumes for several years before developing the symptoms. Five of 21 patients were noted to have preexisting asthma that had remitted.[89] There was no greater incidence of atopy. At their earliest phase, symptoms tended to appear many hours after arriving at work and in 90% tended to persist into the night. As would be expected, wheezing respirations and chest tightness were the most common presenting symptom. Over half of the patients had productive cough with clear-to-opaque sputum. A similar number of affected workers complained of rhinoconjunctivitis, with a smaller number complaining of headache and diffuse myalgias. The majority of workers recovered completely within 2 weeks of having been removed from further exposures. Bronchial provocation studies with flux-cored solder or colophony reproduced asthmatic symptoms in all workers.[89,94] Most patients demonstrated isolated delayed or dual asthmatic reactions. Eleven of 21 patients

purity are dependent on the method of preparation.[78,79] The U.S. produces a slightly lower grade colophony (American WW colophony, Hercules Powder Co.) which causes slightly less reaction in sensitized workers when compared to the Portuguese Y colophony (Socer).[80] Unlike plicatic acid, which has been identified as the principal constituent of western red cedar causing asthma,[21] colophony has actually been measured in ambient pine forest air[81] and in a factory making flux-cored solder and found to be high as 1.92 mg/M[3].[82] Abietic acid and its isomers make up approximately 90% of colophony.[83]

Electronic circuit boards have crept into many aspects of modern life in the last several decades. They are used in computers, and communication and recreational devices. The electronics industry is one of the fastest growing industries worldwide, employing a huge workforce. A number of different soldering processes have been employed in this diverse industry.

Hard soldering is frequently employed by aluminum cable joiners and is carried out at high temperatures (700°C). Aluminum is widely used as a material for electric cables. When heated in the process of soldering, it forms a film of oxide, and the fluxes normally used for copper wire are not satisfactory. A suitable flux contains amino-ethyl ethanolamine mixed with zinc oxide and fluoroborate. In the process of soldering, fumes are liberated

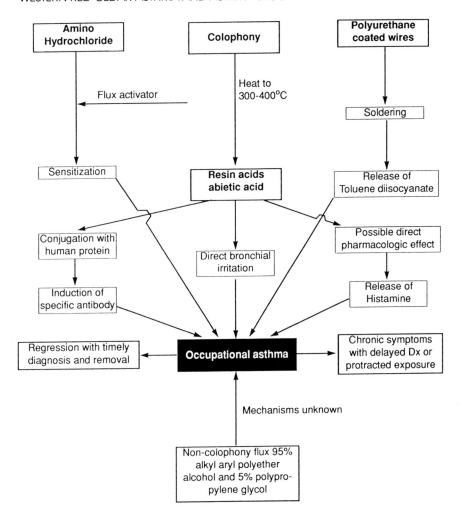

FIGURE 8.   Schematic diagram depicting potential pathogenetic mechanisms in the development of electronic workers' asthma.

continued to have asthmatic symptoms associated with exercise and infections despite removal from work.[85]

Pathogenesis (Fig. 8)

A number of studies were carried out in electronic workers to define the specific agent and pathogenesis of the asthmatic reaction.[92,94] Burge et al. carried out studies comparing all the constituents of two commonly employed flux-cored solders. It was determined that fumes from heated colophony were the principal etiologic agent. Since abietic acid (Fig. 6) was the major resin in colophony, further studies using commercial grade abietic acid reproduced the asthmatic reactions in the workers tested.[94] It was further determined

that fumes from the methyl ester of colophony, which was likely to contain similar breakdown products to the unesterified colophony, produced significantly less reaction than unaltered colophony with similar levels of fume.[94]

The unsaturated double bonds of the resin acids appeared less important for protein binding than the carboxyl groups. This was similar to the mechanisms proposed for toluene diisocyanate sensitivity, in which the tolyl group was felt to be immunogenic.[95] This group of investigators felt that the latent period observed, the relatively small proportion of electronic workers affected, and the low levels of colophony required to induce asthma supported an allergic rather than an irritant mechanism. Despite this, no specific antibody to abietic acid (or a conjugate) has ever been demonstrated. The authors further argued that if colophony fumes were acting as a mere irritant, there would be good correlation between histamine challenge and colophony. This was not the case.

Further evidence implicating intact resin acids in the pathogenesis of work-related asthma was provided by Burge and co-workers in 1986.[96] All prior cases of colophony asthma had occurred in the setting of soldering at temperatures between 350–450°C. The colophony understandably underwent some decomposition, raising the possibility that the occupational asthma was related to a breakdown pyrolytic product. However, a patient was presented who had classic symptoms of occupational asthma that developed while he was crushing colophony at room temperature.[96]

In evaluating patients with possible colophony-induced asthma, one must remember that esters of colophony and phenol-formaldehyde-modified colophony are present in cigarettes, where they are used as adhesives and filter fillings.[89] Colophony is also used as a hot-melt glue, particularly as an adhesive for can labels as well as in hairsprays, paints, and pine-essence cleaners.[49] A few patients have been described as developing symptoms upon exposure to pine dust.[85]

Other Causes of Asthma in Electronic Workers

Polyurethane-coated wires are occasionally used in some electronic factories. This process is especially applicable for coil winding. Fortunately, this represents a very small proportion of wires used and involves only a few workers. When these wires are tinned by dipping them into molten solder or when they are soldered, fumes of toluene diisocyanate (TDI) are liberated. High concentrations of TDI can easily be produced unless good local exhaust ventilation is present.[97,98]

Since the 1930s a variety of activators have been added to colophony to accelerate the reaction. Some electronic workers with nonspecific bronchial hyperreactivity have been found to react to fumes of the flux activator alone. Amine hydrochloride is one of the more popular multicore flux activators. Workers have been described with immediate or delayed asthmatic reactions to this material.[94] Fewer workers reacted to amine hydrobromide.

Stevens reported an electronics assembler who developed reversible bronchospasm to fumes of a flux composed of 95% alkyl aryl polyether alcohol and 5% polypropylene glycol.[99] Inhalation challenge was carried out that reproduced the asthmatic symptoms. The manufacturer of this flux indicated that heating between 400–500°C would pyrolyze aldehydes, ketones, organic esters, and acids that could act as mucosal irritants. The patient was not challenged with isolated pyrolytic products.

VEGETABLE GUM-INDUCED OCCUPATIONAL ASTHMA

(Printers' Asthma)

History and Chemistry

Natural vegetable gums are high-polymer carbohydrate products that are generally insoluble in alcohol and other organic solvents, but generally soluble or dispersible in water.[100,101] When they react with water, they generally produce mucilages. They occur as exudates from various trees and shrubs in tropical areas (Table 4). Their aqueous solutions possess suspending and stabilizing properties, and thus they have been used as protective colloids and emulsifying agents in food and pharmaceutical products, as textile sizers, and as a wet-end additive in paper-making.

TABLE 4.   *Industries Employing Vegetable Gums*

Common Names	Derivation	Industrial Application
Gum acacia	*Acacia senegal*	Food processing
Gum arabic	Bark of African tree	Pharmaceuticals, printing
Babal gum	*Acacia verek*	Inferior gum acacia
Gum Amritsar	*Acacia modesta*	Calico printing, textiles
Gum lini	Linseed	Substitute for gum arabic
Gumthus	French pine resin	Frankincense
Gum tragacanth	*Astragalus gummifer*; Asian vegetable	Printing industry
Guar gum Guaran Guarin	*Cyamopsis tetragonolobus*; Bush-like plant found in tropical regions of Africa, Arabia, India, North Australia, as well as Texas and Arizona	Pharmaceuticals, food processing, emulsions, cosmetics, paper, fracturing aid in oil wells, interior coat of fire nozzles, thickener
Karaya gum	*Sterculia urens*; Indian vegetable	Tragacanth substitute, colostomy paste

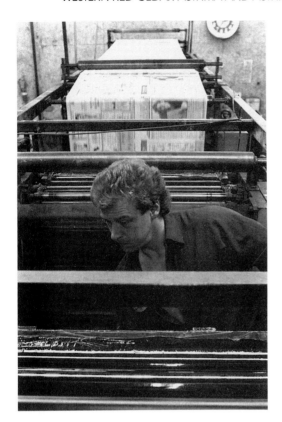

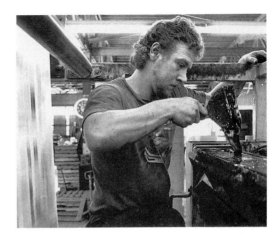

FIGURE 10. Worker shown adding ink to a large printing press.

FIGURE 9. Worker in a newspaper printing facility. Typically, no respiratory protection is being used.

The vegetable gums were initially introduced into the industrial revolution within the printing industry. The most popular material was derived from the bark of a tree, *Acacia senegal*. The juice obtained from the bark formed a viscous colloidal solution. It was extensively used in the printing trade to prevent freshly printed sheets from sticking to each other (Fig. 9). It also served to stabilize the ink from running (Fig. 10). It was applied in the form of a fine spray, which permeated the work area. In addition to gum acacia or gum arabic, gums obtained from the *Astragalus* genus (tragacanth) and from the *Sterculia* genus (karaya) are also employed in the printing industry (*Sterculia* is from the Latin for manure, which alludes to the odor of some species).

The initial case of occupational asthma secondary to gum acacia was reported by Spielman and Baldwin.[102] The mechanism appeared to be clearly IgE-mediated. Both direct and passive skin testing were positive. A year later Bullen and Stearns reported a hairdresser with chronic rhinoconjunctivitis secondary to Karaya gum.[103] In 1938 Humperdinck recorded

34 cases of printers' asthma due to allergy to gum arabic.[104] From this point forward, vegetable gum-induced asthma became a growing problem in this group of workers. Because of the manner in which it was applied, all workers were exposed, and within 5 years up to 30% of those exposed were noted to have developed symptoms. Asthma appeared sooner in those with atopic backgrounds. The allergic basis of the process was supported by the characteristic latent period, prominent immediate (type I) skin reactivity, ability to passively transfer, and confirmatory bronchial provocation studies.[105-107]

Gelfand described a tragacanth-induced asthma in an individual in the import business, among others.[108] Cross-reactivity between tragacanth and acacia was noted by skin testing and Prausnitz-Küstner transfer. Each of the individuals with vegetable-gum induced asthma was shown to have positive skin tests except one. Karaya was not shown to share antigens with either tragacanth or acacia.[108]

Although vegetable gums were phased out of the printing trade in the 1950s, there has been some resurgence of their use in the last decade, and the clinician should be on the alert. Recently, there has been a marked increase in the use of guar gum in the pharmaceutical industry. It has enjoyed an expanding role as a substrate for timed-release formulations, to encapsulate sensitive vitamins and enhance storage capacity, and as a possible hypocholesterolemic agent. It has also found some use in diabetics to influence postprandial glucose adsorption.[109] Kanerva et al. described three cases of work-related allergic rhinitis from guar gum powder. Two of these occurred in a rubber cable insulator factory and another in a paper factory.[109] The diagnosis was confirmed with skin testing and a nasal provocation study. The authors advise proper respiratory protection and optimum ventilation to protect workers.

Recently, Lagier et al. described three additional cases who developed occupational asthma upon exposure to guar gum.[110] The individual had been exposed in a pharmaceutical firm using guar gum as a tablet hardener. There was a 7-year latent period before developing the asthma, but after the symptoms began, the individual also noted angioedema of lips when eating ice cream and salad dressings containing guar gum. Two other subjects worked at a carpet manufacturing plant where guar gum was used to fix colors. Each of the affected individuals had strongly positive skin tests to guar gum, but negative reactions to karaya, tragacanth, and acacia. Bronchial challenge studies were also positive. Preliminary epidemiologic studies in a carpet manufacturing plant have indicated a 5% prevalence of skin reactivity and a 2% prevalence of occupational asthma.[111]

There are some interesting observations relating to potential cross-reactivity among various plant constituents. There are some data suggesting that gum acacia cross-reacts with tragacanth, but neither shares antigens with karaya.[108] Recent studies suggest guar gum does not cross-react with acacia, tragacanth, or karaya.[110] One patient who had classic IgE-mediated reactions to quillaia bark extract was found to have positive RAST reactivity to gum acacia and tragacanth.[67]

WOOD DUST-INDUCED IRRITATION AND HYPERSENSITIVITY PNEUMONITIS

Although beyond the scope of this text, brief mention of the capacity of wood dusts to induce hypersensitivity pneumonitis will be made.[56-57] In most instances, the etiologic agent has been traced to contamination of bark or wood dust by a variety of fungal species. In this respect, *Thermoactinomyces* have been frequently isolated from samples of damp sawdust from many parts of the world.[58]

Maple bark strippers' disease was first described by Tower et al. in 1932.[112] Individuals whose job it was to strip bark from maple logs developed the disease due to inhalation of *Cryptostroma corticale* (coniosporum). The latter grows in the bark of both the maple and sycamore tree, appearing as blackened areas underneath the bark. Further studies elucidating the pathogenesis were published by Emanuel and his group.[113-114]

An individual with advanced allergic alveolitis due to California redwood *(Sequoia sempervirens)* was reported by Cohen and his colleagues in 1967.[56] The patient had worked for 17 years as a sawyer in a redwood lumber mill. He had significant interstitial lung disease when first seen, with a biopsy showing septal thickening, plasma cell infiltrates, and granulomatous pneumonitis. Skin tests with redwood extracts failed to elicit a reaction. However, the patient's serum contained precipitins to this extract. Culture of the sawdust grew several species of fungi, but only *Graphium* and *Aureobasidium pullulans (Pullularia)* showed antigens with immunologic identity to redwood. Based on this rather tenuous observation, these fungi were incriminated as the cause of the illness.

Wood pulp workers' disease has been described in a number of workers within the paper mill industry.[3,14,115] In the most recent report,[115] two patients were challenged with extracts of *C. corticale* without response. A subsequent challenge with *Alternaria* recreated the symptoms and resulted in a dual response. There were significant precipitins in both patient sera against *Alternaria*.

Suberosis was initially described in 1968 by Avila and Villar in Portuguese workers exposed to the bark dust of cork *(Quercus suber)* that was found to be contaminated with *Penicillium frequentans.*[116] Many workers demonstrated a dual reaction, with bronchospasm associated with an allergic alveolitis not dissimilar to allergic bronchopulmonary aspergillosis.[116] A similar process was described in farmers handling wood fuel chips contaminated with *Penicillium species.*[117]

A number of other investigators have reported hypersensitivity pneumonitis in wood trimmers and forest workers (woodman's disease) as well as sawmill workers. A variety of fungi have been incriminated including *Rhizopus, Paecilomyces, Aspergillus,* and *Thermoactinomyces vulgaris.*[118-121]

Hypersensitivity pneumonitis secondary to wood dust without apparent fungal contamination has been reported but is clearly an unusual process.[14,122] The authors have seen significant irritation when chips are milled to a fine powder (wood flour) used as a filler in a variety of products. The dust levels in these mills reach extraordinarily high levels.

OCCUPATIONAL ASTHMA CAUSED BY MISCELLANEOUS PLANT MATERIALS

Numerous isolated reports of work-related asthma secondary to plant-derived materials have been published.[123] These have included dusts from plants, especially cotton and grain dusts.[124] Sensitivity has also been reported to the fruits, seeds, leaves, and pollens of various plants. Frequently, instances of plant-related allergy occur in the setting of an occupation, and a few of these work-related allergies will be described below.

Instances of occupational allergy to plant pollens have been reported. The majority involve one of the 30,000 species of the *Compositae* family. This large number of species has been grouped into 14 tribes, most of which are insect pollinated. Many pollens from this family share cross-reacting allergens.[125] A common example from this family is the sunflower *(Helianthus)*, whose pollen is imperfectly insect pollinated so that a portion has airborne dissemination. Sunflower pollen has been incriminated in the development of work-related dermatitis.[126] Bousquet et al. reported a case of occupational rhinitis and asthma caused by both inhalation and ingestion of sunflower pollen.[127] Similar observations have been made in Japan among chrysanthemum cultivators.[128]

Several unique causes of work-related asthma have been reported in the floral industry. Among the incriminated allergens in florists is the plant *Gypsophila paniculata*, commonly referred to as baby's-breath (from the profusion of small white or pink flowers). Twiggs et al. reported the first case of allergic conjunctivitis, rhinitis, and bronchial asthma in a florist.[129] A second patient was recently evaluated by the same group and specific sensitivity was confirmed by skin tests, bronchial challenge, and the demonstration of specific IgE antibodies to baby's-breath by the direct RAST.[130] The latter was felt to be quite specific by virtue of a lack of inhibition of the RAST by other plant-derived proteins. These investigators felt that baby's-breath may be an important occupational allergen in the floral industry.

Axelsson et al. have reported on a large series of sensitized indoor plant handlers to dust generated by weeping fig *(Ficus benjamina)*.[131] A total of 78 employees from four plant-leasing firms with significant exposures to this plant were studied. Eighteen had developed allergic rhinoconjunctivitis and/or bronchial asthma. Thirty patients (13 from the sensitized and 17 from the non-sensitized group) demonstrated contact urticaria. The principal allergen appeared to reside in the sap (latex) of the plant. All but two of the sensitized handlers were shown to have positive RAST and skin tests to the isolated antigen. Four patients with asthma had positive bronchial challenge tests to the antigen.

Occupational asthmas secondary to plant-related dust are covered in other chapters. These include such substances as grain dust (Chapter 9), wheat and rye flour dust (Chapter 9), castor bean and coffee bean dust (Chapter 10) and garlic dust (Chapter 11).

REFERENCES

1. Seki K: American cedar-induced asthma. J Jap Soc Intern Med 13:884, 1926.
2. Ordman D: Bronchial asthma caused by inhalation of wood dust. Ann Allergy 7:492, 1949.
3. Michaels L: Lung changes in woodworkers. Can Med Assoc J 98:1150, 1967.
4. Eaton KK: Respiratory allergy to exotic wood dust. Clin Allergy 3:307, 1973.
5. Gardner JA: Chemistry and utilization of western red cedar. Department of Forestry Publication No. 1023. Ottawa: Dept. of Forestry, 1963.
6. Barton GM, MacDonald BF: The chemistry of utilization of western red cedar. Dept. of Fisheries and Forestry. Canadian Forestry Service, Publication No. 1023, 1971.
7. Hillis W (ed): Wood Extractives and Their Significance to the Pulp and Paper Industry. New York, Academic Press, 1962.
8. Belleau B, Burke J: Occupancy of adrenergic receptors and inhibition of catechol O-methyl transferase by tropolones. J Med Chem 6:755, 1963.
9. Tagawa J: On western red cedar asthma. J Jap Soc Intern Med 17:420, 1929.
10. Doig AT: Other lung diseases due to dust. Postgrad Med J 25:639, 1949.
11. Komatsu F: Respiratory allergy in woodworkers. In 14th Int. Cong. of Occup. Health, Madrid, 1963. Exc. Medica Intern. Cong. Series No. 62, p 1748.
12. Aoki M: Asthma due to western red cedar among carpenters making furniture. J Allerg 17:428, 1968.
13. Mitsui S, Shi Karai K, Komatsu J, et al: Study on so-called "Beisugi asthma." J Allerg 19:182, 1970.
14. Sosman AJ, Schlueler DP, Fink JN, et al: Hypersensitivity to wood dust. N Engl J Med 281:977, 1969.
15. Milne J, Gandevia B: Occupational asthma and rhinitis due to western red cedar *(Thuja plicata)*. Med J Aust 2:741, 1969.
16. Gandevia B: Ventilatory capacity during exposure to western red cedar *(Thuja plicata)*. Arch Environ Health 20:59, 1970.
17. Gandevia B, Milne J: Occupational asthma due to western red cedar *(Thuja plicata)* with special reference to bronchial reactivity. Br J Indust Med 27:235, 1970.
18. Mitchell C: Occupational asthma due to western red cedar *(Thuja plicata)*. Med J Aust 2:233, 1970.
19. Chan-Yeung M, Barton GM, McLean L, et al: Bronchial reactions to western red cedar *(Thuga plicata)*. Can Med Assoc J 105:56, 1971.

20. Pickering CAC, Batten JC, Pepys J: Asthma due to inhaled wood dust: Western red cedar and iroko. Clin Allergy 2:213, 1972.

21. Chan-Yeung M, Barton GM, McLean L, et al: Occupational asthma and rhinitis due to western red cedar *(Thuja plicata)*. Am Rev Respir Dis 108:1094, 1973.

22. Chan-Yeung M: Maximal expiratory flow and airway resistance during induced bronchoconstriction in patients with asthma due to western red cedar. Am Rev Respir Dis 108:1103, 1973.

23. Ishizaki T, Shida T, Miyamoto T, et al: Occupational asthma from western red cedar dust *(Thuja plicata)* in furniture factory workers. J Occup Med 15:580, 1973.

24. Mitchell JC, Chan-Yeung M: Contact allergy from Frullania and respiratory allergy from Thuja. Can Med Assoc J 110:653, 1974.

25. Mue S, Ise T, Yasuo O, et al: A study of western red cedar-induced asthma. Ann Allergy 34:297, 1975.

26. Chan-Yeung M: Fate of occupational asthma: A follow-up study of patients with occupational asthma due to western red cedar *(Thuja plicata)*. Am Rev Respir Dis 116:1023, 1977.

27. Chan-Yeung M, Ashley MJ, Corey P, et al: A respiratory survey of cedar millworkers. I. Prevalence of symptoms and pulmonary function abnormalities. J Occup Med 20:323, 1978.

28. Ashley MJ, Corey P, Chan-Yeung M, et al: A respiratory survey of cedar millworkers. II. Influence of work-related and host factors on prevalence of symptoms and pulmonary function abnormalities. J Occup Med 20:328, 1978.

29. Hamilton RD, Crockett AJ, Ruffin RE, et al: Bronchial reactivity in western red cedar-induced asthma. Aust NZ Med 9:417, 1979.

30. Cockcroft DW, Cotton DJ, Mink JT: Non-specific bronchial hyperreactivity after exposure to western red cedar. Am Rev Respir Dis 119:505, 1979.

31. Cockcroft DW, Ruffin RE, Dolovich J, et al: Allergen-induced increase in non-allergic bronchial reactivity. Clin Allergy 7:503, 1977.

32. Cartier A, Thomson NC, Frith PA, et al: Allergen-induced increase in bronchial responsiveness to histamine: Relationship to the late asthmatic response and change in airway caliber. J Allergy Clin Immunol 70:170, 1982.

33. Orehek J, Massari JP, Gayrard P, et al: Effect of short-term low-level NO_2 exposure on bronchial sensitivity of asthmatic patients. J Clin Invest 57:301, 1976.

34. Islam MS, Vastag E, Uemer WT: Sulfur dioxide-induced bronchial hyperreactivity against acetylcholine. Int Arch Arbeits Med 29:221, 1972.

35. Empey DW, Laitinen LA, Jacobs L, et al: Mechanisms of bronchial hyperreactivity in normal subjects after upper respiratory tract infection. Am Rev Respir Dis 113:131, 1976.

36. Chan-Yeung M, Grzybowski S: Occupational asthma due to western red cedar *(Thuja plicata)*. In Frazier CA (ed): Occupational Asthma. New York, Van Nostrand, Reinhold, 1980, pp 79–90.

37. Chan-Yeung M, Gicias PC, Henson PM: Activation of complement by plicatic acid, the chemical responsible for asthma due to western red cedar *(Thuja plicata)*. J Allergy Clin Immunol 65:333, 1980.

38. Brooks SM, Edwards JJ, Edwards FH: An epidemiologic study of workers exposed to western red cedar and other wood dusts. Chest 80(Suppl):30S, 1981.

39. Tse KS, Chan H, Chan-Yeung M: Specific IgE antibodies in workers with occupational asthma due to western red cedar. Clin Allergy 12:249, 1982.

40. Butcher BT, O'Neil CE, Reed MA, et al: Radioallergosorbent testing of toluene diisocyanate-reactive individuals using p-tolyl isocyanate antigen. J Allergy Clin Immunol 66:213, 1980.

41. Maccia CA, Bernstein IL, Emmett EA, et al: In vitro demonstration of specific IgE in phthalic anhydride hypersensitivty. Am Rev Respir Dis 113:701, 1976.

42. Zeiss CR, Patterson R, Pruzanski JJ, et al: Trimellitic anhydride-induced airway syndromes: Clinical and immunologic studies. J Allergy Clin Immunol 60:96, 1977.

43. Chan-Yeung M, Lam S, Koener S: Clinical features and natural history of occupational asthma due to western red cedar *(Thuja plicata)*. Am J Med 72:411, 1982.

44. Chan-Yeung M: Immunologic and nonimmunologic mechanisms in asthma due to western red cedar *(Thuja plicata)*. J Allergy Clin Immunol 70:32, 1982.

45. Davies RJ, Pepys J: Occupational asthma. In Clark TJH, Godfrey S (eds): Asthma. Philadelphia, W.B. Saunders, 1977, pp 190–213.

46. Vedal S, Enarson DA, Chan H, et al: A longitudinal study of the occurrence of bronchial hyperresponsiveness in western red cedar workers. Am Rev Respir Dis 137:651, 1988.

47. Shimoda T, Lockey R, Altman LC, et al: Studies on the contractile effects of western red cedar extracts on canine tracheal smooth muscle strips. J Allergy Clin Immunol 79:142, 1987.

48. Chan-Yeung M, Chan H, Tse KS, et al: Histamine and leukotrienes release in bronchoalveolar fluid during plicatic acid-induced bronchoconstriction. J Allergy Clin Immunol 84:762, 1989.

49. Ayars GH, Altman LC, Frazier CE, et al: The toxicity of constituents of cedar and pine woods to pulmonary epithelium. J Allergy Clin Immunol 83:610, 1989.

50. Foresi A, Mattoli S, Corbo GM, et al: Late bronchial response and increase in methacholine hyperresponsiveness after exercise and distilled water challenge in atopic subjects with asthma and with dual asthmatic response to allergen inhalation. J Allergy Clin Immunol 112:829, 1975.

51. Chan-Yeung M: Prognosis in occupational asthma (editorial). Thorax 40:241, 1985.

52. Welliver RC: Upper respiratory infections in asthma. J Allergy Clin Immunol 72:341, 1983.

53. Slavin RG: Relationship of nasal disease and sinusitis to bronchial asthma. Ann Allergy 47:76, 1982.

54. Walker IC: Bronchial asthma. Oxford Med 2:128, 1939.

55. Birmingham DJ, Key MM: Occupational dermatoses. In U.S. Public Health Service: Occupational Diseases. Publ. No. 1097, Washington, D.C., 1964, p 27.

56. Cohen HI, Merigan K, Kosek JC, et al: Sequoiosis: A granulomatous pneumonitis associated with redwood sawdust inhalation. Am J Med 43:785, 1967.

57. Schlueter DP, Fink JN, Hensly GT: Wood-pulp workers' disease. A hypersensitivity pneumonitis. Ann Intern Med 77:914, 1972.

58. Emmanuel DA, Wenzel FJ, Lawton BR: Pneumonitis due to *Crytostroma corticale* (maple bark disease). N Engl J Med 274:1413, 1966.

59. Becker B, Snyder G: Sawdust: A health hazard. JAMA 238:1150, 1977.

60. Ordman D: Wood dust as an inhalant allergen: Bronchial asthma caused by kejeat wood *(Pterocorpus angolensis)*. S Afr Med J 23:973, 1949.

61. Booth BH, Lefoldt RH, Moffitt EM: Wood dust hypersensitivity. J Allergy Clin Immunol 57:352, 1976.

62. Chan-Yeung M, Abboud R: Occupational asthma due to California redwood *(Sequoia sempervirens)* dusts. Am Rev Respir Dis 114:1027, 1976.

63. Greenberg M: Respiratory symptoms following brief exposure to cedar of Lebanon *(Cedra libani)*. Clin Allergy 2:219, 1972.

64. Hinojosa M, Losada E, Moneo I, et al: Occupational asthma caused by African maple (obeche) and ramin: Evidence of cross reactivity between these two woods. Clin Allergy 16:145, 1986.

65. Bush RK, Yunginger JW, Reed CE: Asthma due to African zebra wood *(Microberlinia)* dust. Am Rev Respir Dis 117:601, 1978.

66. Girard JP, Surber R, Guberan E: Allergic manifestations due to wood dusts. In Frazier CA (ed): Occupational Asthma. New York, Van Nostrand, Reinhold, 1980, pp 91–101.

67. Raghu Prasad PK, Brooks SM, Litwin A, et al: *Quillaja* bark (soapbark)-induced asthma. J Allergy Clin Immunol 65:285, 1980.

68. Paggiaro PL, Cantalupi R, Filieri AM, et al: Bronchial asthma due to inhaled wood dust *Tanganyika aningre*. Clin Allergy 11:605, 1981.

69. Hinojosa M, Moneo I, Dominquez J, et al: Asthma caused by African maple *(Triplochiton scleroxylon)* wood dust. J Allergy Clin Immunol 74:782, 1984.

70. Innocenti A, Angotzi G: Occupational asthma due to sensitivity to *Triplochiton scleroxylon* (Samba, obeche). Med Lav 3:251, 1980.

71. Hinojosa M, Subiza J, Moneo I, et al: Contact urticaria caused by obeche wood *(Triplochiton scleroxylon)*: Report of eight patients. Ann Allergy 64:476, 1990.

72. Maestrelli P, Marcer G, Dal Vechhio L: Occupational asthma due to ebony wood *(Diospyros crassiflora)* dust. Ann Allergy 59:347, 1987.

73. Malo JL, Cartier A: Occupational asthma caused by exposure to ash wood dust *(Fraxinus americana)*. Eur Respir J 2:385, 1989.

74. Azofra J, Olaguibel JM: Occupational asthma caused by iroko wood. Allergy 44:156, 1989.

75. Weber N, Haussinger K: Bronchial asthma due to allergy to African maple. Prax Klin Pneumol 42:759, 1988.

76. Plinyu Naturalis Historica, Book 33, Chapter 30, 77 A.D. (Cited by Burge PS, et al, Thorax 34:13, 1979).

77. Mappae Clavicula (circa 1150) Phillipe-Corning Manuscript. Transactions of the Am Philosophical Soc 64:108, 1974 (Cited by Burge PS, et al, Thorax 34:13, 1979).

78. Lawrence RV: Oxidation of resin acids in wood chips. TAPPI 42:867, 1959.

79. Enos HI, Harris GC, Hendrick GW: Rosin and rosin derivatives. In Encyclopedia of Chemical Technology. London, John Wiley & Sons, 1968.

80. Burge PS, Harries MG, O'Brien I, et al: Bronchial provocation studies in workers exposed to fumes of electronic soldering fluxes. Clin Allergy 10:137, 1980.

81. Burge PS: Colophony and asthma. Lancet ii:591, 1979.

82. Burge PS, Edge G, Hawkins R, et al: Occupational asthma in a factory making flux-cored solder containing colophony. Thorax 36:828, 1981.

83. Fisher AA: Allergic contact dermatitis in a violinist. The role of abeitic acid, a sensitizeer in rosin (colophony), as the causative agent. Cutis 27:466, 1981.

84. McCann JK: Health hazard from flux used in joining aluminum electricity cables. Ann Occup Hyg 7:261, 1964.

85. Sterling GM: Asthma due to aluminum soldering flux. Thorax 22:533, 1967.

86. Pepys J, Pickering CAC: Asthma due to inhaled chemical fumes—aminoethyl ethanolamine in aluminum soldering flux. Clin Allergy 2:197, 1972.

87. Weir DC, Robertson AS, Jones S, et al: Occupational asthma due to soft corrosive soldering fluxes containing zinc chloride and ammonium chloride. Thorax 44:220, 1989.

88. Fawcett IW, Newman Taylor AJ, Pepys J: Asthma due to inhaled chemical agents—fumes from "multicore" soldering flux and colophony resin. Clin Allergy 6:577, 1976.

89. Burge PS, Harries MG, O'Brien IM, et al: Respiratory disease in workers exposed to solder flux fumes containing colophony (pine resin). Clin Allergy 8:1, 1978.

90. Burge PS, Perks W, O'Brien IM, et al: Occupational asthma in an electronics factory. Thorax 34:13, 1979.

91. Perks WH, Burge PS, Rehahn M, et al: Work-related respiratory disease in employees leaving an electronics factory. Thorax 34:19, 1979.

92. Burge PS, Perks WH, O'Brien IM, et al: Occupational asthma in an electronics factory: A case control study to evaluate etiological factors. Thorax 34:300, 1979.

93. Burge PS, O'Brien IM, Harries MG: Peak flow rate records in the diagnosis of occupational asthma due to colophony. Thorax 34:308, 1979.

94. Burge PS, Harries MG, O'Brien I, et al: Bronchial provocation studies in workers exposed to the fumes of electronic soldering fluxes. Clin Allergy 10:137, 1980.

95. Karol MH, Ioset HH, Alarie YC: Tolyl-specific IgE antibodies in workers with hypersensitivity to toluene diisocyanate. Am Ind Hyg Assoc J 39:454, 1978.

96. Burge PS, Wieland A, Robertson AS, et al: Occupational asthma due to unheated colophony. Br J Ind Med 43:559, 1986.

97. Paisley DPG: Isocyanate hazard from wire insulation; an old hazard in a new guise. Br J Ind Med 26:79, 1969.

98. Pepys J, Pickering CAC, Breslin ABX, et al: Asthma due to inhalation of chemical agents—toluene diisocyanate. Clin Allergy 2:225, 1972.

99. Stevens JJ: Asthma due to soldering flux: A polyether alcohol-polypropylene glycol mixture. Ann Allergy 36:419, 1976.

100. Hawley GG (ed): The Condensed Chemical Dictionary, 8th ed. New York, Van Nostrand Reinhold, 1971.

101. Smith F, Montgomery R: The chemistry of plant gums and mucilages. New York, Reinhold, 1959.

102. Spielman AD, Baldwin HS: Atopy to acacia (gum arabic). JAMA 101:466, 1933.

103. Bullen SS, Stearns S: Perennial hayfever from Indian gum (karaya gum). J Allergy 5:484, 1934.

104. Humperdinck K: Untersuchung-sergebnisse von drukern und hilfsarbeiterinnen an maschinen mit druckbestaubern. Arch Gewerbepath 9:559, 1938.

105. Bohner CB, Sheldon JM, Trenis JW: Sensitivity to gum acacia with a report of ten cases of asthma in printers. J Allergy 12:290, 1940.

106. Schwarting HH: Occupational allergy in printers. In Occupational Allergy. Leiden, H.E. Stenfert Kroese, 1958, p 278.

107. Fowler PBS: Printers' asthma. Lancet ii:755, 1952.

108. Gelfand HH: The allergenic properties of vegetable gums: A case of asthma due to tragacanth. J Allergy 14:203, 1943.

109. Kanerva L, Tupasela O, Jolanki R, et al: Occupational allergic rhinitis from guar gum. Clin Allergy 18:245, 1988.
110. Lagier F, Cartier A, Somer J, et al: Occupational asthma caused by guar gum. J Allergy Clin Immunol 85:785, 1990.
111. Malo JL, Cartier A, L'Archeveque J, et al: Prevalence of guar gum allergy in carpet manufacturing (submitted for publicaton and cited by Lagier, et al. in ref. 106).
112. Tower JW, Sweaney HC, Huron HC: Severe bronchial asthma apparently due to fungus spores found in maple bark. JAMA 99:453, 1932.
113. Emanuel DA, Wenzel FJ, Lawton BR: Pneumonitis due to cryptostroma corticale (maple bark disease). N Engl J Med 274:1413, 1966.
114. Wenzel FJ, Emanuel DA: The epidemiology of maple bark disease. Arch Environ Health 14:385, 1967.
115. Schlueter DP, Fink JN, Hensley GT: Wood-pulp workers' disease: A hypersensitivity pneumonitis caused by alternaria. Ann Intern Med 77:907, 1972.
116. Avila R, Villar TG: Suberosis respiratory disease in cork workers. Lancet i:620, 1968.
117. Van Assendelft AH, Raitio M, Turkia V: Fuel chip-induced hypersensitivity pneumonitis caused by penicillium species. Chest 87:394, 1985.
118. Wimander K, Berlin L: Recognition of allergic alveolitis in the trimming department of a Swedish sawmill. Eur J Respir Dis 61(Suppl 107):163, 1980.
119. Berlin L: Clinical and immunological data on "wood trimmer's disease" in Sweden. Eur J Respir Dis 61(Suppl 107):169, 1980.
120. Terho E, Husman K, Kotimaa M, et al: Extrinsic allergic alveolitis in a sawmill worker: A case report. Scand J Work Environ Health 6:153, 1980.
121. Dykewicz MS, Laufer P, Patterson R, et al: Woodman's disease: Hypersensitivity pneumonitis from cutting live trees. J Allergy Clin Immunol 81:455, 1988.
122. Howie AD, Boyd G, Moran F: Pulmonary hypersensitivity to ramin (Gonystylus bancanus). Thorax 31:585, 1976.
123. Butcher BT, Salvaggio JE: Occupational asthma. J Allergy Clin Immunol 78:547, 1986.
124. Dosman JA, Cotton DJ (eds): Occupational Pulmonary Disease: Focus on Grain Dust and Health. New York, Academic Press, 1980.
125. Leiferman KM, Gleich GJ, Jones RT: The cross-reactivity of IgE antibodies with pollen allergens. II. Analyses of various species of ragweed and other fall weed pollens. J Allergy Clin Immunol 58:140, 1976.
126. Moussitou FM, Cordero AA: Allergic dermatitis caused by sunflower. Pressa Med Argent 38:1052, 1951.
127. Bousquet J, Dhirert H, Clauzel AM, et al: Occupational allergy to sunflower pollen. J Allergy Clin Immunol 75:70, 1985.
128. Suzuki S, Kuroume T, Todokoro M, et al: Chrysanthemum pollenosis in Japan. Int Archs Allergy Appl Immun 48:800, 1975.
129. Twiggs JT, Yuninger JW, Agarwal MR, et al: Occupational asthma in a florist caused by the dried plant, baby's breath. J Allergy Clin Immunol 69:474, 1982.
130. Shroeckenstein DC, Meier-Davis S, Yuninger JW, et al: Allergens involved in occupational asthma caused by baby's breath (Gypsophila paniculata). J Allergy Clin Immunol 86:189, 1990.
131. Axelsson IGK, Johansson SGO, Zetterstrom O: Occupational allergy to weeping fig in plant keepers. Allergy 42:161, 1987.
132. Speelberg B, Panis EAH, Bijl D, et al: Late asthmatic responses after exercise challenge are reproducible. J Allergy Clin Immunol 87:1128, 1991.
133. Herold DA, Wahl R, Maasch HJ, et al: Occupational wood-dust sensitivity from Euonymus europaeus (spindle tree) and investigation of cross-reactivity between E.e. wood and Artemisia vulgaris pollen (mugwort). Allergy 46:186, 1991.

Chapter 9

BAKERS' ASTHMA AND REACTIONS SECONDARY TO SOYBEAN AND GRAIN DUST

Mark T. O'Hollaren, MD

It has long been known that exposure to grain dust and flour may cause respiratory symptoms of rhinitis and asthma. "Bakers' asthma" is caused by the occupational exposure to flour and/or grain dust in bakeries. Others may also suffer from grain dust-induced asthma, such as grain handlers, mill workers, or those employed in loading and unloading grain.[1] There are multiple potential allergens in both bakers' flour and in grain dust capable of inducing respiratory symptoms. These include not only various components of the grains themselves, but also contaminants of the flour or grain dust, including mold spores, insect parts, rat hairs and protein, pesticides, cellulose hairs and spikes, pollens, mineral particles, bacteria, mites, and other dust particles that may act as mechanical respiratory tract irritants. Because of distinct differences in pathogenesis of bakers' asthma and grain handlers' asthma, these diseases will be discussed separately.

BAKERS' ASTHMA

Historical Perspective

Ramazzini observed in 1713 that grain handlers were "almost all short of breath and rarely reached old age."[2] In 1908, Epstein reported 52 of 98 bakers studied had signs of pulmonary disease.[3] Immediate skin reactivity to wheat was demonstrated in bakers with reactive airway disease as early as 1909.[4] The association of positive skin tests to wheat

extracts in patients with flour allergy was followed by successful Prausnitz-Kustner (P-K) tests with the sera of workers allergic to wheat flour.[3,5] In 1927, Ancona attributed an epidemic of asthma to the presence of *Tinea granella* and *Pediculoides ventricosus* in the flour of a small village.[6] The concept of bakers' asthma as an occupational disease was introduced by DeBesche in 1929.[7] Occupational asthma mediated by soybean flour was first described over 50 years ago.[8]

Epidemiology and Etiology

Bakers' asthma is defined as an allergic sensitivity to inhaled flour dust. Progress on the delineation of all allergenic constituents of flour has been slow.[9] Rhinitis and asthma have long been known to be related to baking, and both have been shown to be IgE-mediated.[10,11] Numerous potential allergens have been implicated, including wheat and other cereals,[4,9-17] grain storage mite,[18] grain weevil,[19] dough improvers,[20] and *Alternaria* and *Aspergillus* organisms[21] (Table 1). Generally it is assumed that in addition to duration and intensity of exposure to the cereal antigen, specific working conditions are important in contributing to the sensitization of individuals to flour. These include ventilation and dust concentration, and inadequate machinery (especially in small bakery trades), as well as differing allergenic potencies of antigens themselves.[22]

Soybean flour has multiple antigens.[8] One of the soybean antigens appears identical to a

TABLE 1.   *Potential Allergens Present in Flour*

Wheat (albumin, globulin, gliadin, glutenin)

Soy, rye, barley

Grain storage mites

Grain weevil

Dough improvers

Alternaria and *Aspergillus* species

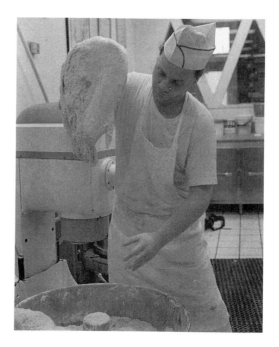

FIGURE 1.   Dough maker at French bakery.

component of green pea extract.[8] Occupational allergic symptoms of sneezing, coughing, and wheezing, accompanied by positive skin tests and radioallergosorbent test (RAST) sensitivity to soy extract, in addition to positive mecholyl challenge and positive bronchoprovocation tests to soy flour, have been noted in symptomatic soy flour workers.[8]

Longer workplace exposures to flour and cereal antigens are associated with an increased risk of acquiring asthma.[23] In one study, the incidence of positive skin tests to wheat antigen increased with the duration of exposure, whereas the incidence of skin test positivity to other allergens decreased with increased baking duration. This suggested that subjects who were sensitized to common allergens were leaving the baking industry, whereas those who stayed increased their risk of becoming sensitized to wheat.[10] Herxheimer reported that the prevalence of positive skin tests to wheat increased from 9% in bakers' recruits to over 30% by the fifth year of baking,[13] and both positive skin test reactivity to wheat antigen and nonspecific bronchial hyperreactivity increased with baking duration.[4]

Flour allergy has been reported to occur in between 10 and 30% of bakers.[13,24,25] However, these data may be biased, because individuals with severe work-related disease may leave the trade. An earlier report found that 44% of bakers in a small bakery were sensitized to flour compared with 25% in a larger, more hygienically organized establishment.[7]

The location within a bakery where one works may also play a role in the incidence of asthmatic symptoms. One study identified oven handlers as having more wheezing and dyspnea, lower random FEV_1 measurements, a higher incidence of positive skin prick tests to cereal antigens, and increased bronchial hyperresponsiveness when compared with either dough makers or general bakers[10] (Figs. 1 and 2). They also found that bakers had more frequent attacks of dyspnea and wheezing than did slicers and wrappers.[10] One

review demonstrated that rhinitis appears usually to precede the onset of reactivity airway disease in bakers, and that the mean age of onset of respiratory symptoms in bakers was 40 years.[23] All subjects in this study were older than 33 years at the onset of their respiratory symptoms.[23]

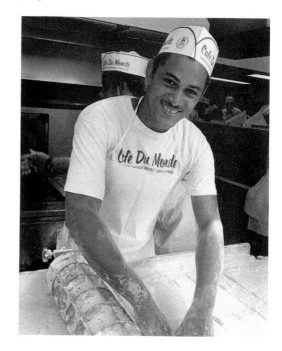

FIGURE 2.   Baker in a French bakery.

Clinical Presentation

A typical clinical history would include rhinitis followed by asthma, which tends to develop after exposure at work and improves on weekends and vacations.[1] It has been the experience of a number of clinicians that many patients with bakers' asthma will wheeze within 30 minutes of exposure to flour, and most within several hours.[25] It appears that a personal or family history of atopic disease may place a bakery worker at greater risk of developing occupational rhinitis and asthma from baking or exposure to flour antigens.[10,26,27] One review of 234 bakery workers in Finland showed that the incidence of atopic disease (allergic rhinitis, asthma, and atopic dermatitis) in this group was 25%.[27] Some patients had more than one manifestation of allergic disease. The incidence of allergic rhinitis was 23%, 9% had asthma, and 5% were noted to have atopic dermatitis. The study showed that every worker who had allergic rhinitis or asthma before undertaking bakery work developed aggravated symptoms after working in a bakery. Ninety percent (19/21) of the bakery employees who developed asthma did not develop asthmatic symptoms until they started work in the bakery. The average time of exposure to flour dust before asthma symptoms developed in this group was 4.2 years.[27] These authors also demonstrated that 71% of bakers suffering from an atopic disease had a positive family history of allergic disorders, compared with only 17% of healthy bakery workers. They concluded by strongly cautioning anyone with a personal or family history of atopic disease about employment in a bakery where there would be direct exposure to flour dust.[27]

Cereal flour antigens may cause occupational asthma in a variety of settings in addition to bakeries. A published report noted evidence of occupational asthma developing in those working with cereals present in animal feed.[28] The patients had positive prick skin tests to cereal flours (wheat, rye, and barley), with negative skin tests to other components of the cereals. Specific IgE to wheat, rye, and barley was found by RAST, and bronchoprovocation studies showed immediate asthmatic responses to wheat flour in two patients and barley flour in one patient.[28] Flour mill operators are also at risk of developing cereal flour-associated asthma.[22,28]

As noted above, in addition to flour as an aeroallergen, there are numerous substances in grain dust that may cause asthma. These will be reviewed later in the chapter.

Antigen Identification and Cross-reactivity

Although much investigation has been done on allergens responsible for the symptoms of bakers' asthma, there is much yet to be learned. Wheat, rye, and barley are three closely related grass species, belonging to the tribe Triticeae.[29] Rye grass has little cross-reactivity with wheat and barley.[30] The relationship between the wheat allergens and those of oat, rice, and maize is less clear.[29] RAST-inhibition studies have been used to investigate the degree of cross-reactivity of the various grain antigens.[29,31] The degree of cross-antigenicity between extracts made from wheat, triticale (a rye-wheat hybrid), rye, barley, oat, rice, and corn closely follows their taxonomic relationship.[31] Closely related species such as wheat, rye, and triticale are shown to have a high degree of cross-antigenicity, and even more distantly related species such as rye, barley, and oat show some significant cross-reactivity[31] (Table 2).

There are four major protein fractions present in wheat: albumin, globulin, gliadin, and glutenin. Sensitivity to any one, or a combination, may be responsible for bakers' asthma in any particular individual.[9] There are multiple characteristics of these various fractions that may be important in the pathogenesis and diagnosis of bakers' asthma; among these are antigenicity and water solubility.

Different components of wheat flour appear to cause symptoms, depending on the disease state and route of exposure. For example, in one study investigating pediatric patients with asthma and/or eczema, serum-specific IgE bound most avidly to the globulin and glutenin fractions.[30] In coeliac disease (gluten-induced enteropathy), there is an immune response

TABLE 2. *Cross-Reactivity of Different Grain Antigens by RAST Inhibition Testing*

Species with a high degree of cross-antigenicity
Wheat
Rye
Triticale (a rye-wheat hybrid)
Species with less cross-antigenicity
Rye
Barley
Oat

with antibodies of the IgG, IgA, and IgD classes directed against gluten.[32] Bakers' asthma is notable for IgE antibodies directed predominantly against the albumin fraction.[30] Albumins are important, albeit diverse, allergens in bakers' asthma.[9] Wheat antigens may also become allergenic after they have been altered in the processing of the wheat. Typical asthma and rhinoconjunctivitis have been reported in a worker after 13 years of employment in a company producing biscuits following inhalation of an alkaline hydrolysis derivative of gluten. Her symptoms began after 8 years of employment, and evaluation showed an immediate strong bronchoconstrictor response to inhalation of the alkaline hydrolysis derivative of gluten and negative bronchial challenges to native gluten.[32]

At least 40 different wheat antigens have been identified by using crossed immunoelectrophoresis, starting with a water soluble extract of wheat flour.[33] In one study, 18 of these antigens bound IgE from sera of allergic bakers, and only six of these were present in one water-soluble, commercially prepared extract of gliadin.[33] The finding of water-insoluble wheat antigens raises the question of whether these antigens may not be present in sufficient amounts in aqueous solutions used for skin testing.[9]

Sensitization to soy is usually via the oral route, but inhalation resulting in IgE-mediated sensitization and asthma has been well described.[8] Separation of soy flour extract by dodecyl sulfate-polyacrylamide gel electrophoresis showed 24 protein bands detected in crude soy flour extracts. After immunoblotting and autoradiography, nine proteins with molecular weights ranging from 14,875 to 54,500 daltons were found, indicating the presence of multiple soy antigens.[8]

Pathophysiology

Bakers' asthma appears to be caused, in most instances, by a classic type I IgE-mediated response.[34] In one study, bakers with bakers' asthma were shown to have immediate skin-test hypersensitivity, positive leukocyte histamine release, passive transfer skin-test reactivity (successfully blocked by heat inactivation and specific IgE immunoadsorption), and immediate bronchoconstriction after provocation with the patient's own bakery flour.[34] As noted above, almost any one (or combination) of the four major protein fractions in

wheat (albumin, globulin, gliadin, and glutenin) may be responsible for bakers' asthma in any particular individual. There does not appear to be one unique allergen in initiating bakers' asthma.[9]

It appears that serum IgE binds to a much greater degree to the albumin and globulin fractions of wheat than to the less soluble gluten (gliadin and glutenin) components.[29] It is not clear how important insoluble allergens may be in the pathogenesis of bakers' asthma. One author has postulated that insoluble proteins may trigger mast cell mediator release directly, or that enzymes present on mucosal surfaces may aid in the extraction of less-water-soluble antigens.[9] This phenomenon may help explain some delayed reactions characteristic of grain-dust fever.[9] Immediate skin-test reactivity to *Alternaria* and *Aspergillus* has been noted in two cases, with a dual response to bronchial provocation with *Aspergillus* and an immediate response to *Alternaria* thought to contribute to the workers' symptoms.[1]

Several studies have looked at the possible role of IgG in the pathogenesis of bakers' asthma.[12,35] Allergic bakers were noted to have high levels of specific IgG to wheat, and binding to solid phase was inhibited with wheat antigen; the importance of this finding is unclear.[35] Popp et al. compared 17 bakers with a 100% increase in specific airways resistance following rye dust provocation with 16 bakers who showed neither symptoms of reactive airway disease nor an increase in specific airways resistance following rye dust provocation. Fifteen of 17 bakers with a positive immediate bronchoconstrictor response had IgG-4 specific for rye grain by indirect immunofluorescence, whereas none of the 16 controls had rye-specific IgG-4. The heaviest concentration of rye-specific IgG-4 by indirect immunofluorescence was in the protein-rich frame between starch granules.[12]

Diagnosis of Bakers' Asthma

The first step in the accurate diagnosis of bakers' asthma is a thorough history and physical examination. The incidence of bakers' asthma clearly increases with duration of employment in a bakery.[4,10,22,23] Symptoms may occur at work, clearing on weekends and vacations.[1] A history of rhinitis almost always antedates the onset of symptoms of bakers' asthma.[23] A prior history of atopy appears to increase the risk of acquiring bakers' asthma, and patients with atopic disease should be counseled accordingly.[10,26]

Physical examination may be completely normal. Although an office examination of the lungs may not be helpful, lung auscultation and pulmonary function studies in the workplace setting may aid in diagnosis.[1] Chest radiographs are usually normal.[1] Pulmonary function studies show typical findings of reactive airway disease.[10]

When evaluating patients with suspected bakers' asthma, both allergen skin testing and RAST have been shown to be reliable methods for demonstration of specific IgE to the cereal antigens.[4,10,12,29,36] The combination of both a positive skin test and RAST to a cereal antigen, as well as an elevated total IgE, was highly predictive in one series of bakers who had bakers' asthma confirmed by bronchial provocation.[12] In that same series, elevated levels of rye-specific IgG-4 had a predictive value of 88% for later positive bronchial provocation challenges;[12] however, the value of this test remains to be determined.

Both skin testing and RAST using water soluble extracts have shown similar relationships with indices of respiratory disease, and bakers with positive prick tests to wheat extracts have been reported to have an increased incidence of respiratory symptoms in general, and increased bronchial hyperresponsiveness in particular.[4] Positive skin tests are seen more commonly in those with a longer duration of baking,[4] and there is a correlation between the level of serum IgE levels specific for cereal antigens, the degree of bronchial hyperreactivity, and an individual baker's bronchial response to an inhalational challenge with an extract of cereal flour.[31] Borderline positive RAST values have been seen in asymptomatic bakers, but strongly positive RAST values have correlated well with history and bronchial provocation challenge.[29] In one study of seven symptomatic bakers, no serum precipitating antibodies were found.[36]

Utilizing a RAST assay to quantify specific IgE directed against wheat may be somewhat complex because of the diversity and varying water solubility of different wheat antigens. Covalent coupling of water-soluble proteins to a solid phase may sometimes be unsatisfactory, and one investigator recommends 1% potassium hydroxide as the best overall solvent to dissolve wheat proteins for maximum adherence of wheat antigens to a RAST solid-phase material.[9] If water alone is used as the solvent, albumins bind the most IgE and glutenins will bind the least, leading some investigators to conclude that the water-soluble fractions (albumins and globulins) are the most allergenic components.[4,9] Using appropriate solvents to enhance glutenin binding to nitrocellulose membranes in the RAST assay has, however, demonstrated significant IgE binding to that particular wheat antigen as well.[29]

As noted above, bakers with pre-existing sensitivity to common allergens have an increased risk of developing wheat flour sensitization. In addition, there is a significant association between skin test reactivity to whole wheat and to other inhalant allergens.[4] Consistent correlation between any specific inhalant allergen and flour antigens in those with bakers' asthma has been lacking,[4] although one small series showed that a significant percentage of patients with bakers' asthma had positive allergen skin tests to mites compared with a general population control.[36] It is clear that allergens other than the cereal may contribute to or cause asthmatic symptoms in bakers, and these need to also be included in the skin-test battery used in the evaluation for bakers' asthma; these include at least house dust mites, grain storage mites, rodents, insects (e.g., cockroach), and fungal antigens.[29]

TREATMENT OF BAKERS' ASTHMA

The best and most advisable treatment of bakers' asthma is the avoidance of future exposure by changing professions. If this is not possible, the use of special masks or respirators is recommended.[1] If the patient chooses to continue working despite the possible risks involved, the pharmacotherapy of bakers' asthma does not necessarily differ from other types of asthma.[9] Many patients have been reported to successfully continue their work by pretreatment on a regular basis with inhaled sodium cromoglycate.[1,22,29] Successful control has also been reported with bronchodilators and inhaled steroid aerosols, although pretreatment with inhaled steroid aerosols alone has been shown to inhibit the late, but not the immediate, asthmatic response.[1] There have not been adequate trials conducted to evaluate the potential role of immunotherapy in patients with bakers' asthma. If possible, changing the patient's exposure pattern is clearly the most advisable course of treatment; however, if that is not possible, medical treatment is effective.

GRAIN DUST-ASSOCIATED RESPIRATORY SYMPTOMS

Historical Perspective

Ramazzini in his discourse on diseases of "Sifters and measurers of grain" appreciated that the fine dust associated with stored grains comprised "not only the dust they pick up from the threshing floor, but also another less innocent sort which is shed from the grain itself when it is kept too long." He also described the complex health effects from exposure, indicating "the throat, lungs, [and] eyes are keenly aware of serious damage," and "intense itching over the whole body of the sort sometimes observed in nettle rash." He also outlines the chronic effects: "Almost all who make a living by sifting or measuring grain are short of breath, cachectic, and rarely reach old age."[2]

Epidemiology and Etiology

Workers may be exposed to grain dust in a number of settings (Fig. 3, Table 3). Outbreaks of asthma have been reported in residents of a community exposed to windborne grain dust from neighboring mills.[37] Swanson and colleagues have analyzed airborne soybean allergens in the dust produced while loading and unloading soybeans in Barcelona, Spain. Asthma epidemics in that city had been noted, and the major allergen responsible was a glycopeptide present in soybean dust weighing less than 14,000 daltons. This allergen is

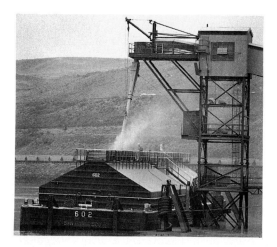

FIGURE 3.   Grain barge being loaded on the Columbia River in Oregon.

TABLE 3.   *Occupations and Individuals with Exposure to Grain Dust*

Farmers during harvest, loading, and unloading of grain
Mill workers
Grain elevator/storage agents and workers
Dock workers and longshoremen
Grain processing workers
Workers manufacturing cereals and feeds
Grain seed workers
Bakers
Individuals living downwind from grain-unloading facilities

present in all parts of the soybean plant at all stages of growth, but the telae (hulls) and pods are the richest source. Further investigation in this area is needed.[38] Because of the complex nature of grain dust, any one of several respiratory problems may arise from grain-dust exposure (Table 4).

Grain-elevator operators are not only exposed to grain particles themselves, but also to multiple other contaminants of grain dust (Table 5). The proportion of grain handlers' respiratory symptoms that are secondary to chemical, mechanical, and/or allergic mechanisms is not yet clear.[39] Grain handlers have been shown to have a higher prevalence of eye, nasal, and chest symptoms, including cough, sputum production, wheezing, and dyspnea.[40] They have also been shown to have lower mean spirometry values than a control population of civic workers and non-cedar sawmill workers.[40] A survey of farmers in England involved with harvesting grain demonstrated that one-quarter complained of respiratory symptoms after working near grain driers and elevators, or on combine harvesters. Their symptoms included cough, wheezing, and dyspnea, sometimes severe enough to prevent work.[41]

The reported incidence of respiratory symptoms in grain handlers varies significantly and ranges from 27–88%.[39,40,42-46] There is conflicting evidence about whether or not respiratory symptoms of grain handlers increase with increasing duration of employment.[39,46] One survey of 300 grain elevator workers showed that 88% complained of eye or respiratory symptoms, and that symptoms on

TABLE 4.   *Adverse Health Effects Reported with Grain-dust Exposure*

Grain-dust asthma
Extrinsic allergic alveolitis
Grain fever
Skin rashes
Eye irritation
Nasal and sinus irritation

TABLE 5. *Potential Antigens Present in Grain Dust*[49,50,52,53,60]

Grain and cereal antigens, including plant matter of various grains (such as durum and spring wheat, oats, barley, rye, corn) and seeds (such as rapeseed, flax, sunflower)

Non-grain plant matter

Insect parts and excreta

Rat hairs and other rodent matter, including excreta

Pesticides and fertilizers in various stages of chemical degradation

Fungal matter, including fungal spores of *Penicillium, Aspergillus, Alternaria, Rhizopus,* and *Cladosporium*

Silica dust

Soil and trace elements

Bacteria

Starch granules

Cellulose hairs and spikes

Pollens

Mineral particles

Wheat weevil debris *(Sitophilus granarius)*

Grain storage mites *(Tyroglyphus farinae)*

Mechanical (dust particles)

Grain rusts, smuts

TABLE 6. *Reported Incidence of Symptoms in Workers Exposed to Grain Dust*[47]*

Cough	34.9%
Wheezing	18.5%
Dyspnea	15.5%
Dermatitis	13.9%
Grain fever	6.1%

* Statistics reporting symptoms in reference to an occupational disease may be swayed by the "survivor effect," in which higher incidence figures are not seen because affected workers may leave the workplace that produced their symptoms.[41]

exposure were independent of age and duration of employment.[39] Another study of 502 grain elevator agents showed that the incidence of respiratory symptoms, especially cough, increased with longer duration of service.[46] In the latter study, the incidence of symptoms on exposure to grain dust is shown in Table 6.[40,46] Another survey of 80 dock workers showed that 86% noted chest symptoms on exposure to barley dust, with 16% experiencing feverish evening episodes after handling barley. No gross deficits in lung function were identified.[43] Barley grain dust was cited in one survey of over 500 grain handlers as the grain dust most likely to cause cough and breathlessness.[46]

Antigen Identification and Pathophysiology

Identification of agents responsible for the production of symptoms in grain handlers has been difficult. Possible etiologic agents responsible include bacteria and/or bacterial endotoxins, fungi, storage mites, grain and cereal antigens, grain weevil, and numerous other antigens as outlined in Table 5.[43] Precipitating antibodies to grain dust extracts have been difficult to find and were not identified in any patients with grain dust-associated symptoms in two large series.[43,47] Various measurements of C-3, C-4, and CH-50 do not appear to

change despite the appearance of respiratory symptoms after grain dust exposure.[43,44,48] There are likely to be multiple etiologic agents for the different types of grain dust-induced respiratory disease.

One investigator has suggested that airflow obstruction may be caused by two different mechanisms; the first is asthma induction via immunologic mechanisms, and the second is by causing an industrial irritant bronchitis.[47] The effects of inhalation of grain dust are thought to be primarily on the bronchial airways and not the lung parenchyma. This supposition is based on the observation that chest radiographs and diffusion capacity of carbon monoxide remain normal after challenge with grain dust, whereas pulmonary function parameters may fall.[44]

The highest concentration of airborne dust particles appears to occur during loading and unloading of grain.[39] In one Canadian study the mean particle size of airborne dust collected during oat and wheat loading was 1.7–3.1 microns; the particles are therefore able to reach the alveoli (organic and inorganic sized particles were similar).[46] Free-silica content of the dust was found to be 8% for oats and 7.4% (by weight) for wheat dust. One-third of the silica was in the organic fraction, and two-thirds in the inorganic fraction (reflecting the fraction of soil in the grain shipments). The authors concluded that the small amount of silica was unlikely to lead to any symptoms of silicosis.[46]

It is not clear whether a prior history of atopic disease predisposes one to grain handlers' asthma, because multiple studies have shown conflicting results.[40-43,46] Several studies have found no relationship between atopy and the prevalence of respiratory symptoms or pulmonary function abnormalities in grain workers.[40,43,44] In contrast, a number of studies have noted a clear relationship between atopic status and grain dust-associated asthma.[41,42,46]

Although the mechanism of grain dust-associated asthma is unknown, an allergic pathogenesis is supported in some patients, because the immediate asthmatic reaction, maximum reaction, and timing of recovery from bronchospasm are similar to that seen in allergen-induced bronchospasm.[47] In addition, one study of 22 grain workers with respiratory symptoms found that the immediate asthmatic reaction could be successfully blocked in one patient by disodium cromoglycate, and the late (not immediate) asthmatic response could be blocked by cromolyn in one patient who experienced a dual asthmatic response.[47]

Another study noted that a history of allergic disorders (defined as asthma, seasonal rhinoconjunctivitis, urticaria, or eczema) was found nearly twice as often in grain-elevator workers with related respiratory symptoms.[46] Another case report of a grain worker with asthmatic symptoms confirmed immediate and delayed asthmatic reactions to the grain weevil, *Sitophilus granarius*, and fever and a delayed positive skin test were also noted.[42] It has been shown that millworkers may have a significantly higher percentage of cutaneous allergen skin test sensitivity to the grain weevil than a nonexposed control group.[49]

Bronchial provocation testing in a farmer using dust from his own stored grain led both to immediate and late asthmatic reactions, which recurred on subsequent nights despite no further exposure to the grain dust. A grain sample disclosed that the predominant mold was comprised of *Penicillium* species, and the predominant mite was *Glyphagus destructor*; there was no grain weevil present, nor was any *Micropolyspora faeni* identified.[48] The grain storage mite *Glyphagus destructor* was thought to be an important allergen.[48] It is noteworthy that the majority of stored grain has been shown to be infested with mites, and farmers more commonly complain of dyspnea after handling old grain than freshly harvested grain.[45,48]

Farmers may also be exposed to grain dust and other contaminants during the harvest procedures, as well as exposure during loading, unloading, and in storage bins and silos. Exposures to airborne dust around combine harvesters have been shown to contain up to 200 million fungus spores/M^3 of air, with drivers exposed to up to 20 million spores/M^3 of air.[41] Mold species identified include *Cladosporium, Verticillium lecanee, Paecilomyces bacillosporus,* and *Aphanocladium.* Extracts of the above species produced immediate wheal reactions in skin tests and, when inhaled

by the affected workers, rapid falls in FEV_1. No delayed reactions were noted. In this case precipitin reactions with the patients' sera were demonstrated.[41] Skin tests to fungal antigens in symptomatic grain workers in Saskatchewan showed positive allergen skin tests in the following percentages of workers: *Aspergillus,* 78%; *Penicillium,* 43%; *Alternaria,* 29%; *Helminthosporium,* 24%; *Hormodendrum,* 20%; and *Candida,* 14%.[52]

The diversity of opinions concerning the role of allergic mechanisms in producing respiratory symptoms in grain handlers is most likely not the result of faulty analysis of data, but more likely is a mirror of the wide spectrum of disease that falls under the heading of "grain handlers" respiratory disease.

The nature of pulmonary disease resulting from chronic exposure to grain remains controversial, as does the origin of "grain fever" and the accompanying leukocytosis.[42] "Grain fever," as contrasted with grain-dust asthma, is characterized by general malaise, fever, and shivering following exposure to grain dust.[46] This may occur following first exposure, following an exposure after being away from work for some time (e.g., more than 1 week), or after a particularly heavy exposure.[46] Systemic symptoms, including fever, have been shown to occur in control patients inhaling grain dust, raising the possibility of bacterial or fungal endotoxins in the dust.[42]

Several studies have failed to find any association with grain dust-associated respiratory disease and cigarette smoking in the grain workers,[40,50] whereas others have noted an increase in lower respiratory symptoms such as cough, dyspnea, and sputum production with these associated factors.[1,39,45,46,51]

Evaluation and Treatment

All patients suspected of having grain dust-associated asthma or grain fever should have a thorough history and physical examination, a complete blood count with differential and eosinophil count, erythrocyte sedimentation rate, chest radiograph, pulmonary function studies with diffusion capacity, and allergy skin testing with suspected allergens, including mites, insects, fungi, etc. Home (and workplace) peak flow monitoring and/or spirometry may be useful in establishing the diagnosis as well.

Treatment is best accomplished through avoidance of the environment known to produce symptoms. Farmers with symptoms upon exposure to grain dust are more likely to wear a protective mask, but overall the compliance of grain workers wearing masks is low.[45,52] Smokers appear to be less likely to wear respiratory protective masks than nonsmokers.[45] Because the precise mechanism of disease is unknown and is probably extremely varied in individual patients, a program of pharmacotherapy needs to be individualized in each patient based on the findings in the evaluation. Smoking cessation, as well as proper respiratory protection, is strongly recommended in those who are unable to change occupations. Adequate trials of storage-mite desensitization to assess its benefit do not appear to have been undertaken in this population of patients. Inhaled bronchodilators combined with aerosol steroids and/or cromolyn may be tried in those with grain-dust asthma. Oral glucocorticoids may be needed in more severe cases. As noted above, because of the wide range of potential etiologies of this disorder, avoidance is clearly the preferred strategy for management.

REFERENCES

1. Tedtse CS, Raghuprasad PK: Baker's asthma (grain-dust-induced asthma). Drug Intelligence and Clinical Pharmacy 16:14–18, 1982.
2. Ramazzini B: Disease of bakers and millers. In De Morbis Artificum (Diseases of Workers; Latin text of 1713 revised and translated by Wilmer Cave Wright). Chicago, University of Chicago Press, 1940, pp 235–252.
3. Bonnevie P: Occupational allergy in bakeries. In Stenfort-Kroese (ed): Occupational Allergy. Springfield, IL, Charles C Thomas, 1958, pp 161–168.
4. Prichard MG, Ryan G, Walsh BJ, et al: Skin test and RAST responses to wheat and common allergens and respiratory disease in bakers. Clin Allergy 15:203–210, 1985.
5. de Besche A: Serologische untersuchungen uber allergische kraukherten. Acta Pathol Immunol Microb Scand 6:115, 1925.
6. Jimenez-Diaz C, Laboz C, Cauto G: The allergens of mill dust. Ann Allergy 5:519, 1947.
7. Von Dishoeck HAE, Roux DJ: Sensitization to flour and flour illnesses amongst flour workers. J Hyg 39:674, 1939.
8. Bush RK, Schroekenstein D, Meier-Davis S, et al: Soybean flour asthma: Detection of allergens by immunoblotting. J Allergy Clin Immunol 82:251–255, 1988.
9. Walsh BJ, Wrigley CW, Musk AW, et al: A comparison of the binding of IgE in the sera of patients with bakers' asthma to soluble and insoluble wheat-grain proteins. J Allergy Clin Immunol 76:23–28, 1985.
10. Prichard MG, Ryan G, Musk AW: Wheat flour sensitization and airways disease in urban bakers. Br J Ind Med 41:450–454, 1984.
11. Bonnevie P: Occupational allergy in bakery. In Stenfort-Kroese WF (ed): Occupational Allergy. Springfield, IL, Charles C Thomas, 1958, pp 161–168.

12. Popp W, Zwick H, Rauscher H: Short-term sensitizing antibodies in bakers' asthma. Int Arch Allergy Appl Immunol 86:215–219, 1988.
13. Herxheimer H: The skin sensitivity to flour of baker's apprentices. Acta Allergologica 28:42, 1973.
14. Thiel H, Ulmer WT: Bakers' asthma: Development and possibility for treatment. Chest 78:400, 1980.
15. Napolitano J, Weiss NS: Occupational asthma of bakers. Ann Allergy 40:258–261, 1978.
16. Block G, Kijek K, Chan H, et al: Pathogenic mechanisms in baker's asthma (abstract). Am Rev Respir Dis 125:74, 1982.
17. Hendrick DJ, Davies RJ, Pepys J: Baker's asthma. Clin Allergy 6:241–250, 1976.
18. Popescu IG Ulmeanu V, Muraniv D: Atopic and non-atopic sensitivity in a large bakery. Allergol Immunopathol 9:307–312, 1981.
19. Frankloud AW, Luan JA: Asthma caused by the grain weevil. Br J Ind Med 22:157–159, 1965.
20. Popa V, George SAL, Gavanoscu O: Occupational and non-occupational respiratory allergy in bakers. Acta Allergol 25:159–177, 1970.
21. Klaustermeyer WB, Bardana EJ, Hale FC: Pulmonary hypersensitivity to *Alternaria* and *Aspergillus* in baker's asthma. Clin Allergy 7:227–233, 1977.
22. Thiel H, Ulmer WT: Bakers' asthma: Development and possibility for treatment. Chest 78:400–404, 1980.
23. Popa V, George SAL, Gavanescu O: Occupational and non-occupational respiratory allergy in bakers. Acta Allergologica 25:159–177, 1970.
24. Blands J, Diamant B, Kailos P, et al: Flour allergy in bakers. Int Arch Allergy Appl Immunol 52:392, 1976.
25. Schwartz M: Flour allergy. J Allergy Clin Immunol 18:341, 1947.
26. Jarvinen KAJ, Pirila V, Bjorkstein E, et al: Unsuitability of bakery work for a person with atopy: A study of 234 bakery workers. Ann Allergy 42:1928, 1979.
27. Jarvinen KAJ, Pirila V, Bjorkstein F, et al: Unsuitability of bakery work for a person with atopy: A study of 234 bakery workers. Ann Allergy 42:192–195, 1979.
28. Valdivieso R, Pola J, Zapata C, et al: Farm animal feeders: Another group affected by cereal flour asthma. Allergy 43:406–410, 1988.
29. Sutton R, Skerritt JH, Baldo BA, et al: The diversity of allergens involved in bakers' asthma. Clin Allergy 14:93–107, 1984.
30. Sutton R, Hill DJ, Baldo BA, et al: Immunoglobulin E antibodies to ingested cereal flour components: Studies with sera from subjects with asthma and eczema. Clin Allergy 12:63–74, 1982.
31. Block G, Tse KS, Kijek K, et al: Baker's asthma: Studies of the cross-antigenicity between different cereal grains. Clin Allergy 14:177–185, 1984.
32. Lachance P, Cartier A, Dolovich J, et al: Occupational asthma from reactivity to an alkaline hydrolysis derivative of gluten. J Allergy Clin Immunol 81:385–390, 1988.
33. Blands J, Diamant B, Kallos-Deffner L, Lowenstein H: Flour allergy in bakers. I. Identification of allergenic fractions in flour and comparison of diagnostic methods. Int Arch Allergy Appl Immunol 52:392, 1976.
34. Wilbur RD, Ward GW: Immunologic studies in a case of baker's asthma. J Allergy Clin Immunol 58:366–372, 1976.
35. Walker CL, Grammer LC, Shaughnessy MA, et al: Baker's asthma: Report of an unusual case. J Occup Med 31:439–442, 1989.

36. Block G, Tse KS, Kijek K, et al: Baker's asthma: Clinical and immunological studies. Clin Allergy 13:359-370, 1983.

37. Parkers WR: Occupational Lung Disorders. London, Butterworth, 1974, pp 450-456.

38. Swanson MC, Li JTC, Wentz-Murtha PE, et al: Source of the aeroallergen of soybean dust: A low molecular mass glycopeptide from the soybean tela. J Allergy Clin Immunol 87:783-788, 1991.

39. Do Pico GA, Reddan W, Flaherty D, et al: Respiratory abnormalities among grain handlers. A clinical, physiologic, and immunologic study. Am Rev Respir Dis 115:915-927, 1977.

40. Chan-Yeung M, Schulzer M, MacLean L, et al: Epidemiologic health survey of grain workers in British Columbia. Am Rev Respir Dis 121:329-338, 1980.

41. Darke CS, Knowelden J, Lacey J, Ward AM: Respiratory disease of workers harvesting grain. Thorax 31:294-302, 1976.

42. Davies RJ, Blainey AD, Pepys J: Occuaptional Asthma. In Middleton E, Reed CE, Ellis EF (eds): Allergy: Principles and Practice. St. Louis, C.V. Mosby, 1983, p 1043.

43. Cockcroft AE, McDermott M, Edwards JH, McCarthy P: Grain exposure-symptoms and lung function. Eur J Respir Dis 64:189-196, 1983.

44. Do Pico GA, Jacobs S, Flaherty D, Rankin J: Pulmonary reaction to durum wheat, a constituent of grain dust. Chest 81:55-61, 1982.

45. Warren CPW, Manfreda J: Respiratory symptoms in Manitoba farmers: Association with grain and hat handling. Can Med Assoc J 122:1259-1264, 1980.

46. Williams N, Skoulas A, Merriman JE: Exposure to grain dust. I. A survey of the effects. J Occup Med 6:319-329, 1964.

47. Chan-Yeung M, Wong R, MacLean L: Respiratory abnormalities among grain elevator workers. Chest 75:461-467, 1979.

48. Davies RJ, Green M, Schofield N: Recurrent nocturnal asthma after exposure to grain dust. Am Rev Respir Dis 114:1011-1019, 1976.

49. Lunn JA: Millworkers' asthma: Allergic responses to the grain weevil (Sitophilus granarius). Br J Ind Med 23:149-152, 1966.

50. Broder I, Mintz S, Hutcheon M, et al: Comparison of respiratory variables in grain elevator workers and civic outside workers of Thunder Bay, Canada. Am Rev Respir Dis 119:193-203, 1979.

51. Dosman JA: Chronic obstructive pulmonary disease and smoking in grain workers. Ann Intern Med 87:784, 1977.

52. Skoulas A, Williams N, Merriman JE: Exposure to grain dust. II. A clinical study of the effects. J Occup Med 6:359-372, 1964.

53. Becklake MR: Grain dust and health. In Dosman JA, Cotton DJ (eds): Occupational Pulmonary Disease. New York, Academic Press, 1980, pp 189-199.

Chapter 10

OCCUPATIONAL ASTHMA DUE TO COFFEE, TEA, AND CASTOR BEAN DUST

Mark T. O'Hollaren, MD

ASTHMA DUE TO COFFEE BEAN DUST

The coffee plant (*coffea arabica* and *C. liberica*) is a tropical evergreen shrub of African origin that has been cultivated in many parts of the world for its beans, which are roasted, ground, and sold for brewing coffee. The relationship of coffee to asthma dates back hundreds of years.[1] Coffee has been used as treatment for asthma for generations, and its benefit has been ascribed to the properties of caffeine, a xanthine whose bronchodilator effect is approximately 40% of that of theophylline on a mole-for-mole basis.[1,2] One large Italian population study even suggested that those who drank coffee on a regular basis had a lower chance of developing asthma.[3]

It is interesting, then, that some workers who process coffee beans may develop occupational asthma as a result of inhalation of the dust from these beans. After the green coffee bean is picked from the coffee plant, it is shipped to a coffee processing mill where it is unloaded, usually from burlap-type bags weighing approximately 60 kg each[4] (Fig. 1). Workers in the coffee industry, especially those workers who handle green coffee beans, may develop occupational asthma, rhinitis, or dermatitis from coffee-bean dust in the processing plant[5] (Fig. 2). Bernton surveyed coffee production and found that over 20 million bags of green coffee beans were roasted per year in the United States.[4] He identified 335 coffee mills in which green coffee beans are transformed into finished products by roasting and grinding, employing approximately 9,000 workers in coffee production.[4] A diagram summarizing coffee production is shown in Figure 3.

Historical Perspective

Figley and Rawling in 1950 initially described asthma from both green coffee-bean dust and contaminating castor-bean dust in used burlap bags.[6] Castor beans are the fruit of the castor-oil plant (*Ricinus communis*). Because castor-bean antigen is such a potent allergen, it was initially thought that the cause of coffee workers asthma was castor-bean pomace (the fine dust remaining after castor oil has been extracted from the castor bean) contaminating the bags used to ship the green coffee beans.[4] Investigations revealed that patients who were allergic to green coffee beans also frequently reacted to citrus fruits and castor beans.[5,7] This finding was initially attributed to cross-reactivity among these different food products due to the presence of a common substance, chlorogenic acid. However, this was later shown by Layton et al. not to be the case.[5,7,8] Although selected coffee workers may react to castor antigen contaminating burlap bags used to ship coffee, green coffee beans have distinct allergens that do not cross-react with castor beans.

Chemistry and Antigen Identification

All areas within a coffee-bean processing plant do not report similar incidences of occupational asthma. There is a distinct difference in the allergenicity of green coffee beans compared to those that have been roasted.[9,10] In addition, coffee-bean workers who are sensitized to green coffee beans do not react to roasted coffee-bean products.[9,10] Obtaining

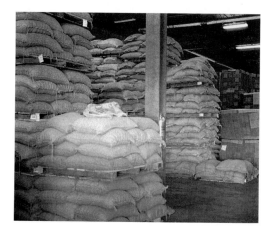

FIGURE 1.   Green coffee bean warehouse in a plant that produces 15,000 lbs/day.

dust samples from coffee processing mills has been useful for testing, but the dust contents vary widely because of differences in cleaning standards, safety precautions, and ventilation in the facilities.[11]

Lehrer and coworkers at Tulane have extensively investigated the nature of allergens present in coffee.[5] After gel filtration, they noted that green coffee-bean extract revealed three peaks, all possessing allergenic activity, as determined by challenge in a sensitized murine model. Further fractionation in a Sephadex column demonstrated four peaks, each with immunochemically similar antigens as judged by antigen inhibition studies. The heterogeneity of green coffee-bean allergens throughout the molecular size range raises the question of polymerization or agglutination of the allergenic coffee protein.[5]

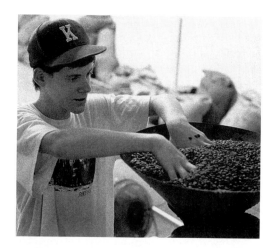

FIGURE 2.   Young coffee worker handling green coffee beans in coffee processing plant.

Lehrer et al. also investigated the allergenicity of several different possible antigens within a coffee processing facility. These included Ethiopian green coffee beans, roasted coffee beans, green coffee-bean debris in the cleaner cans, chaff, coffee dust from the burlap-sack opening area, and raw castor beans. He found that these extracts varied considerably in their ability to elicit a reaginic antibody response, and that roasted coffee beans, cleaner can debris, and chaff were not active. Green coffee beans and coffee dust were the most antigenic coffee constituents. Interestingly, castor-bean extract was also highly allergenic, eliciting the highest passive cutaneous anaphylaxis titer of all the extracts tested (approximately 32 times greater than that of coffee antigens.[5]

Cross-reactivity between coffee- and castor-bean antigens has not been demonstrated by either RAST inhibition studies or by gel diffusion.[9,12,24] In one study rabbit antiserum made to coffee manufacturing plant dust reacted to coffee-bean antigen but not to castor-bean,[24] whereas another study identified both green coffee bean- and castor-bean antigen in coffee factory dust.[12]

Questions have been present for some time regarding the relative importance of castor-bean antigen in those with symptoms on exposure to bags of green coffee beans. It is clear that some coffee workers are reacting to castor-bean allergen alone, which may be present as a dust contaminant of the coffee bags.[9,12] These sacks may be contaminated if used previously to ship castor beans or castor-bean pomace, or by being exposed to castor-bean antigen in the holds of ships or in railroad freight cars that had contained castor beans or pomace.[4] A recent study continues to suggest that castor-bean contamination remains a problem in the coffee-processing industry.[35]

Many coffee workers seem to react to both coffee- and castor-bean antigens, and the relative importance of these two antigens in this population of patients is not clear.[9,12] Symptomatic factory workers in one coffee-processing mill had more allergic symptoms when unloading Brazilian coffee beans compared with those from Africa or Mexico, and the possibility of castor-bean contamination of the Brazilian coffee bags was raised.[11]

Epidemiology and Etiology

Initially, studies of coffee workers showed that approximately 10% of those working with

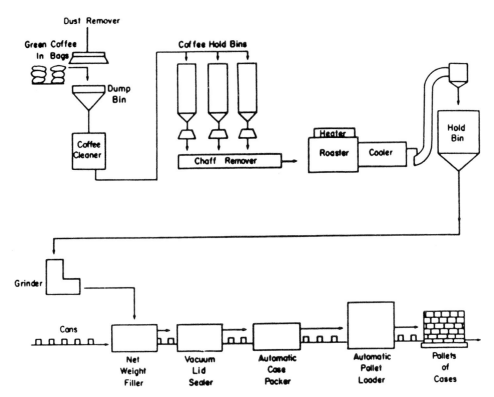

FIGURE 3.   Vacuum-packed coffee processing. Bags of green coffee beans are emptied into a large dump bin, which feeds the beans to the coffee cleaner. Jets of air clean away stems, sack remnants, and other large debris. After storage in hold bins, the beans are passed into the chaff remover. They are then roasted, allowed to cool, and stored in another hold bin. Further processing may include grinding, extraction and freeze-drying, decaffeination, or direct packaging. (From Karr RM: Bronchoprovocation studies in coffee workers' asthma. J Allergy Clin Immunol 64:650–654, 1979, with permission.)

the green coffee-bean dust and chaff developed allergic symptoms, with about half of those having asthma.[9,13] It was noted that about 70% of symptomatic workers in this study had positive intradermal skin tests to chaff and green coffee-bean extracts, with only 12% of asymptomatic workers showing positive skin tests.[13] Karr et al. describe 12 symptomatic workers in one coffee-processing plant employing 140 workers, which suggested a 9% prevalence of disease.[11]

In a subsequent study, the Tulane University group studied 372 workers in two coffee processing plants. Jobs were categorized as involving exposure to green, roasted, or mixed coffee-bean dust. Symptom prevalence did not differ significantly among exposure categories. Asthma was present in 4% of subjects.[14]

Zuskin studied 45 female nonsmoking employees who worked processing green or roasted coffee; they had a mean age of 31 years and a mean duration of employment of 7 years, and were compared to a similar control group who worked in a soft-drink manufacturing company.[15] Compared to the control group, 24.4% of the coffee workers had an elevated total IgE, compared with 5.9% of controls. The coffee workers were twice as likely to have chronic cough and over three times as likely to have chronic phlegm production. Forty percent of coffee workers had positive skin tests to an extract of dust collected from the area where coffee bags were emptied, compared with 14.7% of controls. No control-group members had positive skin tests to green or roasted coffee-bean dust, compared with 12% and 8.9%, respectively, in the coffee workers. She concluded that exposure to coffee-processing dust might cause the development of chronic respiratory symptoms, particularly in those with positive skin tests to coffee allergens.[15]

In a follow-up study, Zuskin et al. carried out bronchial provocation testing with green coffee-bean allergen in nine symptomatic coffee workers. They observed an immediate asthmatic reaction with an acute reduction in ventilatory capacity in four workers.[16] This same group documented the protective effect of disodium cromoglycate on the immediate bronchoconstriction seen in these exposed workers.[17] In a recent report, Zuskin et al. demonstrated that green coffee extract caused significant bronchoconstriction in selected healthy volunteers and that this response was not inhibited by disodium cromoglycate. The bronchoconstrictor effect of the coffee extract probably depends on the concentration of dust in the work environment as well as the workers susceptibility to the dust.[18]

Coffee workers' asthma is primarily an IgE-mediated disease. However, other factors, as yet poorly elucidated, also probably play a role in the modulation of asthmatic symptoms. An IgE mechanism is suggested by available data, including the immediate wheal-and-flare skin test response, the rapid appearance of symptoms after exposure to green coffee-bean dust in symptomatic workers, and consistent RAST inhibition data using green coffee-bean antigen and the sera of affected workers who suffer from green coffee-bean-associated asthma.[12] Layton et al. showed that allergic coffee workers' sera could successfully passively transfer cutaneous coffee-bean hypersensitivity to nonatopic humans and Macaque monkeys.[12,19] RAST inhibition studies utilizing chlorogenic acid in "significant concentrations" failed to verify common antigens with the castor bean or the green coffee bean, and as noted above this compound does not appear to be an allergen in this setting.[12,14]

In some studies of occupational asthma in coffee workers, a significant number of the subjects have been smokers, so studies of pulmonary function are not without confounding variables.[12]

Clinical Presentation and Diagnosis

Coffee workers have reported symptoms of asthma, rhinitis, conjunctivitis, and pruritis or urticaria with occupational exposure to the dust of the green coffee bean.[12] Asthma from an occupational origin such as coffee-bean dust may frequently present with cough rather than the typical wheezing and shortness of breath as the predominant presenting symptom.[11] This cough may be nocturnal, may be productive of eosinophil-laden yellow sputum, and may occur in the early morning hours, long after the patient has left the workplace.[11] Symptoms may extend over the weekend or short holidays, because occupational asthma has been shown to recur in a rhythmic pattern for several days despite only a single exposure.[11]

The time from initial exposure to onset of symptoms appears to vary widely in the population of exposed workers.[11]

Skin tests using extracts prepared from green coffee beans or their dust may be helpful in establishing the diagnosis of coffee-bean dust-associated asthma, and the procedures for making these extracts have been outlined in detail.[5,12,20] RAST assays using green coffee-bean antigen have also been described and shown to be reliable, but the degree of allergic sensitivity as determined by RAST does not appear to predict the degree of bronchial hyperreactivity (e.g., PD_{20}) values for FEV_1 using green coffee-bean antigen in bronchial provocation studies.[12] Karr et al. have suggested that underlying bronchial hyperreactivity may be more important than total serum IgE in this regard, and that serum IgE may not reflect the concentration of allergen-specific IgE bound to bronchial mast cells.[12] Skin reactivity to green coffee bean and coffee mill dust antigens in concentrations of 1 and 10 $\mu g/ml$, respectively, and serum RAST indices of greater than twice control values (with green coffee-bean antigens) were of most help to differentiate the allergic from the nonallergic workers (or controls).[12]

Karr has outlined one method for bronchial provocation studies with green coffee-bean antigen.[20] In his protocol, green coffee beans are homogenized alone and later with phosphate-buffered saline. This recipe is mixed for 24 hours, filtered, centrifuged, dialyzed, centrifuged again, and stored at $-20°C$ after sterility is proven by culture. Bronchial provocation is done using a nebulizer, and spirometry is performed 2 and 8 minutes after 20 breaths of the extract, beginning with a concentration of 0.1 mg/ml and proceeding to a maximum dose of 10 mg/ml if needed. Spirometry is continued for 24 hours to detect any late asthmatic reactions.[20]

Treatment

The recommended treatment for occupational asthma due to coffee-bean dust is removal of the affected worker from the workplace. There are case reports that clearly describe coffee production workers who continue to have significant symptoms despite the use of filter masks.[11] Davies comments on the difficult problem of comparing medical treatment for asthma despite continued work exposure versus avoidance of the antigen altogether.[11]

He recommends transfer of the worker to a different area of the mill, or change to a different occupation altogether. He states that a trial using preventative and therapeutic medications may be undertaken, but strict clinical follow-up, including regular examinations, pulmonary function studies including lung volume and diffusion capacity determinations, and chest radiographs, is needed to ensure that there is not development of airway obstruction or parenchymal lung disease.[11]

OCCUPATIONAL ASTHMA DUE TO TEA DUST

The true tea plant (genus *Thea*) is a group of Asiatic evergreen shrubs and trees, although the word tea is applied to many other cultivated plants. *Thea* is the Latinized version of the Chinese name for tea.

Asthma due to occupational exposure to tea dust was described in 1970, but respiratory symptoms among tea workers have been described since approximately 1920.[21,22] Although there is scant literature on this topic, tea-associated asthma appears to be a significant problem for the country of Sri Lanka, the largest exporter of tea in the world.[21] Those individuals or companies involved in the export of tea will buy different grades of tea leaves in bulk at tea auctions and blend them in such a way as to appeal to foreign clients.[21]

This blending may be done manually by hand-mixing tea leaves or by a mechanical process. When the blending takes place, the tea workers may be exposed to a fine dust referred to as "tea fluff," a waste product that adheres to the tea leaves and becomes airborne during the blending process.[21] Those involved with manual blending may be covered with a fine coating of this golden-colored tea fluff by the end of the day, and bronchial provocation with tea fluff in a symptomatic tea manufacturing supervisor reproduced his work-associated asthmatic symptoms.[21,22]

Mechanical vats used in the blending process are preferred, since they may be equipped with "fluff extractors" that carry the tea fluff through large air ducts away from the workers, where it may be collected in large bags or precipitated using jets of water. In this way, the workers would have minimal exposure to the tea fluff, and presumably significantly decrease their risk of developing occupational asthma in this setting.[21]

OCCUPATIONAL ASTHMA DUE TO CASTOR BEAN DUST

Castor oil was used in the past primarily as a cathartic, although its role as a pharmaceutical agent now accounts for no more than 1% of the world's production.[23] It is obtained from the castor bean and is now used industrially in the production of cosmetics, hair oils, nylons, explosives, paints, varnishes, fungistatic preparations, hydraulic fluids, jet plane lubricants, dyeing aids, plastics, textile finishing materials, and inks.[23,24] The castor bean is the seed of the castor-oil or castor-bean plant of Palmer Christi (*Ricinus communis*), a species belonging to the *Euphorbiaceae* family. It is originally from Africa but is now grown widely in other warm climates as well.[23] In tropical regions the castor-bean plant commonly reaches 20–40 feet in height and has large, smooth, multilobed leaves that may measure 3 feet in diameter.[23] Brazil and India are important producers of castor beans and oil, and the United States is the largest user of castor oil in the world, buying more than 50% of the world's production.[23] Increased petroleum prices have led to some increase in demand for this nonpetroleum oil.[24]

Although the seeds of the castor-bean plant are highly toxic for both man and animals by virtue of the toxin ricin, castor oil is nontoxic, nonallergenic, and is extracted manually by crushing or by solvent extraction. Castor oil is typically clear and light-colored, with a characteristic paint-like odor and slightly acidic and nauseating aftertaste. The oil contains the glyceride of ricinoleic acid, which has several double bonds, thus permitting easy polymerization. Turkey red oil is sulfonated castor oil, which is used in the preparation of cotton textiles, soaps, and certain cutting fluids. The process of oil extraction is enhanced through the use of an organic solvent such as hexane or heptane.[23,24] The dry, powdery residue that remains after extraction of castor oil from the castor bean is known as "pomace," and its high nitrogen content has made it useful as a fertilizer.[25] Most allergic problems are associated with the pomace rather than the whole castor beans.[24]

Historical Perspective

Allergy associated with castor beans was initially recognized in laboratory workers in 1914, in a U.S. Department of Agriculture worker in 1923, and later in industrial workers in 1928.[24,26] In 1928, Figley and Elrod investigated an outbreak of asthma in a neighborhood of Toledo, Ohio.[25] Both children and adults living near a linseed and castor oil processing plant were noting symptoms of asthma. School children near the plant had asthmatic symptoms while at school, as did mothers who lived near the plant and were home during the day. Those traveling away from the area to work had their symptoms predominantly at night upon returning home. These symptoms were initially thought to be secondary to linseed because the odor of linseed was noticeable to the members of the neighborhood; however, skin testing later verified that the essentially odorless castor-bean pomace was the inciting agent.[25]

Similar epidemic reactions were noted by other investigators. The same year, Grimm reported 30 cases in Germany in which scratch tests made with dust from castor beans gave strongly positive reactions.[27] In August 1952, the public health department of the state of Sao Paulo, Brazil was informed that in the town of Bauru there had appeared an epidemic of 150 cases of acute asthma appearing over a few days. Ultimately nine deaths were attributed to the illness, and the origin was found in the dust from a large castor-bean crushing mill in the town of Bauru.[28] Similar episodes were described by Ordmann in 1955 in South Africa and Panzani in 1962 in Marseille, France.[29,30]

The toxic properties of castor beans have been identified for many years. Ricin is the toxin present in castor beans, and it is composed of a number of isotoxins that are lectins.[24] Reports as far back as 1928 describe workmen in castor-bean mills who note the toxic effects of castor bean dust if it contacts an abrasion in the skin.[25] Over the years, numerous occupations have had difficulty with occupational exposure to castor-bean dust.

Chemistry and Antigen Identification

Castor-bean-associated asthma appears to be an IgE-mediated response to inhaled castor-bean antigen and may elicit an immediate or delayed bronchospastic reaction.[24,25,31,32] Davison et al.[24] have prepared various extracts of castor bean including whole-castor-bean extract, ricin extract, and dericinated extract. Specific IgE has been connected to each of these extract preparations, as evidenced by an

inability to cross-inhibit IgE binding by one of the other three extracts using a RAST inhibition assay.[24] Thus, evidence exists that multiple antigens in castor-bean dust are capable of eliciting an IgE response. Castor bean-sensitive asthmatics had evidence of IgE directed against castor-bean antigens, which was also shown by a red cell-linked antigen-antibody reaction, using passive sensitization of red blood cells with castor-bean antigen.[32] Basophil-associated IgE specific for castor bean has been shown cytologically via rosette formation with castor-bean allergen coated erythrocytes.[10] The active allergenic fraction in castor-bean dust is water soluble, and this property has been used to trap allergen prior to exhausting it into the air in castor-bean plants.[23]

Epidemiology

As noted above, there are many different professions in which individuals may contact castor-bean antigens and experience allergic symptoms. In contrast to coffee beans, in which most of the reported allergic reactions occur with the green coffee bean, most of the allergenicity exists in the pomace residue that remains after extraction of the castor oil from the bean.[24] Castor-bean-associated asthma has been seen in castor-oil mill workers,[24] communities surrounding castor-bean mills,[9,25] farmers who may use castor bean pomace residue as a part of fertilizer,[33] seamen and dock workers who load and unload shipments of castor beans,[24] laboratory workers making castor-bean extract,[24] and those who may contact the hessian bags that were previously used to ship castor bean pomace[6] (Table 1).

Clinical Presentation

Asthma is the usual allergic manifestation that has been associated with castor-bean exposure; however, urticaria, conjunctivitis, and rhinitis have been reported.[24,33] Clinical historical findings identified as risk factors in castor-bean workers have typically included excessive castor-bean dust exposure. Examples include exposure to spillage of beans during loading and unloading, particulate exposure to pomace from sacks that leak the fine powder, and poor ventilation of working areas and crews quarters on ships carrying castor beans.[24] Prior atopic history is often present but not a necessary prerequisite to development of asthma. One study demonstrated that 38.5% of patients who developed community-acquired castor-bean dust asthma had no prior atopic history.[23] As noted above, the clinical history may also include proximity of the patient's home or place of employment to a castor-bean mill.[9,23,25] The majority of patients who develop castor-bean associated asthma have a latent period of 6–18 months from first contact with the dust until appearance of symptoms.[9]

Diagnosis

Diagnosis is accomplished through a combined approach of a thorough history, physical examination, pulmonary function tests, and, in selected cases, skin testing and bronchial provocation. Because of the ricin toxin that is a part of castor-bean extracts, great caution needs to be taken when performing skin tests with castor-bean antigens.[25] Not only must the toxin be excluded, but the antigen has great potency.[25] Scratch skin tests using a 1:100 extract of castor-bean dust have demonstrated large reactions (2.5–8 cm wheals) in patients with castor-bean asthma. If possible, in vitro diagnostic tests using castor-bean antigens would be preferable. Lehrer et al. and others have heated castor-bean extract at 100°C to denature the ricin prior to skin testing, and this approach is advised if the risks of skin testing are outweighed by the potential benefits.[5,23] Many of the skin test reactions in one study were delayed in nature.[25] Intradermal skin tests using 0.01 ml of a 1:100 extract of castor-bean dust have resulted in a severe reaction, including widespread lymphangitis of the entire arm lasting for days, and therefore cannot be recommended.[25]

Mendes reported blood eosinophilia of up to 43% on white blood cell differential count, sputum eosinophilia, leukocytosis, an elevated erythrocyte sedimentation rate, fever, and transient splenomegaly in some patients during an "asthma epidemic" due to community exposure to castor-bean dust from a castor-oil plant.[23] During this period multiple patients required hospitalization, and chest x-rays in this group showed a diffuse interstitial reaction that cleared after 2 weeks. In this group of Brazilian patients precipitins to castor bean by gel-diffusion were negative, but others have demonstrated antibodies by both passive hemagglutination and by radioimmunoelectrophoresis using I-131 labeled castor-bean extract.[23,34]

TABLE 1. *Occupations Associated with Reported Cases of Castor-bean-associated Asthma*

Castor-oil mill workers
Coffee workers
Communities surrounding castor-bean mills
Farmers
Leather workers
Seamen and dock workers
Hydraulic oil production
Laboratory workers
Paint production
Polyurethane resin production
Workers exposed to Hessian bags previously used to ship castor-bean pomace
Textile workers
Soap production

Bronchial provocation tests have been done with the dust from shipments of castor beans, and late asthmatic responses have been reported.[24] A surreptitious bronchial challenge was also done in one study, in which castor-pomace antigen was nebulized into an entire room where patients suffering from potential community exposure to castor-bean dust from a neighboring castor-bean processing plant were exposed.[23] Typical asthma ensued and was persistent; the doctors and nurses in the same room served as the negative controls and did not develop symptoms.[23]

Treatment

The mainstay of treatment of castor-bean-associated asthma is avoidance of the antigen. In those involved in shipping of castor beans and/or pomace, the use of airtight shipping containers has been advised.[24] Proper respiratory protection in those unable to avoid the antigen is recommended, and proper filtering of exhaust from castor-oil mills and other processing areas is necessary to prevent asthmatic sensitization from exposure to the antigen of those living in areas surrounding these manufacturing plants. If patients sensitized from community-wide exposure to castor-bean pomace dust move from the surrounding areas, it appears that the symptoms may often clear, if castor-bean pomace was the only antigen precipitating their asthma.[23] Pharmacologic management would be identical to that for reactive airway disease in general.

Positive skin test reactions persisted in one group of patients 4 years after the factory source of community airborne castor-bean dust was eliminated, indicating the persistence of allergic sensitization in many individuals.[23] However, 80% of individuals in that study were symptom-free promptly after the processing of castor beans was stopped and appropriate filtering procedures implemented, indicating the efficacy of appropriate public health measures in this disease.[23]

REFERENCES

1. Persson CG: On the medical history of xanthines and other remedies for asthma: A tribute to H.H. Slater. Thorax 40:881–886, 1985.
2. Gong H Jr, Simmons MS, Tashkin DP, et al: Bronchodilator effects of caffeine in coffee. Chest 89:335–342, 1986.
3. Pagano R, Negri E, Decarli A, et al: Coffee drinking and prevalence of bronchial asthma. Chest 94:386–389, 1988.
4. Bernton HS: On occupational sensitization—a hazard to the coffee industry. JAMA 223:1146–1147, 1973.
5. Lehrer SB, Karr RM, Salvaggio JE: Extraction and analysis of coffee bean allergens. Clin Allergy 8:217–226, 1978.
6. Figley KD, Rowling FFA: Castor bean—an industrial hazard as a contaminant of green coffee dust and used burlap bags. J Allergy 20:545, 1950.
7. Freedman SO, Krupey J, Sebron AH: Chlorogenic acid: An allergen in green coffee bean. Nature 192:241, 1961.
8. Layton LL, Greene FC, Panzani R: Allergy to green coffee: Failure of patients allergic to green coffee to react to chlorogenic acid, roasted coffee, or orange. J Allergy 36:84, 1965.
9. Davies RJ, Blainey AD, Pepys J: Occupational asthma. In Middleton E, et al (eds): Allergy: Principles and Practice, 2nd ed. St. Louis, C.V. Mosby, 1983.
10. Jones RN, Hughes JM, Lehrer SB, et al: Lung function consequences of exposure and hypersensitivity in workers who process green coffee beans. Am Rev Respir Dis 125:199, 1982.
11. Karr RM, Davies RJ, Butcher BT, et al: Allergy grand rounds: Occupational asthma. J Allergy Clin Immunol 61:54–65, 1978.
12. Karr RM, Lehrer SB, Butcher BT, et al: Coffee workers' asthma: A clinical appraisal using the radioallergosorbent test. J Allergy Clin Immunol 62:143–148, 1978.
13. Kaye M, Freedman SO: Allergy to raw coffee. An occupational disease. Can Med Assoc J 84:469, 1961.
14. Jones RN, Hughes JM, Lehrer SB, et al: Lung function effects of exposure and hypersensitivity to green coffee beans. In Gee JB, Morgan WKC, Brooks SM (eds): Occupational Lung Disease. New York, Raven Press, 1984, p 190.
15. Zuskin E, Valic F, Kanceljak B: Immunological and respiratory changes in coffee workers. Thorax 36:9–13, 1981.
16. Zuskin E, Kanceljak B, Skuric Z, et al: Bronchial reactivity in green coffee exposure. Br J Ind Med 42:415, 1985.
17. Zuskin E, Valic F, Skuric Z: Respiratory function in coffee workers. Br J Ind Med 36:117, 1979.
18. Zuskin E, Kanceljak B, Witek JJ, et al: Acute ventilatory response to green coffee dust extract. Ann Allergy 66:219, 1991.
19. Layton LL, Panzani R, Cortese TA: Coffee-reaginic human sera tested in human volunteers and macaque monkeys. Absence of reactions to chlorogenic acid. Int Arch Allergy 33:417, 1968.
20. Karr RM: Bronchoprovocation studies in coffee workers' asthma. J Allergy Clin Immunol 64:650–654, 1979.
21. Vragoda CG: Respiratory disease in tea workers in Sri Lanka. Thorax 35:114–117, 1980.
22. Vragoda CG: Tea makers' asthma. Br J Ind Med 27:181–182, 1970.
23. Mendes E: Asthma provoked by castor-bean dust. In Frazier CA (ed): Occupational Asthma. New York, Van Nostrand Reinhold, 1980, pp 272–282.
24. Davison AG, Britton MG, Forrester JA, et al: Asthma in merchant seamen and laboratory workers caused by allergy to castor beans: Analysis of allergens. Clin Allergy 13:553–561, 1983.
25. Figley KD, Elrod RH: Epidemic asthma due to castor bean dust. JAMA 90:79–82, 1928.
26. Beruton HS: On occupational sensitization to the castor bean. Am J Med Sci 165:196–202, 1923.
27. Grimm V, Veroffeutl a.d.Geb. d. Med Verwalt 26:5, 1928. Quoted in Hansel K. Tratado de Alergia. Madrid, Editoriale Labor, 1946.
28. Mendes E: Asthma provoked by castor bean. In Frazier CA (ed): Occupational Asthma. New York, Van Nostrand Reinhold, 1980, p 272.
29. Ordman D: An outbreak of bronchial asthma in South Africa affecting more than 200 persons caused by castor bean dust from an oil processing factory. Int Arch Allergy 7:10, 1955.
30. Panzini R: Etude de l'allergie entre. lagraine de ricin et spondylocladium. Int Arch Allergy 21:288, 1962.
31. Wilson AB, Marchand RM, Coombs RRA: Passive allergisation in vitro of human basophils with serum containing IgE reaginic antibodies to castor allergen, demonstrated by Rosette-formation. Lancet i:1325–1329, 1971.
32. Coombs RRA, Hunter A, et al: Detection of IgE (IgND) specific antibody (probably reagin) to castor-bean allergen by the red-cell-linked antigen-antiglobulin reaction. Lancet i:1115–1118, 1968.
33. Panzini R, Layton LL: Allergy to dust of *ricinus communis* (castor beans): Clinical studies upon human beings and passively sensitized workers. Int Arch Allergy 22:350, 1963.
34. Strauss A: Collective asthma due to castor bean allergy. In Ourinhous SP: Follow-up Study After Industrial Processing of Castor Bean Was Stopped. Rev Inst Med Trop, Sao Paulo, 1975, NF 79.
35. Thomas KE, Trigg CJ, Baxter PJ, et al: Factors relating to the development of respiratory symptoms in coffee process workers. Br J Ind Med 48:314, 1991.

Chapter 11

ASTHMA IN THE FOOD INDUSTRY

Anthony Montanaro, MD

Although food allergy has been recognized for decades, occupational sensitization to foods has only recently been adequately described. Although the incidence of occupational asthma to foods is reasonably low, the number of workers at risk in the food processing industry is immense. A review of the available literature with regard to specific food agents will be presented in this chapter. While baker's asthma can be considered an occupational condition secondary to inhalation of a food, it is presented in a separate chapter (Chapter 9) because of its epidemiologic importance and the large amount of available data. In addition, coffee is discussed more extensively in the previous chapter.

EGG

Hypersensitivity to egg constituents are common and well recognized. Indeed, ovalbumin has been considered by many allergists to be one of the most important food antigens. Despite the ubiquitous nature of egg in the food industry and the widespread use of "egg washes" in the pastry industry, the first report of occupational asthma secondary to inhaled egg proteins did not appear until 1983.[1] In this study of workers who used a spray system to coat meat rolls with an egg solution, 8 of 13 workers developed symptoms suggestive of occupational asthma. Reported symptoms included cough, dyspnea, and wheezing occurring ½ to 2 hours following initial workday exposure. None of the workers developed late febrile or flu-like responses that would have indicated hypersensitivity pneumonitis. There was no correlation between the presence of respiratory symptoms and skin tests to egg, serum IgE levels, or precipitating antibody

levels. Although bronchial provocation studies were not undertaken, the investigators suggested sensitization had occurred, because respiratory symptoms ceased when a different coating method was introduced.

Subsequently more detailed studies of egg-processing workers have appeared.[2,3] Twenty-five workers were evaluated at a plant where raw eggs were processed into powdered egg yolk and whole egg. Personal total dust exposures were measured to be 12.8 and 7.3 mg/M^3 on 2 successive days. Fifty percent of the dust was determined to be protein with an amino acid profile similar to egg yolk. Five of the 25 workers were determined to have occupational asthma based on the appearance of typical workplace-related symptoms and a decrease in peak expiratory flow rate of 20% or more from the day's maximum reading. These same workers were further detailed immunologically in a follow-up study. All workers with definite asthma demonstrated epicutaneous reactivity to one or more egg allergens, whereas only 3 of 20 without asthma had positive tests. Radio-allergosorbent testing to egg antigens was positive in only 4 of the 25 workers and was positive only in workers with definite asthma. All RAST-positive workers demonstrated significant binding to factory whole egg extract, egg white, ovalbumin, and ovomucoid, with the highest binding occurring to ovomucoid. Specific IgG responses were found to be higher in workers than in nonexposed controls, but they did not correlate with clinical responses.

A follow-up study has recently been undertaken by the same authors to estimate the prevalence of IgE-mediated occupational asthma in egg-processing workers.[4] One hundred-eighty-eight workers in two additional plants were surveyed. Eighty-eight of these workers were further evaluated clinically. Fifty-eight of 188 respondents complained of work-related shortness of breath or chest pain. Peak flow variability occurred in 18 of 37 workers who were suspected as having bronchial asthma. Thirty-four percent of the 86 workers who underwent skin testing displayed cutaneous hypersensitivity to one or more egg allergens. On the basis of these findings, 10% of workers in one plant and 5% from the second were diagnosed as egg-induced asthma. There was no association between underlying atopy and the prevalence of egg-induced asthma.

These studies demonstrate definite IgE-mediated hyperresponsiveness in a significant number of workers exposed to inhaled egg allergens in occupational settings. Since sensitization may occur through oral ingestion in atopic as well as nonatopic individuals, there are many workers in the egg and food processing industry who are potentially at risk. Due to the relatively small size of individual companies in the industry, environmental control measures may be inadequate or nonexistent. Physicians caring for at-risk workers must pay particular attention to respiratory complaints and pulmonary function of at-risk individuals to avoid any potential long-term health effects.

SHELLFISH

Allergic reactivity to shellfish constituents has been recognized for centuries. While hypersensitivity reactions most commonly follow ingestion of shellfish, asthmatic responses following inhalational exposures are well described. Seafood processing remains a major industry in the United States, employing an estimated 350,000 workers in 1986.[5] The occurrence of occupational asthma to shellfish antigens is not surprising, given their antigenicity and airborne exposure through the substantial amounts of steam and water vapor released during processing. Leher has previously documented significant antigen present in the processing fluid following boiling, as well as cross-reactivity among shrimp, crab, crawfish, and lobster antigens.[6]

An additional mode of inhalational exposure to seafood is through the generation of dust in processing the dried product. An interesting report of a laboratory worker exposed to powdered marine sponge appeared in 1982.[7] In this report an atopic laboratory worker with a previous history of non-work-related asthma developed severe occupational asthma following operation of a grinding mill processing freeze-dried marine sponge. Subsequent evaluation indicated the presence of sponge-specific IgE by skin testing and RAST. Interestingly, these antibodies appeared to cross-react with extracts of soft corral. Other cases of hypersensitivity following inhalation of marine invertebrates have been reported in letter form. A single case of occupational asthma was reported by Karlin[8] following inhalation of clam liver extract, whereas Clarke[9] described a case of respiratory hypersensitivity to abalone. While these observations are limited, they support the concept of seafood allergenicity in the workplace by virtually any mode of exposure.

There are a limited number of studies in the literature regarding the incidence of occupational asthma in the seafood-processing industry. An investigation of 50 workers employed in a prawn-processing factory in Norway in 1980[12] suggested that 36% of workers had symptoms of allergic hyperresponsiveness to prawn extract, with 24% of workers displaying specific cutaneous reactions. These 50 workers were employed in a unique method by which whole prawns were processed through air jets that removed the meat from the shell but also generated small fragments of meat and droplets. Twenty-four percent of these workers demonstrated positive skin prick tests to freeze-dried prawn extracts, which were confirmed by RAST studies. Thirty-six percent complained of asthmatic symptoms within 15 minutes of exposure to the processing environment. Two workers demonstrated significant decrements in FEV_1 following bronchial provocation to the prawn extract.

Cartier and others first described the occurrence of occupational asthma in workers processing snow crab in 1984.[10] These same authors more recently studied 303 workers in two snow crab-processing plants.[11] Surprisingly, a diagnosis of occupational asthma was made in 15.6% of the workforce. Subsequently the presence of crab-specific IgE antibody was found to be significantly correlated with the presence of occupational asthma. These findings highlight the potential for prominent antigenicity of seafood in processing workers and confirm the occurrence of IgE-mediated occupational asthma. Although many seafood-processing workers have limited seasonal exposures, these observations suggest more aggressive use of respiratory protective devices in this industry and highlight the need for employers to identify high-risk employees.

ASCIDIAN (Sea Squirt)

The ascidian is a lower animal that is a member of the Protochordate family. Larvae-like tadpoles attach themselves to rocks and oyster shells. When they are removed from water, their body fluid is expelled through an exhalant orifice, thus explaining the derivation of their common name of sea squirt. Inhalation of this aerosolized material may take place during oyster processing. Following the Second World War, oyster farmers in Japan used an offshore raft system that promoted oyster growth and sea squirt breeding. Subsequently this trend has continued and has provided opportunity for observation and study of sea squirt-induced asthma in oyster workers. Jyo and co-workers in Hiroshima, Japan have been the major contributors to the scientific literature in this area and have summarized their findings in a recent book chapter.[13] In 1964 these authors estimated that the incidence of sea squirt asthma was in excess of 20%, ranging from 19 to 46% among 1,416 oyster farm workers in various locations. They confirmed cutaneous and RAST sensitivity by utilizing a glycoprotein antigen that is found in the fleshy portion as well as the body fluid of the sea squirt. Interestingly, a trial of hyposensitization therapy utilizing the purified antigen was found to be successful in 97% of workers who undertook this therapy within 3 months of its institution. Although IgE levels remained high, they were able to continue their seasonal employment. This represents one of the few reported instances where patients with occupational asthma have benefited from occupational allergen-specific immunotherapy. These unique observations have not been reproduced by other groups in other parts of the world.

COFFEE (See also Chapter 10)

Coffee consumption worldwide has promoted a major industry, with more than 20 million workers. Although the United States is the major importer of coffee beans, the number of potentially exposed workers is relatively small. In 1982 it was estimated that approximately 150 coffee companies employed a total of 11,800 workers nationwide.[14] Observations of occupational allergic reactions to coffee beans were made as early as 1950.[15] Initially the major coffee bean allergen was suspected to be chlorogenic acid, but this simple chemical alone was subsequently found to be nonallergenic in atopic individuals.[16] Jones and co-workers undertook studies of 372 coffee workers. Lower respiratory symptoms such as cough and wheeze were found in 37% of workers, but occupational asthma was not documented in any of the workers studied. Upper respiratory symptoms suggestive of rhinitis or sinusitis were reported in 43%. Immunologic reactivity to coffee bean antigens was never demonstrated, although positive castor-bean radioallergosorbent testing correlated with highest green coffee bean exposure. It has been suggested that the castor bean may be an important allergen in this occupational setting with exposure occurring through handling of coffee bean sacks which had previously contained castor bean.

GARLIC DUST

Occupational asthma due to inhalation of garlic dust was first reported by Henson in 1940.[17] Subsequently well documented cases confirmed by skin testing and bronchial provocation have appeared. One study reported development of respiratory sensitization following occupational inhalation of garlic dust in an individual who could ingest garlic without difficulty.[18] Subsequently an electrician at a spice-processing plant was described who developed typical signs and symptoms of garlic dust occupational asthma.[19] Bronchial provocation studies as well as skin testing were positive to garlic dust and garlic extract. Subsequent garlic extract challenges in non-garlic-sensitive asthmatics failed to reveal any significant changes in pulmonary function, indicating a lack of potential irritant effect. Interestingly, oral challenge was associated with a 21% reduction in FEV_1 and associated systemic symptoms. These observations confirm an IgE mechanism in this form of occupational asthma. Because garlic is a member of the Liliaceae (lily) family, which includes onion, asparagus, and chives with proven antigenic cross-reactivity, clinicians should be aware of potential for immunologic reactivity to inhalation or ingestion of these food substances.

CINNAMON

Cinnamon is the bark of the *Cinnamomum zeylanicum* tree, which is native to and almost exclusively found in Sri Lanka. Its characteristic taste and fragrance have led to its widespread use in foods, cosmetics, and pharmaceuticals. Powdered cinnamon contains only 1% cinnamic aldehyde which is a potent irritant of skin and mucous membranes. Although to our knowledge no systematic study has been undertaken of cinnamon-processing workers, a single report from Sri Lanka questioned 40 workers in a cinnamon store.[20] Using the British Medical Research Council respiratory questionnaire, this study indicated a significant number of respiratory complaints in these workers. Although 35 of 40 (87.5%) workers reported some symptoms ascribed to their work environment, 9 (22.5%) complained of symptoms compatible with bronchial asthma. Whereas a limited bronchial provocation study to cinnamon was undertaken and interpreted as positive in one worker, seven workers had developed asthma since beginning work, and four had attributed their asthma to work exposures. While this study does not address the potential mechanism of cinnamon-induced asthma, clinicians should be aware of the potential for cutaneous and respiratory irritation from this ubiquitous spice.

HONEYBEE DUST

Although inhalant insect allergy has been recognized for decades,[21] it was not generally appreciated as a cause of occupational asthma other than in beekeepers.[22] More recently occupational asthma to honeybee-body dust in a honey-processing worker has been described by Yunginger and colleagues at the Mayo Clinic.[23] The worker had developed severe asthma during the July to October honey-packing season. Interestingly, during the handling of wood frames that contained honeycombs the worker was exposed to dead honeybees. Subsequent medical evaluation failed to reveal any predisposing factors such as underlying atopy or pulmonary disease. The worker had previously sustained honeybee stings without systemic reactions. Bronchial provocation, skin test, and RAST with honeybee whole-body extract were positive. Insecticide bronchial challenges and skin testing to seasonal outdoor aeroallergens were negative. The patient's positive RAST could be inhibited by preincubation from an air sample eluate from inside the packing plant, but not from air sample eluates from outside the patient's home. These observations document an IgE-mediated seasonal occupational asthma to honeybee-body dust. At-risk workers would include not only beekeepers, but honey-processing workers as well.

MUSHROOMS

Mushrooms have been described as being a source of immunologically mediated pulmonary disease for many years. The first case of mushroom-induced extrinsic allergic alveolitis was described in 1959.[24] Subsequent reports of similar disease were confirmed by British investigators in agricultural workers.[25] These investigators termed this form of extrinsic allergic alveolitis "mushroom workers lung." While these cases represented nonreagin-induced disease, subsequent reports in the Japanese literature documented bronchial asthma in individuals raising greenhouse grain mushrooms. These individuals did not develop a clinical picture of hypersensitivity pneumonitis but were felt to have immediate hypersensitivity to mushroom spores.[26] More recently, Scottish investigators have reported immediate onset occupational asthma and rhinitis in food-processing workers exposed to dried mushroom soup.[27] Mixed species of mushrooms were dried, mixed, and emulsified, resulting in significant particulate aerosolization. Eight of 400 employees presented with lower respiratory or nasal complaints. Five of eight of these workers displayed cutaneous reactivity to the dried extract. Four of the eight workers demonstrated a greater than 30% decline in FEV_1 following breathing zone inhalational provocation with the dried mushroom extract. An additional two workers who were skin-test negative displayed profuse rhinorrhea. These cases represent further examples of potential respiratory sensitization that can occur in the food processing industry. These observations should lead to increased awareness within the industry and to promotion of improved industrial hygiene measures in areas where potential airborne allergens are encountered.

HOT PEPPER WORKERS (Capsaicin)

Capsaicin is the active chemical contained in cayenne peppers *(Capsicum)*. This chemical accounts for the hot characteristic of hot chilies, which are the dried pods of these peppers (usually *Capsicum frutescens*). There has been renewed interest in the mechanism of action of capsaicin since the isolation and characterization of the neurotransmitter substance P. Capsaicin's chemical actions appear to be mediated through the release of this neurotransmitter, as well as other potential neurotransmitters from nociceptive afferent nerve endings.[28] Interestingly, these same capsaicin-sensitive nerves located in the airways have been felt to be initially involved in the inflammatory process that underlies increased airway hyperreactivity and cough.[29] Recently, spice workers' inhalational exposure to capsaicin through the processing of capsaicin-containing peppers was studied.[30] Twenty-two capsaicin-exposed and 19 non-capsaicin-exposed administrative workers in a spice-processing plant were studied. Fifty-nine percent of the capsaicin-exposed workers reported cough as compared to 21% of the nonexposed administrative workers. Baseline spirometric parameters did not differ between these two groups. Cough threshold was determined by assessing the lowest concentration of inhaled capsaicin that elicited a cough. The capsaicin-exposed workers compared to the administrative workers displayed a bimodal pattern of higher and lower cough threshold to capsaicin. A higher cough threshold in the exposed group was significantly related to male gender, cigarette smoking, and dietary preference for hot food. These findings suggested that chronic occupational exposure to chili peppers is associated with subjective complaints of cough but apparently does not alone lead to decreased responsiveness of capsaicin-sensitive nerve endings. Given the recent observations with regards to the effects of angiotensin-converting enzyme inhibitors and increased cough, which appear to be mediated by substance P mechanisms,[31] it would appear that individuals should be cautious when potentially exposed to capsaicin-containing substances in and away from the workplace. Clinicians should be aware of this potential mechanism of cough in a small but significant workforce.

REFERENCES

1. Edwards JH, McConnochie K, Trotman DM, et al: Allergy to inhaled egg material. Clin Allergy 13:427–432, 1983.
2. Smith AB, Berstein DI, Aw T, et al: Occupational asthma from inhaled egg protein. Am J Ind Med 12:205–218, 1987.
3. Bernstein DJ, Smith AB, Moller DFR, et al: Clinical and immunologic studies among egg processing workers with occupational asthma. J Allergy Clin Immunol 80:791–799, 1987.
4. Smith AB, Bernstein DJ, Landan M, et al: Evaluation of occupational asthma from airborne egg exposure in multiple settings. Chest 98:398–404, 1990.
5. Baunan O (ed): Fisheries of the United States. Washington, D.C., U.S. Dept. of Commerce, 1987.
6. Lehrer SB: Hypersensitivity reactions in seafood workers. Allergy Proc 11:69–70, 1990.
7. Baldo BA, Krilis S, Taylor KM: IgE-mediated acute asthma following inhalation of a powdered marine sponge. Clin Allergy 12:179–186, 1982.
8. Karlin JM: Occupational asthma to clam's liver extract. J Allergy Clin Immunol 63:197, 1979.
9. Clarke PS: Immediate respiratory hypersensitivity to abalone (letter). Med J Aust 1:623, 1979.
10. Cartier A, Malo JL, Fevest F: Occupational asthma in snow crab processing workers. J Allergy Clin Immunol 74:261–269, 1984.
11. Cartier A, Malo JL, Ghezzo H, et al: IgE sensitization in snow crab processing workers. J Allergy Clin Immunol 78:344–348, 1986.
12. Gaddie J, Legge JS, Friend JAR: Pulmonary hypersensitivity in prawn workers. Lancet 20/27:1350–1353, 1980.
13. Jyo T, Katsutani T, Tsuboi S, et al: Hoya (sea squirt) asthma. In Frazier CA (ed): Occupational Asthma. New York, Von Nostrand Reinhold, 1980.
14. Jones RN, Hughes JM, Lehrer SB: Lung function consequences of exposure and hypersensitivity in workers who process green coffee beans. Am Rev Respir Dis 125:199–202, 1982.
15. Figley KD, Rawlings FFA: Castor bean: An industrial hazard as a contaminant of green coffee dust and used burlap bags. J Allergy Clin Immunol 21:545–553, 1950.
16. Layton LL, Green FC, Corse JW, Panzani R: Pure chlorogenic acid not allergenic in atopy to green coffee: A specific protein probably is involved. Nature 203:188–189, 1964.
17. Henson CE: Garlic: An occupational factor in the etiology of bronchial asthma. J Fla Med Assoc 27:86–88, 1981.
18. Falleroni AI, Zeiss CR, Lentz D: Occupational asthma secondary to inhalation of garlic dust. J Allergy Clin Immunol 68:156–160, 1981.
19. Lybarger JA, Gallagher JS, Pulver DW, et al: Occupational asthma induced by inhalation and ingestion of garlic. J Allergy Clin Immunol 69:448–453, 1982.
20. Urogoda CG: Asthma and other symptoms in cinnamon workers. Br J Ind Med 41:224–227, 1984.
21. Perlman F: Insects as inhalant allergens. Consideration of aerobiology, biochemistry, preparation of material and clinical observations. J Allergy 29:302, 1958.
22. Feinberg AR, Feinberg SM, Benaim-Pinto C: Asthma and rhinitis from insect allergens. Clinical importance. J Allergy 27:437, 1956.
23. Ostrom NK, Swanson MC, Agarwal MK, Yunginger JW: Occupational allergy to honeybee-body dust in a honey-processing plant. J Allergy Clin Immunol 77:736–740, 1986.
24. Bringhurst LS, Byrne RN, Gershan-Cohen S: Respiratory disease of mushroom workers. JAMA 171:15, 1959.
25. Sakula A: Mushroom workers lung. Br Med J 3:708, 1967.
26. Kando O: A case of cartinellis shiitake spore asthma. Jap J Allergy 18:81, 1969.
27. Symington IS, Kerr JW, McLean DA: Type I allergy in mushroom soup processors. Clin Allergy 11:43–47, 1981.

28. Buck SH, Burks TF: The pharmacology of capsaicin: A review of some recent observations. Pharm Rev 38:180–226, 1986.

29. Barnes PJ: Neuropeptides in human airways: Function and clinical implications. Am Rev Respir Dis 136:S77–S83, 1987.

30. Blanc P, Liu D, Juarez C, Boushey HA: Cough in hot pepper workers. Chest 99:27–32, 1991.

31. O'Hollaren MTO, Porter G: Angiotensin converting enzyme inhibitors and the allergist. Ann Allergy 64:503–506, 1990.

Chapter 12

ISOCYANATE ASTHMA

Anthony Montanaro, MD

The isocyanates are a group of highly reactive, low molecular weight chemicals used primarily in the polyurethane industry. Worldwide use of the chemicals exceeds several billion pounds. Due to its highly unsaturated isocyanate group, this chemical group has numerous and varied industrial applications. Monoisocyanates are used in agricultural herbicide and insecticide products, whereas polyisocyanates are used for production of polyurethane. Specific products made from these chemicals include adhesives, paints, and coatings as well as rigid and flexible foams (Figs. 1–3). A partial listing of the industries in which isocyanate exposure may take place is summarized in Table 1. Although toluene-diisocyanate (TDI) is the principal isocyanate used in industry, methylene diphenyl-diisocyanate (MDI) and hexamethylene-diisocyanate (HDI) are widely used and well documented causes of occupational lung disease.

Since the original description in 1951 of occupational asthma following isocyanate inhalation,[1] there have been numerous reports that have detailed immunologic and clinical aspects of this disorder. Although the precise pathophysiologic events underlying this condition remain uncertain, this chapter will review the clinical toxicologic and immunologic data that have accumulated.

HISTORY OF ISOCYANATES

Polyurethane foams were first produced in Germany during the Second World War, principally using toluene diisocyanate. The initial technology had been developed by Dr. Otto Bayer in 1937. Isocyanates were initially employed as curing agents for polyurethane resins.[2] Polyurethane polymers were first produced in the United States in 1953.[2] The initial application was in the production of rigid foam. These early foam systems used MDI because of its lower volatility and subsequent diminished capacity for human toxicity. Over the subsequent 40 years, the use and applications of the isocyanates have dramatically risen worldwide. In 1975, 300 million pounds of MDI and 400 million pounds of TDI were manufactured. In 1980, worldwide use of polyurethane resins exceeded 7 billion pounds.[2a] The U.S. Public Health Service estimated that between 1972 and 1974 50,000 to 100,000 workers were potentially exposed to isocyanates in the U.S. alone[3] (Table 1).

CHEMISTRY OF ISOCYANATES

The isocyanates are a group of highly reactive, low molecular weight compounds (Fig. 4). The polyfunctional isocyanates (more than one isocyanate group, e.g., TDI) are extremely reactive, particularly those having active hydrogen. It is this reactivity that allows them to be used in the production of polymeric structures. Their reactive nature enables them to *self-react*, leading to the formation of dimers, trimers, and unpredictable and sometimes very large structures that may be dissimilar both sterically and antigenically. This high degree of reactivity to most organic and many inorganic substances such as proteins, carbohydrates, and even water results in the formation of a wide variety of compounds with different biochemical and immunologic properties. The unpredictable nature of the

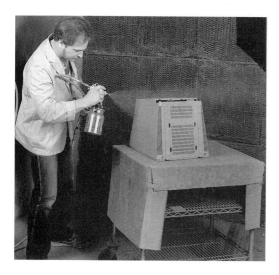

FIGURE 1. Electronics worker spraying isocyanate-containing coating.

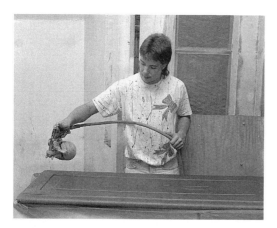

FIGURE 2. Truck painter applying isocyanate-containing enamel paint.

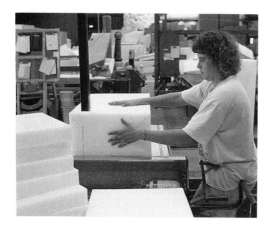

FIGURE 3. Worker cutting polyurethane foam to be used in packaging application.

TABLE 1. *Partial List of Occupations with Possible Exposure to Isocyanates*

Adhesive workers	Organic chemical
Artists	synthesizers
Boat builders	Plastic industry
Carpet layers	Polyurethane
Chemists	manufacturing
Electricians	Resin workers
Enamelers	Rubber manufacturing
Furniture makers	Sculptors
Insulation workers	Spray painters
Lacquer workers	Textile manufacturing
Laminators (wood	Upholsterers
and plastic)	Wire coating workers

chemical reactivity has made it difficult to identify compounds involved in the chemical processes resulting from isocyanate exposure. Because of their biologic reactivity, isocyanates are capable of respiratory tract toxicity as well as immunologic sensitivity. It must be stressed that, although the polyfunctional isocyanates are well-known immunologic sensitizers, the aliphatic isocyanates such as hydrogenated diphenylmethane diisocyanate (HMDI) have not been established as sensitizing agents.[4] Aliphatic isocyanates have found industrial importance because of their "light, stable" characteristics. Although the vapor pressures of TDI and HDI are similar, when HDI exists in the biuret form, i.e., three molecules of HDI bound together, the size of the molecule results in a decrease in vapor pressure. When employed in the biuret form in HDI-based paints, the risk of respiratory disease is much reduced. In these formulations, monomeric HDI comprises at most 1% of the isocyanate composition. In addition, MDI exerts only a fraction of the vapor pressure of TDI or HDI and therefore is markedly less volatile. Pure MDI is solid at room temperature and is frequently stored as a liquid combination of polymerized MDI and acetone.

TOXICITY OF ISOCYANATES

A number of important medical consequences of isocyanate exposure have been well detailed[3,4] and are outlined below:

Neurologic Sequelae. Neurologic sequelae of acute and chronic isocyanate exposure have been difficult to quantify. Acute isocyanate exposure has not been associated with specific predictable neurologic signs, but subjective symptoms such as euphoria and ataxia have been recorded. The occasional loss of consciousness has been described following extreme exposures. The effects of chronic low-dose exposure are difficult to verify and incompletely studied. Nevertheless, symptoms such as chronic headache, memory defects, and difficulty concentrating have all been attributed to high-dose chronic exposure.[3,4]

Pulmonary Toxicity. Pulmonary toxicity can arbitrarily be separated into (1) acute irritative responses; (2) occupational asthma; (3) chronic respiratory effects, and (4) hypersensitivity pneumonitis. Pulmonary symptomatology may occur through irritant, pharmacologic, or immunologic mechanisms (Fig. 5). Symptoms such as cough, chest pain or tightness, and shortness of breath may occur immediately following a single exposure. Exposures to greater than 100 parts per billion (ppb) are likely to result in symptoms from a primary irritant effect.[3–5] When considering primary irritation of the lung, it is important to consider nonrespiratory chemical irritant symptoms, such as headache, sore throat, nasal congestion, ocular irritation, and nausea or vomiting, that may occur. Respiratory irritation is unlikely to occur at exposure levels of less than 30 ppb.[5] Documentation of irritant exposures and resultant symptomatology are critical, because the medical consequences are significant.

In a small proportion of exposed workers immunologic sensitization may occur. The incidence of sensitization to TDI has been estimated to be 5–10%.[6] Sensitization of the respiratory tract may occur at extraordinarily low levels of exposure. There are some data that suggest that sensitization is very unlikely at ambient levels at or below 20 ppb.[7] Respiratory sensitization characteristically begins following high-dose exposure to TDI.[3–5] Following initial sensitization, symptoms such as cough, chest tightness, wheezing, and shortness of breath may occur within minutes on subsequent subirritant exposures or 4–8 hours following such exposure. Some patients will have a dual response following exposure, with both immediate and delayed responses. A recurrent late pattern of occupational asthma has been observed in selected workers with TDI asthma. This may begin 12 to 24 hours after initial exposure and is followed by recurrent patterns of recovery and bronchoconstriction lasting up to 12 hours.[8] Because sensitization can result in prolonged symptoms with chronic exposures, recognition of this symptom pattern and complex is important. Because there is virtually no safe level of

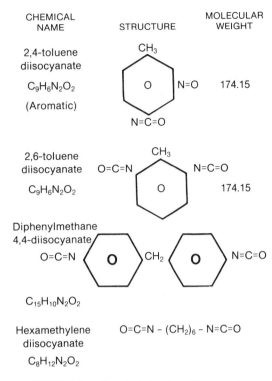

ISOCYANATES
CHEMICAL AND PHYSICAL DATA

CHEMICAL NAME	STRUCTURE	MOLECULAR WEIGHT

2,4-toluene diisocyanate

$C_9H_6N_2O_2$

(Aromatic)   174.15

2,6-toluene diisocyanate

$C_9H_6N_2O_2$ 174.15

Diphenylmethane 4,4-diisocyanate

$C_{15}H_{10}N_2O_2$

Hexamethylene diisocyanate $O=C=N - (CH_2)_6 - N=C=O$

$C_8H_{12}N_2O_2$

FIGURE 4.   Chemical structure of isocyanates.

exposure in individuals who have become sensitized, these individuals must be completely removed from the workplace.

Although primary irritation may result in significant symptomatology, the effects of respiratory irritation are short-lived in most cases and do not result in long-term impairment.

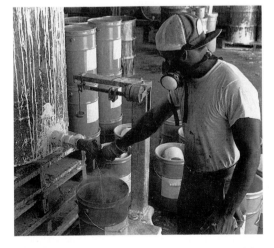

FIGURE 5.   Production worker filling barrels containing isocyanate resins, demonstrating the potential for spills and the need for adequate respiratory protection.

Unlike those individuals who have been sensitized, subsequent low-dose exposures may not result in symptoms or changes in pulmonary function in those individuals who have sustained irritant reactions. While these individuals do not necessarily need to be removed from the workplace, they should be provided adequate respiratory protection to avoid future possibility of sensitization.

DOSE RESPONSE

In an early attempt to establish a dose-response association between chronic isocyanate exposure and pulmonary function decrements, Wegman and Peters studied 57 workers in a polyurethane cushion manufacturing plant.[9] These workers were arbitrarily divided into three groups based on the results of personal breathing zone isocyanate measurements for periods of 20 to 90 minutes (group I less than 0.0015 ppm; group II, 0.0020–0.0030 ppm; and group III, equal to or greater than 0.0035 ppm). Those workers in group I revealed normal declines in FEV_1 over the 2 years of the study. Group III experienced an average loss of 103 ml/year, and group II 42 ml/year. The group III workers were felt to have a three- to fourfold excessive loss of pulmonary function when compared to a control population. On the basis of these findings, the authors suggested that chronic exposure to TDI at 0.003 ppm or higher was unsafe. The authors pointed out that a large dropout rate of 45% was a methodologic problem in this study. Nevertheless, the study population did not differ in age, sex, size, or smoking history, which are all variables that may affect the extent and rate of pulmonary function decline.

INDUSTRIAL STUDIES

Adams and co-workers were one of the first groups of investigators to study the long-term respiratory effects of TDI exposure.[10] In 1975 they reported on a long-term prospective study of 76 workers in a TDI manufacturing plant followed over 9 years. Respiratory questionnaires revealed no significant differences in the respiratory complaints in TDI-exposed workers compared to control workers without exposure. In addition, annual pulmonary function studies in 180 asymptomatic exposed workers did not differ from nonexposed controls. When selected symptomatic TDI-exposed

workers who had left the manufacturing plant were evaluated, their FEV_1 and FVCs appeared approximately 260 ml lower than nonexposed controls. These findings suggest that there may be a "safe" level of exposure to TDI below which no respiratory compromise will develop. Nevertheless, these findings also highlight the importance of removing or adequately protecting the worker from exposure when symptoms develop that may be related to TDI exposure.

Chan Yeung and colleagues reported their retrospective experience with MDI occupational asthma in a steel foundry in British Columbia.[11] Workers were exposed to an MDI-containing product used as a chemical binder in a mold fabrication process. Ambient levels of MDI were determined to be 0.008 ppm at the time of study. Seventy-eight workers were surveyed. Respiratory complaints were found to be common in these surveyed workers. Twelve of the 78 workers were found to have abnormal methacholine challenge studies. Eleven of these 12 subjects subsequently underwent formaldehyde and MDI bronchial provocation studies. Formaldehyde was included in these studies because it was a by-product in the manufacturing process. No worker had a positive challenge to formaldehyde, whereas six workers were determined to have positive responses to MDI bronchial provocation. Specific IgE to MDI was detected in only two of the responsive workers. Importantly, there were no differences in age, smoking history, or atopy between responders and nonresponders.

The extent of the MDI asthma problem in foundry workers was further detailed by this same group in 1985.[12] In this report the same 78 foundry workers were compared with 372 railway yard workers who presumably were not exposed to airborne contaminants. Compared to these control workers, the foundry workers complained of a greater incidence of respiratory symptoms, such as cough, shortness of breath, and episodic wheezing. In addition, the foundry workers appeared to have significantly lower FEV_1 and FEF_{25-75} in comparison to controls. As expected, the rate of respiratory symptoms as well as a decrement in pulmonary function appeared to be more notable in cigarette smokers as well as ex-cigarette smokers. It was noted that positive methacholine challenges were present in approximately 20% of the workers. When smoking history was considered, 30% of currently smoking workers had positive methacholine studies, with only 9.7% of the nonsmoking workers positive. Although specific bronchial provocation studies were not undertaken in this report, 12 of the 78 patients were considered to have a "sensitivity to MDI as a probable cause of their asthma." These studies highlight the difficulty in interpreting retrospective industrial studies where very little preemployment information is known. Although many smoking workers may deny previous respiratory complaints, it is clear that they are predisposed not only to recurrent respiratory difficulties, but to an increased rate of decline in pulmonary function when compared to the nonsmoking population.

In a recent British report, Venables and co-workers at the Brompton Hospital in London examined an outbreak of occupational asthma in a plant in which steel was coated with a plastic covering.[13] The plastic coating was made of isocyanate-containing epoxy resins, phenol formaldehyde, and polyvinyl chloride, and was cured to 400°C. Two hundred and twenty workers were studied. Of these workers, 84 reported work-related respiratory complaints. On more detailed questioning, 21 (9.5%) had symptoms suggestive of occupational asthma. Interestingly, symptomatic workers who had been exposed to the cleaning process had similar pulmonary function to the other groups studied, including an entirely asymptomatic group. Eight-hour time-weighted averages for TDI were measured and found to vary from 0.001 ppm to 0.026 ppm. Bronchial provocation testing was undertaken with the two-part varnish substance in only two subjects and found to be positive in both of these individuals. Importantly, the latent period from the initial exposure to the onset of symptoms was approximately 3 years in these workers. When surveyed 1 year after discontinuation of the use of isocyanate, 40% of the affected workers with presumed occupational asthma reported no work-related symptoms. An additional 45% continued to have work-related symptoms with no exposure to TDI but reported that their symptoms were improved. While this paper details important observations, it has a number of methodologic problems. It is a retrospective cross-sectional study with less than 50% follow-up. No preexposure, pulmonary function, or smoking data are available on reported workers with presumed occupational asthma. We find only two workers actually had bronchial provocation studies, thus truly confirming occupational asthma in only these two. Nevertheless, the authors do highlight important clinical findings of a 3-year latent period from the time of exposure to TDI to the actual development of symptomatic airway obstruction; other authors have reported this in the past. Another important observation in this report is that the majority of individuals, following cessation of TDI exposure, actually had no symptoms or improving symptoms despite continuation of work with no observed change in pulmonary function.

The pulmonary effects of chronic inhalational isocyanate exposures are controversial. Wegmen et al.[14] studied workers exposed to up to 20 ppb TDI over a 2-year time period. Their results suggested that chronic exposure to this previously considered "safe" level resulted in significant declines in FEV_1. Concern about the validity of lung function measurements in this series of observations was made later by Gee and Morgan.[15] In contrast, Diem and co-workers at Tulane University have prospectively assessed the long-term effects of isocyanate exposure in workers exposed to variable levels of isocyanate in the manufacturing process.[16] In a 5-year longitudinal study of workers in a TDI manufacturing plant, they found this group's mean annual decline in FEV_1 to be no different than age-matched controls. In a nonsmoking high-exposure group, there was a small decline in FEV_1 noted. Similar observations were made by Musk et al. in a retrospective study.[17]

Although cases of MDI asthma have been reported, it occurs less frequently due to its low vapor pressure and infrequent high-dose exposure. Unfortunately, there are no prospective, longitudinal studies available of workers chronically exposed to MDI. In 1986, Banks et al. noted that there had been no acute toxic exposures to MDI resulting in acute respiratory distress or long-term respiratory impairment.[18] This continues to be the case at this time.

HYPERSENSITIVITY PNEUMONITIS

Although hypersensitivity pneumonitis is classically ascribed to inhalation of organic dusts, there have been many case reports of hypersensitivity pneumonitis occurring following exposure to TDI, MDI, and HDI.[3,4,18,19] Characteristic clinical findings of fever, cough, malaise, pulmonary infiltrates, leukocytosis, and hypergammaglobulinemia may be associated with exposure to these low molecular weight compounds. Subsequent inhalation challenge studies have reproduced symptoms confirming the association in selected cases. In some patients, wheezing may occur in association with this syndrome, which may make differentiation of hypersensitivity disease from pure occupational asthma difficult. In a recent report, Mapp et al.[20] documented the coexistence of allergic alveolitis due to MDI, as well as occupational asthma documented by bronchial provocation studies. Interestingly, the two individuals reported in this study who had been exposed to MDI for over 2 years in an athletic shoe manufacturing plant did not react to TDI when challenged. This observed lack of cross-reactivity between MDI and TDI conflicts with observations claiming shared antigenicity or reactivity.[21,22] The lack of cross-reactivity to challenge testing may be explained by the relative purity of the antigens used in the challenge studies or technical difficulties inherent in the challenge procedure itself.

PATHOPHYSIOLOGY

Since the initial description of isocyanate asthma, investigators have attempted to attribute the physiologic events underlying bronchial hyperresponsiveness to a specific etiology. Although a great deal of valuable information has been learned in the study of this disease, multiple possibilities have been explored. The potential mechanisms that have been studied include nonimmunologic (irritant) as well as immunologic and pharmacologic mechanisms. At the present time, it remains to be determined whether there in fact is a single mechanism of isocyanate asthma or if it is multifactorial in its pathogenesis.

Immunologic Hypotheses

Clinical descriptions of immediate asthmatic responses to isocyanates led to investigations for isocyanate-specific IgE in affected workers. The results have been variable and disappointing in many instances, primarily because of the difficulties in identifying an appropriate etiologic substance with which to study the pathophysiology of the disorder.

Karol and colleagues at the University of Pittsburgh examined newer technology for determining isocyanate-specific IgE antibodies.[23] In their report, they outlined the methodologies that are currently available for isocyanate-specific IgE RAST determinations.

Their findings indicated binding to nitrocellulose appeared to be superior to binding to paper disks in the measurement of isocyanate-specific antibodies. In addition, the nitrocellulose methodology appeared by inhibition studies to be more specific than the paper disk methodology, thus eliminating chances for false-positive tests. While nitrocellulose immunoblotting has become the standard in immunology testing in many settings, further study will be required to determine its role in the diagnosis of isocyanate asthma.

Recently Wass and Belin[24] evaluated the immunologic specificity of isocyanate-induced IgE antibodies in previously occupationally sensitized patients. They describe a procedure for the preparation of radioallergosorbent testing (RAST) disks in which the number of isocyanate molecules could be varied when added to human serum albumin (HSA) conjugate. Their findings indicate optimal binding when 10 or less molecules of isocyanate are bound to each molecule of HSA. This is less than half the number of molecules that had been previously described as optimal by Baur[25] and Karol.[23,26] Importantly, all asymptomatic control subjects were negative by this methodology. Unfortunately, only 4% of patients with suspected isocyanate hypersensitivity were found to be positive. Although these authors chose a RAST ratio of greater than 3.0 as indicating a positive reaction to eliminate false-positive tests, their findings indicate a much lower rate of positivity than the previously reported rates of up to 75%.[26] Substantial immunologic cross-reactivity was demonstrated among TDI, HDI, and MDI by RAST inhibition studies.[21-26] These findings highlight the continuing difficulty of establishing immunologic hypersensitivity in patients suspected of having isocyanate asthma.

Controversy and uncertainty surrounding specific IgE responses to isocyanates and their role in the pathogenesis of isocyanate asthma has led to the development of new animal models. Bernstein and colleagues at the University of Cincinnati have studied immune responses in mice immunized with TDI conjugated to heterologous albumin.[27] In this study, homocytotropic antibodies developed to unconjugated albumin as well as to TDI-conjugated albumin. Interestingly, antibody titers to the TDI conjugates were approximately four times lower compared to those raised against albumin alone. Inhibition of the antibody activity by mono- and diisocyanate suggest the antibody responses were specific. The authors further speculated that the O-tolyl side chain may be important in the antigenic specificity of these conjugates. While this model allowed for the use of well-standardized and controlled antigens, its potential application to the human disease remains to be established.

A subsequent report on immunologic and respiratory responses to airway challenges of TDI in animals was made in 1983 by Patterson et al.[28] In their study, dogs were exposed to inhaled TDI on a twice-weekly basis for 4 months. The concentration of 1 mg/kg had been established to be equivalent to two to three times that of a potentially exposed human worker. A systemic immune response was subsequently noted in all three dogs studied, with measurable specific IgG, IgA, and IgM antibodies. IgE responses were determined by skin titration and found in two of the three dogs, but in fluctuating degrees of reactivity that ultimately became negative. Responsiveness of the peripheral blood lymphocytes was increased. Mild early and late airway responses occurred but were limited. One animal died following the challenge, suggesting that the dose chosen was indeed significant. These observations provide provocative data indicating a complex array of physiologic and immunologic changes that may occur following isocyanate exposure. While some of these changes have been described in humans, further investigation is necessary to determine their clinical significance.

To determine the significance of IgE antibodies to isocyanates in occupational asthma, Butcher and colleagues utilized a RAST methodology with a P-tolyl isocyanate side chain conjugated to HSA.[29] This hapten had previously been used by Karol[26] to obviate possible difficulties with self-complexing. Twenty-six workers were studied who had been previously documented to have positive TDI bronchial provocation studies. In this group of workers, positive RAST studies were obtained in only 15 to 19%. These findings again support the theory that isocyanate asthma is not solely IgE-mediated.

Recent insights into the potential role of specific IgE in isocyanate asthma have been provided by Patterson and colleagues.[30] Fifty-five isocyanate workers who had reported respiratory symptoms compatible with occupational asthma were studied. Isocyanate-specific antibody was measured by ELISA methodology and results were reported as an index to minimize false-positive conjugate reactivity.

Workers who were positive to bronchial provocation studies had statistically significant greater isocyanate-specific IgG indices and a non-statistically significant trend to higher IgE indices. Those workers demonstrating significant IgE or IgG indices were then used for in vitro ELISA inhibition studies. Preincubation with the isocyanate human serum albumin conjugate to which they were exposed by bronchial provocation completely inhibited IgG responses. Preincubation with human serum albumin alone, isocyanate dog serum albumin, or isocyanate ovalbumin resulted in partial or no inhibition. These data support the hypothesis that antibody response is not directed against the isocyanate or its conjugate, but against new antigenic determinants formed against the combination of the highly reactive isocyanates and serum proteins. While these observations do not establish isocyanate immunoresponsiveness as the sole etiology in isocyanate asthma, they provide further insights into previous findings of variable seropositivity among affected workers.[30]

The lack of clearly defined IgE-mediated mechanisms of isocyanate asthma led to the search for alternative explanations. Atkins and others have described the release of neutrophil chemotactic factors in immediate hypersensitivity responses to other antigens in 1977.[31] Subsequently Caroll et al. reported the activation of neutrophils in allergen and histamine-induced bronchospasm.[32] These apparently nonspecific pathophysiologic events were further studied by Valentino and colleagues in 12 workers with isocyanate asthma confirmed by bronchial provocation studies.[33] In their study, an increase in serum leukocyte chemotactic activity was seen after a late-phase TDI-induced asthmatic response, but *not* following an acute phase response. Although a presumed mast cell releasing factor was biochemically defined in this study, the findings are consistent with the hypothesis that late-phase TDI asthma is associated with inflammatory changes of the airways.

Recently Sastre and co-workers have described neutrophil chemotactic activity (NCA) in patients who were undergoing bronchial provocation studies with subirritant levels of TDI.[34] Their findings suggest that a rise in serum NCA paralleled a decline in FEV_1 in TDI-sensitive patients following bronchial challenge in both early and late asthmatic responses. NCA was not increased following methacholine challenge alone. Since similar high molecular weight NCA has been described in non-IgE-mediated asthmatic responses such as exercise-induced bronchospasm, this observation supports the participation of nonimmunologic mechanisms in isocyanate asthma. However, since NCA appears to be derived from mast cells and basophils, it would appear that activation of these cells may be important in the pathogenesis of specific asthmatic responses. While it is unlikely that the neutrophil activity described is responsible for the initiation of all isocyanate-induced changes, these findings support a multifactorial etiology in this condition.

Pharmacologic Studies

Butcher and colleagues at Tulane University first suggested the association of altered beta-adrenergic function in isocyanate asthma.[35] In this study, selected isocyanate-sensitive workers underwent immunologic, pharmacologic, and bronchial provocation studies. The findings indicated that TDI exposure did not affect lymphocyte cyclic 3_1, 5_1 adenosine monophosphate (cAMP) levels of clinically sensitive or nonsensitive workers, but did inhibit stimulation of cAMP by the beta-agonist isoproterenol. The inhibitory effect was seen in both clinically sensitive and nonsensitive controls, suggesting a beta receptor blocking action of TDI. They further demonstrated that TDI did not cause a nonspecific release of histamine from peripheral leukocytes. Methacholine hyperresponsiveness was demonstrated in 7 of the 10 clinically sensitive workers and 1 of 10 non-clinically sensitive workers. These were important observations, because these results suggested an alternative explanation other than a direct IgE response for isocyanate-induced pulmonary disease.[35]

Further support for a biochemically mediated mechanism of action of TDI in the induction of hyperreactivity was proposed by Davies in 1977.[36] In this in vitro study, human lymphocyte intracellular cAMP was measured after incubation with TDI. TDI was found to have a stimulatory or a beta-agonist-like effect on intracellular cAMP at a concentration of 10^3M. More importantly, incubation with TDI appeared to have an inhibitory effect on cAMP stimulation induced by isoproterenol and prostaglandin E_1. These findings suggested that TDI may in fact cause asthma by a "pharmacologic" interference with mediator release or control mechanisms. No effect of TDI was noted on histamine-induced lymphocyte cAMP production. Unfortunately, neither the nature nor the site of the TDI direct stimulatory effect or its interference with mediator-induced secretion of lymphocyte cAMP is known. Nonetheless, these are very provocative findings that may help to explain the multiple factors involved in the pathogenesis of isocyanate asthma.

Davies' findings on lymphocyte cAMP inhibition by TDI and its apparent mixed effect on beta adrenergic-like activity led to further study of the effects of isocyanates on beta adrenergic receptor function. McKay and Brooks recorded their initial observations in 1981.[37] In their in vitro model, TDI was shown to inhibit frog erythrocyte beta adrenergic receptors when stimulated by isoproterenol in a dose-dependent fashion. Interestingly, MDI and HDI had similar inhibitory effects. These responses suggested that the highly reactive N-C-O ligand may mediate this inhibition. They did not find that partial beta agonist effect as Davies had previously reported. Possible mechanisms to explain these results were speculated as: (1) a nonspecific toxic effect on the membrane due to covalent binding of isocyanate to the receptor; (2) inhibition of adenylate cyclase due to covalent modification; (3) modification of guanyl nucleotide regulatory site, or (4) a combination of any of these mechanisms. Again, this area of investigation has led to new insights into the multifactorial pathogenesis of isocyanate asthma and has underscored that further clarification will be required in human models.

NATURAL HISTORY AND OUTCOME

Although the natural history of isocyanate asthma has classically been one of resolution after removal of the worker from the offending exposure, reports of persistent asthma and pulmonary function declines have appeared in the literature. Many of these reports have significant methodologic problems. Nevertheless, these observations highlight the importance of removing or protecting any potentially sensitized worker from any further isocyanate exposures.

Newman Taylor and co-workers have reported on the outcome of isocyanate occupational asthma in 50 workers followed at the Brompton Hospital in England, which has an international reputation in the care of patients with respiratory diseases.[38] Outpatients had reportedly undergone confirmatory bronchial provocation testing to MDI, TDI, and HDI. These 50 patients comprised 89% of all cases of isocyanate-induced asthma documented in Brompton Hospital between 1971 and 1979. Outpatients had avoided exposure to isocyanate for at least 4 years. At the time of follow-up, 82% of patients reported respiratory symptoms, with 54% requiring treatment at least once per week. Pulmonary function data indicated mild obstructive deficits at the time of follow-up that were similar to those obtained at the time of initial diagnosis. Interestingly, of the nine patients who had undergone histamine provocation initially and at the time of follow-up, only one remained hyperresponsive, with two developing hyperresponsiveness since the time of diagnosis. Importantly, 39% of their study group were determined to be atopic. Furthermore, 35 of the 50 workers were either current or former smokers. These are very important observations but are limited by the large number of cigarette smokers, former smokers, or atopic workers, as well as the limited preemployment respiratory history available. None of these workers had undergone preemployment pulmonary function studies of any kind. There were no precise data relating to the timeliness of the diagnosis in relation to the onset of their symptoms. Nevertheless, these observations highlight the possibility for persistent airways dysfunction in workers who may have a predisposition for bronchial hyperresponsiveness and who are felt to have developed isocyanate-induced asthma.[38]

A large study of patients with isocyanate occupational asthma from Italy was more recently reported.[39] This study was unique in that it included 162 workers with a low proportion of cigarette smokers (7.5%) and an incidence of atopy similar to the general population (21.5%). Of the 162 subjects, positive bronchial provocation studies were documented at 57.1%. The potential for prolonged latency between exposure and diagnosis was documented to range from 9 to 12.9 years, with the duration of symptoms prior to diagnosis ranging from 2.5 to 3.9 years. Late asthmatic responses occurred in 71% of patients and were associated with greater methacholine responsiveness in longer duration of exposures in these patients. Only one subject had evidence of specific IgE to isocyanate by RAST. These findings support the possible unique characteristics of prolonged latency and predilection for late asthmatic responses in isocyanate asthma. The observations are especially important in Italy where a large number of small furniture factories utilize isocyanate-containing varnish with multiple possibilities for poorly protected inhalational exposures.

The potential for recurrence was recently highlighted in a case report by Banks and Rando.[40] In this unique case study, a chemical plant worker who had developed well-documented isocyanate asthma in 1974 was described. Eleven years after leaving the chemical plant he underwent reevaluation, which indicated no respiratory symptoms, no methacholine hyperresponsiveness, and a negative bronchial provocation to subirritant levels of TDI. He subsequently returned to the workplace where he once again developed classic symptoms of occupational asthma associated with low levels of isocyanate exposure. Repeat methacholine and TDI bronchial provocation studies were positive. This report emphasizes the need for complete and indefinite removal of workers with isocyanate asthma from any potential exposure.

In another unique observation on the natural history of TDI asthma, Butcher et al. correlated immunopharmacologic changes associated with the loss of bronchial hyperresponsiveness. In this report, a 32-year-old atopic chemical worker with TDI asthma was followed longitudinally for 2 years following his removal from the workplace. Methacholine responsiveness normalized 17 months following removal. Tolyl-mono-isocyanate RAST ratios decreased from 11.5 during his exposure to 3.5 approximately 2 years following cessation of exposure. Interestingly, following suppression of isoproterenol, prostaglandin E_1-induced lymphocyte cAMP levels persisted for approximately 2 years. Importantly, no excess decline in pulmonary function was noted over 3 years. Although it is difficult to generalize these findings to all patients, they suggest that in some patients immunopharmacologic events underlying bronchial hyperresponsiveness may persist for significant periods of time. Nevertheless, this report also details the absence of permanent respiratory physiologic sequelae of isocyanate asthma. The nature and extent of any long-term sequelae remain to be defined in larger, future, prospective studies. These observations are similar to the prospective study done at Tulane University where the majority of patients who developed TDI sensitivity either improved or became normal after removal from the workplace.[16] Similar observations were noted by Burge and his co-workers.[42,43]

DIAGNOSIS

The diagnosis of isocyanate asthma, as with all occupationally induced asthma, largely relies on a comprehensive history and physical examination. In addition to obtaining a detailed occupational history, specific laboratory tests can be helpful. As previously discussed, there is very little value in serologic testing. Unfortunately, there is no specific immunologic marker of isocyanate-induced disease. When present, a positive RAST test to isocyanate can be helpful, but because it may be negative in many patients with demonstrated sensitivity, its value is certainly limited. Methacholine bronchial provocation testing remains the standard of establishing nonspecific bronchial hyperresponsiveness. It is axiomatic that most patients with asthma, occupationally induced or otherwise, will have positive methacholine tests. The methacholine challenge can also be helpful in establishing the level of responsiveness prior to specific bronchial provocation studies.

Recently, there have been a number of reports in the literature that indicate that isocyanate-induced asthma may exist in the absence of methacholine hyperresponsiveness. After the initial description of a case by Smith in 1980,[44] a subsequent report was detailed by Hargreave et al. in 1984.[45] A recent report by Banks in 1986[46] describes a 29-year-old nonatopic male cigarette smoker who was exposed to MDI in loading a railroad tank car. A methacholine challenge test before and after specific MDI bronchial provocation was negative. MDI challenge was positive and well controlled. The patient did not develop asthmatic symptoms during the challenge, but did have periorbital edema, pruritus, and rhinitis associated with the decline in FEV_1. The presumed MDI-induced occupational asthma resolved within 2 months. This is a unique case report that challenges the methacholine provocation study as the standard for diagnosing asthma in this setting.[46] This report certainly does not question the usefulness of methacholine provocation studies in evaluating patients with occupational asthma, but it does suggest that there may be a rare patient with mild bronchial hyperresponsiveness who does not respond to methacholine. The key to these observations is the fact that patients without demonstrable bronchial hyperresponsiveness tend to have mild or subclinical forms of isocyanate asthma.

The difficulty of interpreting methacholine challenges in occupational asthma is highlighted in a recent report from Italy.[50] In this interesting study 113 workers with a history of work-related respiratory complaints following exposure to TDI underwent methacholine and TDI bronchial provocation. Only 40% of those studied had positive TDI provocation. Interestingly, 46% of the workers with negative TDI provocation had positive methacholine challenges, whereas only 78% of the workers with positive TDI challenges had methacholine hyperresponsiveness. These findings highlight the importance of considering factors such as the time interval between occupational exposure and specific challenge, which was significantly larger in the workers with negative TDI challenges.

As previously detailed, isocyanate inhalation may result not only in occupational asthma, but in occupationally induced hypersensitivity pneumonitis. Again, the diagnosis of hypersensitivity pneumonitis is based on the history and physical exam. In addition to developing cough, most patients with hypersensitivity pneumonitis will develop constitutional symptoms of fever, malaise, and arthralgias. Many of these patients will demonstrate immune hyperresponsiveness with elevated acute phase reactants, elevated erythrocyte sedimentation rate, and hypergammaglobulinemia. A report by Bascom et al.[47] suggests that there may be additional value in bronchial alveolar lavage in hypersensitivity pneumonitis for MDI. In this interesting report, Bascom details the case of a 57-year-old male who developed hypersensitivity pneumonitis from exposure to MDI. MDI was encountered while using polyurethane foam insulation in the construction of a modular home. The worker underwent bronchial alveolar lavage and was found to have not only elevated levels of lymphocyte in the fluid, but MDI-specific involvement of an IgG class. In addition, MDI-specific IgG was demonstrated in the patient's serum. While the authors did not suggest that this test be used as a routine diagnostic study, the findings do add further support to the existence of non-IgE immunologically mediated lung disease following isocyanate exposure. Similar observations were made by Malo and Zeiss.[19]

There is no accurate biochemical method for diagnosing isocyanate asthma.[18] The diagnosis can only be established with certainty if asthma is demonstrated to occur following subirritant exposures to the isocyanate moiety implicated. There are several different ways to challenge a worker. The first is to return the patient to work (or a work-like setting) and to reproduce the exposure and symptoms and record them

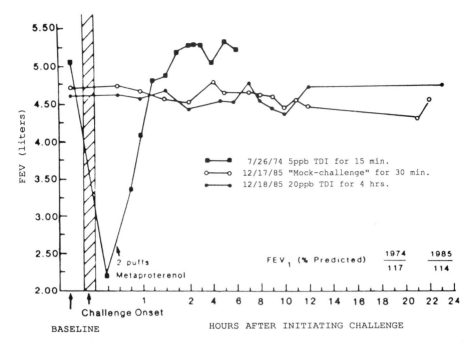

FIGURE 6.   Spirometric results of a controlled bronchial provocation study to TDI, indicating a positive immediate response. (From Banks DE, et al: Isocyanate-induced respiratory disease. Ann Allergy 57:389, 1986,[18] with permission.)

objectively with physiologic measurements. The second is to recreate the work exposure in a challenge chamber by specifically challenging the individual to known subirritant levels of the specific isocyanate.[48] These studies are costly, time-consuming, and potentially hazardous, but they constitute the only reliable diagnostic method. A protocol for such challenge studies has been developed and proven to be extremely useful in the clinical setting.[18] An example of a positive challenge is illustrated in Figure 6.

SPECIFIC INDUSTRIAL HYGIENE RECOMMENDATIONS

As previously stated, a worker proven to have been immunologically sensitized or who has demonstrated decline in pulmonary function following isocyanate exposure should be completely removed from potential exposures. This is most easily done by finding the worker a new job or job site. To protect nonsensitized, but potentially exposed, individuals, general engineering controls of airflow should be used. Where this is not feasible, use of supplied air has traditionally been recommended. In those instances where engineering controls and fresh-air-supply respiratory protective devices are not available or feasible, other respiratory

protective devices have been studied. Dharmarajan et al. in 1986[49] reported on their experience with various cartridge respiratory protective devices. Each cartridge was tested in triplicate at 0.2 ppm TDI for more than 40 hours and once for 20 hours or more at concentrations of 1.5 ppm TDI. These levels were well beyond the ACGIH- and NIOSH-recommended time-weighted average exposure limit of 0.005 ppm and the 0.02 ppm short-term exposure limit, as well as the current OSHA PEL of 0.02 ppm as a ceiling (Table 2). At these high levels,

TABLE 2.   *Occupational Exposure Limits to 2,4-Toluene Diisocyanate*

Organization	Year	ppm	Concentration mg/M³	
ACGIH	1986	0.005	0.04	TLV-TWA
		0.02	0.15	TLV-STEL
NIOSH	1978		0.035	TWA
			0.14	Ceiling
OSHA	1983		0.14	Ceiling

ACGIH: American Conference of Government Industrial Hygienists
NIOSH: National Institutes of Occupational Safety & Health
OSHA: Occupational Safety and Health Administration
TWA: Time-weighted average
STEL: Short-term Exposure Limit

there was no breakthrough of TDI up to 40 hours with any of the respirators or cartridges tested. Even at extraordinary levels of TDI, breakthrough was not noted with the Survivair cartridge. Though not recommended by NIOSH or OSHA, cartridge respirators, if used properly, can protect against potential exposure to TDI vapors. Although cartridge respiratory protective devices may suffer from improper fitting and discomfort in some workers, they may be useful in certain settings.

REFERENCES

1. Fuchs S, Valade P: Etude clinique et experimentale sur quelques cas d'intoxication par de desmodur T (diisocyanate de toluyene 1-2-4 et 1-2-1). Arch Maladies Prof 12:191, 1951.
2. Ulrich H: Urethane polymers. In Kirk-Othmer: Encyclopedia of Chemical Technology, Vol 23, 3rd ed. New York, John Wiley & Sons, 1983, pp 577–608.
2a. Chemical and Engineering News. June 20, 1983, p 19.
3. Occupational Exposure to Diisocyanates. NIOSH Criteria Document for a Recommended Standard. Publication Number 78-215. Washington, D.C., U.S. Department of Health, Education and Welfare, 1978.
4. Karol MH: Respiratory effects of inhaled isocyanates. CRC Critical Reviews in Toxicology 16:349–379, 1986.
5. Hama GM: Symptoms in workers exposed to isocyanates: Suggested exposure concentrations. Arch Ind Health 16:232, 1957.
6. Butcher BT, Salvaggio JE, Weill H, Ziskind M: Toluene diisocyanate pulmonary disease: Immunologic and inhalational challenge studies. J Allergy Clin Immunol 58:89, 1976.
7. Porter CV, Higgins RL, Scheel LD: A retrospective study of clinical, physiologic and immunologic changes in workers exposed to toluene diisocyanate. Am Ind Hyg J 36:159, 1975.
8. Bernstein IL: Isocyanate-induced pulmonary diseases: A current perspective. J Allergy Clin Immunol 70:24, 1982.
9. Wegmen DH, Peters JM, Pagnotto LD, Fine LC: Chronic pulmonary function loss from exposure to toluene diisocyanate. Br J Ind Med 34:196–200, 1977.
10. Adams WGF: Long-term effects on the health of men engaged in the manufacture of toluene diisocyanate. Br J Ind Med 32:72–78, 1975.
11. Zammit-Tabona M, Sherkin M, Kijek K, et al: Asthma caused by diphenylmethane diisocyanate in foundry workers: Clinical, bronchial provocation and immunologic studies. Am Rev Respir Dis 128:226–230, 1983.
12. Johnson A, Chan-Yeung M, Maclean L, et al: Respiratory abnormalities among workers in an iron and steel foundry. Br J Ind Med 42:94–100, 1985.
13. Venables KN, Daily MB, Burge PS, et al: Occupational asthma in a steel coating plant. Br J Ind Med 42:517–524, 1985.
14. Wegmen DH, Pagnotto LD, Fine LJ, Peters JM: A dose-response relationship in TDI workers. J Occup Med 16:258, 1974.
15. Gee JB, Morgan WKC: A 10-year follow-up study of a group of workers exposed to isocyanates. J Occup Med 27:15, 1985.
16. Diem JB, Jones RN, Hendrick DS, et al: Five-year longitudinal study of workers employed in a new toluene diisocyanate manufacturing plant. Am Rev Respir Dis 126:420–426, 1982.
17. Musk AW, Peters JM, DiBernardinis L, et al: Absence of respiratory effects in subjects exposed to low concentrations of TDI and MDI. J Occup Med 24:746, 1982.
18. Banks DE, Butcher BT, Salvaggio JE: Isocyanate-induced respiratory disease. Ann Allergy 57:389, 1986.
19. Malo JL, Zeiss CR: Occupational hypersensitivity pneumonitis after exposure to diphenylmethane diisocyanate. Am Rev Respir Dis 125:113, 1982.
20. Mapp CE, Boschetto P, Dalvecchio L, et al: Occupational asthma due to isocyanates. Eur Respir J 1:273–279, 1988.
21. Gallagher JS, Tse T, Brooks SM, Bernstein IL: Diverse profiles of immunoreactivity in toluene diisocyanate asthma. J Occup Med 23:610–616, 1981.
22. Liss GR, Moller DR, Bernstein DI, et al: Immunologic evaluation of methylene diphenyl diisocyanate (MDI)-exposed foundry workers. J Allergy Clin Immunol 73(Part 2):173, 1984.
23. Grunewalder E, Karol MH: Nitrocellulose-based RAST to detect IgE antibodies in workers hypersensitive to diphenylmethane 4-4'diisocyanate. Allergy 41:203–209, 1986.
24. Wass U, Belin L: Immunologic specificity of isocyanate-induced IgE antibodies in serum from 10 sensitized workers. J Allergy Clin Immunol 83:126–135, 1989.
25. Baur X, Dewarr M, Fruhmann G: Detection of immunologically sensitized isocyanate workers by RAST and intracutaneous skin test. J Allergy Clin Immunol 73:610–618, 1984.
26. Karol MH, Ioset HH, Alarie YC: Tolyl-specific IgE antibodies in workers hypersensitivity to toluene diisocyanate. Am Ind Hyg Assoc J 39:454–458, 1978.
27. Tse CST, Chen SE, Bernstein IL: Induction of murine reaginic antibodies by toluene diisocyanate. An animal model of immediate hypersensitivity reactions to isocyanates. Am Rev Respir Dis 120:829–835, 1979.
28. Patterson R, Zeiss CR, Harris KE: Immunologic and respiratory responses to airway challenges of dogs with toluene diisocyanate. J Allergy Clin Immunol 71:604–611, 1983.
29. Butcher BT, O'Neil CE, Reed MA, Salvaggio JE: Radioallergosorbent testing of toluene diisocyanate-reactive individuals using p-tolyl isocyanate antigen. J Allergy Clin Immunol 66:213–216, 1980.
30. Grammer LC, Harris KE, Malo J, et al: The use of an immunoassay for antibodies against isocyanate human protein conjugates and application to human isocyanate disease. J Allergy Clin Immunol 86:94–98, 1990.
31. Atkins PC, Norman M, Weiner H, Zweimann B: Release of neutrophil chemotactic activity during immediate hypersensitivity reactions in humans. Ann Intern Med 86:415–418, 1977.
32. Caroll MP, Durham SR, Walsh G, Kay AB: Activation of neutrophils and monocytes after allergen- and histamine-induced bronchoconstriction. J Allergy Clin Immunol 75:290–296, 1985.
33. Valentino M, Governa M, Fiorini R: Increased neutrophil leukocyte chemotaxis induced by release of a serum factor in toluene-diisocyanate (TDI) asthma. Lung 166:317–325, 1988.
34. Sastre J, Banks DE, Lopez M, et al: Neutrophil chemotactic activity in toluene diisocyanate-induced asthma. J Allergy Clin Immunol 85:567–572, 1990.

35. Butcher BT, Salvaggio JE, O'Neil CE, et al: Toluene diisocyanate pulmonary disease: Immunopharmacologic and mecholyl challenge studies. J Allergy Clin Immunol 59:223–227, 1977.
36. Davies RJ, Butcher BT, O'Neil CE, Salvaggio JE: The in vitro effect of toluene diisocyanate on lymphocyte cyclic adenosine monophosphate production by isoproterenol, prostaglandin and histamine. J Allergy Clin Immunol 60:223–229, 1977.
37. McKay RT, Brooks SM, Johnson C: Isocyanate-induced abnormality of beta adrenergic function. Chest 80(Suppl 1):61S–63S, 1981.
38. Newman Taylor AJ, Lozewicz S, Assouti BK, Hawkins R: Outcome of asthma induced by isocyanates. Br J Dis Chest 81:14–22, 1987.
39. Fabbri LM, Mapp CE, Boschetto P, et al: Occupational asthma due to isocyanates. Eur Respir J 1:273–279, 1988.
40. Banks DE, Rando RJ: Recurrent asthma induced by toluene diisocyanate. Thorax 43:660–662, 1988.
41. Butcher BT, O'Neil CE, Reed MA, et al: Development and loss of toluene diisocyanate reactivity: Immunologic, pharmacologic and provocative challenge studies. J Allergy Clin Immunol 70:231–235, 1982.
42. Burge PS: Non-specific bronchial hyperreactivity in workers exposed to TDI, MDI and colophony. Eur J Respir Dis 123:91, 1982.
43. Burge PS, O'Brien OM, Harries MG: Peakflow rate records in the diagnosis of occupational asthma due to isocyanates. Thorax 34:317, 1979.
44. Smith AB, Brooks SM, Blanchard J, et al: Absence of airway hyperreactivity to methacholine in a worker sensitized to toluene diisocyanate (TDI). J Occup Med 22:237–241, 1980.
45. Hargreave FE, Ramsdale EH, Pugsley SO: Occupational asthma without bronchial hyperresponsiveness. Am Rev Respir Dis 130:513–515, 1984.
46. Banks DF: Absence of hyperresponsiveness to methacholine in a worker with methylene diphenyl diisocyanate (MDI)-induced asthma. Chest 89:389–392, 1986.
47. Bascom R, Kennedy TP, Levitz D: Specific bronchoalveolar lavage IgG antibody in hypersensitivity pneumonitis from diphenylmethane diisocyanate. Am Rev Respir Dis 131:463–465, 1985.
48. Barkman HW Jr, Banks DE: Bronchoprovocation testing in occupational asthma. Folia Allergol Immunol Clin 32:45, 1985.
49. Dharmarajan V, et al: Evaluation of air-purifying respirators for protection against blue toluene diisocyanate vapors. Ann Ind Hyg J 47:393, 1986.
50. Moscato G, Dellabianca A, Vinci G, et al: Toluene diisocyanate-induced asthma: Clinical findings and bronchial responsiveness studies in 113 exposed subjects with work-related respiratory symptoms. J Occup Med 33:720–725, 1991.

Chapter 13

ASTHMA SECONDARY TO ACID ANHYDRIDES

Anthony Montanaro, MD

CHEMISTRY AND PHYSICAL PROPERTIES OF ACID ANHYDRIDES

Acid anhydrides are highly reactive, low molecular weight compounds that are used widely in industry. Because of their biochemical reactivity, they are used as polymerizing agents in many epoxy resin systems. Since the initial recognition of phthalic anhydride-induced occupational asthma in 1939,[1] a great deal of new information has accumulated. This chapter will review the important clinical and immunologic data that have developed over the past 50 years.

Since these compounds have such low molecular weights, they are unable to induce antibody responses without conjugating with human proteins. The acid anhydrides may act as haptens when conjugated with ubiquitous proteins such as human serum albumin (HSA). While there are many commercially important acid anhydrides (Fig. 1), the best studied compounds have been phthalic anhydride and trimellitic anhydride.

HISTORICAL PERSPECTIVE

The acid anhydrides are used as "hardeners" in the production of many epoxy resin systems. A typical resin is produced by condensation of epichlorhydrin with a diphenol in the presence of a curing agent. Curing agents are referred to as hardeners or plasticizers and represent nonvolatile solvents that become incorporated with substances of greater molecular size to improve workability, flexibility, and distensibility. Typical hardeners or plasticizers are the polyamines (diethylenetriamine or piperazine) or the acid anhydrides and polybasic acids (phthalic anhydride, dibutyl phthalate).

Prior to 1941 plasticizers were principally employed for the manufacture of surface coating and safety glass. The first plasticizer was camphor. It was used as early as 1870 for making celluloid from nitrocellulose. The phthalates became prominent in the 1920s. Since that time the varieties of phthalates have increased rapidly, and some are produced in volumes over 100 million lbs/year and are widely used in the manufacture of adhesives, paints, varnishes, shellacs, and glass. In the production of safety glass, special laminates of polyvinyl copolymer are linked with a phthalate plasticizer. Dibutyl phthalate is extensively used in the manufacture of polyvinyl chloride resins. The relevant chemicals and sources of potential occupational exposures are listed in Table 1.

PHTHALIC ANHYDRIDE

Phthalic anhydride (PA) is the anhydride of benzene orthodicarboxylic acid. It is a moderately flammable crystalline solid that solubilizes in ether or alcohol. PA is widely used in the production of chemicals and dyes, including phthaleins, benzoic acid, polyester resins, alizarin dye, and sulfathaladine (Table 1). It may be found in some herbicides and pesticides. PA's widest application is in the plastics industry, including its use as a cross-linker in epoxy resins, adhesives, surface coatings, reinforced plastics and epoxy paints. Exposed workers may be exposed by contact, ingestion,

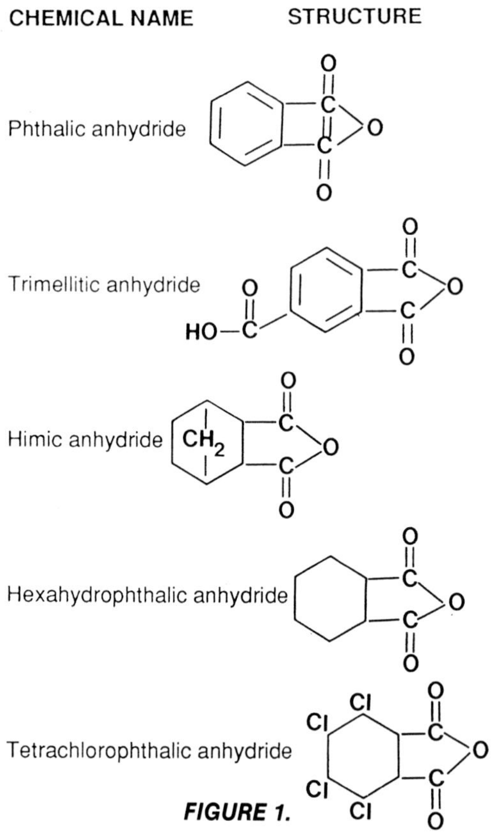

CHEMICAL NAME   STRUCTURE

Phthalic anhydride

Trimellitic anhydride

Himic anhydride

Hexahydrophthalic anhydride

Tetrachlorophthalic anhydride

FIGURE 1.

or inhalation. The incidence of sensitization and the precise level of exposure required for sensitization are unknown, but recent evaluations of exposed workers have begun to address these questions.

TABLE 1. *Acid Anhydrides*

Chemical	Source
Phthalic anhydride	Chemical production
	Benzoic acid
	Polyester resins
	Sulfathalidine
	Dye production
	Phthaleins
	Alizarin red
	Epoxy resins
	Adhesives
	Surface coatings
	Reinforced plastics
	Paints
	Safety glass
Trimellitic anhydride	Plastic production
	Epoxy resins
	Alkyl surface coatings
	Curing agents
Hexahydrophthalic anhydride	Epoxy resins
Tetrachlorophthalic anhydride	Epoxy resins
Dibutyl phthalate	Polyvinyl chloride resins

The first reported case of PA-induced occupational asthma and rhinitis was in a chemist exposed to PA dust and was described in 1939 by Kern.[1] Positive cutaneous scratch test and successful passive transfer study confirmed the presence of PA-specific IgE. In the 1960s, polyvinyl chloride (PVC) films with thermo-activated labels became the predominant form of meatwrapping. While numerous anecdotal reports of meatwrapper's asthma appeared in the early 1970s, Andrasch and co-workers[2,3] were the first to perform work-simulated bronchial provocation studies. These studies indicated that inhalational exposure to the thermally activated label was responsible for immediate and severe bronchospastic responses in 9 of 14 affected subjects, as opposed to the heating of the PVC film alone. They also noted that workers with chronic bronchitis or those who smoked cigarettes appeared to have an augmented response. Further automation and extensive revision of the labeling process led to decreased or abandoned use of PA-containing adhesives. Fortunately, this led to a decrease in the incidence of meatwrappers asthma in the late 1970s. Subsequent bronchial provocation studies by Pauli[4] and others confirmed PA as an important product of label thermoactivation and the probable inducer of bronchospasm. Further observations of immunologic reactivity in meatwrappers and others have led to important advances in the understanding of occupational asthma induced by acid anhydrides.

Similar observations on phthalic anhydride-induced occupational asthma have been made in Sweden. Wernfors and colleagues reported their findings on 118 workers employed in four separate plants producing alkyd and/or polyunsaturated polyester resins.[5] Workers who had potential PA exposure for more than 2 months were studied. A surprisingly large proportion of exposed workers reported work-related symptoms, with 24% presenting with work-related rhinitis, 11% chronic bronchitis, and 28% reporting work-associated asthma. Asthma appeared to be preceded by rhinitis, but only 3 of 11 asthmatics studied revealed dermal reactivity to PA. Interestingly, 16% of 25 heavily exposed workers without clinical asthma displayed nonspecific bronchial hyper-responsiveness by methacholine challenge. Additionally, two workers who were PA skin test positive and methacholine positive underwent specific bronchial provocation studies with PA. Both workers demonstrated significant dual responses to 0.5 mg/M³ and 6 mg/M³, respectively, with breathing zone time-weighted average PA levels having been measured in two of the plants between 3 and 13 mg/M[3]. These important and well-documented observations confirm previous reports on the hazard of sensitization to PA in unprotected or poorly protected workers.

Bernstein and co-workers have undertaken numerous studies documenting immunologic reactivity to acid anhydrides.[6,7] Using methylcellulose radioallergosorbent testing (RAST) and RAST-inhibition studies to PA, to hexahydrophthalic (HHPA), or to himic anhydride (HA) human serum albumin conjugates, they have demonstrated significant haptenic cross-reactivity as well as specific responses to these related compounds.[6] Interestingly, significant allergenic cross-reactivity was not observed between these compounds and trimellitic anhydride. In the workers with symptoms of occupational asthma in this study, there appeared to be a good correlation between high levels of RAST binding and symptoms. These observations led to further study of workers exposed to HHPA by Moller et al.[8] In this study, 27 workers exposed to HHPA in an epoxy resin molding system underwent RAST screening for HHPA-HSA specific Ig and IgE antibodies. In addition, detailed questionnaires and pulmonary function studies were undertaken. Seven workers reported symptoms of asthma or rhinitis, although no workers demonstrated significant changes in pulmonary function during exposures at work. Twelve of the 27 workers studied had significantly elevated levels of IgE directed against HHPA, with 11 forming specific anti-HHPA IgG. The degree of exposure correlated with degree of elevation of antibody.

TRIMELLITIC ANHYDRIDE

Trimellitic anhydride (TMA) is a commonly used material in the plastics and resin industry (Table 1). This relatively simple chemical is highly active biologically and is used in the production of plastics, alkyl resin-based surface coatings, and as a curing agent for epoxy resins. Workers may be exposed to TMA by direct inhalation of fumes during TMA production or by use of a TMA-containing product. In addition, workers involved with the processing, storage, or transportation of TMA in the form of powder or flakes may have substantial inhalational exposures. Inhalational exposure to TMA may produce a wide

TABLE 2. *TMA Associated Respiratory Syndromes**

Syndrome	Onset Symptoms	Latent Period	Antibody Response
Asthma-rhinitis	Immediate (min)	Weeks-months	Elevated, total, *and* IgE
Late respiratory systemic syndrome	4–12 hr	Weeks-months	Elevated total Ab-IgE
Pulmonary disease anemia	Progressive	Weeks-months	Markedly elevated total Ab-IgE
Irritant	Variable	Occurs on first high-dose exposure	May have elevated IgE

*Adapted from ref. 8.

spectrum of immunologically mediated pulmonary disease (Table 2). Zeiss, Patterson and others at Northwestern University have provided detailed clinical and immunologic observations of TMA-induced pulmonary disease. Over the previous decade, they have noted that in addition to TMA acting as a potent respiratory irritant, exposure to TMA dust or fumes may result in several distinct respiratory syndromes, including an IgE-mediated occupational asthma, a hypersensitivity pneumonitis (which they termed the "late respiratory systemic syndrome"), and a restrictive lung disease associated with pulmonary infiltrates and anemia, designated the pulmonary disease-anemia syndrome.[9-12] Since this compound is so widely used in industry, it is important to consider the spectrum of pulmonary disease that may occur when encountering a potentially exposed individual.

Longitudinal studies undertaken at a TMA manufacturing plant have indicated a correlation between development of immunologic syndromes and significant IgE responses to TMA.[13] Of 61 workers who had detailed clinical and immunologic assessments, 20% developed immunologically related respiratory disorders. Forty-one percent of exposed workers developed significant antibody response that did not correlate with the duration of exposure. Two-thirds of patients with high antibody levels developed an asthma-rhinitis syndrome, the late respiratory syndrome, or both. Interestingly, no workers without antibody responses developed immunologic respiratory syndromes.

Of these 61 longitudinally studied workers, six have developed a classic immediate IgE-mediated asthma-rhinitis syndrome, characterized by wheezing, dyspnea, cough, or rhinitis on exposure to TMA fumes or dust. Only two of these six workers were identified as atopic. All six presented with occupational asthma or rhinitis at the beginning of the study, although one patient developed asthma 6 years after his initial exposure. Those workers who developed significant IgE responses tended to have lower total antibody to TMA than those who developed a syndrome clinically more suggestive of hypersensitivity pneumonitis. Despite low levels of TMA-specific IgE detected by in vitro assays in some patients, all patients with an occupational asthma-rhinitis syndrome had significant immediate skin test reactivity. Importantly, all patients who developed significant total and IgE antibody responses to TMA in association with respiratory disease had dramatic reductions in antibody following removal from exposure.

Very few data are available on specific TMA exposure levels of patients who have developed TMA-induced respiratory syndromes. Many of the inhalational exposures to TMA are to particulates that contain TMA bound to resin materials. In order to accurately measure TMA in these particulate samples, the resin must be separated, leaving small amounts of measurable material. In one group of workers in whom exposure levels were measured, TMA-induced symptoms and TMA-specific antibody levels diminished with decreasing exposure levels.[14] Improvements in ventilation in the studied work environment led to a fall in TMA dust levels from 0.82–2.1 mg/M^3 to 0.01–0.03 mg/M^3. Despite this improvement, intermittent low-level exposure in one worker led to a small increase in TMA-specific IgE antibodies and persistent presumed TMA-induced rhinitis. Thus, while the current TLV-TWA of 0.005 ppm (0.04 mg/M^3) appears safe in most workers, there may be some previously sensitized workers in whom no exposure can be entirely safe.

The late respiratory systemic syndrome appears to be clinically and immunologically distinct from the classic occupational asthma that may occur in response to TMA.[9] This syndrome is characterized by cough, shortness of breath, fever, and myalgias/arthralgias, which occur several hours following exposure. Affected workers may have wheezing, which may mimic typical occupational asthma. These symptoms have prompted the designation of "TMA-flu." This syndrome typically occurs 4–12 hours after exposure and may occur following a latent period after initial exposure of many weeks to months before the appearance

of symptoms. This syndrome is associated with high levels of IgG and IgA directed against TMA-human serum albumin conjugates, but absent IgE responses.

A serious disorder termed the pulmonary disease-anemia syndrome has been described in workers who have been exposed to high-dose TMA fumes, especially during spraying of TMA-containing anticorrosives onto heated surfaces.[13] This syndrome is characterized by the appearance of cough, hemoptysis, and progressive dyspnea. Radiographically, one may see pulmonary infiltrates that are characteristically absent in other TMA syndromes. The presence of anemia in these patients indicates the serious systemic nature of this illness. Immunologically, these workers may have high levels of total antibody directed against TMA human sera conjugates, primarily of the IgG class, but no measurable TMA-specific IgE.

As with many chemical exposures, inhalation of high doses of TMA vapors or dust may result in acute irritational injury.[13] Patients may present with acute irritational symptoms such as cough or chest pain following their first high-dose exposure. Although workers with this syndrome may have elevated levels of total antibody directed against TMA, these levels are not as high as those seen in the late respiratory systemic syndrome (LRSS). TMA-specific IgE antibodies are characteristically absent. Whereas the severity of this syndrome is variable, it is important to consider that it is likely that the most severe cases have been those that have been reported. Minor irritational symptoms may in fact be important and more common than any of the described syndromes.

Recently Zeiss and co-workers have reported on the ongoing evaluation of 196 workers involved in the manufacturing of TMA.[15] Occupational exposures occurred through inhalations of fumes from the molten product or of dust from the dried product being bagged, transported, or warehoused. Most workers experienced respiratory irritant (113 of 196) or no symptoms (46 of 196). Thirty-three of the 196 (17%) workers developed immunologically mediated syndromes. Occupational asthma and/or rhinitis was the most common immunologically mediated syndrome, occurring in 17 of 196 workers. An asymptomatic latent period of months to years preceded the appearance of immediate hypersensitivity responses in all cases. All workers with this syndrome displayed positive immediate prick tests and IgE RAST to TM-HSA. Late respiratory systemic syndrome was noted in seven workers.

Three workers had late-onset asthma, and one displayed mild pulmonary disease and anemia syndrome. These authors reconfirmed the potential importance of measuring the total antibody (predominantly IgG) responses in potentially affected workers. Ninety-two percent of workers without symptoms lacked IgG antibody response, while 97% of workers with presumed immunologic clinical syndromes had elevated levels. Fortunately, the incidence of these syndromes had decreased in their study population due to increased awareness, use of personal respiratory devices, and improvement in industrial hygiene measures.

HIMIC ANHYDRIDE

Himic anhydride (3,6 endomethylene-,4 tetrahydrophthalic anhydride) is an acid anhydride that is used in the production of brominated fire retardants. As can be seen in Table 1 himic anhydride is structurally closely related to the other clinically relevant acid anhydrides. Although the data are limited, there have been important observations made by Rosenman and colleagues that suggest IgE-mediated bronchial hyperresponsiveness to himic anhydride in chemical plant workers.[16] In this report, 20 of 32 potentially exposed workers were evaluated. Of the 20 workers evaluated, 8 (40%) complained of symptoms compatible with occupational rhinitis or asthma. Four workers (20%) presented with symptoms of wheezing related to himic anhydride exposure. Limited immunologic evaluations were undertaken in only seven workers. Three of these seven (43%) exhibited significant RAST binding to himic anhydride-human serum albumin conjugate, which appeared to cross-react with hexahydrophthalic anhydride-albumin conjugates. While these observations are limited, they are important in supporting the wide range and significant antigenicity of the acid anhydrides. These observations further support the need for stringent industrial hygiene measures in production environments using these substances in powdered or volatile form.

TETRACHLOROPHTHALIC ANHYDRIDE

Apparent tetrachlorophthalic anhydride (TA)-induced asthma was initially described in 1978 in five workers.[17] Unfortunately, TA-specific IgE was not demonstrated in these workers. Since the acid anhydrides had previously been shown to be a prominent respiratory irritant, it was important to document specific TA-immunologic reactivity to prove TA as a cause of occupational asthma. In 1983 Howe and co-workers in the United Kingdom described seven workers in an electronics assembly plant who had developed occupational asthma.[18] These workers had been exposed to TA in an epoxy resin powder used in a protective coating. None of these workers presented with clinical histories, which suggested pre-TA exposure bronchial hyperresponsiveness. These seven workers were part of a 400-worker work force and were referred with typical symptoms of occupational asthma. Immediate skin test reactivity to a TA human serum albumin conjugate was positive in all seven workers and was confirmed by positive RAST studies. RAST studies were negative in asymptomatic exposed and nonexposed control groups. Specific TA bronchial provocation studies were positive in four of four workers who were tested with up to 0.96 mg/M³ (less than 1/10 the manufacturers recommended PEL). Although these observations were limited to seven workers, the findings provide compelling evidence that exposure to TA may result in the formation of specific IgE-mediated bronchial asthma. That the findings of specific reactivity existing at concentrations below the PEL suggests this value may need to be reevaluated.

SUMMARY

In summary, the acid anhydrides are an important group of highly reactive low molecular weight compounds. They are widely used throughout the world in the manufacturing and application of plastics and epoxy resins. The data presented in this chapter define the clear risk of occupational asthma to workers exposed primarily to dusts containing these compounds. The mechanism of induction of immediate and late bronchial hyperresponsiveness to the acid anhydrides appears to be at least in part mediated by IgE antibodies. Other clinical syndromes such as the pulmonary disease-anemia syndrome associated with TMA exposure appear to be associated with IgG antibodies to TMA as well as IgE. While specific IgE has been described to all of the acid anhydrides, significant cross-reaction occurs. More recent RAST inhibition studies have further illuminated the nature of the human IgE response to inhaled acid anhydrides.[19]

These studies indicate that for patients sensitized to TMA or TA, the antibody combines with the specific anhydride *and* the spatially related albumin conjugate that serves as a hapten in inducing an immunologic response. In patients sensitized to PA, it appears that the IgE antibody is more specifically directed at the hapten, suggesting that the PA-hapten binding has resulted in the formation of new antigenic determinants. These findings are analogous to previously reported findings in studies of human IgE response to the highly reactive isocyanates, which also may induce new antigenic determinants resulting in immunologic hypersensitivity. The clinical immunology of the acid anhydrides has recently been reviewed in the context of other highly reactive industrial chemicals by Zeiss, who has been a prominent leader in this area.[20] Regardless of the final accepted mechanism, it is abundantly clear that inhalational exposure to the highly reactive acid anhydrides may result in significant pulmonary disease and that adequate protection in potentially exposed workers and removal from exposure of affected workers is essential.

REFERENCES

1. Kern RA: Asthma and allergic rhinitis due to sensitization to phthalic anhydride. Report of a case. J Allergy 10:164, 1939.
2. Andrasch RH, Bardana EJ, Kloster F, Pirofsky B: Clinical and bronchial provocation studies in patients with meatwrappers asthma. J Allergy Clin Immunol 58:291, 1976.
3. Bardana EJ, Anderson CJ, Andrasch R: Meatwrapper's asthma: Clinical and pathogenetic observations. In Frazier CA (ed): Occupational Asthma. New York, Van Nostrand Reinhold, 1980, pp 14–32.
4. Pauli G, Bessot MC, Kopferschmitt MC, et al: Meatwrappers asthma: Identification of the causal agent. Clin Allergy 10:263–269, 1980.
5. Wernfors M, Nielsen J, Schutz A, Skerfving S: Phthalic anhydride-induced occupational asthma. Int Arch Allergy Appl Immunol 79:77–82, 1986.
6. Bernstein DI, Gallagher JS, D'Souza L, Bernstein IL: Heterogeneity of specific IgE responses in workers sensitized to acid anhydride compounds. J Allergy Clin Immunol 94:794–801, 1984.
7. Bernstein DI, Patterson R, Zeiss CR: Clinical and immunologic evaluation of trimellitic anhydride and phthalic anhydride exposed workers using a questionnaire with comparative analysis of enzyme linked immunosorbent and radioimmunoassay studies. J Allergy Clin Immunol 69:311–318, 1982.
8. Moller DR, Gallagher JS, Bernstein DI, et al: Detection of IgE mediated respiratory sensitization in workers exposed to hexahydrophthalic anhydride. J Allergy Clin Immunol 75:663–679, 1985.
9. Zeiss CR, Patterson R, Pruzansky JJ, et al: Trimellitic anhydride-induced airway syndromes: Clinical and immunologic studies. J Allergy Clin Immunol 60:96–103, 1978.
10. Sale SR, Roach DE, Zeiss CR, Patterson R: Clinical and immunologic correlations in trimellitic anhydride airway syndromes. J Allergy Clin Immunol 68:188–192, 1981.
11. Patterson R, Zeiss CR, Pruzansky JJ: Immunopathology of trimellitic anhydride pulmonary reactions. J Allergy Clin Immunol 70:19–23, 1982.
12. Zeiss CR, Wolkansky P, Pruzansky JJ, Patterson R: Clinical and immunologic evaluation of trimellitic anhydride workers in multiple industrial settings. J Allergy Clin Immunol 70:15–18, 1982.
13. Zeiss CR, Wolkansky P, Chacan R, et al: Syndromes in workers exposed to trimellitic anhydride. Ann Intern Med 98:8–12, 1983.
14. Bernstein DJ, Roach DE, McGrath KG, et al: The relationship of airborne trimellitic anhydride concentrations to trimellitic anhydride-induced symptoms and immune responses. J Allergy Clin Immunol 72:709–713, 1983.
15. Zeiss CR, Mitchell JH, Van Peenen PFD, et al: A twelve year clinical and immunologic evaluation of workers involved in the manufacture of trimellitic anhydride. Allergy Proc 11:71–77, 1990.
16. Rosenman KP, Bernstein DJ, O'Leary K, et al: Occupational asthma caused by himic anhydride. Scand J Work Environ Health 13:150–154, 1987.
17. Schleuter DP, Banaszak EF, Fink JN: Occupational asthma due to tetrachlorophthalic anhydride. J Occup Med 20:183, 1978.
18. Howe W, Venables K, Topping M, et al: Tetrachlorophthalic anhydride asthma. Evidence for specific IgE antibody. J Allergy Clin Immunol 71:5–11, 1983.
19. Topping MD, Venables KM, Luczynska CM, et al: Specificity of the human IgE response to inhaled acid anhydrides. J Allergy Clin Immunol 77:834–842, 1986.
20. Zeiss CR: Reactive chemicals in industry. J Allergy Clin Immunol 87:755–761, 1991.

Chapter 14

FORMALDEHYDE ASTHMA

Emil J. Bardana, Jr., MD

Formaldehyde is a low molecular weight substance with significant chemical and industrial applications. It is extensively used as a raw material in the production of foam insulation, plywood, chipboard, textiles, paper, plastics, resins, paints, glues, and cosmetics. It is also used as a fulgurant and as a disinfectant in the health care industry. Formaldehyde's presence in building materials catapulted it into prominence following the energy crisis of the mid-1970s, which focused attention on conservation of energy. Many older buildings were retrofitted with urea-formaldehyde foam insulation (UFFI), and new buildings were tightly constructed. These conservation efforts resulted in a spectrum of problems related to indoor air quality. Formaldehyde was at the apex of many of these indoor pollution problems. Its potential adverse health effects triggered considerable public debate, widely covered by the national media. Early scientific reports were largely uncontrolled anecdotal observations,[1-18] or tentative extrapolations from animal models.[19-22] In 1979 an attempt was made to analyze the scientific literature to determine potential harmful effects of this chemical.[23] Based on the data that were available at that time, it was felt that formaldehyde had the potential to act as both a respiratory irritant and immunogen. Since that time there has been a literal explosion of scientific information on formaldehyde. This information will be summarized in this chapter.

HISTORICAL PERSPECTIVE

The aldehydes were initially identified in 1826 and referred to as oxyethers because of their properties. Two years previously urea had been synthesized by Friedrich Wohler, a German chemist (1800–1882), which opened new vistas relating to organic chemistry. Further, the availability of urea and the discovery of formaldehyde by A.M. Butlerov, a Russian chemist (1828–1886), in 1859 facilitated the later development of many synthetic resins. The history of formaldehyde's discovery and its potential as a polymer precursor has been well described by Walker.[24]

The evolution of synthetic resins started soon after Wohler synthesized urea. Synthetic resins are a group of chemical compounds that includes most of the common plastics. They are composed of many simple molecules linked together to form large, complex materials called polymers. There are basically two major groups of plastics or resins: *thermosets*, which cure or harden on exposure to heat and cannot be reset or reshaped after curing; and *thermoplastics*, which can, on heating, be reset or reshaped repeatedly. In 1872 Adolf Baeyer, a German organic chemist (1835–1917), reported that formaldehyde reacted with phenols resulting in a resinous solid. Some 5 years later Goldschmidt began his studies on urea formaldehyde.

The first commercially important, synthetic thermoset resin was a phenol formaldehyde condensation product developed by Dr. Leo Balkeland in 1909. The original trade name for this synthetic resin was Bakelite. It is a transparent material that is unaffected by organic solvents and dilute acids, but is affected by alkalis. Phenol-formaldehydes have been used extensively as adhesives in the wood, sandpaper, linoleum, fiberglass, and brake-lining industries, as well as for coatings in the metal, textile, and wood industries (Fig. 1). More recently applications have been extended

151

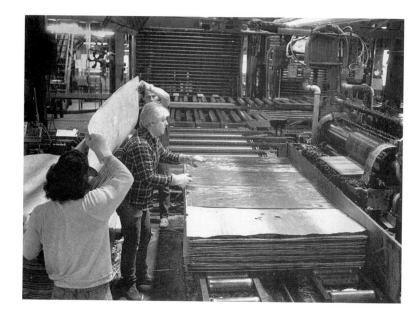

FIGURE 1.   Northwest plywood mill where phenol-formaldehyde is extensively used as an adhesive.

to ion-exchange resin systems, paints, enamels, thermal and acoustical insulation, and rubber adhesives.

In 1929 Vierling and his associates described the use of aqueous urea formaldehyde resins as a thermosetting resin for plywood.[25] The original trade name for this material was Kaurit. It became the preferable bonding material in the manufacture of particle board, chipboard, and plywood (Fig. 2). It has also been used as an economic foam resin with excellent insulating properties.

In 1939, the melamine-formaldehyde resin was introduced commercially. Melamine, first studied by Justus von Liebig, a German chemist (1803–1873), in 1834, is a triazine and offers six active hydrogen atoms for reaction with formaldehyde. This provided improved cross-linking and better water-resistant adhesives. This resin has found extensive application in the textile industry. It has also been mixed with wood pulp products.

Resorcinol-formaldehyde resin was commercially introduced in 1943 as a major modification of the phenolic resins. Resorcinol-formaldehyde natural rubber latex was one of the earliest systems employed in the tire industry for bonding rayon to rubber. A recent innovation has been to add resorcinol and a formaldehyde donor directly into the rubber

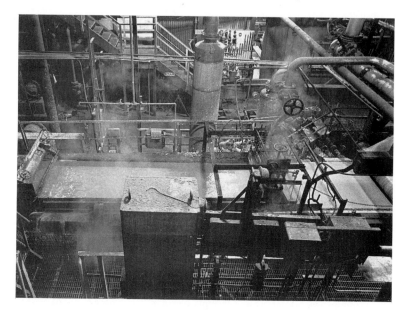

FIGURE 2.   Large particleboard manufacturing facility where urea formaldehyde is extensively utilized as a bonding material.

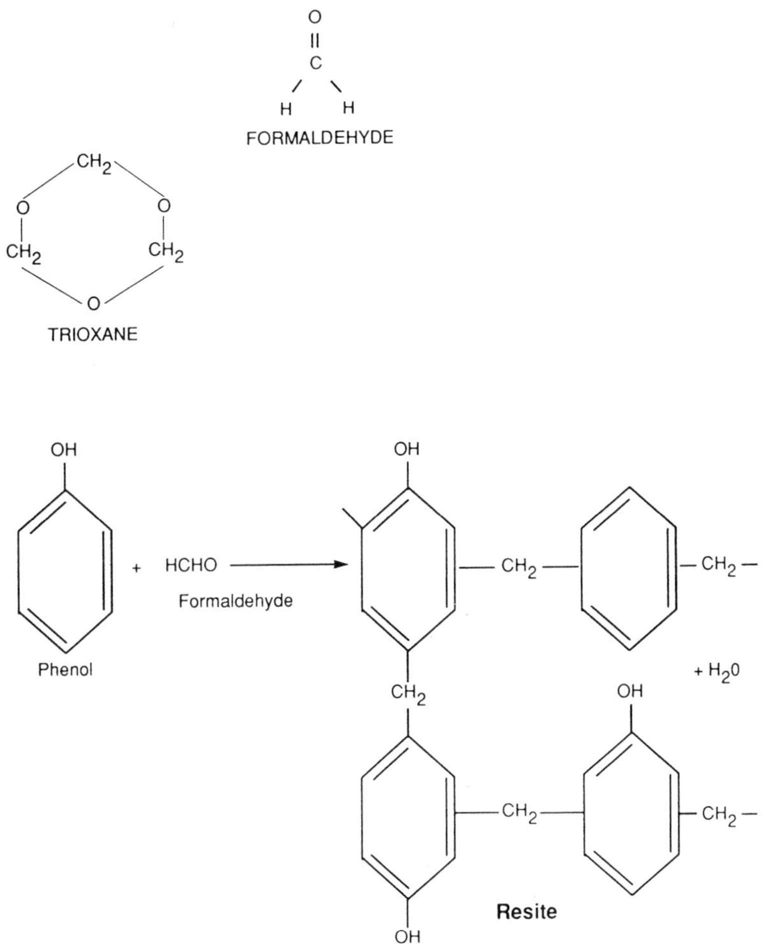

FIGURE 3. Structural formulas for formaldehyde, trioxane, and phenol-formaldehyde (Resite).

stock. It is also frequently used as an adhesive in the production of marine and plywood glues. Even later modifications of the phenolic resin systems included the use of para-tertiarybutylphenol formaldehyde in the production of certain neoprene adhesives. The latter have been extensively employed in the shoemaking and automotive industries.

CHEMICAL AND PHYSICAL PROPERTIES

In its pure monomeric form, formaldehyde is one of the simplest of organic molecules (Fig. 3). Monomeric formaldehyde is a colorless gas with a characteristic suffocating, pungent odor. Pure formaldehyde can exist only as a dilute vapor. It has a molecular weight of 30.03, a high vapor pressure, and a boiling point of -19°C. The pure gas is relatively stable at 80° to 100°C, but at lower temperatures it

spontaneously polymerizes. Above 300°C, it decomposes to carbon monoxide and water. Aqueous solutions contain less than 0.1% of formaldehyde in monomeric form. At normal temperatures it is readily soluble in polar solvents, water, alcohol, and ether. It is commonly marketed as formalin, an aqueous solution (37% to 50% formaldehyde by weight). Usually 10 to 15% methyl alcohol is added to prevent polymerization. The aqueous solution of formalin contains complex equilibrium mixtures of methylene glycol, hemiformol, polyoxymethylene glycols, and so forth (Table 1).

Due to its natural reactivity, formaldehyde can combine with itself to form trioxane, a cyclic trimer, or paraformaldehyde from the linking of eight monomer units (Fig. 3, Table 1). Pure trioxane is a colorless, water-soluble solid with a chloroform-like odor. When ignited, it burns easily and cleanly, and thus it is used as a lightweight, easy-to-carry fuel source.

TABLE 1. *Summary of the Major Formaldehyde Species and Their Application*

Common Designation and Formula	Chemical Synonyms	Properties	Commercial Application
Formaldehyde gas (CH_2O)	Methanol Oxomethane Oxymethylene Methylene oxide Methylaldehyde	Flammable; highly soluble in water, alcohol, and ether; MW 30.03	The natural gas is used to manufacture paraformaldehyde
Formalin solution (CH_2O)	Formal Morbicid Formal-chloral	Cooling leads to turbidity, and very low temperatures to a precipitate of trioxymethylene; oxidizes to formic acid in atmosphere	Disinfectant, concrete, plastic, resin, cosmetic & dye manufacture, textiles, inks, embalming fluid
Formacin (CH_3CONCH_2OH)	Formaldehyde Acetamide Methylol acetamide	Colorless, hydroscopic, soluble in water and insoluble in ether	Disinfectant
Paraformaldehyde ($HO(CH_2O)nH$)*	Paraform Formagene Triformal Trioxymethylene	Requires heating to solubilize in alkaline solution; insoluble in ether & alcohol; average MW 600	Active ingredient in many contraceptive creams; used in manufacture of resins
Trioxane	Metaformaldehyde 1,3,5-Trioxane	Colorless, water-soluble solid with a chloroform-like odor; MW 90.08	Used in preparing intermediates for resin manufacture; light-weight fuel source

* n = 8 to 100

Paraformaldehyde is a solid formaldehyde polymer that has a molecular weight of 600 and comes as a white crystalline powder. It contains a mixture of short-chain linear polyoxymethylene glycols (Table 1). When heated at around 100°C, it decomposes to formaldehyde gas, providing numerous applications in resin production and other industrial and sterilant uses.

Formaldehyde vapor solubilizes upon contact with mucous membranes. It combines easily with a number of organic compounds and functional groups, including nucleic acids, histones, proteins, and amino acids of many biological systems. This occurs by virtue of formaldehyde's capacity to form methylol adducts with amines, which can react further to form methylene linkages.[26,27] It appears that before formaldehyde reacts with amino groups in RNA, the hydrogen bonds forming the coiled RNA are broken.[28,29] Formaldehyde reacts with DNA less frequently than with RNA, because the hydrogen bonds holding DNA in its double helix are more stable.[30] Presumably, it is the reversible bonding of formaldehyde to proteins that accounts for its antigenicity. The immunogenicity of formaldehyde-modified protein was initially reported by Landsteiner and Jablons[31] and Horsfall.[32]

The biochemical transformation of endogenous and exogenous formaldehyde is essentially the same and is present in all animals and bacteria.[33,34] Normal endogenous tissue

levels of formaldehyde in man range from 3 to 12 ng/g of tissue, about 10 to 40% of which is free formaldehyde. The principal reaction is an oxidation to formic acid in the liver and erythrocytes.[35,36] This reaction is catalyzed by formaldehyde dehydrogenase. Formic acid can then undergo three possible reactions: (1) oxidation to carbon dioxide and water; (2) elimination in the urine as a sodium salt (urinary formate or formic acid levels do not reflect formaldehyde exposure)[37]; or (3) entrance into the metabolic one-carbon pool. Formaldehyde disappears very rapidly from the plasma, with a half-life of 1 to 1.5 minutes.[38,39]

DISTRIBUTION AND EXPOSURE ESTIMATES

There are many potential sources of exposure to formaldehyde, both for the consumer and the worker. The earth's troposphere contains 0.12 to 0.39 ppb of formaldehyde.[40] It is ubiquitous in our everyday indoor and outdoor environment.[41] In fact, aldehydes are among the most abundant of the carbon-containing pollutants in most urban atmospheres. Only the hydrocarbons, carbon monoxide, and carbon dioxide are present at higher concentrations.[36]

Important sources of public exposure include automotive exhaust, incinerators, photochemical smog, woodburning stoves, and degassing of formaldehyde resins (Table 2). The incomplete combustion of hydrocarbons

TABLE 2. *Range of Formaldehyde Concentrations in Selected Environments**

Industry or Faculty	Range of Exposure Levels (ppm)
Iron foundry	0.02–18.3
Biology laboratories	2.75–14.8
Laminating plants	0.04–10.9
Autopsy room	0.06– 7.9
Dyestuff production	0.1 – 5.8
Houses with urea-F	0.01– 4.0
Funeral homes	0.09– 5.26
Clothing store	0.9 – 3.3
Urea F resin plant	0.2 – 0.74
Mobile homes†	0.0 – 1.77
Dialysis unit	0.27– 0.63
Hospital	0.37– 0.73
Offices (3 locations)	0.20– 0.12
House without urea-F	0.01– 0.10
Ambient urban air	0.004– 0.002
Rural pasture	0.0005– 0.002

* Compiled and modified from references 36, 58 and 63.
† Complaint homes in which residents had complained of symptoms putatively associated with exposure to formaldehyde. Alternative sources of formaldehyde not sought.

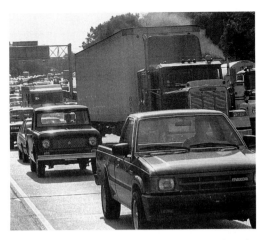

FIGURE 4. Vehicular emissions account for the principal source of outdoor formaldehyde. Approximately 6 pounds of formaldehyde are produced during the combustion of 1000 pounds of gasoline.

accounts for much of the formaldehyde generated in the atmosphere.[42] Approximately 6 pounds of formaldehyde are produced during the combustion of 1000 pounds of gasoline.[43] Mobile sources (automobiles, trucks, and aircraft) emit about 666 million pounds of formaldehyde in the U.S. annually[42] (Fig. 4). Stationary combustion sources emit an additional 200 million pounds[42] (Fig. 5). Local concentrations may vary with traffic patterns and vehicular density. Stupfel reported formaldehyde levels ranging between 0.05 to 0.12 ppm in Los Angeles over a 26-day period.[44] In Houston, levels of formaldehyde up to 0.081 ppm have been noted, with ranges between undetectable to 0.048 in other cities.[42] Significant aldehyde levels have been reported in ambient clean air, e.g., up to 0.01 ppm in Antarctica.[41]

In certain parts of the country increasing numbers of private individuals are using wood as a fuel source.[45,46] During the decade of the 1970s, the shipment of woodstoves increased 10-fold, with the current inventory estimated to exceed 11 million units. Residential wood-burning typically occurs under oxygen-starved conditions that increase emission rates for

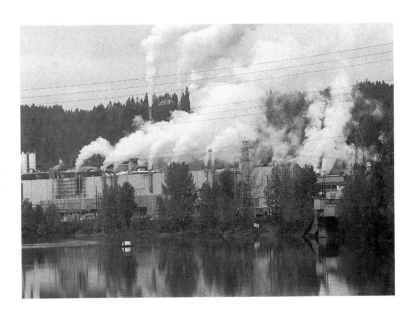

FIGURE 5. Significant combustion emissions from a pulp mill in the Pacific Northwest. Stationary combustion sources are the second major contributor of formaldehyde in the atmosphere.

carbon monoxide, respirable particulates, and polycyclic aromatic hydrocarbons.[47] Formaldehyde, acetaldehyde, and p-tolualdehyde are the primary aldehydes emitted from the experimental burning of cedar, jack pine, red oak, and ash. The amounts of aldehydes and particulates released relate to the burn rate and type of wood. It has been established that between 14 and 54 billion grams of total aldehydes yearly (21 to 42% of which is formaldehyde) are produced nationwide from residential burning of wood.[48]

Perhaps the largest and most direct exposure individuals have to formaldehyde worldwide derives from the use of tobacco products (Table 3).[49] Tobacco smoke affects both the active and the involuntary smoker who shares work space or living quarters. The exposures to involuntary and active tobacco smoke differ quantitatively and, to some extent, qualitatively.[47,50-53] Because of the lower temperature in the burning cone of the smoldering cigarette, most partial pyrolytic products are enriched in the sidestream as compared to the mainstream smoke. Sidestream cigarette smoke can contain as much as 30 to 40 ppm (by volume) of formaldehyde as compared to between 5 and 8 ppm in the mainstream smoke of a filtered cigarette.[50,51,54] It has been observed that a pack-a-day smoker (filtered cigarettes) inhales approximately 1400 ppm total aldehydes (the majority of which is formaldehyde) in the course of a single day.[55] With 95% retention from ten 40 ml puffs on each of 20 cigarettes, a smoker could receive a total daily burden of 0.38 mg of formaldehyde.[42]

Chronic exposure to formaldehyde can also result from involuntary smoking. Nonsmokers in an average room containing an active smoker could have a chronic exposure of between 0.23 and 0.27 ppm.[56] Smoking five cigarettes in a 30 M^3 chamber resulted in a formaldehyde concentration of 0.23 ppm.[57]

In addition to cigarette smoke, there are many other indoor sources of formaldehyde.[56] Formaldehyde may be released from UFFI, particleboard, fiberboard, and plywood (Fig. 6). Elevated concentrations of formaldehyde can be generated by woodburning in fireplaces, inserts, and various types of woodburning stoves.[47,48] It is also emitted from upholstery, drapes, rugs, wallpaper, clothing, and other articles. Contamination may also follow the use of cooking oil or from gas burners, ovens, and space heaters.[58]

The Occupational Safety and Health Administration (OSHA) believes that about 1.3 million workers are exposed to formaldehyde (Table 4). About one-third of them work in medical and health services. About 88% of these workers are exposed to levels below 1 ppm, 8% are exposed to levels between 1 to 3 ppm, and about 4% to levels above 3 ppm.[59] Industries with potentially high exposure levels include fertilizer production, dyestuffs, textile manufacture, foundries for resin production, bronze and iron foundries, pathology/autopsy suites, and the plywood and paper industries (Table 5). Recent application of industrial hygiene principles in these industries has reduced ambient levels significantly.

In addition to industrial exposures, a large segment of the population may be exposed to formaldehyde in its daily experiences. The Environmental Protection Agency (EPA) estimates the mean conventional home level to be 0.03 ppm.[60] Offices and day-care centers have been reported to have mean formaldehyde

TABLE 3.   *Selected Species of Aldehydes Identified in Tobacco Smoke*[49]

Aromatic
Formaldehyde
Acetaldehyde
Propanol
Isobutanol
Benzaldehyde
Olefinic
Acrolein
Crotonaldehyde
Cyclic
Furfural

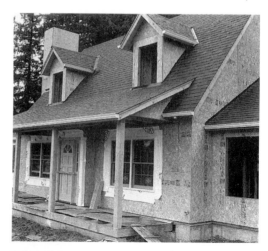

FIGURE 6.   Housing stock where particleboard has been extensively used in the construction.

TABLE 4. *Occupations with Significant Formaldehyde Exposure**

Anatomists	†Foundry workers	Mobile homes
Beauticians	Fumigants	Paints
Biologists	Furniture	†Paper industry
Cellulose industry	Germicides	Photography
Chemicals	Hide preservers	Pest control
Concrete	Home building	Plastics
Contraceptives	Ink makers	Printing
Dentistry	Insulations	†Resin makers
Dialysis	Ivory makers	Rubber
Drycleaning	Latex makers	†Textiles
†Dye industry	Laundry	Shoe industry
Embalming	Mechanics	Silk industry
Explosives	†Medicine	Silk screeners
Farmers	Mining	†Wood industry
†Fertilizer	Mirror industry	

* Modified from Bardana EJ, ref. 23.
† Industries with potential exposures over 1 ppm.[58]

levels of 0.37 and 0.55 ppm, respectively.[61,62] The EPA further believes some 28 million people are living within 12.5 miles of factory sources and may be exposed to continuous low levels of formaldehyde. Many of the 1.5 million medical, nursing, and biology students are also exposed to formaldehyde during their training. A spectrum of formaldehyde concentrations in various environments is summarized in Table 2.

TABLE 5. *Product Uses of Formaldehyde*

Adhesives	Lubricants
Baby shampoos	Mascara
Baby lotions, oils, creams	Makeup bases
Bath soaps	Makeup foundation
Bubble baths	Mouthwash
Cosmetics	Mothballs
Cuticle softeners	Nail creams/lotions
Deodorants	Paints
Dry cleaning solutions	Paper
Dyes	Polishes
Embalming fluids	Photographic solutions
Explosives	Pharmaceuticals
Face powders	Plastics
Feminine hygiene deodorants	Plywood
Fertilizers	Room deodorizers
Food	Rubber
Food packaging materials	Sachets
Fuels	Shaving preparations
Fungicides	Starch
Furniture	Suntan lotions
Hair conditioners	Talcs
Hair rinses	Textiles
Hair shampoos	Toothpaste
Hair dyes	Wave sets
Insulation and fiberglass	Wood preservatives
Laminates	Varnishes
Leathers	

PHYSICAL EFFECTS

Formaldehyde has been reported to cause a variety of problems in exposed individuals. Most of the earlier reports were anecdotal in nature and focused on formaldehyde's capacity to irritate the mucous membranes.[1-17] It is so soluble and rapidly metabolized that it rarely reaches the lower respiratory tract to inflict damage, except when actively inhaled by the cigarette smoker.[63,64] Formaldehyde may, on rare occasions, induce bronchial asthma at relatively high exposure doses.[10,12,16,17] Although many claims have been made that formaldehyde may lead to sensitization,[1,9] the only controlled and convincing scientific data in this regard relate to the skin, e.g., contact dermatitis.[32,65]

A number of recent studies have demonstrated formaldehyde's capacity to induce specific antibodies to formaldehyde-protein complexes.[66,67] However, no one has yet shown that these antibodies have any clinical relevance.[68] Formaldehyde has been implicated in severe systemic reactions when administered parenterally.[69,70] A number of reports have alluded to formaldehyde's capacity to induce neuropsychiatric disorders.[71,72] For the most part, these observations have serious deficiencies of design, exposure assessment, and outcome measurement. Formaldehyde has been classified as possibly carcinogenic by a number of federal agencies.[73,74]

These diverse health effects will be discussed in some detail below.

Annoyance Reactions

Inhaled formaldehyde primarily affects the upper airways and eyes. The severity and precise physiological response depend on its ambient concentration. Exposures to lower levels of formaldehyde may result in annoyance complaints associated with a heightened sense of olefactory awareness. The odor threshold for recognition of formaldehyde vapor in air has been variously reported between 0.1 to 1 ppm. The most likely threshold value is about 0.5 ppm. One can predict that within the population some individuals will tolerate the odor of formaldehyde less well than others. The capacity to cope with a nonirritating, yet undesirable, odor may relate to genetic factors or acquired traits that blunt olefactory capacity. It has been shown that a large variety of odors can aggravate the symptoms of reactive airway disease.[75] Congenital familial dysautonomia and Turner's syndrome are both associated with an increased detection and lowered recognition threshold, whereas hypothyroidism, sinusitis, polyposis, and many rhinoplastic procedures result in anosmia, hyposmia, or parosmia.[76] Cigarette smoking, inhalation of cocaine, and chronic use of nasal decongestants all lead to variable abnormal decreased sensitivity to odors (hyposmia).

Chronic exposure to formaldehyde may be associated with the development of short-term tolerance.[11,21,77,78] Nasal hyperirritability is commonly associated with viral coryzas and symptomatic allergic rhinitis. The pathophysiology of annoyance reactions has encompassed the deposition of formaldehyde on the outer surface of the nasal mucous blanket. The chemical is present in small amounts and does not penetrate the nasal mucous blanket to reach the underlying periciliary fluid. Thus, the patient is aware of a disagreeable odor but suffers no physiologic harm.

Ocular and Mucous Membrane Irritation

Exposures to higher ambient levels of formaldehyde may result in transient irritation of the eyes and mucous membranes. Because of the considerable overlap in the effects of different formaldehyde concentrations in different individuals, it is not possible to draw a single line of demarcation between concentrations that are simply annoyances and those that induce mucous membrane irritation. This was well documented in a study in a controlled environmental chamber of symptoms and pulmonary function associated with a 3-hour exposure to 0–3.0 ppm of formaldehyde.[79] The latter study showed wide variations in individual response.

Studies that were reviewed and summarized by the National Research Council suggested that formaldehyde caused eye irritation at ranges between 0.1 to 2.0 ppm. Upper airway irritation of the nose and throat was reported at concentrations as low as 0.1 ppm, but more likely at levels between 1.0 and 11 ppm. Lower airway and pulmonary effects were said to occur at levels between 5 and 30 ppm.[42] At the time the federal standard in the U.S. allowed a 3 ppm exposure as an 8-hour time-weighted average (TWA), with a ceiling of 5 ppm.[80] In 1987 OSHA revised its standard by reducing the 8-hour TWA to 1 ppm and introduced a 15-minute, short-term exposure limit of 2 ppm. The American Conference of Governmental Industrial Hygienists (ACGIH) adopted a 1 ppm TWA with a 2 ppm short-term exposure limit.[81]

Our review of the literature indicates that the threshold of irritation for individuals ranges between 0.3 and 3.0 ppm. Irritant reactions are most likely to occur at values in excess of 0.8 ppm.[82] In irritant reactions, formaldehyde actually penetrates the mucous blanket into the periciliary area. It can affect olefactory and trigeminal nerve endings, causing transient burning sensation of the eyes, nasal passages, and the throat. This may be followed by lacrimation and reduced flow in the secretion of mucous in nose and throat. These symptoms are temporary and abate entirely with removal from exposure. Though low ambient concentrations of formaldehyde result in stimulation of mucociliary function, higher concentrations result in inhibition of mucociliary function and ultimately complete mucostasis and ciliastasis.[83]

Three mechanisms have been proposed to explain how low molecular weight chemicals induce sensory irritation: (1) nucleophilic addition, (2) disulfide bond cleavage, and (3) physical interaction.[78] Nucleophilic addition or direct binding is probably the most applicable mechanism with regard to formaldehyde. Formaldehyde reacts with SH and NH_2 groups in a reversible manner.[84] It is unlikely that ambient concentrations of formaldehyde at or below 5 ppm will stimulate bronchial receptors via either sensory or inflammatory mechanisms. Because of its extraordinary solubility, most inhaled formaldehyde is retained in the upper respiratory tract.[64,85] A number of studies indicate that levels of approximately 15 ppm on a chronic, long-term basis would be required to produce irreversible damage to the upper respiratory tract.[86,87] However, ambient concentrations of formaldehyde above 5 ppm are generally very disagreeable and would cause most individuals to immediately avoid these potentially harmful circumstances.

Dermatologic Reactions

The best known industrial hazard of formaldehyde is the induction of a dermatitis. This can occur as a result of an irritational mechanism or via a delayed hypersensitivity mechanism. Skin irritation or sensitivity to airborne formaldehyde has not been recently reported. Because threshold levels for both irritant and allergic reactions are quite high, it would be unlikely that ambient formaldehyde vapor alone would result in dermatitis. A single application of 1% formalin in water will produce an irritant response in about 5% of the population. In 1966, Epstein and Maibach reported their findings with patch-testing for formaldehyde sensitization of the skin.[65] Prior to their studies the indiscriminant use of terms "contact dermatitis" and "allergic contact dermatitis," together with a frequent failure to separate irritant from immunologic responses, produced both confusion and erroneous conclusions. The threshold point for induction of delayed hypersensitivity contact dermatitis has only been imprecisely determined to be less than 5% formalin in water.[89] In sensitized subjects, the approximate thresholds for elicitation of contact dermatitis from exposure to formaldehyde ranges from 30 ppm for patch-testing to 60 ppm for actual use concentrations of formalin.[88] The establishment of true contact dermatitis in an individual can pose a very significant avoidance problem because of its ubiquitous occurrence in home and work environments.[89] Sensitized patients may react to a variety of paper products, photographic materials, clothing, textile products, cosmetics, and medicaments, including the plaster of orthopedic casts.

Early reports describing formaldehyde-induced dermatitis suggested possible induction by contact, inhalation, or both.[90,91] Unfortunately, the majority of these reports were anecdotal and failed to support their observations with careful immunologic testing. In addition, many of these reports dealt with formaldehyde resin products as opposed to pure formaldehyde. The earliest of these benchmark studies was the work of Horsfall. He showed that inhalation of formaldehyde vapor (at about 10 ppm) through a respirator by a formaldehyde-sensitive individual resulted in the delayed appearance at 15½ hours of typical hand dermatitis.[92] The response was accentuated when the individual inspired 40 ppm of formaldehyde. In other experiments, Horsfall also demonstrated immediate skin reactions in formaldehyde-sensitized rabbits.[32] The immunologic nature of the response was confirmed by positive immunodiffusion responses and the anaphylactoid responses of guinea pig uterine strips sensitized to a formaldehyde conjugate.

Formaldehyde has also been reported to cause contact urticaria.[93-100] The mechanism of the urticarial reaction has never been clearly demonstrated. Mechanisms may involve true IgE-mediated release of mast cell inflammatory mediators, activation of the complement pathway by either immune or nonimmune triggers, or by direct release of mast cell mediators. Rappaport and Hoffman described a unique patient who developed contact urticaria with as small a topical exposure as a 1×10^{-7} formalin solution (3.7 ppm) during his work.[95] He was a nonatopic histology technician whose lesions progressed from localized itching and hives on the fingers to generalized lesions. His problem continued after removal from work and was ascribed to formaldehyde in the aromatic fraction of cigarette smoke. He was noted to have a positive epicutaneous skin test to formaldehyde as well as all the nonconjugated aldehydes and acrolein. Other as yet unexplained but unique reports involve the development of urticaria from vaporized formaldehyde,[101] and delayed urticarial reaction secondary to formaldehyde in solutions.[102] A rare example of formaldehyde-induced photodermatitis has also been reported.[103]

Respiratory Symptoms

Sufficiently well-controlled and reproducible scientific studies are not yet available to definitively establish the development of respiratory tract allergy to formaldehyde vapor.[63,68,104] Many earlier reports of formaldehyde-induced respiratory disease invoked an irritative mechanism.[2-8,10-12,105-111] Some of these observers did attempt to conduct immunologic studies to shed light on potential mechanisms.[1,8,9,13,109] Nevertheless, conclusive data were not generated. Almost all these reports dealt with a cause-and-effect relationship based on an assumption. There are several reports suggesting the association between inflammatory bronchitis and formaldehyde is likely to be due to an excessive exposure level.[10,12,112]

Perhaps the earliest report of asthma attributable to formalin sensitivity was published in 1939 by Vaughn and Black.[1] They described a match-factory worker who developed work-related asthma secondary to formalin exposure. Vaughn conducted some uncontrolled skin tests with formalin, which supported his suspicion of sensitivity. Similarly Popa et al.[9] used dilute saline solutions of formalin to conduct skin tests for immediate and delayed reactions, as well as inhalation provocation and other serologic studies, to demonstrate sensitivity. Most of their cases were felt to be irritative in nature. One subject with a positive inhalation challenge test to UFFI resin fumes associated with peripheral eosinophilia was felt to have features consistent with an allergic mechanism.

The contemporary era of investigation into the possibility of bona fide respiratory allergy was started in 1975 by Hendrick and Lane.[13] In a series of articles these investigators reported the results of a survey of 12 nurses, 10 nursing aides, and two domestic assistants who spent most of their working hours in a small, temporary, poorly ventilated hemodialysis unit.[13,17] Each of the subjects was interviewed and underwent baseline studies of lung function. Subsequently, each underwent bronchial provocation studies, with blood being drawn before and after each test. Exposure to formalin was simulated by painting different concentrations of formalin solution on a piece of cardboard in a confined space. Unfortunately, ambient concentrations of formaldehyde were not measured. Studies showed that prior episodes of recurrent wheezing and productive cough appeared to be related to formalin hypersensitivity in two nurses. Three others with similar, but less frequent, symptoms failed to develop symptoms on bronchial provocation. The positive reactions were characterized by delayed onset of bronchial obstruction 3 to 4 hours after initial exposure, with maximal response between 6 and 20 hours later. Reactions persisted for between 10 hours and 10 days, depending on the degree of exposure. During the height of the reaction, productive cough was the most prominent symptom and peripheral eosinophilia was striking.[17]

In 1982, Hendrick and Lane restudied the two nurses with the most significant reactions. The initial provocative exposures were recreated and measured. The resultant ambient formaldehyde levels were 3–6 ppm.[113] One of these nurses had transferred away from the renal dialysis unit and had no further exposure to formaldehyde. Her asthma had resolved completely, and a duplicated challenge test provoked no adverse response. The remaining nurse had continued to work with formalin in significantly improved conditions. This individual developed a mild, late asthmatic response, with eosinophilia following the duplicated provocation.[113] No further studies were carried out to elucidate immunologic hyperresponsiveness, but the investigators believed some form of sensitization was involved. However, an irritative mechanism could not be excluded, especially with the high exposure levels involved.[113,114]

At about the same time, Wallenstein and Rebble attempted to correlate nasal symptoms with intracutaneous and epicutaneous skin tests in 180 individuals with a history of formaldehyde exposure. Approximately 10% reacted in a dose-response manner to between 0.02 and 0.1% formaldehyde intracutaneously. Nasal provocation was then carried out, with about half showing positive reactions. Serum antibody studies were not performed.[115]

Several groups have studied and reported the development of bronchial asthma related to the domestic exposure to UFFI. Frigas and his associates carried out bronchial provocation studies with UFFI dust and formaldehyde alone at 3 ppm.[116] Only the UFFI provoked an immediate asthmatic reaction. These observations were criticized because they lacked appropriate controls.[117] It was suggested that the observed responses were nonspecific irritant reactions. Frigas et al. published additional data supporting their initial report, but they emphasized there was no evidence that incriminated formaldehyde as an immunogen.[118] Day et al. studied the responses of human volunteers to controlled exposures of formaldehyde and offgassing from UFFI. Ten of the subjects were alleged to have symptoms related to UFFI—nine were asthmatics and nine were normal adults. None of the 10 individuals complaining of UFFI-induced illness developed significant changes in pulmonary function or in any other variable studied. There were no significant differences between the UFFI or formaldehyde-challenged groups. In 1986, Pross et al. reported a comprehensive study of 23 subjects with a history of asthmatic symptoms attributed to UFFI and four non-UFFI-related control subjects.[120] The main objective of the study was to examine a spectrum of immunologic tests that could conceivably be affected by long- or short-term exposure to formaldehyde or other UFFI off-products. The results demonstrated minimal increases in total eosinophils, basophils, and T-8 positive cells after controlled short-term exposure. These changes were felt to be of doubtful significance. The long-term exposure to UFFI off-products had no apparent effect on the immunologic parameters studied.[120]

Cockcroft et al. reported the development of work-related asthma in two carpenters exposed to urea-formaldehyde used as an adhesive in particleboard.[121] One developed immediate and another a dual asthmatic response to sawdust from cedar urea-formaldehyde wood dust. Both complained of upper respiratory symptoms as well. Provocation studies used cedar urea formaldehyde sawdust with plain cedar and spruce dust as controls. Provocation with formaldehyde was not carried out. Attempts to demonstrate IgE-specific antibody to a formaldehyde-protein conjugate were negative.

Kwong and associates described the clinical presentation of a pathology resident who developed immediate hoarseness, sore throat, and chest tightness on exposure to formaldehyde.[122] Symptoms peaked at 24 hours and regressed with topical corticosteroids. Edematous vocal cords were evident on exam, and an eczematoid dermatitis was noted over the fingers. IgE- and IgG-specific antibodies were not found in the serum. Specific bronchial provocation studies were not done.

To assess the effects of low-level formaldehyde exposure, Main and Hogan compared a group of police workers exposed to ambient formaldehyde in two mobile home trailers being used as temporary office facilities with a group of 18 employees who had not worked in the trailers.[123] The exposed group inhaled formaldehyde at levels between 0.12 and 1.6 ppm. Irritational symptoms of the upper and lower respiratory tract were found to be more common among the exposed group. The authors concluded that the significant increase in frequency of symptoms in the exposed group resulted from formaldehyde.[123] This study was limited by its dependence on subjective parameters and the presumption that formaldehyde was emanating from particleboard subflooring and paneling. There were alternative sources of formaldehyde and other chemicals, the most important of which was active and passive cigarette smoking.[124] Unfortunately, the same observations could be made for many other studies on the subject.

Frigas et al. carried out a seminal, single-blind, bronchial provocation study of 13 selected patients with symptoms suggestive of asthma in whom formaldehyde was felt to be a major trigger or cause.[125] Bronchial challenges of 0.1, 1.0, and 3.0 ppm of formaldehyde gas and randomly interspersed room-air placebos were administered via a dynacalibrator. The period of bronchial challenge was 20 minutes. Pulmonary function was measured before and for 24 hours after each bronchial challenge. Based on changes in FEV_1, the authors were unable to substantiate that exposure to formaldehyde gas at 3 ppm or less was either causing or aggravating asthmatic symptoms. A relatively short exposure time and the fact that subjects were kept at rest were cited as shortcomings of the study.[126] However, this study made some very valid observations regarding the fragility of an individual's perception regarding severe "sensitivity."

Schachter and associates conducted several studies of 15 laboratory workers routinely exposed to formaldehyde as their work.[127,128] A double-blind, random exposure sequence from zero to 2 ppm formaldehyde for 40 minutes in a climate-controlled environmental chamber was employed. Exposures were repeated on two or more occasions, with 10 minutes of exercise after 5 minutes in the provocation chamber. Mild mucous membrane irritation was noted. No lower airway symptoms were noted and pulmonary function remained unchanged. The authors concluded that no acute or delayed pulmonary function changes occurred.

Sheppard et al. conducted studies to determine whether mild asthmatics would experience evidence of bronchoconstriction when exposed to modest levels of formaldehyde.[129] Chamber exposure levels were 1–3 ppm for 10 minutes and included exposure during moderate exercise. None of the subjects developed respiratory symptoms within 24 hours of exposure. The authors did not feel that ambient levels of formaldehyde up to 3 ppm would provoke bronchospasm in patients with mild bronchial asthma.

Nordman et al. carried out bronchial provocation studies in 230 individuals with asthma-like symptoms who had been exposed to formaldehyde in their work.[130] The authors made a diagnosis of formaldehyde-induced asthma on the basis of history and a positive 30-minute inhalation test to concentrations of 1 and 2 ppm in a 10 M^3 exposure chamber. Challenges were not blinded, and a positive ventilatory response was based on a 15% decrease in the peak expiratory flow by a Wright peak-flow meter. This study was limited in several areas. The Wright peak-flow meter is an instrument that is eminently patient-dependent, particularly when parameters for reproducibility were not included in the report. In addition, the investigators failed to elaborate on the potential role of alternative pulmonary immunogens or irritants at the workplace.[131] Detailed smoking histories were neither included in the original illustrative cases nor in their reply to a critique, e.g., active versus former versus never-smokers.[132]

Further industrial studies were carried out by Burge and his associates, who tested 15 symptomatic workers with formaldehyde challenge.[133] Each had symptoms of tight chest and cough felt to be related to formaldehyde in the workplace. Ambient levels of formaldehyde at the workplace were generally higher than is usually found, e.g., about 3 ppm. The nature of the occupation was never defined. The authors conclude that 3 of the 15 workers had "classic" work-induced asthma (late asthmatic response) caused by formaldehyde fumes. Six of the 15 workers had immediate asthma-like reactions felt to be due to irritation. Unfortunately, this study suffers from the same limitations of several others in that it was retrospective, uncontrolled, and with an unclear description of alternative potential causations. No direct studies were carried out to implicate immunologic mechanisms.

Kilburn and his associates reported both respiratory and neurobehavioral effects in 45 technicians and workers exposed to formaldehyde in a manufacturing process involving the embedding of fiberglass in a phenol-formaldehyde plastic foam matrix (batt makers).[72,134,135] The thrust of this investigation focused on the central nervous system. Unfortunately, no information related to smoking habits, atopy, airway hyperreactivity, or other immunologic studies is provided. Norman et al. reported their observations on 29 children exposed to UFFI in a home setting. Nine reported lower respiratory tract symptoms in relation to a presumed home exposure. No changes were observed on pulmonary function studies.[136]

Trasher et al. reported on a spectrum of individuals chronically exposed to formaldehyde at relatively low indoor ambient concentrations.[137,138] These individuals were compared to normal "unexposed" subjects. A large number of tests, including antibodies to formaldehyde-conjugated human serum albumin and percentage of T and B lymphocytes, as well as mitogenic response, were carried out. In the exposed cohort, three of eight were active smokers, but there is no information as to passive smoking. The majority of the exposed group are reported to have had immunologic changes that are putatively linked to formaldehyde. Four of seven exposed individuals had altered respiratory values.[137]

Sauder et al. studied nine nonsmoking asthmatic volunteers to evaluate the acute pulmonary response to 3 ppm of formaldehyde over a 3-hour exposure. Symptoms, pulmonary function, and bronchial hyperreactivity were assessed before and after the exposure. No significant changes in pulmonary function or nonspecific airway reactivity were observed. There was a significant increase in eye and mucous membrane symptoms during the exposure.[139]

Horvath and his colleagues studied 109 workers and 254 control subjects to evaluate the effects of formaldehyde on the mucous membranes and lungs.[140] A history was obtained from and spirometry administered to all study participants before and after their work shift. Information related to smoking habits and alternative work irritants was obtained. Formaldehyde levels were determined for each test subject. The results suggested that formaldehyde could contribute to short-term declines in pulmonary function in some occupational settings, but that dose-response relationships were not always strong. Only a small portion of cross-shift changes in lung function could be attributed to measured airborne formaldehyde levels, which was found to exert a dose-dependent irritation of the eyes and mucous membranes at low level exposures. However, after a mean exposure of 10 years, formaldehyde was not related to any permanent respiratory impairment.

Holmstrom and Wilhelmsson evaluated the effects of formaldehyde alone (in 70 chemical workers), and formaldehyde and wood dust (in 100 furniture workers), as well as 36 control individuals described as government clerks.[141] The authors felt there were no significant differences in tobacco use among the groups, but did not specify the incidence. The authors report a reduced nasal mucociliary clearance and sense of smell in the exposed groups when compared against the "controls." A number of flaws in study design make it difficult to derive significant conclusions from this report.

Alexandersson and Hedenstierna recently reported a prospective study of 47 woodworkers and 20 control subjects initially studied in 1980 and again 5 years later.[142] About half the study group were active smokers. Exposure levels of formaldehyde were reported between 0.42 and 0.50 mg/M^3, with small amounts of respirable wood dust. A dose-response relationship was noted between exposure to formaldehyde and decreased lung function. The authors point out, however, that smoking was a confounding factor in evaluating industrial exposure to formaldehyde. As well, the decreased lung function essentially reverted to normal during a 4-week holiday period during which no industrial exposure took place.[142]

Conclusion

It appears reasonably clear that formaldehyde is capable of acting as a respiratory irritant. There is no consistent or convincing evidence that it acts as a respiratory immunogen. There is no evidence that formaldehyde is capable of inducing transient or permanent bronchial hyperreactivity that is associated with ozone or nitrogen dioxide. The best model of this potential effect would be the inhalation of cigarette smoke known to contain rather significant quantities of formaldehyde. However, recent studies in smokers without fixed airway obstruction demonstrated only 3 of 13 showed any transient airway constriction secondary to tobacco smoke.[143]

PATHOPHYSIOLOGIC REACTIONS TO FORMALDEHYDE

Formaldehyde as an Immunogen

It has been known for some time that low-molecular-weight reactive chemicals can combine with human self-protein to form antigenic conjugates capable of inducing hypersensitivity reactions. A number of such chemicals have been well described[144,145] and some are covered in detail in Chapter 12 (Isocyanates) and Chapter 13 (Acid Anhydrides). Initial descriptions of the antigenicity of formaldehyde-altered proteins were made over 75 years ago by Landsteiner and Jablons[31] and expanded in 1934 by Horsfall.[32,92] It appeared that many of these initial observations were reinforced by the initial studies of formaldehyde as a skin sensitizer.[88] Patterson and his associates developed an enzyme-linked immunosorbent assay (ELISA) to measure antibody response to formaldehyde-albumin conjugates.[66,67] Initial studies conducted in a parenterally immunized canine model demonstrated IgG and IgA antibodies.[66] However, the antibodies lacked specificity for either formaldehyde or dog serum albumin alone, and seemed most reactive with a new antigenic ligand on the albumin molecule.

Later studies were carried out in sera from 18 asymptomatic hemodialysis patients and four individuals with formaldehyde-associated upper and lower respiratory symptoms.[67] Low titers of IgG antibodies to a formaldehyde-albumin determinant were universally present in the dialysis patients. IgE antibodies were also noted in two of these 18 patients with no clinical signs of immediate hypersensitivity to formaldehyde exposure. Of the four patients with formaldehyde-associated upper and lower respiratory symptoms, two subjects with acute rhinitis had no detectable antibodies to formaldehyde or to its albumin conjugates. However, sera from two previously reported dialysis nurses with formaldehyde-induced asthma[13,114] were observed to have IgE antibody against a determinant in the formaldehyde-albumin conjugate and the human serum albumin alone, but not the formaldehyde alone.[67] More recently, this same group studied 61 serum samples for IgG-specific antibodies against formaldehyde-albumin conjugate.[68] Again, IgG-specific antibodies were noted to be most prevalent in subjects who had received intravenous formaldehyde. In no case did these authors verify a correlation of serologic results with symptoms. In the same study the authors reviewed inhalational respiratory disease caused by proteins or chemicals acting as immunogens. They concluded that there was no evidence that gaseous formaldehyde met characteristic criteria for medical problems associated with IgG antibodies to inhaled antigens.[68]

These observations are in stark contrast to reports by Thrasher et al.[138,139,146] These authors have published several studies suggesting that the presence of antibodies to formaldehyde conjugates and changes in T-cell lymphocyte subsets demonstrated "immune activation" that correlated with patient complaints. Criticism was directed to the journal editors by Greenberg.[147] This investigator pointed out that the immunologic measures in these reports represented "an unproven tool proposed to evaluate an undocumented pathogenesis for an undefined disease." Similar cogent points were raised by Beavers.[148]

Kramps et al. conducted measurements for formaldehyde-specific IgE antibodies in four groups of individuals exposed to formaldehyde.[149] One group[28] was exposed to formaldehyde offgassing from construction materials, a second group[18] to high dose occupational exposure, a third group[12] consisted of paramedical employees in a dialysis unit, and finally a group of 28 subjects undergoing hemodialysis. Formaldehyde-specific IgE antibodies were detected in only one of 86 serum samples. This individual had been exposed to high levels of formaldehyde but had not history of symptoms. It was concluded that even high concentrations of formaldehyde rarely evoke production of IgE-specific antibodies and that their presence is unassociated with symptoms.[149]

In a collaborative study between Northwestern University and the University of Washington, 37 aircraft workers with an exposure history to formaldehyde were evaluated to determine whether their respiratory and ocular symptoms were the result of formaldehyde sensitivity.[150] After comprehensive clinical and serologic evaluation, none of the workers was found to have IgE or IgG antibody to formaldehyde-albumin conjugate, or evidence of an immunologically mediated respiratory or ocular disease caused by formaldehyde. However, some of the workers appeared to experience irritant symptoms caused by workplace exposure to either formaldehyde or other irritant chemicals at their plant.[150]

In a recent investigation, 55 subjects with a history of exposure to gaseous formaldehyde in laboratory environments, cigarette smokers and nonsmokers without known occupational exposure to gaseous formaldehyde were studied. The study was focused on two major questions: (1) whether exposure to gaseous formaldehyde was associated with the development of antibodies to formaldehyde-albumin conjugate, and (2) whether the presence of antibodies correlated with a history of respiratory and conjunctival symptoms from gaseous formaldehyde. The study failed to uncover any immunologic basis for respiratory or conjunctival symptoms from gaseous formaldehyde exposure. The authors concluded that IgE allergy to gaseous formaldehyde either does not exist, or if it does exits, it is extremely rare.[151]

In summary, formaldehyde has the capacity to bind to human protein and act as an immunogen. Routes of potential antigen exposure include dermal contact, ingestion, and inhalation. Whether each or all of these routes of exposure are capable of inducing de novo antibodies is currently unknown. Specific antibody to the conjugate (but not formaldehyde alone) has been demonstrated within the IgG, IgA, IgM, and IgE classes of immunoglobulin. Demonstration of serum antibody to formaldehyde-albumin conjugates has not been shown to have any relation to concentration or route of exposure, and its presence has never been conclusively linked to a symptomatic state. In fact, it can be said that measurement of such antibody has an extraordinarily limited role in the evaluation of patients with putative formaldehyde-induced disease.

Systemic Formaldehyde Reactions

Sensitization arising from release of formaldehyde into the circulation during renal dialysis has been reported. Although the antigenicity of formaldehyde-protein complexes has been known for many years,[31,32,92] contemporary observations of autoimmune hemolytic anemia in dialysis patients have affirmed these old observations.[69,152-159] In contrast to the relatively low doses associated with inhalation of formaldehyde, even in active cigarette smokers, patients on hemodialysis may be infused with as much as 126 mg of formaldehyde during a single dialysis.[69] It is quite plausible that such a comparatively large exposure would be sufficient to yield potentially antigenic functional groups with nucleic acids, histones, and proteins. Subsequent re-exposure could result in development of circulating immune complexes and a serum sickness-like syndrome. Rarely, systemic sensitivity has been associated with peripheral eosinophilia and associated sensitivity or asthma-like reactions.[69,160]

Maurice et al. reported the development of anaphylactic shock secondary to formaldehyde exposure in a 20-year-old female undergoing chronic hemodialysis.[70] Interestingly, this patient had a history of formaldehyde contact sensitivity prior to dialysis-associated formaldehyde infusion. Evaluation included positive epicutaneous test with 0.1 and 1.0% formaldehyde. Similar tests were reportedly negative in 30 atopic and 30 nonatopic control individuals. Patch-testing with 1% solution was also strongly positive, but produced anaphylaxis 26 hours after application. Contact urticaria was not observed. Significant amounts of IgE-specific antibody to formaldehyde conjugate was observed. The observations are consistent with formaldehyde-induced anaphylaxis mediated by an IgE mechanism. However, one cannot exclude participation by other class-specific antibodies, with or without cell-mediated mechanisms.[63]

Neurotoxic Formaldehyde Reactions

Several epidemiologic studies have attempted to relate subjective complaints of fatigue, forgetfulness, headache, inability to concentrate, inability to sleep, nausea, etc. on the environmental or occupational exposure to formaldehyde.[15,71,72,134,135,138,146,161-163] Many of these studies proport to demonstrate a neurobehavioral deficit in exposed individuals.[71,72,134,135,164] All of these studies suffer from serious deficiencies of design, assessment of exposure, and outcome measurement. Data are usually derived from questionnaires without verifiable objective measures of the neurobehavioral symptoms. Generally there was no attempt to measure dose-response–mean-symptom scores with measured levels of formaldehyde. In fact, in some cases, the exposure data are based on self-reported exposure to formaldehyde fumes.[164] Carefully case-controlled studies have failed to show significant differences in the occurrence of nonspecific symptoms in residents of homes with UFFI as compared to controls.[165,166] Considering the fact that formaldehyde is so ubiquitous in our environment, it seems unlikely that we have overlooked these neurologic and behavioral symptoms so long. Active and involuntary cigarette smokers have the largest continuous exposure to this chemical, and such neurobehavioral impairment has not yet been reported in this group. Aside from this, formaldehyde is so rapidly metabolized that it is difficult to imagine any deleterious effect from low-level exposures. It seems more likely that many of these systemic complaints relate to anxiety and a strong public perception of harmful effects.[104,166,167]

Formaldehyde as a Carcinogen

Much of the public concern and media attention to formaldehyde relates to its classification as a carcinogen.[73,74] Indeed, formaldehyde vapor has been found to be carcinogenic in two strains of rats (Fischer-344 and Sprague-Dawley). Squamous cell carcinoma of the nose occurred when 14.3 ppm of formaldehyde was inhaled 6 hr/day, 5 days/week, up to 2 years. Only two of 215 mice developed nasal cancer after 24 months of exposure at 14 ppm.[168,169] The marked difference in susceptibility between the rat and the mouse is felt to be due to the fact that the mouse's respiratory minute volume is greatly reduced when compared to the rat when exposed to 14 ppm of the chemical.[169] Despite the ubiquity of formaldehyde in our society, epidemiologic surveys have not convincingly demonstrated an increased rate of cancer that is dose-related to formaldehyde in an exposed population. A complete review of this subject is beyond the scope of this chapter. However, the issue has been succinctly reviewed by AMA's Council on Scientific Affairs.[166] This report aptly summarized the present situation by indicating that the evidence in humans is limited and controversial. Nevertheless, both the EPA and OSHA, in consideration of the available epidemiologic and toxicologic studies, regard formaldehyde as a possible human carcinogen.[166]

CLINICAL EVALUATION

As can be discerned by the considerable controversy surrounding this low molecular weight chemical, the evaluation of any patient with suspected formaldehyde-induced disease must be approached with considerable care. A number of items are essential to a complete evaluation. A visit to the putative site should be made, with application of industrial hygiene methods. Measurement of formaldehyde by qualified individuals and methods should be conducted under conditions that were likely to exist when complaints arose. A detailed evaluation of the ventilation system may prove useful in determining the cause of nonspecific symptoms. Particular attention should be paid to tobacco smoking in the area.

In evaluating the patient, a meticulous history and examination are critical. Emphasis should be placed on elucidating any preexisting medical condition in all prior medical records. Any incidental exposure to formaldehyde should be recorded, including tobacco abuse; use of marijuana; the presence and use of woodstoves, inserts and fireplaces; room deodorants; cat litter; and both avocational and occupational exposures (Table 5). In addition to active smoking, all opportunities for involuntary smoking should be recorded, e.g., family members or co-workers who smoke. Laboratory evaluations have a limited scope of usefulness. Determination of formic acid blood levels is not useful in assessing exposure or adsorption.[33-35]

Skin testing has had limited application but has proven helpful. Patch testing with nonirritating concentrations of formalin is useful in determining delayed hypersensitivity reactions.[65,88,89] In testing for delayed hypersensitivity, it is well to remember that a significant number of individuals will react to 2% aqueous solution, e.g., 3–6%.[170] The incidence of positivity is quite low in children under 10 and increases steadily with age until the seventh decade and beyond, when it decreases.

An open test, or a 15-minute closed test, with 1 or 2% aqueous formaldehyde will provoke a wheal-and-flare response in contact urticaria.[92,101,171] Similarly, epicutaneous skin testing with similar concentrations of formaldehyde should react by the same mechanism and has been reported to demonstrate "immediate-type" reactions.[1,8,9,70,93,113] Maurice et al. reported the prick test with 0.1 and 1.0% aqueous formaldehyde to be er.tirely negative in 30 atopic and 30 nonatopic individuals with no regular contact to formaldehyde. These investigators successfully employed the prick test to demonstrate what they felt to be skin-sensitizing antibodies in a uniquely sensitive patient.[70] In a review of formaldehyde, Imbus describes skin testing to be useless and potentially dangerous, without providing the background.[172] In cases of immunologically mediated urticaria, passive antibody transfer has been demonstrated for some contact allergens, but this phenomenon has only been described without details for formaldehyde.[99]

Patterson et al. have described and employed an ELISA system for measurement of IgG-, IgM-, IgA-, and IgE-specific antibodies to formaldehyde conjugates.[66, 68, 150,151] The presence of antibody to such conjugates cannot by itself be interpreted as representing a symptomatic hypersensitivity disorder. The observations thus far support this conclusion,[68,149] which also has ample precedent in the studies associated with other low molecular weight antigens.[144,145]

The comparison of any physiologic parameter that can be recorded pre- and post-exposure would be very desirable, e.g., measurement of both upper and lower airway resistance by rhinomanometric measurements and pulmonary function, respectively. Perhaps the most reliable objective measurement lies in the application of controlled nasal and bronchial provocation tests. Standardized chambers with laminar flow delivery of precise concentrations of chemicals have become available in many centers throughout the country.[173] Controlled provocation studies are becoming an integral part of such evaluations.[174]

REFERENCES

1. Vaughn WT, Black JH: The Practice of Allergy. St. Louis, C.V. Mosby, 1939, p 677.
2. Harris DR: Health problems in the manufacture and use of plastics. Br J Ind Med 10:255, 1953.
3. Herzog H, Pletscher A: Die Wirkung von industriellen Reizgasen auf die Bronchialschleimhaut des Menschen. Schweizerische medizinische Wochenschrift 85:477, 1955.
4. Bourne HG, Seferian S: Insufficiently polymerized resins used for wrinkle-proofing clothing may liberate toxic quantities of formaldehyde. Ind Med Surg 28:232, 1959.
5. Coulant MP, Lopes G: L'allergie au formal et a ses derives. Archives des Maladies Professionelles, de Medicine du Travail et de Securite Sociale (Paris) 22:769, 1961.
6. Fuchs E, Gronemeyer W: Zur Frage der Entschädigung beim Asthma-bronchiale, insbesondere beim Gewerbeasthma. Deutsche medizinische Wochenschrift 86:298, 1961.
7. Gervais P: L'asthme professionel dans industrie des matieres plastiques. Poumon et le Coleur 22:2199, 1966.
8. Tara MS: Intolerance? Sensibilisation? Allergie pulmonaire an formol. Archives des Maladies Professionelles, de Medicine du Travail et Securite Sociale (Paris) 17:66, 1966.
9. Popa V, Teculescu D, Stanescue D, et al: Bronchial asthma and asthmatic bronchitis determined by simple chemicals. Dis Chest 65:395, 1969.
10. Sakula A: Formalin asthma in hospital laboratory staff. Lancet ii:816, 1975.
11. Kerfoot E, Mooney T: Formaldehyde and paraformaldehyde study in funeral homes. Am Ind Hyg Assoc J 36:533, 1975.
12. Porter JAH: Acute respiratory distress following formalin inhalation. Lancet ii:603, 1975.
13. Hendrick DJ, Lane DJ: Formalin asthma in hospital staff. Br Med J 1:607, 1975.
14. Gamble JF, McMichael AJ, Williams T, et al: Respiratory function and symptoms: An environmental-epidemiological study of rubber workers exposed to a phenol-formaldehyde type resin. Am Ind Hyg Assoc J 37:499, 1976.
15. Breysse PA: Formaldehyde in mobile and conventional homes. Environmental Health Safety News Seattle, WA, Univ. of Washington, 26 (Nos. 1–6), 1977.
16. Editorial: Formalin asthma. Lancet i:790, 1977.
17. Hendrick DJ, Lane DJ: Occupational formalin asthma. Br J Ind Med 34:11, 1977.
18. Morin NC, Kubinski H: Potential toxicity of materials used for home insulation. Ecotoxicology and Environmental Safety 2:133, 1978.
19. Horton AW, Tye R, Stemmer KL: Experimental carcinogenesis of the lung. Inhalation of gaseous formaldehyde or an aerosol of coal tar by C_3H mice. J Natl Cancer Inst 30:31, 1963.
20. Murphy SD, Davis MV, Zaratzian VL: Biochemical effects in rats from irritating air contaminants. Toxicol Appl Pharmacol 6:520, 1964.
21. Kane LE, Alaire Y: Sensory irritation to formaldehyde and acrolein during single and repeated exposures in mice. Am Ind Hyg Assoc J 38:509, 1977.
22. Ionescu J, Marinescu D, Tapu V, et al: Experimental chronic obstructive lung disease. I. Bronchopulmonary changes induced in rabbits by prolonged exposure to formaldehyde. Morphol Embryol (Bucuk) 24:233, 1978.
23. Bardana EJ: Formaldehyde: Hypersensitivity and irritant reactions at work and in the home. Immunol Allergy Pract 2:60, 1980.

24. Walker JF: Formaldehyde. New York, Rinehold Publishing, 1964.
25. Meyer B: Urea-formaldehyde resins. Reading, MA, Addison-Wesley, 1979, p 14.
26. Auerbach C, Moutschen-Dahmen M, Moutschen J: Genetic and cytogenetical effects of formaldehyde and related compounds. Mutat Res 39:317, 1977.
27. Doenecke D: Digestion of chromosomal proteins in formadehyde-treated chromatin. Hoppe-Seyler's Z Physiol Chem 359:1343, 1978.
28. Feldman MY: Reactions of nucleic acids and nucleoproteins with formaldehyde. Prog Nucleic Acid Res Mol Biol 13:1, 1973.
29. Palecek E: Premelting changes in DNA conformation. Prog Nucleic Acid Res Mol Biol 18:151, 1976.
30. Shikama K, Miura KI: Equilibrium studies on the formaldehyde reaction with native DNA. Eur J Biochem 63:39, 1976.
31. Landsteiner K, Jablons B: Ueber die Bildung von Antikoerpern gegan verändertes arteigenes Serumeiweiss. V. Mitteilung ueber Antigene Ztschr fuer Immunitätsforsch und Exper Therap 20:618, 1914.
32. Horsfall FL Jr: Formaldehyde and serum proteins: Their immunological characteristics. J Immunol 27:553, 1934.
33. Karlson P: Introduction to Modern Biochemistry, 2nd ed. New York, Academic Press, 1965, Ch. 6, 8, 11, and 12.
34. LaDu BN, Mandel HG, Way HL (eds): Fundamentals of Drug Metabolism and Drug Deposition. Baltimore, Williams & Wilkins, 1971, pp 169–171, 206–208, 292–294.
35. Einbrodt HJ: Formaldehyde and formic acid level in blood and urine of people following previous exposure to formaldehyde. Zentralbl Arbeitsmed Arbeitsshutz Prophyl 26:154, 1976.
36. Martin-Amat G, McMartin KE, Hayreh SS, et al: Methanol poisoning. Ocular toxicity produced by formate. Toxicol Appl Pharmacol 45:201, 1978.
37. Gottschling LM, Beaulieu HJ, Melvin WW: Monitoring of formic acid in urine of humans exposed to low levels of formaldehyde. Am Ind Hyg Assoc J 45:417, 1984.
38. National Research Council: Formaldehyde and other Aldehydes, Washington, D.C., National Academy of Sciences, 1981.
39. Rietbrock N: Kinetics and pathways of methanol metabolism. Naunym-Schmiedsbergs Arch Pharmakol Exp Pathol 263:88, 1969.
40. Warneck P, Klippel W, Moortgat GK: Formaldehyd in tropospharischer Reinluft. Der Bundesgesellschaft Phys Chem 82:1136, 1978.
41. Breeding RJ, Lodge JP Jr, Pate JB, et al: Background trace gas concentration in the central United States. J Geophys Res 78:7057, 1973.
42. National Research Council: Formaldehyde: An Assessment of its Health Effects. Washington, D.C., National Academy Press, 1980.
43. Kitchens JF, Casner RE, Edwards GS, et al: Investigation of selected potential environmental contaminants: Formaldehyde. Final Technical Report. Alexandria, VA, Atlantic Research Corp., Rept. No. ARC 49-5681, EPA/560/2-76/009.
44. Stupfel M: Recent advances in investigations of toxicity of automotive exhaust. Environ Health Perspect 17:253, 1976.
45. Office of Technology Assessment: Wood Use: U.S. Competitiveness and Technology, Vol 11. Washington, D.C., U.S. Government Printing Office, 1984, OTA-M-224.
46. Cooper JA: Environmental impact of residential wood combustion emissions and its implications. J Air Pollution Control Assoc 30:855, 1980.
47. Samet JM, Marbury MC, Spengler JD: Health effects and sources of indoor air pollution, Parts 1 and 2. Am Rev Respir Dis 136:1486, 1988 and 137:221, 1988.
48. Lipari F, Dasch JM, Scruggs WF: Aldehyde emissions from wood-burning fireplaces. Environ Sci Technol 18:326, 1984.
49. Groedel TE: Chemical Compounds in the Atmosphere. New York, Academic Press, 1979.
50. U.S. Dept. of Health and Human Services, Public Health Service, Office on Smoking and Health: The Health Consequences of Smoking: Chronic Obstructive Lung Disease. A Report of the Surgeon General. Washington, D.C., U.S. Government Printing Office, 1984, DHHS (PHS) 84-50205.
51. U.S. Dept. of Health and Human Services, Public Health Service, Office on Smoking and Health: The Health Consequences of Involuntary Smoking: A Report of the Surgeon General. Washington, D.C., U.S. Government Printing Office, 1986.
52. National Research Council, Committee on Passive Smoking: Environmental Tobacco Smoke: Measuring Exposures and Assessing Health Effects. Washington, D.C., National Academy Press, 1986.
53. Sterling TD, Kobayashi D: Indoor byproduct levels of tobacco smoke: A critical review of the literature. J Air Pollution Control Assoc 32:250, 1982.
54. Kensler CJ, Battista SP: Components of cigarette smoke with ciliary-depressant activity; their selective removal by filters containing activated charcoal granules. N Engl J Med 269:1161, 1963.
55. Rickert NS, Robinson JC, Young JC: Estimating the hazards of "less hazardous" cigarettes. I. Tar, nicotine, carbon monoxide, acrolein, hydrogen cyanide and total aldehyde deliveries of Canadian cigarettes. J Toxicol Environ Health 6:351, 1980.
56. Gammage RB, Gupta KC: Formaldehyde. In Walsh PJ, Dudney CS, Copenhaven ED (eds): Indoor Air Quality. Boca Raton, FL, CRC Press, 1984, Ch. 7.
57. Weber-Tschopp A, Fischer T, Grandjean E: Air pollution and irritation due to cigarette smoke. Soz Proerentimed 21:101, 1976.
58. Feinman SE: Formaldehyde Sensitivity and Toxicity. Boca Raton, FL, CRC Press, 1988, p 29.
59. Occupational Health & Safety Letter 15:2, 1985.
60. Environmental Protection Agency: Formaldehyde: Determination of significant risks; advance notice of proposed rulemaking and notice. Fed. Register 49:21870, 1984.
61. Konopinski VJ: Formaldehyde in office and commercial environments. Am Ind Hyg Assoc J 44:205, 1983.
62. Olsen JH, Dassing M: Formaldehyde-induced symptoms in day care centers. Am Ind Hyg Assoc J 43:336, 1982.
63. Bardana EJ, Montanaro A: Formaldehyde: An analysis of its respiratory, cutaneous, and immunologic effects. Ann Allergy 66:441–452, 1991.
64. Engle JL: Retention of inhaled formaldehyde, propionaldehyde and acrolein in the dog. Arch Environ Health 25:119, 1972.
65. Epstein E, Maibach HI: Formaldehyde allergy. Arch Dermatol 94:186, 1966.
66. Patterson R, Harris KE, Grammer LC: Canine antibodies against formaldehyde-dog serum albumin conjugates: Induction, measurement and specificity. J Lab Clin Med 106:93, 1985.

67. Patterson R, Pateras V, Grammer LC, et al: Human antibodies against formaldehyde-human serum albumin conjugates or human serum albumin in individuals exposed to formaldehyde. Int Arch Allergy Appl Immunol 79:53, 1986.
68. Patterson R, Dykewicz MS, Evans R, et al: IgG antibody against formaldehyde human serum proteins: A comparison with other IgG antibodies against inhalant proteins and reactive chemicals. J Allergy Clin Immunol 84:359, 1989.
69. Goh KO, Cestero RVM: Health hazards of formaldehyde. JAMA 247:2778, 1982.
70. Maurice F, Rivory J-P, Larsson PH, et al: Anaphylactic shock caused by formaldehyde in a patient undergoing long-term hemodialysis. J Allergy Clin Immunol 77:594, 1986.
71. Cripe LI, Dodrill CB: Neuropsychological test performances with chronic low-level formaldehyde exposure. Clin Neuropsychol 2:41, 1988.
72. Kilburn KH, Warshaw R, Boylen CJ, et al: Pulmonary and neurobehavioral effects of formaldehyde exposure. Arch Environ Health 40:254, 1985.
73. Occupational Safety and Health Administration: Preliminary assessment on the health effects of formaldehyde. Occup Saf Health Rep 14:476, 1984.
74. EPA says formaldehyde likely a carcinogen. Chem Engineer News 65:18, 1987.
75. Shim C, Williams MH: Effect of odors in asthma. Am J Med 80:18, 1986.
76. Scott AE: Clinical characteristics of taste and smell disorders. Ear, Nose, Throat J 68:297, 1989.
77. Anderson I, Molhave L: Controlled human studies with formaldehyde. In Gibson JE (ed): Formaldehyde Toxicity. Washington, D.C., Hemisphere, 1983, pp 154-165.
78. Nielsen GD, Alarie Y: Sensory irritation, pulmonary irritation, and respiratory stimulation by airborne benzene and alkylbenzenes. Prediction of safe industrial exposure levels and correlation with their thermodynamic properties. Toxicol Appl Pharmacol 65:459, 1982.
79. Kulle TJ, Sauder LR, Hebel JR, et al: Formaldehyde dose-response in healthy nonsmokers. JAPCA 37:919, 1987.
80. OSHA Safety and Health Standards—General Industry (29CFR 1910). Washington, D.C., Superintendent of Documents, Office of the Federal Register, National Arch. and Record Admin., 1983.
81. Threshold Limit Values and Biological Exposure Indices for 1985-1986. Cincinnati, Am Conf Govern Ind Hyg, 1985.
82. Pierson WE, Koenig JQ, Bardana EJ: Potential adverse health effects of wood smoke. West J Med 151:339, 1989.
83. Morgan KT, Patterson DL, Gross GA: Frog palate mucociliary apparatus; structure and response to formaldehyde gas. Fundam Appl Toxicol 4:58, 1984.
84. Heck Hd'A, Casanova-Schmitz M: The relevance of disposition studies to the toxicology of formaldehyde. CIIT Act 4:2-5, 1984.
85. Chang JCF, Gross EA, Swenberg JA, et al: Nasal cavity deposition, histopathology, and cell proliferation after single and repeated formaldehyde exposures in B6C3F$_1$ mice and F344 rats. Toxicol Appl Pharmacol 68:161, 1983.
86. Swenberg JA, Barrow CS, Boneiko CJ, et al: Nonlinear biological responses to formaldehyde and their implications for carcinogenic risk assessment. Carcinogenesis 4:945, 1983.
87. Dolbey WE: Formaldehyde and tumors in hamster respiratory tract. Toxicology 24:7, 1982.
88. Maribach H: Formaldehyde: Effects on animal and human skin. In Gibson JE (ed): Formaldehyde Toxicity. Washington, D.C., Hemisphere Publishing, 1983, pp 163-174.
89. Hatch KL: Textile dermatitis from formaldehyde. In Feinman SE (ed): Formaldehyde Sensitivity and Toxicity. Boca Raton, FL, CRC Press, 1988, pp 92-101.
90. Schwartz L: Dermatitis from synthetic resins and waxes. Am J Public Health 26:586, 1936.
91. Pirila V, Kilpio O: On dermatitis caused by formaldehyde and its compounds. Am Med Intern Fenn 38:38, 1949.
92. Horsfall FL: Formaldehyde hypersensitiveness: An experimental study. J Immunol 27:569, 1934.
93. Pisati G, Brini D, Carla AM: Formaldehyde allergy in a synthetic resins factory (Ital). Med Lav 71:88, 1980.
94. Guyot JD: Report on formalin urticaria. South Med J 14:115, 1921.
95. Rappaport B, Hoffman MH: Urticaria due to aliphatic aldehydes. A clinical and experimental study. J Am Med Assoc 164:2656, 1941.
96. McDaniel W, Marks J: Contact urticaria due to sensitivity of spray starch. Arch Dermatol 115:628, 1979.
97. Key MM: Some unusual allergic reactions in industry. Arch Dermatol 83:3, 1961.
98. Glass WI: Outbreak of formaldehyde dermatitis. NZ Med J 60:423, 1961.
99. Fabry H: Formaldehyde sensitivity: Two interesting cases. Contact Dermatitis Newsletter 3:51, 1968.
100. Hilander I: Contact urticaria from leather containing formaldehyde. Dermatologica 113:1443, 1977.
101. Lindskov R: Contact urticaria to formaldehyde. Contact Derm 8:333, 1982.
102. Anderson KE, Malbach MI: Multiple application delayed onset contact urticaria: Possible relation to certain unusual formalin and textile relations. Contact Derm 10:227, 1984.
103. Shelley WB: Immediate sunburn-like urticarial dermatitis in a patient with formaldehyde photosensitivity. Arch Dermatol 118:117, 1982.
104. Bardana EJ, Montanaro A: "Chemically sensitive" patients: Avoiding the pitfalls. J Respir Dis 10:32, 1989.
105. Kratochvil I: Effects of formaldehyde on the health of workers in the crease-resistant clothing industry. Pracovni Lekarstri 23:374, 1971.
106. Schoenberg J, Mitchell CA: Airway disease caused by phenolic (phenol-formaldehyde) resin exposure. Arch Environ Health 30:574, 1975.
107. Spassovski M: Health hazards in the production and processing of some fibers, resins and plastics in Bulgaria. Environ Health Perspec 17:199, 1976.
108. Baur X, Fruhmann G: Bronchial asthma of allergic or irritative origin as an occupational disease. Prox Klin Pneumol 33(Suppl 1):317, 1979.
109. Burge PS, Pepys J: Berufsbezogner brochialer provokation stest. Allergologie 2:7, 1979.
110. Granati A, Calsini'e P, Lenzi R: Criteri di valutuzione di pericolosita di agenti chimici richerche nell'industria dell'abbigliamento. Med Lavoro 1:22, 1981.
111. Skelfving S, Akesson B, Simonsson BG: Meat wrappers' asthma caused by thermal degradation products of polyethylene. Lancet i:211, 1980.
112. Trinkler H: Working with formaldehyde. Medizinche Laboratorium (Stuttgart) 21:283, 1968.
113. Hendrick DJ, Rando RJ, Lane DJ, et al: Formaldehyde asthma challenge exposure levels and late reactions after 5 years. J Occup Med 24:893, 1982.

114. Hendrick DJ: The formaldehyde problem: A clinical appraisal. Immunol Allergy Pract 5:97, 1983.
115. Wallerstein G, Rebohle E: Sensitization to formaldehyde in occupational exposure by inhalation (German). Allerg Immunol 22:287, 1976.
116. Frigas E, Filley WV, Reed CE: Asthma induced by dust from urea-formaldehyde foam insulating material. Chest 79:706, 1981.
117. Newhouse MT: UFFI dust. Non-specific irritant only? Chest 82:511, 1982.
118. Frigas E, Filley WV, Reed CE: UFFI dust. Non-specific irritant only? Chest 82:511, 1982.
119. Day JH, Lees REM, Clark RH, et al: Respiratory response to formaldehyde and off-gas of urea formaldehyde foam insulation. Can Med Assoc J 131:1061, 1984.
120. Pross HF, Day JH, Clark RIT, et al: Immunologic studies of subjects with asthma exposed to formaldehyde and UFFI off-products. J Allergy Clin Immunol 79:797, 1987.
121. Cockcroft DW, Hoeppner VA, Dolovich J: Occupational asthma caused by cedar urea formaldehyde particle board. Chest 1:49, 1982.
122. Kwong F, Kraske G, Nelson AM, et al: Acute symptoms secondary to formaldehyde exposure in a pathology resident. Ann Allergy 50:326, 1983.
123. Main DM, Hogan TJ: Health effects of low level exposure to formaldehyde. J Occup Med 25:896, 1983.
124. Bardana EJ: Effect of cigarette smoke on formaldehyde data. J Occup Med 26:410, 1984.
125. Frigas E, Filley WV, Reed CE: Bronchial challenge with formaldehyde gas: Lack of bronchoconstriction in 13 patients suspected of having formaldehyde-induced asthma. Mayo Clin Proc 59:295, 1984.
126. Hyatt RE: Formaldehyde exposure: A case in point. Mayo Clin Proc 59:350, 1984.
127. Schachter EN, Witek TJ, Tosun T, et al: Respiratory effects of exposure to 2.0 ppm of formaldehyde in asthmatic subjects. Am Rev Respir Dis 131:A170, 1985.
128. Witek TJ, Schachter EN, Brody D, et al: A study of lung function and irritation from exposure to formaldehyde in routinely exposed laboratory workers. Chest 88:65, 1985.
129. Sheppard WL, Eschenbacher WL, Epstein J: Lack of bronchomotor response in up to 3 ppm formaldehyde in subjects with asthma. Environ Res 35:133, 1984.
130. Nordman H, Keskinen H, Tuppurainen M: Formaldehyde asthma: Rare or overlooked? J Allergy Clin Immunol 75:91, 1985.
131. Bardana EJ, Montanaro A: Formaldehyde asthma. J Allergy Clin Immunol 77:384, 1986.
132. Nordman H, Keskinen H, Tuppurainen M: Formaldehyde asthma. J Allergy Clin Immunol 77:384, 1986.
133. Burge PS, Harries MG, Lam WK, et al: Occupational asthma due to formaldehyde. Thorax 40:255, 1985.
134. Kilburn KH, Warshaw R, Boylen CT, et al: Toxic effects of formaldehyde and solvents in histology technicians. J Histochem 6:73, 1983.
135. Kilburn KH, Seidman BC, Warshaw R: Neurobehavioral and respiratory symptoms of formaldehyde and xylene exposure in histology technicians. Arch Environ Health 36:220, 1985.
136. Normal GR, Pengelly LD, Kerigan AT, et al: Respiratory function of children in homes insulated with urea formaldehyde foam insulation. Can Med Assoc J 134:1135, 1986.
137. Thrasher JD, Wojdani A, Cheung G, et al: Evidence for formaldehyde antibodies and altered cellular immunity in subjects exposed to formaldehyde in mobile homes. Arch Environ Health 42:347, 1987.
138. Broughton A, Thrasher JD: Antibodies and altered cell mediated immunity in formaldehyde exposed humans. Comments Toxicol 2:155, 1988.
139. Sauder LR, Green DJ, Chatham MD, et al: Acute pulmonary response of asthmatics to 3.0 ppm formaldehyde. Toxicol Ind Health 3:569, 1987.
140. Horvath EP, Anderson H Jr, Pierce WE, et al: Effect of formaldehyde on the mucous membranes and the lungs. JAMA 259:701, 1988.
141. Holmstrom M, Wilhelmsson B: Respiratory symptoms and pathophysiological effects of occupational exposure to formaldehyde and wood dust. Scand J Environ Health 14:306, 1988.
142. Alexandersson R, Hedenstierna G: Pulmonary function in wood workers exposed to formaldehyde: A prospective study. Arch Environ Health 44:5, 1989.
143. Higgenbottam T, Feyerdband C, Clark TJH: Cigarette smoke inhalation and acute airway response. Thorax 35:246, 1980.
144. Patterson R, Zeiss CR, Pruzansky JJ: Immunology and immunopathology of trimellitic anhydride pulmonary reactions. J Allergy Clin Immunol 70:19, 1982.
145. Bardana EJ, Andrasch RM: Occupational asthma due to low molecular weight antigens. Eur J Respir Dis 64:241, 1983.
146. Thrasher JD, Boughton A, Micevich P: Antibodies and immune profiles of individuals occupationally exposed to formaldehyde: Six case reports. Am J Ind Med 14:479, 1988.
147. Greenberg GN: Formaldehyde case reports. Am J Ind Med 16:479, 1988.
148. Beavers JD: Formaldehyde exposure reports. Am J Ind Med 16:331, 1989.
149. Kramps JA, Peltenburg LTC, Kerklaan PRM, et al: Measurement of specific IgE antibodies in individuals exposed to formaldehyde. Clin Exp Allergy 19:509, 1989.
150. Grammer LC, Harris KE, Shaughnessy MA, et al: Clinical and immunologic evaluation of 37 workers exposed to gaseous formaldehyde. J Allergy Clin Immunol 86:177, 1990.
151. Dykewicz MS, Patterson R, Cugell DW, et al: Serum IgE and IgG to formaldehyde-human serum albumin: Lack of relation to gaseous formaldehyde exposure and symptoms. J Allergy Clin Immunol 87:48, 1991.
152. Boettcher B, Nanra RS, Roberts TK, et al: Specificity and origin of anti-N antibodies developed by patients undergoing chronic hemodialysis. Vox Sang 31:408, 1976.
153. Howell ED, Perkins HA: Anti-N-like antibodies in sera of patients undergoing chronic dialysis. Vox Sang 23:291, 1972.
154. MeLeish NA, Brathwaite AF, Peterson PM: Anti-N-antibodies in hemodialysis patients. Transfusion 15:43, 1975.
155. Crosson JT, Moulds J, Comty CM, et al: Clinical study of anti-N in the sera of patients in a large repetitive hemodialysis program. Kidney Int 10:463, 1976.
156. Fussbunder W, Seidl S, Koch KM: The role of formaldehyde in the formation of hemodialysis-associated anti-N-like antibodies. Vox Sang 35:41, 1978.
157. Sandler SG, Sharon R, Buch M, et al: Formaldehyde-related antibodies in hemodialysis patients. Transfusion 19:682, 1979.

158. Lyen R, Rothe M, Gallaseh E: Characterization of formaldehyde-related antibodies encountered in hemodialysis patients at different stages of immunization. Vox Sang 44:81, 1983.
159. Hoy WE, Cestero RVM: Eosinophilia in maintenance hemodialysis patients. J Dialysis 3:73, 1979.
160. Dally KA, Hanrahan LP, Woodbury MA, et al: Formaldehyde exposure in non-occupational environments. Arch Environ Health 36:277, 1981.
161. Sardinas AV, Most RS, Guiletti MA, et al: Health effects associated with urea-formaldehyde foam insulation in Connecticut. J Environ Health 41:270, 1979.
162. Garry VF, Oatman L, Preus R, et al: Formaldehyde in the home: Some environmental disease perspectives. Minn Med 91:107, 1980.
163. Kilburn KH, Warshaw R, Thornton JC: Formaldehyde impairs memory, equilibrium, and dexterity in histology technicians: Effects which persist for days after exposure. Arch Environ Health 42:117, 1987.
164. Thun MJ, Lakat MF, Altman R: New Jersey urea-formaldehyde foam insulation study. Trenton, NJ, New Jersey Health Department, 1983.
165. Bracken JJ, Leasa DJ, Morgan WKC: Exposure to formaldehyde: Relationship to respiratory symptoms and function. Can J Public Health 76:312, 1985.
166. Council on Scientific Affairs: Formaldehyde. JAMA 261:1183, 1989.
167. Dallas CE, Theiss JC, Fairchild EJ: Effects of subchronic inhalation of formaldehyde. Ind Hyg News Rept 27:2, 1984.
168. Kerns WD, Parkov KL, Donofrio DJ, et al: Carcinogenicity of formaldehyde in rats and mice after long-term inhalation exposure. Cancer Res 43:4382, 1983.
169. Bloom M: Populations predisposed to allergic contact sensitivity. In Feinman SE (ed): Formaldehyde Sensitivity and Toxicity. Boca Raton, FL, CRC Press, 1988, pp 116–122.
170. Adams R: Patch testing—1982. Sem Dermatol 1:1, 1982.
171. Noceto JB, Laffont H: A case of asthma from sensitization to formalin (Fr). Arch Mol Prof 23:314, 1962.
172. Imbus HR: Clinical evaluation of patients with complaints related to formaldehyde exposure. J Allergy Clin Immunol 76:831, 1986.
173. McKay RT: Bronchoprovocation challenge testing in occupational airways disorders. Sem Respir Med 7:287, 1986.
174. Selner JC, Staudenmayer H: The practical approach to the evaluation of suspected environmental exposures: Chemical intolerance. Ann Allergy 55:665, 1985.

Chapter 15

OCCUPATIONAL ASTHMA DUE TO PROTEOLYTIC ENZYMES

Anthony Montanaro, MD

Occupational asthma due to inhalation of proteolytic enzymes is a rare but well-documented event in many occupational settings. The major proteolytic enzymes that have been implicated include alcalase, papain, chymopapain, bromelains, and trypsin. The sources, biochemical characteristics, and major industrial applications of these enzymes are reviewed in Table 1. A large number of potentially exposed workers exists in a variety of industries. In addition to the detergent industry, in which many workers have been exposed in the past, others continue to be exposed in the medical research, pharmaceutical, food and beverage, cosmetic, and textile industries. The applications of these enzymes in these industries and the workers potentially at risk are reviewed in Tables 2 and 3. This chapter will review the medical literature that has documented the extent of this problem and will then focus on practical diagnostic and treatment issues.

ALCALASE *(Bacillus subtilis)*

Historical Background

In 1920 the German government granted Dr. Otto Rohm a patent for the addition of trypsin to washing soaps to facilitate the eradication of protein stains in clothing. Trypsin, however, was not especially effective in the alkaline setting of the soap. It never achieved any popularity. In 1959, Dr. Jaag of Switzerland discovered in a strain of *Bacillus subtilis* a proteolytic enzyme that was stable under conditions of heat and alkalinity. The enzyme,

alcalase, was well accepted throughout Europe. By the mid-1960s it was widely distributed in all detergent powders in Europe. By 1967, it had gained wide acceptance in the United States as well.

In the 1960s and 1970s proteolytic enzymes were widely used in the detergent industry. These enzyme-containing products were found to be effective as prewashing or soaking agents for heavily soiled clothing. Alcalase was found to be particularly effective. The enzyme preparation was manufactured by the submerged fermentation of *B. subtilis*. The early enzymes preparations contained 10 to 15% organic matter consisting primarily of protein and carbohydride. Alcalase is an alkali-stable endopeptidase with a broad spectrum of proteolytic activity. Since alcalase preparations are such a fine dusty powder, they were further diluted with sodium sulfate and 2% mineral oil. Commercial products were further diluted with standard detergents to yield a final alcalase concentration of 0.5 to 1%.

The initial reports from manufacturers and consumers focused on irritative-type dermatitis at sites of heavy contact, e.g., hands and face.[3,4] The skin lesions were felt to be the result of a digestive process. Later work revealed that mixtures of the enzyme and detergent were probably much more allergenic than the enzyme alone.[3]

Since the original descriptions of occupational asthma in laundry workers by Flindt and by Pepys et al. in 1969,[1,2] further understanding and awareness of the hazards of alcalase inhalation have led to marked decrease in the incidence of this disorder. The original cases were described in British laundry detergent

TABLE 1. *Occupational Asthma Due to Proteolytic Enzymes*

Enzyme	Source	Biochemical Characteristics	Major Industrial Applications
Alcalase	Bacterial (*Bacillus subtilis*)	Endopeptidase, heat and alkalai stable	Soap/detergent
Papain, chymopapain	Fruit, latex of *Carica papaya*	Sulfhydryl proteases	Pharmaceutical, food/beverage, tanning
Bromelains	Fruit (bromeliacael pineapple stems)	Glycoprotein protease with active site amino acid sequence similar to papain	Food processing, biomedical
Trypsin, chymotrypsin	Pancreas, bovine/porcine	Protease	Plastics/rubber manufacturing, biomedical research

workers who were exposed to dried enzyme products of *B. subtilis*. Subsequently, the scope of the problem increased when the great majority of household detergents contained 0.5 to 3% concentrations of this bacterial enzyme product. While topical application of alcalase resulted in digestive and irritative changes of the skin, respiratory allergy was found to occur on the basis of IgE sensitization.

Shortly after the initial descriptions of enzyme sensitivity in detergent workers, further awareness led to more comprehensive investigation of this industry. Mitchell and Gandevia[5] began a formal investigation with a survey of 98 workers periodically exposed to high concentrations of proteolytic enzymes. Unfortunately, the determinations of industrial exposure levels were arbitrary, because chemical and dust concentrations were never measured. A striking incidence of respiratory complaints was documented. Sixty percent of workers complained of sneezing, nasal obstruction, and rhinorrhea. These symptoms characteristically appeared within 2 hours of the initial work exposure and resolved within 2 hours of discontinuation of the exposure. Lower respiratory complaints of cough, chest tightness, or shortness of breath occurred in 50% of workers.

Many heavy smokers reported that they were unable to smoke. In 13 of the 49 affected workers the symptoms occurred within 30 minutes of exposure. The remaining 36 affected workers had the onset of their complaints delayed 4 to 5 hours following exposure or during sleep following an asymptomatic period. A history of atopy or cigarette smoking was not associated with an increased incidence of respiratory complaints. Immediate or delayed skin reactivity to epicutaneous or intracutaneous skin testing to proteolytic enzyme extracts was not more frequent in symptomatic workers. Pulmonary function studies revealed no evidence of permanent impairment in symptomatic or asymptomatic workers. Although this study did not establish an allergic mechanism for the complaints, the authors' observations were important in highlighting the need for careful workplace surveillance and investigation of detergent workers.[5]

Slavin and co-workers[6] subsequently studied 238 workers in a detergent factory who had potential inhalational exposure to *B. subtilus* alcalase. Sixty-six of the 238 workers studied developed presumed allergic respiratory complaints. Five workers developed rhinitis, 35 developed occupational asthma, and 26 developed both conditions. As in other studies, these workers tended to develop symptoms within minutes to hours following their

TABLE 2. *Protease-exposed Workers*

Occupation	Application
Medical research	Proteolytic capacity, immunoglobulin analysis
Food/food additive industry	Meat tenderizer
Beverage industry	Clearing of beer
Textile industry	Treatment of wool and silk
Tanning	Hide preparation
Cosmetic industry	Additive
Pharmaceutical industry	Common proprietory drug additive, primary digestive aid, toothpaste
Detergent industry	Proteolytic "cleaning"

TABLE 3. *Enzyme-induced Occupational Asthma*

Enzymes	Potential At-risk Workers
Pancreatic extracts	Pharmaceutical workers
Bacillus subtilis (alcalase)	Detergent manufacturing
Papain	Food processors
Trypsin	Plastics and rubber workers
Flaviastase	Pharmaceutical workers
Bromelain	Food processors
Pectinase	Food processors

initial exposures. Prominent respiratory complaints tended to occur in patients with high level, brief exposures to enzyme-containing dusts.

A typical biphasic reaction to alcalase inhalation has been described by Franz et al.[7] Upper respiratory symptoms appear initially, followed by some improvement, and then the development of occupational asthma. These authors also described instances of hypersensitivity pneumonitis in detergent factory workers that were later confirmed by others.[8] Immunologic testing in these workers documented definite IgE responses to alcalase. Fifty-six of 66 affected workers had immediate prick test reactions to 0.05 to 0.5 mg of protein/ml of solution. Importantly, 58 of the 172 unaffected workers also displayed cutaneous reactivity of up to 5 mg/ml of solution. This skin sensitivity was successfully passively transferred in three negative control workers. Additionally, systemic sensitivity could be passively transferred to a monkey who had undergone inhalational provocation studies. Atopic workers in this study and others have appeared to be particularly at risk, with 60 of the 66 affected workers having been identified as atopic. Early epidemiologic studies indicated that approximately 21% of exposed workers were affected 6 months after production had started. There was a clear relationship between sensitization and exposure to alcalase.[9]

Because of the wide distribution of alcalase-containing laundry products in the U.S. in the 1970s, Bernstein et al. studied homemakers for possible allergy to alcalase.[10] These individuals had prolonged, long-term low-level exposure of laundry products in the household. Ambient concentrations were not determined. Three-hundred-fifty-three patients attending allergy clinics in Ohio were studied. Twenty-five percent of these patients exhibited positive skin tests either to alcalase or to amylase protein contained in these detergents. The incidence of positive tests correlated with degree of preexisting allergic history. Positive passive transfer studies were observed in 5 of 10 patients studied. Nasal and bronchial provocations were undertaken in 14 patients who had complained of upper or lower respiratory symptoms. Positive nasal provocations were observed in seven patients with upper respiratory complaints, while positive bronchial provocations were observed in seven patients with lower respiratory symptoms. Bronchial and nasal provocations were undertaken during asymptomatic periods. The provocation studies used stock solutions of 1:100,000 to 1:1000 (alcalase 10 mg/ml, amylase 3.75 mg/ml). These concentrations had been determined to have no nasal or bronchial irritant effects in healthy, asthmatic, or rhinitic controls. Unfortunately, we have no information of how these concentrations compare to ambient levels found in the home environment.

Under the leadership of Dr. Hans Weill of Tulane University and Dr. John Gilson, the Director of the British Medical Research Council Pneumoconiosis Unit, a symposium was convened in 1976 on the biologic effects of proteolytic enzyme detergents.[11] The symposium was co-sponsored by the Soap and Detergent Industries Association, which had become concerned with the industrial hygiene aspects of this manufacturing process. Under the auspices of The Procter & Gamble Company and the Colgate-Palmolive Company, several industrial hygiene investigations led to recommended operating procedures for the production of enzyme-containing detergents.[12,13] These new operating procedures focused on the use of "closed systems," which minimized inhalational exposures to the particulate enzyme-containing dust. It was felt that these industrial hygiene measures were responsible for achieving enzyme dust levels in the industry below which sensitization would not occur.

Although industry acted responsibly in reducing the use and exposure to this enzyme, this information provides an important historical lesson in occupational allergy. Enzymes of the ubiquitous *B. subtilis* can be potent sensitizers in industrial workers and consumers. Atopic individuals appeared to have a predisposition to develop sensitivity. Clearly, most of the sensitized individuals, as determined by skin testing or RAST, were asymptomatic, but allergic respiratory symptoms of rhinitis and reactive airways disease were common. Rarely, hypersensitivity pneumonitis was also noted in exposed workers. Removal of affected individuals has resulted in total disappearance of symptoms and return to normal pulmonary function. As of the early 1980s, only three or four commercial all-fabric household laundry bleaches sold in the U.S. contained proteolytic enzymes.[14]

PAPAIN AND CHYMOPAPAIN

Papain and chymopapain are proteolytic enzymes derived from the latex of the papaya fruit *(Carica papaya)*. Papain is a sulfhydryl protease that is composed of a single polypeptide chain of molecular weight 23,000.[15] Three-dimensional x-ray studies have shown this enzyme to be folded into two distinct parts that are separated by a cleft containing the active enzymatic site. Because of its wide range of substrate sensitivity, this enzyme has been used extensively in the pharmaceutical, biomedical research, tanning, and food and beverage industry (Table 1). In the food and beverage industry, papain is employed to tenderize meat and clarify beer (Fig. 1). Papain continues to be a standard tool in the structural analysis of immunoglobulins because of

its ability to cleave disulfide bonds. Human consumption of papain is common, whether as a natural ingredient of foods or as an additive to medications. While most of the crude extract is prepared in Africa, India, and Sri Lanka, the U.S. is the major importer of the extract. (*Carica* is Latin for Caria, a division of southwestern Asia Minor, but the papaya is not native there.)

Although anecdotal reports of papain-induced allergy have been described in consumers, the majority of information available is from occupational studies in which workers had inhalational exposure during manufacturing or processing of this enzyme.[16-18] Novey

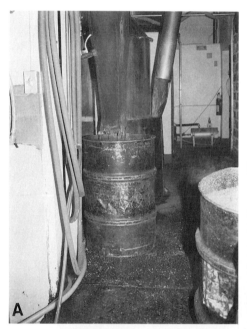 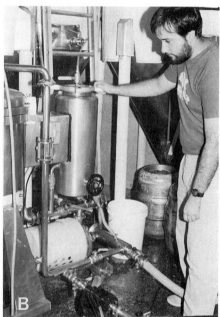

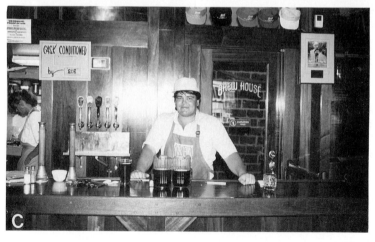

FIGURE 1, A to C.   The microbrewery industry has proliferated throughout the U.S. Proteolytic enzymes are used as clarifying agents in the brewing industry and may result in significant adverse health effects.

and co-workers made important observations in their study of 23 employees at a pharmaceutical plant manufacturing a papain-containing tablet designed for external use.[16] Twelve of these workers developed symptoms of cough, wheezing, dyspnea, or chest pain. Although 9 of these 12 workers had a personal or family history of atopy, none had experienced symptoms of asthma prior to their industrial exposures. In this study there was no correlation between the duration of exposure and the appearance of symptoms, pulmonary function abnormalities, or immunologic reactions. No specific ambient levels of this enzyme in the workplace were documented. Pulmonary function data were difficult to interpret because of concomitant cigarette smoking, but a trend of lower respiratory flow rates was observed in patients with significant IgE responses to papain. Bronchial provocation studies were not undertaken in these workers.

Subsequent bronchial provocation studies in papain manufacturing workers were undertaken by Baur and Fruhmann.[15] These investigators studied 11 workers who had been exposed to airborne papain over a period of time ranging from 2 months to 10 years. Seven out of 11 workers studied developed respiratory hypersensitivity responses. Epicutaneous skin testing and RAST to papain were positive in all seven symptomatic patients and in none of the exposed asymptomatic workers. Five of the six workers who had described asthmatic symptoms underwent bronchial provocation studies. Specific airways conductance (SG_{aw}) was measured following inhalation of 0.15 to 0.5 mg of papain solution. An immediate fall of at least 50% in SG_{aw} was seen in all five workers. One late asthmatic response was documented. Symptoms resolved or significantly diminished following removal from exposure or use of a more granular enzyme product that lessened the likelihood of respiratory tract deposition.

Immunologic studies indicated both IgE and IgG responses to papain in exposed workers. Eight of 11 workers with pulmonary complaints demonstrated IgE antibodies to papain, whereas nine of the 11 had papain precipitins. Of the 11 workers without respiratory complaints, two had specific IgE and three had precipitating IgG antibody. In 52 nonexposed controls, only one patient demonstrated IgE or precipitating antibody to papain. Interestingly, atopic workers appeared to develop IgE antibodies earlier and following less intense exposures than did

nonatopic exposed workers. Further study of papain sensitivity in atopic patients revealed apparent low incidence of sensitivity. Haverly and co-workers reported their findings on papain skin testing in an allergic population.[19] Epicutaneous testing with 1 mg/ml of papain was positive in 12 of 412 patients. Systemic hyperresponsiveness was confirmed by double-blind oral challenges in five of these patients for an incidence of 1.2%.

In the early 1980s chymopapain became the agent of choice for the nonoperative chemonucleolysis of intervertebral disc disease. Chymopapain, like papain, is a sulfhydryl protease derived from *Carico papaya*. It differs from papain in its electrophoretic mobility, stability, and solubility. It had been noted by early investigators that 1% of all patients undergoing chemonucleolysis experienced severe allergic reactions.[20-22] Subsequently, Travenol Laboratories studied the allergenic cross-reactivity of papain and chymopapain.[23] Their investigators studied six patients 2 weeks following chymopapain disc infusions who were determined to have 4+ skin reactions to papain. Cross-antigenicity was demonstrated by RAST and RAST-inhibition studies in all patients. This shared antigenicity was thought to be caused by both cross-contamination in product preparation as well as by shared antigenic determinants. This study also emphasized the observation that many individuals have been sensitized to chymopapain or papain by previous ingestion, topical application, or inhalation. This may predispose them to anaphylactic responses on a subsequent administration. Tarlo et al. had previously reported finding seven of 330 workers without known papain exposure to be skin test positive or RAST positive to papain.[24] Previous studies have indicated that 1.2% of an allergic population have been sensitized to papain.[19] Because of these concerns, chymopapain chemonucleolysis has largely been abandoned by neurosurgeons and orthopedists. Nevertheless, the historical lessons are important when considering other related occupational and nonoccupational enzyme exposures.

Since papain can induce specific IgE and IgG responses, immunologic lung disease may develop by multiple mechanisms. In addition to potential immunologic mechanisms, papain has been used to successfully induce emphysematous airways changes in animals. Since it is ubiquitous in industry and society, the clinician must remain aware of the toxicity and immunogenicity of these enzymes.

BROMELAIN

Bromelains are a group of proteolytic enzymes of Bromeliaceae plants (the pineapple family). The highest concentrations of these enzymes are found in the stems of ripe pineapples *(Ananas sativus)*, but are also present in the fruit pulp. (It is perhaps significant that no other cultivated fruit has the stem passing through it.) The enzyme is widely used in medical research laboratories as well as in the pharmaceutical and food industries (Table 1). Bromelains are glycoproteins with active site amino acid sequences very similar to papain. Occupational asthma in response to inhalational exposure is rare but well documented.[25-27]

While sensitivity to orally administered proteolytic enzymes was described in the 1960s, it was not until 1978 that a case report of occupational asthma appeared in the literature.[25] In this report two previously healthy non-smoking pharmaceutical workers processing bromelain were described. Epicutaneous skin testing was positive in both workers. Inhalation of bromelain in 2% lactose powder resulted in markedly significant and immediate declines in FEV_1. Baur[26] subsequently detailed a case of occupational asthma to bromelain in a pharmaceutical worker with positive bronchial and oral challenges. In this case positive epicutaneous skin tests to bromelain were confirmed by RAST. Baur pointed out that five of six workers previously sensitized to papain had positive RAST and skin tests to bromelain. Furthermore, two of these previously papain-sensitized workers had positive bronchial provocation studies to bromelain despite no known airborne bromelain exposure. In 60 asthmatics with no known previous protease exposures, two were skin-test positive and eight were RAST positive to bromelain. This study suggested immunologic cross-reactivity among the protease group of enzymes.[27]

Baur subsequently reported on the apparent immunologic cross-reactivity between these plant proteases.[28] Seven patients clinically hypersensitive to papain were compared to non-papain-sensitive allergic asthmatics. RAST reactions were documented to bromelain and papain in six of the seven patients who had clinically hypersensitivity to papain, whereas no protease RAST reactions were seen in asthmatic controls. Interestingly, these patients also had multiple positive RAST reactions to clinically irrelevant antigens such as grass pollen, birch pollen, or wheat. RAST inhibition studies revealed significant cross-reactivity to papain and bromelain. Furthermore, papain, bromelain, wheat flour, rye flour, grass, and birch pollen all mutually inhibited IgE binding to each antigen. Although the degree of inhibition was variable, this suggests that these plant allergens may share antigenic determinants leading to immunologic cross-reactivity.

These previous observations led an Austrian group of investigators to study laboratory workers in a blood bank who had inhalational exposures while weighing bromelain powder.[19] Four exposed workers from this diagnostic laboratory developed typical symptoms of occupational asthma. None of these workers was shown to be previously atopic or asthmatic. Three of the patients demonstrated positive skin reactions to 0.0001 mg/ml of bromelain. Two of the three had systemic reactions to testing. Subsequent RAST studies to bromelain revealed class 2–4 reactions in all four subjects with no demonstrated reactivity to papain.

Although these observations are limited, the implications are important. Because of the common use of bromelain as a meat tenderizer and beverage-clearing agent, food and beverage industry workers as well as laboratory personnel should be considered at risk for the development of enzyme-induced occupational asthma.

TRYPSIN

Trypsin is a proteolytic enzyme commonly derived from bovine and porcine pancreas that has both industrial and biomedical applications. It is used in the rubber industry in which workers may have contactant or inhalational exposures. Its protein-cleaving and digestive properties have led to its use in research laboratories for many years. Now largely abandoned, inhaled trypsin had been used in the early 1950s as a mucolytic agent.[29]

Despite its therapeutic use in patients with underlying bronchial hyperresponsiveness, reports of asthmatic reactions did not appear in the literature. In addition, although workers employed in trypsin processing had complained of ocular and nasal irritation, only a few documented cases of allergy and occupational asthma were found.[30-32] In one case study, an atopic pharmaceutical worker with unprotected inhalational exposure to trypsin described typical acute and delayed asthmatic symptoms following exposure. Skin-testing and bronchial-provocation studies were positive. Skin testing in 50 atopic controls was negative. Bronchial provocation to 0.3 cc of 1 g percent trypsin was markedly positive initially, with persistent changes for 24 hours. Bronchial provocation with trypsin was undertaken in two unexposed asthmatics and was negative. Marked improvement in respiratory symptoms occurred following cessation of exposure, but persistent pulmonary function abnormalities in vital capacity and maximum midexpiratory flow rates were described.[31]

MISCELLANEOUS ENZYMES

Rare immediate-type hypersensitivity reactions have been reported following inhalational exposure to other enzymes. Respiratory symptoms were reported in a pharmaceutical worker extracting an enzyme material from *Aspergillus flavus*.[33] Asthma and rhinitis have also been reported in the parents of a cystic fibrotic child following inhalation of pancreatic extract.[34] An additional case was recently reported in a pediatric auxillary nurse who mixed pancreatic extract with infant formulas on a cystic fibrosis ward. These unusual observations highlight the potential allergenicity of these ubiquitous enzymes.

REFERENCES

1. Flindt MLH: Pulmonary disease due to inhalation of derivatives of *Bacillus subtilis* containing proteolytic enzymes. Lancet i:1177, 1969.
2. Pepys J, Hargreave FE, Longbottom JL, Faux J: Allergic reactions of the lungs to enzymes of *Bacillus subtilus*. Lancet i:1181–1184, 1969.
3. Little DC: Allergic disease in detergent workers. In Frazier CA (ed): Occupational Asthma. New York, Van Nostrand Reinhold, 1980, pp 186–192.
4. Ducksbury CFJ, Dave VK: Contact dermatitis in home helps following use of enzyme detergents. Br Med J i:535, 1970.
5. Mitchell CA, Gandevia B: Respiratory symptoms and skin reactivity in workers exposed to proteolytic enzymes in the detergent industry. Am Rev Respir Dis 104:1–12, 1971.
6. Slavin RG, Lewis CR: Sensitivity to enzyme additives in laundry detergent workers. J Allergy Clin Immunol 48:262–266, 1971.
7. Franz T, McMurrain KD, et al: Clinical and physiologic observations in factory workers exposed to *Bacillus subtilis* enzyme dust. J Allergy 47:170, 1971.
8. Johnson CL, Bernstein IL, Gallagher JS, et al: Familial hypersensitivity pneumonitis-induced by *Bacillus subtilis*. Am Rev Respir Dis 122:339, 1980.
9. Newhouse ML, Tagg B, Pocock SJ: An epidemiologic study of workers producing enzyme washing powders. Lancet i:689, 1970.
10. Bernstein IL: Enzyme allergy in populations exposed to long term, low level concentrations of household laundry products. J Allergy Clin Immunol 49:219–237, 1972.
11. Gilson JC, Juniper CP, Martin RB, Weill H: Biologic effects of proteolytic enzyme detergents. Thorax 31:621–634, 1976.
12. Soap and Detergent Association: Recommended operating procedures for U.K. factories handling enzyme materials. Ann Occup Hyg 14:71–78, 1971.
13. Soap and Detergent Association: Reports of the Soap and Detergent Industry Association. First report October, 1969; Fifth report April, 1976. Obtainable from the Secretary of the Association, 475 Park Avenue South, New York, NY 10016.
14. Weaver JE, Hermann KW: Evaluation of adverse reaction reports for a new laundry product. J Am Acad Dermatol 4:577, 1981.
15. Baur X, Fruhmann G: Papain-induced asthma: Diagnosis by skin test, RAST and bronchial provocation test. Clin Allergy 9:75–81, 1979.
16. Novey HS, Keenan WS, Forhster RD, et al: Pulmonary disease in workers exposed to papain: Clinicophysiological and immunological studies. Clin Allergy 10:721–731, 1980.
17. Milne J, Brand S: Occupational asthma after inhalation of dust of the proteolytic enzyme papain. Br J Ind Med 32:302–307, 1975.
18. Tarlo SM, Shaikh W, Bell B, et al: Papain-induced allergic reactions. Clin Allergy 8:207, 1978.
19. Haverly RW, Mansfield LE, Ting S: The incidence of hypersensitivity to papain in an allergic population. J Allergy Clin Immunol 73:179, 1984.
20. Rajagopatan R, Tindal S, McNabb I: Anaphylactic reactions to chymopapain during general anasthesia: A case report. Anasth Analg 53:191, 1974.
21. Watts C: Complications of chemonucleolysis for lumbar disc disease. Neurosurgery 1:2, 1977.
22. Bernstein IL: Adverse effects of chemonucleolysis. JAMA 250:1167, 1983.
23. Sagana MA, Bruszer GV, Lin L, et al: Evaluation of papain/chymopapain cross allergenicity. J Allergy Clin Immunol 76:776–781, 1985.
24. Tarlo SM, Shaikh W, Bell B, et al: Papain-induced allergic reactions. Clin Allergy 8:207–215, 1978.
25. Galleguillos F, Rodriguez JC: Asthma caused by bromelin inhalation. Clin Allergy 8:21–24, 1978.
26. Baur X, Fruhmann G: Allergic reactions, including asthma to the pineapple protease bromelain following occupational exposure. Clin Allergy 9:443–450, 1979.
27. Gailhofer G, Wilders-Truschnig, Smolle J, Ludvan M: Asthma caused by bromelain: An occupational allergy. Clin Allergy 18:445–450, 1988.
28. Baur X: Studies on the specificity of human IgE antibodies to the plant proteases papain and bromelain. Clin Allergy 9:451–457, 1979.
29. Unger L, Unger AH: Trypsin inhalations in respiratory conditions with thick sputum. JAMA 152:1109, 1953.
30. Criep LH, Beam LR: Allergy to trypsin. J Allergy 35:425, 1964.
31. Zweiman B, Green G, Mayock RL, Hildreth EA: Inhalation sensitization to trypsin. J Allergy 39:11–16, 1967.
32. Colten HR, Polakoff PL, Weinstein SE, et al: Immediate hypersensitivity to hog trypsin resulting from industrial exposure. N Engl J Med 292:1050, 1975.
33. Panwells R, Devos M, Callens L, et al: Respiratory hazards from proteolytic enzymes. Lancet i:669, 1978.
34. Dolan TF, Meyers A: Bronchial asthma and allergic rhinitis associated with inhalation of pancreatic extracts. Am Rev Respir Dis 110:812, 1974.
35. Hayes JP, Newman Taylor AJ: Bronchial asthma in a pediatric nurse caused by inhaled pancreatic extracts. Br J Ind Med 48:355, 1991.

Chapter 16

ASTHMA DUE TO METALS AND METAL SALTS

Mark T. O'Hollaren, MD

The metal manufacturing industry has been associated with a number of pulmonary health problems.[1] Exposure to some metals and metal processing substances may contribute to the development of disorders such as pulmonary fibrosis, pulmonary edema, carcinoma of the lung, skin sensitization, and occupational asthma. The focus of attention here will be on occupational asthma associated with exposure to these materials.

Fumes from some metals cause health problems in their native form, and others need to be present as the metal salt to induce sensitization and/or produce immediate symptoms. When considering asthma caused by sensitivity to metals or their salts, the heterogeneity of clinical presentations with each metal is quite striking. For this reason, each metal is discussed separately, to emphasize its unique properties.

Metals that have been associated with occupational asthma include platinum, aluminum ("potroom asthma"), nickel, chromium, and cobalt (in hard metal and probably in stainless steel manufacturing). Asthmatic responses to vanadium and uranium as well as metal fume fever will also be covered.

PLATINUM SALTS

Background and Historical Perspective

Platinum is a rare metal in a group that includes rhodium, palladium, ruthenium, osmium, and iridium. Until 1915, the majority of the world's platinum came from Russia and Columbia, where the native metal is usually found alloyed with other metals of the rare metal group and with iron. Recently platinum has also been found in Canada and Alaska.[2] Platinum and its alloys are made into wire and sheets to be used in jewelry, dentistry, and in the electrical and chemical industries. Platinum salts may be used in the manufacture of platinum catalysts, for electroplating, and for photographic applications.[2]

Biagini et al. and others[3,4] noted that the relative inertness of precious metals such as platinum necessitated the use of concentrated acids to solubilize them from rich ores or metal concentrates into metal salts. This may lead to exposure of involved metal workers to both metal aerosols as well as acidic mists and other irritant gases. In sufficient concentrations, the latter could possibly damage the airways, making them more prone to sensitization by platinum.[3]

Platinum workers exposed to the fine dust or spray of platinum salts frequently develop a syndrome consisting of rhinitis, conjunctivitis, and bronchial asthma.[5] Salts implicated include potassium tetrachloroplatinate (K_2PtCl_4), potassium hexachloroplatinate (K_2PtCl_6), ammonium chloroplatinate ($(NH_4)_2PtCl_6$), and sodium (hexa) chloroplatinate (Na_2PtCl_6).[5] These are all potent sensitizers, and sensitization appears to be related to the number of chlorine atoms present.

In addition to metal and photographic workers, platinum sensitivity has also been reported in a university chemistry teacher who, after 10 years of exposure, was eventually not able to enter his own laboratory without experiencing rhinitis and asthma.[5] On one occasion, a co-worker inadvertently splashed some ammonium chloroplatinate in his face, resulting in acute, severe angioedema and generalized urticaria requiring epinephrine and steroids.[5]

Platinum compounds have been used in a myriad of applications. Prevost utilized platinum in the treatment of epilepsy in 1833, and Hotler proposed sodium chloroplatinate and platinum perchloride to treat syphilis.[2] Pedler, in 1878, demonstrated platinum perchloride's ability to inactivate cobra venom in vitro; however, this was later shown to be of no use clinically.[2] In 1911, Karasek examined 40 photographic workers in Chicago and found eight cases of "platinum poisoning" characterized by pronounced irritation of the nasal passages and throat, sneezing, coughing, and other respiratory difficulties.[2] However, it was Hunter and his associates in 1945 who first described a syndrome of rhinorrhea, sneezing, chest tightness, and cough in 52 of 91 workers in a platinum refining plant. Symptoms only occurred on contact with the complex salts of platinum and not with the dust of the metal itself.[2]

Epidemiology and Etiology

Gallagher et al. reported a 14% incidence of positive skin tests in workers exposed to sodium hexachloroplatinate in a platinum refinery.[6] Twenty-six percent of workers that had left the refinery for health reasons were positive on skin-testing to this platinum salt. Sixty and 63% of active workers and former workers, respectively, with positive skin tests had increased bronchial responsiveness determined by cold air challenges.[6] In other studies, symptoms of upper respiratory symptoms and bronchial asthma have been reported in 20–100% of exposed workers.[3]

Both atopic and nonatopic workers may be affected, and positive skin test responses to platinum salts may have a variable time of onset in relation to pulmonary symptoms.[7] In most cases, sensitization occurs within 6 to 12 months from onset of exposure, but it may occur as quickly as 10 days or be delayed by as much as 25 years.[8] There are also instances of wives being sensitized by the dust from their husband's work clothes.[2] In some cases pulmonary reactivity may precede skin test reactivity by over a year, raising the question of either an initial pulmonary pharmacologic mechanism or other factors that predispose some workers to dermatologic and pulmonary sensitization at different rates.[3,9]

Skin tests, RAST studies, and passive transfer experiments in both humans and monkeys support a type I IgE-mediated mechanism in patients with hypersensitivity reactions to platinum salts.[3] Other investigators have also questioned whether or not IgG-4 may play a role, but this is not clear.[3] Positive skin tests to platinum salts have persisted in precious metal refinery workers for over 4 years despite discontinuation of exposure.[3] In addition, persistent bronchial reactivity may persist for years, despite removal from the workplace where exposure to platinum occurred.[3] However, platinum asthma may also occur in workers with negative tests.[8,10,11]

Biagini investigated cynomolgus monkeys *(Macaca fascicularis)* and found that ozone exposure (1 ppm O_3) combind with ammonium hexachloroplatinate [$(NH_4)_2PtCl_6$] for 6 hr/day, 5 days/week for 12 weeks significantly reduced the concentration of platinum salt and methacholine needed to increase average pulmonary flow resistance by 200%. Combined ozone and platinum exposure also increased the incidence of positive skin tests to platinum compared with exposure to platinum or ozone exposure alone.[3] In a different study, he noted an acute bronchoconstrictor effect of a platinum salt (sodium hexachloroplatinate), presumed to be secondary to induced histamine release.[9] The reactivity to this compound increased with the duration of exposure.[9]

Murdoch and Pepys immunized rats with free platinum salt via intraperitoneal, intramuscular, intradermal, subcutaneous, intratracheal, and footpad routes without evidence of induction of specific IgE antibody as measured by skin testing, radioallergosorbent testing, or passive cutaneous anaphylaxis testing.[12] However, when $(NH_4)_2PtCl_6$ was conjugated with ovalbumin (2–10 haptenic platinum groups per ovalbumin molecule), IgE antibody against the platinum moiety was demonstrated by heterologous PCA challenge and by specific RAST. The latter was confirmed by RAST inhibition studies.[12]

In guinea pigs, intravenous infusion of sodium chlorplatinate produces (after only 1 minute of infusion) increased intestinal motility, dyspnea, and asphyxiation via anaphylaxis.[13] Post-mortem examination of these animals revealed pale, distended lungs, and markedly elevated blood histamine levels.[13] Intravenously infused sodium chlorplatinate produces a bronchospasm that is equally severe to that caused by histamine.[13] Interestingly, however, after several doses of the platinum salt, the response disappeared, and the animal was able to tolerate what would have previously been a lethal dose. This tolerance effect did not occur with histamine challenges.[13]

In further experiments involving rats and dogs, intravenous sodium chlorplatinate also caused substantial increases in blood histamine levels; and isolated guinea pig ileum also showed a significant increase in histamine release after introduction of sodium chlorplatinate.[13]

Saindelle postulated the need for a period of time for platinum salts to combine with protein in vivo to form an antigenic molecule capable of eliciting an immune response (i.e., sensitization).[13]

CLINICAL PRESENTATION AND EVALUATION

Patients suspected of having asthma due to sensitivity to platinum salts may exhibit typical signs of wheezing, shortness of breath, and cough in association with workplace exposure. Merget et al.[14] conducted a cross-sectional study of workers in a platinum refinery. They stated that basophil histamine release and RAST were not helpful in establishing sensitivity to platinum, and that those two tests had a low specificity compared with skin tests. He found total serum IgE was higher in those exposed to higher platinum concentrations at work, as well as those non-exposed controls with a history of atopic disease. Basophil histamine release by platinum was found in all groups (i.e., platinum workers and nonexposed controls) with or without symptoms, suggesting a pharmacologic effect on the basophils independent of unique allergic sensitivity to platinum salt clinically.[14]

As noted above, it has been well described that workers may have pulmonary symptoms from platinum salts before they have evidence of sensitivity by skin testing, and some workers with platinum-induced pulmonary disease never develop positive skin tests. Although an IgE mechanism has been shown, few have attempted immunotherapy to platinum salts, although it has been successfully performed (albeit with significant side-effects). Levene[2] described an analytical chemist with rhinoconjunctivitis, asthma and contact urticaria when exposed to complex salts of platinum.[2] He was desensitized using ammonium hexachloroplatinate intradermally several times daily for a month. The course of his desensitization, however, was somewhat stormy, with urticarial reactions, serum sickness-like symptoms,

and arthus reactions at the site of injection at higher doses. The desensitization was eventually successful, however, and appeared to be specific for ammonium hexachloroplatinate, because a chance exposure to tetrachloroplatinate produced symptoms.[2] This modality of therapy is not recommended.

The usual "treatment" of choice is prevention of symptoms through avoidance of the platinum antigens, because persistent positive skin tests and bronchial hyperresponsiveness have been described despite removal from the workplace in those sensitized to complex platinum salts.[3] It would be prudent to remove workers who experience asthmatic symptoms from further exposure to attempt to avoid the possibility of potential life-long asthma.

Hunter et al. have carefully reviewed the workplace in platinum refineries and recommend that platinum salts should not be allowed to reach the workplace atmosphere, either in dust or spray form.[2] Proper exhaust ventilation is suggested. Although masks are suggested, they do introduce the "human factor" and are therefore not completely reliable, because improper fit and noncompliance may interfere with effectiveness. Affected workers should be removed from the workplace.[2]

ALUMINUM ("POTROOM ASTHMA")

Background and Historical Perspective

"Potroom asthma" is a type of occupational asthma found in potroom workers in primary aluminum production.[15] In the review by Abramson et al., the authors report that the first description of respiratory "irritation" in aluminum workers was published by Frostad in 1936.[16] In the aluminum manufacturing process, the fumes from the pots of molten aluminum are likely to be liberated during the breaking of the crust that forms over the molten metal (Fig. 1). In addition, fumes are released when anodes are being changed or liquid aluminum is being tapped off[16] (Fig. 2). The emissions encountered in these settings are: fluorides (gaseous and particulate), alumina, carbon dust, sulfur dioxide, and carbon monoxide.[16] There are two different inhalable materials generated from the smelting of bauxite, the ore from which aluminum is smelted by electrolysis. One is alumina (aluminum oxide, Al_2O_3), and the other is a metallic aluminum dust. There are usually fume hoods that duct the emissions away from the workers

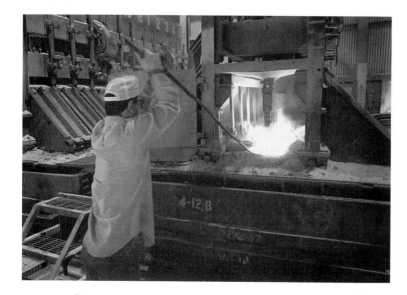

FIGURE 1. Aluminum plant employee working with the molten metal.

and treat the emissions with a wet scrubbing system, electrostatic filtration, or dry scrubbing with substances such as alumina that trap fluorides.[16] Levels of exposure to various contaminants in the work environment depend on the specific job involved and the ambient conditions (e.g., ventilation) in that particular area of the plant.[16]

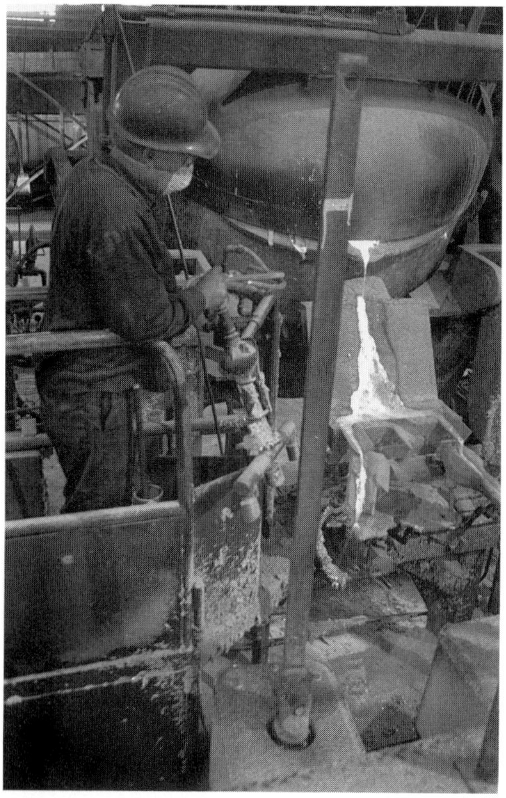

Those investigating the possible pulmonary diseases associated with the aluminum smelting industry have considered four diseases: (1) lung cancer, (2) pulmonary fibrosis (bauxite pneumoconiosis or Shaver's disease), (3) chronic obstructive lung disease (COLD), and (4) an asthmatic syndrome. Recent investigations have not identified pulmonary fibrosis as a significant occupational problem in aluminum potroom workers.[16] However, other observations suggest that more studies will be necessary before the pulmonary effects of aluminum oxide are fully understood.[17] Exposure to volatile materials from coal tar pitch used in anode production has "plausibility" for an association of lung cancer with aluminum smelting.[16] Some authors have questioned the lack of smoking data in the analysis of lung cancer among aluminum workers, as well as exposure to coal tar in aluminum processing.[16] It is difficult to say at this time whether or not aluminum exposure is capable of causing chronic obstructive lung disease. Evidence at this point appears to be inconclusive, but aluminum manufacturing workers are at least as likely as others in dusty occupations to develop COLD.[16,18] Martin found a twofold increase in COLD in exposed aluminum workers, and smoking had an additive effect to workplace exposure.[19]

Mitchell and Abramson have proposed criteria defining "potroom asthma," as outlined in Table 1.

FIGURE 2. Molten aluminum.

TABLE 1. *Criteria for Defining "Potroom Asthma"*

1. No previous history of bronchial asthma
2. An initial period of symptom-free exposure
3. Symptoms such as dyspnea, chest tightness, wheezing, and cough
4. A temporal association to the workplace
5. Improvement away from work
6. Documentation of either reversible airway obstruction or bronchial hyperreactivity.

Epidemiology and Etiology

The estimated incidence of potroom asthma ranges from 0.06% to 4% per year in aluminum potroom workers, depending on the study.[16] Symptoms of potroom asthma in one study of 15 aluminum workers appeared after an average of 3.9 months of exposure (range 1–8 months). All patients had nocturnal dyspnea; eight had cough and eight had exercise-induced asthma.[20] There may be considerable variability, however, in the time of onset of potroom asthma after beginning work in the potroom.

Swedish investigators have reported bronchial asthma in five of seven workers using potassium aluminum tetrafluoride. They state that the particle size of this compound (used as flux for soldering aluminum) is less than 10 microns and therefore in the respirable size range.[21] Provocation with aluminum-fluoride flux did not induce an immediate asthmatic reaction but did result in a late reaction with a prolonged increase in nonspecific reactivity.[21] The mean age of those who acquired potroom asthma in one group of potroom workers was 32.6 years, 5 years younger than the group as a whole.[22]

The pathogenesis of potroom asthma is not known.[43] Suggestions of the etiology include bronchial irritant receptor stimulation by noxious fumes or gases, inflammatory bronchoconstriction due to irritant gas exposure, and pharmacologic and/or allergic bronchoconstriction. The gases present may include sulfur dioxide (SO_2), hydrogen fluoride, chlorine gas (Cl_2), and particulates containing fluorides.[15,16] Vanadium, another metal associated with occupational asthma, may also be found in potroom fumes.[16] It is occasionally used in some aluminum alloys.[16] Further research is needed to clarify the role of each of these possible agents in the genesis of asthma in aluminum potroom workers.

Clinical Presentation and Evaluation

Symptoms of asthma in aluminum potroom workers usually manifest as shortness of breath, cough, chest tightness, and wheezing.[15,16] These may occur as immediate, delayed, and presumably dual asthmatic responses.[16] In potroom asthma due to aluminum, symptoms from airway obstruction may occur either at work or several hours after leaving work.[15]

There may be a large variability among workers regarding the time between onset of workplace exposure and development of symptoms. Although this may range from 1 week to 10 years, most workers become symptomatic within the first 3 years of employment.[16] A history of continued asthmatic symptoms despite discontinuation of work with aluminum does not exclude the diagnosis of potroom asthma, because persistent symptoms and increased bronchial hyperreactivity (as measured by methacholine sensitivity) are well described long after cessation of employment in the potroom.[15,16,20,23–27] Follow-up of 35 aluminum workers with potroom asthma an average of 2.5 years after cessation of work in the plant showed that 28.6% (10/35) still had persistent symptoms of asthma.[15] It should be understood, however, that all these studies were retrospective in nature, and there is no way of knowing how many workers had pre-existing asthma or bronchial hyperreactivity.

Several factors have been suggested as possible predisposing factors for the development of potroom asthma. These include childhood bronchitis, pleurisy, pertussis, and especially smoking.[28] It should be noted, however, that conflicting data have been noted regarding the importance of smoking in the development of potroom asthma.[28] Although "allergies" have been mentioned in passing in the literature regarding risk factors for the development of potroom asthma, skin testing with dust from potroom environments, as well as other aeroallergens, have not been helpful in establishing a diagnosis of potroom asthma.[16,29] A Yugoslavian study by Saric et al. of 227 workers using the Alu-Swiss process for the electrolytic extraction of aluminum did not show that an atopic predisposition led to an increased incidence of potroom asthma.[22] Others have also noted that atopy does not appear to be a predisposing risk factor for developing potroom asthma.[30] Although tested in only a limited number of patients with persistent potroom asthma, total IgE did not appear to be increased in those workers.[15]

In a recent report from Norway, Kongerud and Samuelsen observed that both total fluoride exposure and smoking were related to asthmatic symptoms in potroom workers. However, they also admitted that the causal relationship between fluorides and symptoms deserved further investigation by specific bronchial provocation and other immunologic studies.[53]

The treatment for potroom asthma is prompt removal from the workplace, because persistent symptoms have been reported despite leaving the offending environment. Clearly, if individuals leave the work environment after early diagnosis, their chances of timely improvement are maximized. If potroom asthma can be compared to other models of occupational asthma, such as that from western red cedar, then continued exposure after the onset of symptoms could result in a worse prognosis. Asthmatic symptoms should be treated similarly to asthma from other causes.

HARD METAL AND COBALT

Background

"Hard metal" and "heavy metal" are terms given to a blend of metals that form a particularly hard and durable product. The alloy is 90–95% as hard as diamond.[31] It is used when resistance to heat, as well as strength and rigidity, is necessary, such as in cutting tools, dies, and bits used in cutting rock.[31] Hard metal is an alloy with tungsten carbide (75 to 95%) and cobalt (5 to 20%) as a matrix, with other metals such as titanium, nickel, chromium, niobium, vanadium, and tantalum used for special purposes.[32,33] To form carbides, metals such as tungsten, molybdenum, and niobium are blended with carbon and superheated.[31] Cobalt serves as a matrix in some forms of hard metal, as does nickel.[31] The metals are poured in powder form into steel or rubber forms, then "presintered" in hydrogen furnaces at temperatures ranging from 500–800°C. They are then shaped, and finally sintered at temperatures of approximately 1550°C.[31]

Several steps in the use or manufacture of hard metals have been shown to increase the risk of occupational asthma. These include handling the basic material, processing the mixture after it has been presintered, and grinding the sintered hard metal.[32] Cobalt is known to cause hard-metal worker's asthma and may participate in causing occupational interstitial pneumonitis.[31]

Historical Perspective, Epidemiology, and Etiology

Kusaka et al. note that research regarding the production of hard metal began in 1928, and the product was initially sold in 1931.[31] In 1967, Bruckner reported the first case of occupational asthma in association with hard-metal exposure.[34] Occupational asthma occurred at a prevalence rate of 5.6% in one Japanese hard-metal factory.[31] One study of three diamond polishers with cobalt-induced asthma suggested that the actual level of cobalt dust exposure was more significant than the duration of exposure.[31] In most western countries, the industry threshold standard for airborne cobalt dust is 0.1 mg/M^3, although there is some question whether sensitization may occur below this level.[31]

Asthma associated with cobalt exposure in diamond polishers has been described even when it is not alloyed to tungsten carbide.[32] Although tungsten alone is thought by some authors to be relatively inert, tungsten carbide is thought to possibly potentiate cobalt's toxicity in the lung in hard-metal workers.[32] The latent period between beginning work in a hard-metal factory and the onset of asthmatic symptoms ranged from 3 months to 10 years.[31]

Some investigators have attributed the asthmatic reaction to cobalt to a hypersensitivity reaction, in which cobalt acts as a hapten rather than an irritant.[32] While immunologic mechanisms may play a role in some cases of cobalt-induced asthma, nonimmune mechanisms are also felt to be involved.[33] Despite the significant data base concerning the immunologic basis of cobalt sensitivity, the exact mechanism of hard-metal asthma is unknown.[33]

Interstitial lung disease has been seen in hard-metal workers.[35] Ruttner and Furrer described post-mortem examination findings in two patients who had worked with heavy metals for over 20 years. In the lungs were partially fibrosed, stellate-shaped nodules containing dust and elementary nodules similar to silicosis. These nodules were surrounded by perifocal emphysema.[31] Cobalt may cause interstitial lung disease in diamond polishers and presumably in others exposed to cobalt dust.[36] In addition, tungsten carbide workers have been described with lowered FEV_1, decreased diffusion capacity, mild hypoxemia, and interstitial infiltrates on chest radiographs.[36] Severe exposures to tungsten carbide have been reported to cause an interstitial pneumonitis, with a diffusion capacity of 35%

predicted.[36] Electron probe analysis of lung biopsy specimens in patients with hard-metal worker's lung disease has shown some patients to have tungsten only in diseased areas, and some to have tungsten and cobalt.[46] Thus, there is still much investigation that needs to be done to clarify the relative roles of these various constituents of hard metal in producing the lung disease seen in these workers.

Clinical Presentation and Evaluation

Depending on the patient, asthmatic reactions of the immediate, late, and dual patterns have been seen in cobalt workers.[31] Workers often noted decreased symptoms on weekends, holidays, and after appropriate industrial ventilation measures and/or respiratory masks were provided to the workers.[31] Asthma in cobalt workers has been shown, at least in some patients, to resolve after discontinuation of work in the hard-metal factory. However, some fail to recover despite transfer to nonindustrial areas.[31] This is especially true if timely diagnosis is not made or delay in transfer after the diagnosis is made. Eight patients with hard-metal worker's asthma could not be distinguished from nonasthmatic controls using cobalt chloride skin tests ($CoCl_2$).[33] Bronchial provocation testing with cobalt chloride, however, was positive in all patients with the disease, and negative in controls, showing that cobalt skin testing is not useful in establishing this diagnosis.[33] Positive bronchial provocation testing with cobalt can be followed by extended periods of increased nonspecific bronchial hyperreactivity.[32]

Those workers who exhibit a pattern of interstitial lung injury may have symptoms of progressive dyspnea, fever, weight loss, dry cough, and increased fatigue.[31] Diffuse linear shadows may be seen on chest radiographs in association with a restrictive ventilatory impairment on pulmonary function testing.[31]

NICKEL

In 1973, McConnell and associates reported asthma due to sensitivity to inhaled nickel.[37] Nieboer et al. demonstrated that serum from a patient with asthma secondary to nickel sulfate inhalation contained antibodies of the IgG class against a nickel-human serum albumin (HSA) complex.[38] Ammonium sulfate precipitation as well as anti-IgG co-precipitation were used to demonstrate specific antibodies. There was no such binding in 30 nonallergic control sera. Ligand competition studies demonstrated that the formation of the reactive ligand depends on the selective binding of nickel at the native copper/nickel transport site of HSA.[38]

Dolovich et al. have studied nickel-HSA interactions and observed that cobalt slightly inhibited binding of radiolabeled nickel, whereas zinc and magnesium failed to inhibit it.[39] Copper effectively inhibited the binding. Their conclusion was that the antigenic determinant in nickel sensitivity depends on the combining of nickel with HSA at the specific nickel/copper combining site.[39]

Malo et al. reported a worker who developed occupational asthma from nickel a few months after starting work. Skin prick tests to nickel were negative and a bronchial inhalation test showed an isolated late asthmatic response beginning 3 hours after the challenge.[40] In another study, Malo identified nickel-specific IgE in a patient with nickel sulfate-induced asthma by skin testing, RAST, and immediate asthmatic reactions after bronchial provocation testing with a nickel-HSA complex.[41]

Novey described a previously nonatopic metal plating worker who developed de novo asthma after plating with nickel and chromium, but not other metals.[42] Specific BPT with nickel produced a biphasic asthmatic response. Skin tests to both nickel and chromium salts were negative; however, RAST was positive for both metals with negative RAST to other metals and gold.[42] Other investigators have found that skin tests and antibody screens may be negative in the presence of a positive bronchial provocation test using nickel.[43] Block and Yeung described a 60-year-old metal polisher with nickel-induced asthma who had a positive prick test to nickel sulfate solution and whose FEV_1 fell 28% within 5 minutes of exposure to workplace dust. The FEV_1 normalized within 35 minutes of removal from the exposure. No late asthmatic response was seen in that patient.[44] A manager of a plant manufacturing nickel carbonyl was reported to develop Loffler's syndrome in association with his workplace exposure.[45]

In summary, patients with inhalant sensitivity to nickel may or may not have positive skin tests to nickel solutions, such as nickel sulfate, and laboratory tests such as RAST may occasionally be useful. Specific bronchial provocation testing in the lab or workplace may be needed to confirm the diagnosis.

STAINLESS STEEL

Koskinen et al. noted that welding fumes consist of solid and gaseous pollutants.[46] The solid airborne particles are composed of work-piece metal and electrode coating. The gaseous portion consists of mainly nitrogen, oxides, ozone, fluoride compounds, and carbon dioxide.[46] The concentration of metallic airborne particles depends on both the welding method and the ventilation conditions. Manual metal arc welding on mild (as opposed to stainless) steel produces fumes containing a number of substances, including aluminum, magnesium, fluoride, silicon, potassium, calcium, titanium, manganese, and iron, with trace amounts of cobalt, zinc, and lead.[46] Stainless steel welding, in addition to the above mentioned substances, also releases chromium and nickel.[46]

These welding fume particles are in the respirable size range of 0.3–0.5 microns and may form rings and long chains as seen in transmission electron micrographs.[46] A worker who had asthmatic symptoms in association with welding stainless steel, but not mild steel, had negative bronchial provocation testing after welding mild steel, but a strongly positive response after welding stainless steel.[46] The asthmatic response was blocked by prior inhalation of either cromolyn sodium or beclomethasone. The authors of the study postulated that either the chromium or nickel in stainless steel was responsible for the asthmatic response in that worker.[46]

CHROMIUM

The toxic effects of chromate compounds were first experimentally produced by Gmelin in 1824.[47] Apparent asthma due to chromates was described in four workers by Delpech and Hilairet in 1876.[48] Joules reported chromate-associated asthma in a metal-plating worker in 1932.[49] In 1935, Card reported reproducible asthmatic responses to intradermally injected potassium chromate in a 28-year-old chromium-plating factory worker, which required epinephrine treatment. Orally ingested chromates provoked no symptoms in this worker.[49] Novey et al. described a 32-year-old metal-plating worker with inhalation asthma to chromium and nickel, with a positive bronchial provocation to chromium (immediate response only). Skin tests to chromium salts

were negative in this patient. RAST, however, was positive, with a negative RAST to other common allergens as well as to gold, which served as a control metal.[42]

VANADIUM AND URANIUM HEXAFLUORIDE

Vanadium pentoxide has been associated with occupational asthma.[36,50] Of interest, several of the reported cases were associated with a green tongue discoloration in the affected workers.[50]

Four workers in a vanadium pentoxide refinery in western Australia were noted to have respiratory symptoms after exposure to vanadium pentoxide. The clinical presentation included wheezing, dyspnea, green discoloration of the skin and tongue, headache, nausea, nasal congestion, lethargy, and dry mouth. Three of the four workers were nonatopic by skin testing. Two workers manifested bronchial hyperreactivity by histamine challenge testing. One of the four workers (an atopic smoker) continued to wheeze 8 weeks after leaving the workplace.[50]

Another investigator reported a 25-year-old vanadium pentoxide worker who experienced injected mucous membranes, wheezing, and shortness of breath after exposure to vanadium. Green discoloration of the skin or tongue was not mentioned.[51] Lower respiratory symptoms have been reported soon after exposure to vanadium pentoxide, indicating the potential for inducing asthmatic symptoms within 24 hours after first exposure.[36] This suggests an irritant or pharmacologic mechanism of action.

Uranium hexafluoride, used in some metal coat removers, floor sealants, and spray paint has produced an asthma syndrome accompanied by increased methacholine reactivity.[36]

METAL FUME FEVER AND OTHER MISCELLANEOUS METAL-ASSOCIATED SYNDROMES

Although not considered occupational asthma, there are a number of other pulmonary syndromes associated with metal exposure. The reader is referred to a comprehensive review for further information.[36]

Numerous names have been given to the syndrome referred to as "metal fume fever." These include the following: "monday morning fever, the smothers, brass founders ague, brazier's disease, foundry fever, galvanizer's poisoning, smelters' chills, zinc chills, zinc fume fever, brass chills, and copper fever."[52] It appears that the most common metals causing this syndrome are zinc and copper, although many other metals have been implicated.[52]

Metal fume fever may include symptoms such as cough, pleuritic chest pain, dyspnea, thirst with dry throat, metallic taste, fever, chills, nausea, and myalgias.[52] Physical exam may show a temperature of 102–104°F, sinus tachycardia, and localized or diffuse rales.[52] The condition is usually self-limited and clears within 24–48 hours; treatment consists of bed rest and symptomatic measures. Although two cases have been reported in which serum zinc levels were elevated, that correlation has not been consistently noted by other investigators.[52]

Cadmium may be associated with interstitial pneumonitis and adult respiratory distress syndrome (ARDS), but it is not a known cause of occupational asthma.[52] It has been reported to be a risk factor for the development of emphysema.[36] Acute cadmium pneumonitis in a welder showed a slow, relentless progression, with eventual development of pulmonary fibrosis, stressing the importance of long-term follow-up in patients with cadmium exposure.[36]

Mercury vapor may cause a severe pneumonitis if inhaled in high concentration and has also been reported to cause fever, leukocytosis, and acute depression of FEV_1 and diffusion capacity.[36] Acute exposure to zinc chloride may also cause severe interstitial pulmonary fibrosis, as can exposure to vitallium used in the manufacture of dental prostheses.[36] An engineer was inadvertently sprayed with titanium tetrachloride in an industrial setting and had severe respiratory failure requiring assisted ventilation for 5 weeks. Examination of the bronchial anatomy demonstrated fleshy polypoid lesions in the major bronchi, and his course gradually improved over a year with the aid of steroid therapy.[36]

In summary, there is tremendous variability in the clinical presentation of patients experiencing pulmonary symptoms from metal or metal salt exposure. A high index of suspicion is needed on the part of the evaluating physician. Careful evaluation, considering all alternatives, is essential in arriving at a diagnosis. Although biological tests may be helpful, the only method of establishing the diagnosis is bronchial provocation with subirritant doses of the metal fume suspected. Once a diagnosis is established, the best possible course is to advise strict avoidance of further exposure. Residual symptoms should be treated as in any patient with asthma.

REFERENCES

1. Cullen MR: Respiratory diseases from hard metal exposure. A continuing enigma. Chest 86:513, 1984.
2. Hunter D, Milton R, Perry KMA: Asthma caused by the complex salts of platinum. Br J Ind Med 2:92–98, 1945.
3. Biagini RE, Moorman WJ, Lewis TR, et al: Ozone enhancement of platinum asthma in a primate model. Am Rev Respir Dis 134:719–725, 1986.
4. Biagini RE, Moorman WJ, Lewis TR, Bernstein IL: Pulmonary responsiveness to methacholine and disodium hexachloroplatinate (Na_2PtCl_61). Toxicol Appl Pharmacol 69:377–384, 1983.
5. Freedman SO, Kruupey J: Respiratory allergy caused by platinum salts. J Allergy 42:233–237, 1968.
6. Gallagher JS, Baker D, Gann PH, et al: A cross-sectional investigation of workers exposed to platinum salts (abstract). J Allergy Clin Immunol 69:134, 1982.
7. Dally MB, Hunter JV, Hughes EG, et al: Hypersensitivity to platinum salts: A population study. Am Rev Respir Dis 4(Suppl):120, 1980.
8. Parks WR: Occupational Lung Diseases, 2nd ed. London, Butterworth, 1982, p 433.
9. Biagini RE, Moorman WJ, Smith RJ, et al: Pulmonary hyperreactivity in cynomolgus monkeys *(Macaca fasicularis)* from nose-only inhalation exposure to disodium hexachloroplatinate, Na_2PtCl_61. Toxicol Appl Pharmacol 69:377–384, 1983.
10. Pepys J, Parish WE, Cromwell O, et al: Passive transfer in man and monkey of type 1 allergy due to heat labile and heat stable antibody to complex salts of platinum. Clin Allergy 9:99, 1979.
11. Cromwell O, Pepys J, Parish WE, et al: Specific IgE antibodies to platinum salts in sensitized workers. Clin Allergy 9:229, 1979.
12. Murdoch RD, Pepys J: Immunological responses to complex salts of platinum. I. Specific IgE antibody production in the rat. Clin Exp Immunol 7(1):107–114, 1984.
13. Saindelle A, Ruff F: Histamine release by sodium chloroplatinate. Br J Pharmacol 35:313–321, 1969.
14. Merget R, Schultze-Werninghaus LT, Muthorst T, et al: Asthma due to the complex salts of platinum—a cross sectional survey of workers in a platinum refinery. Clin Allergy 18:569–580, 1988.
15. Wergeland E, Lund E, Waage JE: Respiratory dysfunction after potroom asthma. Am J Ind Med 11:627–663, 1987.
16. Abramson MJ, Wlodarczyk JH, Saunders NA, et al: Does aluminum smelting cause lung disease? Am Rev Respir Dis 139:1042–1057, 1989.
17. Jederlinic PJ, Abraham JL, Churg A, et al: Pulmonary fibrosis in aluminum oxide workers. Am Rev Respir Dis 142:1179, 1990.
18. Martin RR, Durand P, Ghezzo H: Studies on the health of primary aluminum workers in Quebec: Airway obstruction—chronic components. Montreal, Alcon Aluminum, 1986.
19. Johannessen H: The respiratory condition of potroom workers: Norwegian experience. In Hughes JP (ed): Health Protection in Primary Aluminum Production. London, International Primary Aluminum Institute, 1977, pp 87–90.

20. Simonsson BG, Haeger-Aronsen B, Sjoberg A, et al: Bronchial hyperexcitability in workers exposed to aluminum salts. Scand J Respir Dis 138(Suppl):181–188, 1950.

21. Hjortsberg U, Nise G, Orbaek P, et al: Bronchial asthma due to exposure to potassium aluminumtetrafluoride (letter). Scand J Work Environ Health 12:223, 1986.

22. Saric M, Godnic-Cvar J, Gomzi M, et al: The role of atopy in potroom workers' asthma. Am J Ind Med 9:239–242, 1986.

23. Simonsson BG, Sjoberg A, Rolf C, et al: Acute and long-term airway hyperreactivity in aluminum-salt exposed workers with nocturnal asthma. Eur J Respir Dis 66:105–118, 1985.

24. O'Donnell TV, Welford B, Coleman ED: Potroom asthma: New Zealand experience and follow-up. Am J Ind Med 15:43–49, 1989.

25. Wergeland E, Lund E, Waage JE: Respiratory dysfunction after potroom asthma. Am J Ind Med 11:627–636, 1987.

26. Simonsson BG, Sjoberg A, Rolf C, et al: Acute and long-term airway hyperreactivity in aluminum salt. Eur J Respir Dis 66:105–118, 1985.

27. Simonsson BG, Sjoberg A, Rolf C, Haeger-Aronsen B: Acute and long-term airway hyperreactivity in aluminum salt exposed workers with nocturnal asthma. Eur J Respir Dis 66:105–118, 1985.

28. Constantopaidos F: Aluminum respiratory disorders at Saint Nicholas Aluminum de Greece. In Covlon J-P (ed): Seminar on Aluminum Respiratory Disorders. St. Nicholas Aluminum, Greece. Paris, Aluminum Peuchiney, 1980, pp 81–90.

29. Midtun O: Bronchial asthma in the aluminum industry. Acta Allergol 25:208–221, 1960.

30. Saric M, Godnic-Cvar J, Gozmi M, et al: The role of atopy in potroom workers' asthma. Am J Ind Med 9:239–242, 1986.

31. Kusaka Y, Yokoyama K, Sera Y, et al: Respiratory diseases in hard metal workers: An occupational hygiene study in a factory. Br J Ind Med 43:474–485, 1986.

32. Gheysens B, Auwerx J, Van den Eeckhout A, et al: Cobalt-induced bronchial asthma in diamond polishers. Chest 88:740–744, 1985.

33. Shrakawa T, Kusaka Y, et al: Occupational asthma from cobalt sensitivity in workers exposed to hard metal dust. Chest 95:29–37, 1989.

34. Bruckner HC: Extrinsic asthma in a tungsten carbide worker. J Occup Med 9:518, 1967.

35. Davison AG, Haslam PL, Corrin B, et al: Interstitial lung disease and asthma in hard-metal workers: Bronchoalveolar lavage, ultrastructural, and analytical findings and results of bronchial provocation tests. Thorax 38:119–128, 1983.

36. Bates D: Occupational lung diseases. In Bates D (ed): Respiratory Function in Disease, 3rd ed. Philadelphia, W.B. Saunders, 1989, pp 291–336.

37. McConnell LH, Fink JN, Schlueter DP, et al: Asthma caused by nickel sensitivity. Ann Intern Med 78:888–890, 1973.

38. Nieboer E, Evans SL, Dolovich J: Occupational asthma from nickel sensitivity. II. Factors influencing the interaction of NI^{2+}, HSA, and serum antibodies with nickel related specificity. Br J Ind Med 41:56–63, 1984.

39. Dolovich J, Evans SL, Nieboer E: Occupational asthma from nickel sensitivity. I. Human serum albumin in the antigenic determinant. Br J Ind Med 41:51–55, 1984.

40. Malo JL, Cartier A, Gagnon G, et al: Isolated late asthmatic reaction due to nickel sulphate without antibodies to nickel. Clin Allergy 15(2):95–99, 1985.

41. Malo JL, Cartier A, Doepner M, et al: Occupational asthma caused by nickel sulfate. J Allergy Clin Immunol 69:55–59, 1982.

42. Novey HS, Habib M, Wells ID: Asthma and IgE antibodies induced by chromium and nickel salts. J Allergy Clin Immunol 72:407–412, 1983.

43. Malo JL, Cartier A, Gagnon G, et al: Isolated late asthmatic reaction due to nickel sulphate without antibodies to nickel. Clin Allergy 15:95–99, 1985.

44. Block GT, Yeung M: Asthma induced by nickel. JAMA 247:1600–1602, 1982.

45. Sunderman FW, Sunderman FW Jr: Loffler's syndrome associated with nickel sensitivity. Arch Intern Med 107:405–408, 1961.

46. Keskinen H, Kalliomaki PL, Alanko K: Occupational asthma due to stainless steel welding fumes. Clin Allergy 10:151–159, 1980.

47. Gamelin CG: Edin Med Surg J XXVI:133, 1826.

48. Delpech A, Hilairet JB: [article title missing] Ann d'hyg pub XLV:193, 1876.

49. Joules H: Asthma from sensitisation to chromium. Lancet ii:182–183, 1932.

50. Musk AW, Tees JG: Asthma caused by occupational exposure to vanadium compounds. Med J Aust 1:183–184, 1982.

51. Sjoberg SG: Vanadium pentoxide dust: A clinical and experimental investigation on its effect after inhalation. Acta Med Scand 138(Suppl 238):181–188, 1950.

52. Noel NE, Ruthman JC: Elevated serum zinc levels in metal fume fever. Am J Emerg Med 6:609–610, 1988.

53. Kongerud J, Samuelsen SO: A longitudinal study of respiratory symptoms in aluminum potroom workers. Am Rev Respir Dis 144:10, 1991.

Chapter 17

ASTHMA ASSOCIATED WITH AMINE-BASED EPOXY RESINS, LATEX, REACTIVE DYES, AND MISCELLANEOUS CHEMICALS

Emil J. Bardana, Jr., MD

AMINE-BASED EPOXY RESINS

In 1939, both Kern[1] and Vaughn[2] reported instances of occupational asthma due to low-molecular-weight agents phthalic anhydride and formaldehyde, respectively. The multitude of simple chemicals implicated in work-related asthma has expanded considerably since that time. However, the major reason for the increasing prevalence has been the rapid proliferation of complex plastic polymers and resins in our industrialized society.[3,4] The plastics industry, with an annual growth rate of 10 to 15%, has assumed a very visible role in all aspects of manufacturing. Among the plastics, the cured epoxy resins possess excellent resistance to heat and chemicals. The finished product has commendable electrical resistance and the capacity to form a superior bond. Because of these properties epoxy resins are widely employed as glue for metal, rubber, plastics, ceramics, for casting models, concrete repair, electrical insulation, floor covering, paints, and in dentistry (Fig. 1). Epoxy resin is also commercially available as a household glue.

The term "resin" has an imprecise meaning in the plastics industry and occasionally is used interchangeably with the term "plastic." In some instances, resins indicate short-chain uncured polymers that are employed in further polymerization and hardening processes. In other applications, resins are granular, fully cured thermoplastics that can be heated for extrusion and molding.

This chapter will review some of the basic principles of resin chemistry. It will focus primarily on hypersensitivity reactions related to the epoxy resins, including their hardeners, plasticizers, colorants, and fillers. Components of other important resin systems are discussed in separate chapters, including the amino resins formed by the condensation of aldehydes (formaldehyde) with amines (Chapter 14), and with the polyurethanes derived by the poly-addition reactions between a diisocyanate and either a polyhydroxy compound, a polyester, or a polyether (Chapter 12). Because of their importance, the acid anhydrides and polybasic acids are also considered separately (Chapter 13). Also, a number of miscellaneous chemicals that do not logically fit into any particular resin system are reviewed in this chapter.

HISTORICAL PERSPECTIVE

Epoxides or epoxy resins were discovered before the Second World War by a Swiss dentist who sold his patent to CIBA Pharmaceutical Corporation. The resin system was developed in Switzerland in 1938 and first marketed by CIBA-GEIGY in 1946. The trade name for its product was Araldite. Epoxy resins were not introduced into the United States until 1951. The quantity used in the U.S. increased from less than one million pounds in 1951 to more than 360 million pounds in 1979. Their unique combination of toughness, adhesiveness, and chemical and electrical resistance is not found in any other plastic. For this reason, the epoxy resins will remain among the most popular plastics for many years to come. More than

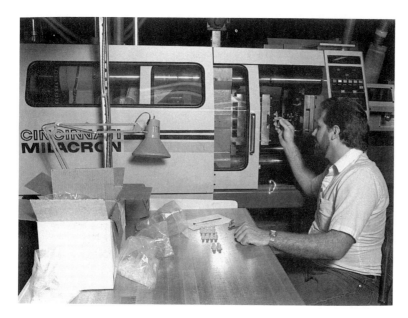

FIGURE 1. Worker shown with a thermoset plastic injection machine used in the manufacture of a plastic part for tennis shoes.

50 resins of this type are currently available. Those of low molecular weight are most commonly employed in industry. In 1978, NIOSH estimated that one million U.S. workers were regularly exposed to epoxy resins in their work.[5]

CHEMISTRY

The plastics can be divided into two major groups, referred to as the thermosets and the thermoplastics. The thermoset plastics cannot be reformed or melted after their initial cure. They include the amino resins (urea and melamine formaldehyde), epoxy resins (ethoxylins), phenolics, polyesters and alkyds, polyurethanes, and the silicones. The thermoset plastics are usually prepared by condensation. The latter process is a polymerization reaction in which two or more molecules unite simultaneously, releasing water and another simple substance, usually an alcohol. This type of reaction proceeds in one direction only and reaches equilibrium as the by-products are continuously removed. The reaction can be stopped at any point, in which case the mixture is called a semi-cured resin. It can be packaged and distributed for final processing at a later time. Restarting the reaction usually requires the addition of an activator—usually termed a hardener or curing agent.

The thermoplastics can be reheated and reshaped repeatedly and are usually formulated using polymerization by addition. The latter process is one in which large molecules

(polymers) are built from smaller molecular units (monomers). Polyethylene from ethylene is an example. No byproduct such as water or alcohol is emitted. However, considerable heat can be generated, which occasionally poses an engineering or structural problem.

Epoxy or epoxy resins are thermoplastics that are characterized by the epoxide group:

$$\overset{\displaystyle O}{\overset{\diagup\;\diagdown}{-CH-CH_2}}$$

They are linear macromolecules with a fairly low molecular weight, and over 90% are generated from the reaction of glycerol epichlorhydrin on a polyphenol, such as bisphenol A or diphenylolpropane (Fig. 2). Depending on the length of the chain, epoxy resin is either a viscous liquid or a solid. Hardeners increase the molecular weight and generate bridges between linear chains. Manufacturers can obtain resins with various molecular weights ranging between 340 to approximately 4000 daltons. Two types of hardeners are generally employed: (1) The **acid anhydrides** (dicarboxylic acids) and polybasic acids require external heat during processing. Commonly used curing agents in this class are phthalic anhydride and adipic acid. These curing agents are used for casting applications. (2) The **diamines** generate their own heat during the curing process. During this thermal reaction, fumes and/or particulates of the curing agents are emitted, leading to exposure by a wide variety of workers (Table 1).[6] Among the most commonly used aliphatic amines are diethylene triamine

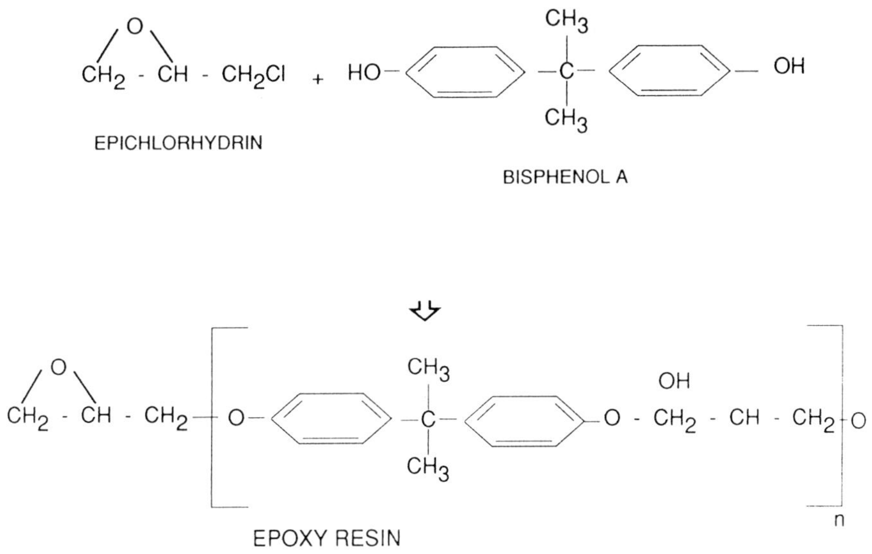

n	MW
0	340
1	624
2	908
3	1192
4	1476
5	1760

FIGURE 2.   Basic chemical structure of epoxy resin. Made by reacting bisphenol A and epichlorhydrin, resins are mixtures of oligomers with different molecular weights. The repeated part has a molecular weight of 284. When n = 0, an oligomer of the lowest molecular weight is obtained (MW 340); when n = 1, the molecular weight is 624.

and triethylene tetramine. Table 2 summarizes selected potential allergens or irritants in the epoxy resin class of chemicals.[7]

HEALTH EFFECTS

Occupational health effects caused by the epoxy resins may result from irritation or allergic mechanisms. Any number of chemical components may be operative and occasionally several may be implicated in the same patient. Although the NIOSH estimated approximately one million workers exposed to epoxy resins,[5] the overall extent of the exposure is probably much greater.

Dermatitis

For many years after the epoxies were introduced, the aliphatic polyamine hardeners were felt to be the principal cause of both irritant and allergic dermatitis.[8-10] The cured resin itself is believed to be the major cause. Completely cured resin is nonallergenic, but material prepared at room temperature, though it appears hardened, may contain from 5 to 25% uncured material.[11] Curing at high temperatures assures complete hardening and essentially eliminates allergenicity. Contact allergy to the epoxy resin usually develops within months of initial exposure. Only rare individuals are sensitized after that time, despite extensive contact. Relatively few individuals have isolated sensitization to the hardener or reactive diluent. The allergic dermatitis is usually localized to the hands and forearms, but may appear over the face and neck. More than 90% of those sensitized react to constituents with molecular weights under 500 daltons. The most highly sensitizing resin is an oligomer, with a molecular weight of 340.[12,13] Oligomers with molecular weights of approximately 900–1000

TABLE 1. *Industries in Which Epoxy Resin Systems Are Likely to Be Encountered*

Abrasive wheel makers	Electricians
Adhesive manufacturing	Floor coverers
Aircraft workers	Garage workers
Artists	Glue manufacture
Automobile workers	Histology technicians
Cabinetmakers	Linoleum makers
Cable splicers	Metal workers
Cast makers	Painters
Cement workers	Resin production
Ceramic workers	Road workers
Chemists	Rubber workers
Dentists	Shoemakers
Electric apparatus makers	Woodworkers

TABLE 2. *Potential Allergens or Irritants Encountered in Common Epoxy Resin Systems**

Hot process hardeners (acid anhydrides)
  Phthalic anhydride
  Maleic acid
  Methyl anhydride
  Hexahydrophthalic anhydride
  Dodecenyl succinic anhydride
  Adipic acid

Hot or cold process hardeners (diamines)
  Diethylenetriamine
  Triethylenetetramine
  Isophoronediamine (IPD)
  Triethanolamine
  Ethylenediamine
  Diethylenediamine (piperazine)
  Hexamethylenetetramine
  Dimethylaminopropylamine
  Tris(dimethylaminomethyl) phenol

Cycloaliphatic polyamines
  Isophorone diamine
  N-Aminoethyl piperazine
  3,3'-dimethyl-4-4'-diaminodicyclohexylmethane

Aromatic amines
  p',p-Diaminodiphenylmethane

Base products
  Bisphenol A
  Epichlorohydrin

Additive/reactive diluents
  Allyl glycidyl ether
  Butyl glycidyl ether
  Phenyl glycidyl ether

Fillers
  Asbestos
  Glass fiber
  Silica
  Dyes
  Tar

*Modified from ref. 7.

daltons were found to express little allergenicity. There are no reliable data on the frequency of dermatitis to epoxy, but prior reports cited a prevalence of 3%.[13] This has placed epoxy resin in the top 20 contact allergens.

The reactive components epichlorohydrin and bisphenol A have both been reported to be irritants. Epichlorohydrin is extremely irritating and capable of causing severe burns.[14] It has been purported to be a potential sensitizer, but finding an acceptable dilution to employ in patch testing has rendered investigation problematic.[15] Recently, van Joost has reported sensitization to epichlorohydrin in six patients with contact dermatitis. In two of these cases an isolated positive patch test was noted. In the remaining cases, concomitant positive reactions were seen to a low molecular weight epoxy resin.[16]

Exposure to the aliphatic polyamine hardeners is also capable of causing primary irritation, as well as contact allergic dermatitis (Fig. 2). Irritation stems from a strong alkaline (pH 13-14) composition with the capacity to induce burns. Cutaneous reactions include erythema, pruritus, facial swelling, and occasionally blistering with subsequent crusting and scaling. These compounds may also act as contact sensitizers. Bourne et al. suggested that the amines might react with body proteins to form potential allergens.[17] However, there has never been any experimental work to confirm this hypothesis.

Respiratory Irritation and Sensitivity

As noted above, the curing process involved in the production of epoxy resins may emit fumes of both resin and curing agents.[6] To date, pulmonary reactions associated with the epoxy resins have all been related to acid anhydrides and the aliphatic polyamine hardeners. These amine curing agents have been reported to cause respiratory tract irritation,[18] bronchitis,[19] and bronchial asthma.[20-22] In Dernehl's overview of health hazards at a Union Carbide production plant,[22] he reported 15 new cases of bronchial asthma among 2600 individuals who had worked 12 years with the ethylene amines. The asthmatic attacks were described as severe and required removal from further contact with amines. With removal from the workplace, the asthmatic attacks ceased in all "but a few workers" who continued to have bronchial asthma after exposure to high concentrations of non-amine irritant chemicals that did not adversely effect nonasthmatic workers.[22]

In 1963 Gelfand reported several cases of occupational respiratory allergy to the diamine compounds in a variety of occupational

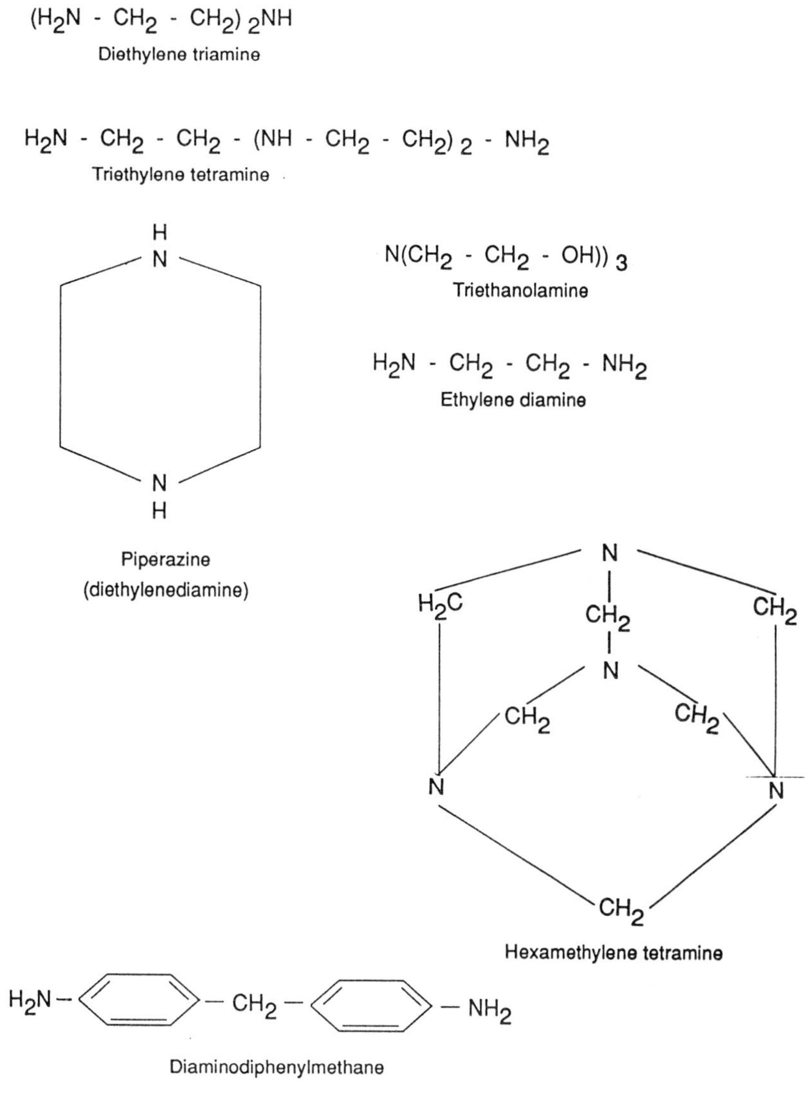

$(H_2N - CH_2 - CH_2)_2NH$

Diethylene triamine

$H_2N - CH_2 - CH_2 - (NH - CH_2 - CH_2)_2 - NH_2$

Triethylene tetramine

$N(CH_2 - CH_2 - OH))_3$

Triethanolamine

$H_2N - CH_2 - CH_2 - NH_2$

Ethylene diamine

Piperazine
(diethylenediamine)

Hexamethylene tetramine

$H_2N -$ ⟨⟩ $- CH_2 -$ ⟨⟩ $- NH_2$

Diaminodiphenylmethane

FIGURE 3. Structural formulas for selected aliphatic polyamine hardeners. Most of these have strong sensitizing potential.

settings.[23] Ethylene diamine, used as a rubber accelerator in the manufacture of rubber products (Fig. 3), was described as inducing bronchial asthma in two workers. Intracutaneous skin tests with 0.02 ml of ethylene diamine and hexamethylenetetramine (Fig. 3) as well as work-simulated bronchial provocation studies with ethylene diamine were positive.

Fourteen individuals from the beauty products industry with bronchial asthma (two also had rhinitis) have demonstrated skin reactivity to monoethanolamine and ethylene diamine in addition to ammonium thioglycolate (Fig. 4). All 14 were also reported to be atopic and sensitive to allergens unrelated to their occupation. All had an immediate wheal-and-flare

reaction to skin testing, and a positive work-simulated bronchial provocation test to work-related amine compounds.[23] Normal controls were reported to be negative.

An additional 14 individuals, half of whom were shellac handlers and the other half lacquer handlers, were also reported. The seven individuals who worked with shellac had come in contact with ethylene diamine used as a solvent. Six had bronchial asthma and one was reported to have allergic rhinitis. All had very positive intracutaneous skin tests to 1:100 dilution of ethylene diamine. Control subjects were negative. Work-simulated bronchial provocation produced either asthma, allergic rhinitis, or allergic skin manifestations. The lacquer

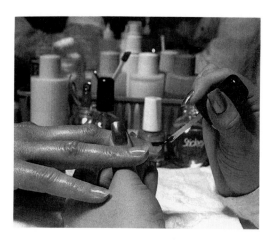

FIGURE 4.   Manicurist applying nailpolish on a client. A variety of resin products are employed, with both cutaneous and respiratory exposure. The most common resin system is a formaldehyde-toluene-sulfonamide resin.

handlers had been exposed to hexamethylenetetramine as a paint thinner. Each had bronchial asthma with a positive intracutaneous skin test response and work-simulated bronchial provocation to hexamethylenetetramine. Perhaps the most convincing evidence of immunologic sensitivity in Gelfand's report is the demonstration of passive transfer of antibody from two patients allergic to ethylene diamine[23] (Fig. 3).

Popa and his associates had an opportunity to study 33 patients with bronchial asthma and 15 said to have "asthmatic bronchitis" caused by occupational exposure to low-molecular-weight chemicals.[24] Asthmatic bronchitis was described as mild paroxysmal dyspnea with wheezing, cough, and some sputum production. Four subjects with exposure history to ethylene diamine were noted to develop dyspnea at work immediately after contact with the chemical. Both bronchial provocation and intracutaneous skin tests were positive, with an immediate wheal-and-flare reaction. Sputum eosinophilia was found in each of the subjects, and the PK reaction confirmed the transfer of antibody in each of the four individuals.[24]

Seven additional individuals also had substantial evidence of bronchial asthma secondary to paraphenylenediamine exposure. In this group the appearance of symptoms was delayed to the end of the workshift. It often reappeared nocturnally as a classic paroxysm of asthma. Similarly, intracutaneous skin test response was delayed (24–48 hrs) with positive patch tests to the chemical. Bronchial provocation

resulted in a delayed obstructive pattern 4 to 12 hours after exposure.[24] This group was felt to demonstrate immune mechanisms of a delayed hypersensitivity type. They postulated that Type-IV delayed hypersensitivity might be operative in bronchial asthma, but they admitted that much work would have to be done before this could be said to represent more than a hypothesis.[24] Although this work has not been repeated recently in other laboratories, one must wonder if these delayed obstructive patterns were a manifestation of an isolated late-phase asthmatic response. These authors also demonstrated the presence of some cross-sensitization by patch testing between paraphenylenediamine and at least one of the related substances—orthophenylenediamine, metaphenylenediamine, and tolulenediamine. They were not able to demonstrate any cross-reactivity between aminophylline and ethylene diamine.[23]

Pepys and Pickering described three patients who developed bronchial asthma due to fumes of aluminum soldering flux containing amino-ethyl ethanolamine.[25] Two patients demonstrated a biphasic asthmatic response to a work-simulated bronchial provocation. The third subject had an isolated delayed response. Immunologic studies were not carried out, but the challenge methodology used to demonstrate sensitivity was similar to that used by Sterling in a similar situation.[26]

Vallieres et al. reported the first case of allergic rhinitis and bronchial asthma secondary to an acquired sensitivity to dimethyl ethanolamine.[27] In this case, the dimethyl ethanolamine was used as a hardener in specially prepared paint. Because the dimethyl ethanolamine triggered an asthmatic response in the subject patient, but not in an asthmatic with greater underlying bronchial hyperreactivity (as demonstrated with histamine challenge), it was inferred that the effect of the amine compound was not an irritant effect analogous to that of histamine. In fact, the histamine inhalation test demonstrated the persistence of bronchial hyperreactivity 6 months after exposure to dimethyl ethanolamine had been discontinued. Because this study was retrospective in nature, it was not known whether the hyperreactivity preceded the occupational disorder or resulted from it.[27]

Fawcett and his colleagues reported on several cases of work-related asthma caused by low-molecular-weight chemicals. Among the seven subjects studied, one was found to react to the fumes of triethylene tetramine[28] (Fig. 2).

Work-simulated bronchial provocation revealed an isolated delayed reaction. The reaction was felt to be immunologic in nature, because traditional criteria for hypersensitivity were present, i.e., it affected only a minority of the workforce and required a latent period before symptoms appeared, and it was demonstrated that reactions were to subirritant concentrations to which other workers, and previously the subjects themselves, did not react.[28]

Lam and Chan-Yeung reported a patient with ethylene diamine-induced asthma in a photographic worker.[29] Other potential chemical sensitizers present at the workplace failed to elicit an asthmatic response. Bronchial provocation studies revealed an isolated delayed reaction without associated elevation in plasma histamine. Skin testing with ethylene diamine was negative. When the worker was removed from further exposure, the observed bronchial hyperreactivity decreased and approached the normal range.

Among the diamine low-molecular-weight chemicals, piperazine or diethylenediamine has been implicated more than any other compound in this class as a cause of respiratory sensitization (Fig. 3). Cutaneous and respiratory sensitivity to piperazine has been known since the mid-1960s. Its capacity to sensitize relates to the presence of two free NH groups in the 1,4 position. Piperazine is widely used in medical and veterinary practice in the treatment of worm infestations (i.e., a vermifuge or antihelmintic agent). It is also used as a component in the manufacture of many widely used phenothiazine tranquilizers (Atarax, Moditen, Isocurine) (Chapter 18). A number of contact allergy cases have also been reported to a cardiac stimulant (Antalby) containing the piperazine moiety.

Hagmar et al. observed that piperazine was the most common cause of asthma in workers in a Swedish chemical plant.[30] He found 29 of 130 workers with probable asthma. The asthma was described as a delayed or dual type. However, inhalational challenge testing was actually done for only one patient. This individual did not react to a nebulized solution of 10 mg piperazine dissolved in physiologic saline. The solution had a pH of 12. After inhalation of 50 mg of piperazine the patient had a delayed bronchoconstrictive reaction with a 50% fall in FEV_1. Two control subjects did not react to a similar challenge with 50 mg of inhaled piperazine solution.[30]

Pepys and Hutchcroft reported on two nonatopic asthmatic chemists who had developed an isolated delayed reaction on work-simulated bronchial provocation to piperazine. These investigators used a 2:1 mixture of lactose powder and piperazine dihydrochloride dust, to which the patient was exposed for 30 minutes.[31]

Hagmar et al. have continued to follow a cohort of 602 chemical workers for evidence of piperazine-induced respiratory disease. In a cross-sectional study using a questionnaire in former and current employees, this group reported a substantial risk of contracting airway symptoms from occupational exposure to piperazine.[32] They reported a correlation between the duration of exposure to piperazine and the incidence of respiratory disease including bronchial asthma and chronic bronchitis. Atopy was not associated with airway symptoms, and except for severe cough, none of the respiratory symptoms appeared to be influenced by smoking.[32] A later study was carried out to determine the pathogenetic role of specific IgE antibodies directed to piperazine. The study involved 140 workers in a chemical plant, some of whom were exposed to piperazine during the course of their work.[33] This group reported increased binding to a piperazine-human serum albumin conjugate in 6 of 72 employees exposed to the chemical. The binding was felt to be immunologic in only five patients, based on nearly complete inhibition with the piperazine conjugate. However, none of the patients with positive RAST studies had an unequivocal history of symptomatic asthma, and the authors were unable to find any association between the presence of IgE-specific antibodies to a piperazine-albumin conjugate and symptomatic asthma.[33]

In summary, the aliphatic polyamine hardeners used to produce the epoxy resins have the capacity to induce both irritant and allergic dermatitis. Their capacity to irritate derives from their strong alkaline composition and the proclivity to cause caustic damage. It has also been suggested that the low-molecular-weight amines might interact with body proteins to form potential allergens. Scientific proof of this hypothesis has never been clearly demonstrated. The polyamine hardeners have been linked to respiratory irritation with development of inflammatory bronchitis. Bronchial asthma has also been reported in workers exposed to the amine hardeners. The earlier descriptions of asthma were associated with positive intracutaneous skin tests, and several investigators reported the ability to passively transfer these immediate reactions to nonsensitized individuals. Bronchial provocation has been shown to produce immediate, delayed, and dual responses in affected workers. Although initial reports of isolated delayed responses were interpreted as having a probable immunologic connotation, there are a number of recent studies that have associated delayed asthmatic responses with nonimmune triggers, i.e., exercise[34] and distilled water.[35] All of the reports associating asthma with the polyamine hardeners have been retrospective in nature, and, interestingly enough, there have been no reports dealing with this association in the past decade. Further studies will be necessary before the pathogenetic mechanisms of polyamine-induced asthma are fully understood and, indeed, verified as authentic.

OCCUPATIONAL ALLERGY TO LATEX

Natural latex (rubber) is a polymer of isoprene and is obtained principally from the rubber tree, *Hevea braziliensis,* which is native to the Amazon region of South America. The British transplanted the tree to Southeast Asia where a plantation rubber industry has flourished. The milky latex in the *H. braziliensis* flows in canals immediately beneath the bark. To harvest this material, a cut is made in the bark and a cup placed beneath it. Approximately one deciliter is obtained with each cutting. Latex is a true excretory product, and the more that is harvested, the more that is formed.

There are a large number of other shrub and tree species within the spurge family (family Euphorbiaceae) that yield natural rubber latex. In addition, the guayule plant *(Parthenium argentatum),* a member of the large Compositae family also produces a natural latex product. The guayule was well known to the Aztecs and is the source of guayule rubber, which also contains an aliphatic hydrocarbon called cispolyisoprene common to natural latex. Despite the world's capacity to manufacture synthetic rubber from a nonrubber source beginning as far back as 1884, there continues to be a considerable demand for the natural product. The production of synthetic rubber developed using butadiene in the case of **Buna** rubber, and chloroprene in the case of **neoprene** rubber (Fig. 5).

In the generation of the final rubber product, vulcanization is used as a hardening process and incorporates sulfur into the matrix. Piperazine is employed as a vulcanization retarder. Thiuram monosulfide and tetramethylthiuram disulfide are two commonly used vulcanization accelerators. Other ingredients are added to improve the quality of the final product, e.g., antioxidants are added to retard aging in air and light, and plasticizers to improve its handling and subsequent shaping.

Commercial applications of latex products are continually expanding, and it has been estimated that more than 40,000 rubber products are in use at the present time.[36] Only a

$$CH_2 = C - CH = CH_2$$
$$|$$
$$CH_3$$

Isoprene

$$CH_2 = C - CH = CH_2$$
$$|$$
$$H$$

Butadine

FIGURE 5. Structural formulas for several rubber materials.

$$CH_2 = C - CH = CH_2$$
$$|$$
$$Cl$$

Chloroprene

limited number are sufficiently encountered to pose a risk to either primary sensitization or a reaction in an already sensitized individual (Table 3). Sensitization to latex can occur as a result of both occupational or non-work-related exposures. Prior to 1979, most of the problems related to natural or synthetic rubbers presented as contact allergic dermatitis.[37-40]

Despite the wide application of natural latex in industry and society (Table 3), reports of immediate hypersensitivity were nonexistent until 1979, when Nutter reported the first case of contact urticaria.[41] Since that time the number of case reports relating to immediate hypersensitivity has virtually exploded.[36] The increased incidence of latex allergy has been associated with the widespread use of latex gloves and condoms to protect against acquired immune deficiency syndrome, infectious hepatitis, and other infectious processes. The clinical presentation of immediate hypersensitivity has taken a spectrum of syndromes, including contact urticaria and angioedema,[42-50] allergic rhinitis and/or bronchial asthma,[51-55] and systemic anaphylaxis.[56-60] Although the reactions described can be quite severe, at the time of this writing there were no published scientific reports of deaths related to latex exposure. However, there have been media reports of at least four deaths in patients undergoing barium enemas linked to an allergic reaction to a latex cuff.[61] The majority of these immediate-type reactions have been associated with latex gloves, anesthesia or radiological equipment, and some isolated cases involving condom use.

Populations appearing to be at greater risk include medical, dental, and janitorial workers who are wearing latex gloves throughout their work day. Patients with ostomies or those requiring repeated bladder catheterizations or surgical procedures are also at higher risk. In addition, a higher incidence of latex allergy has been noted in atopic patients, and especially in those with active atopic dermatitis.[36] The latter is said to disrupt the natural skin barrier, facilitating direct adsorption of latex proteins. In addition to individuals who use latex products for worker protection, latex hypersensitivity has recently been reported in a worker employed by a surgical glove manufacturing plant.[55] A survey of the plant uncovered 6% of the workers who had pulmonary function evidence of latex-related occupational asthma. Similarly, Turjanmaa reported 7.4% of surgeons and 5.6% of operating room nurses manifested clinical symptoms of latex sensitization confirmed by skin prick testing and RAST testing.[62] Although almost all cases of latex hypersensitivity have been in adults, Axelsson has reported instances in children.[56] The latter is interesting given the frequent use of rubber pacifiers, rubber nipples on feeding bottles, and rubberized teething rings that children are exposed to on a daily basis. One wonders if there is any relation between these common exposures and underlying atopic state and sudden infant death syndrome.

Attempts to characterize the relevant allergens in latex have yielded conflicting results. There have been convincing demonstrations that natural latex, products made from latex, and extracts derived from the *H. braziliensis* bind IgE in latex-sensitive patients.[36] A variety of rubber products have been shown to contain soluble antigens that will elicit a wheal-and-flare response in performing an epicutaneous test in a sensitized patient. Significant amounts of reactive proteins can be eluted in minutes from latex products. Carillo et al. attempted to isolate the reactogenic antigen and felt it had a molecular weight greater than 30 kDa.[52] Seaton implicated carene, a bicyclic terpene composed of two molecules of isoprene (Fig. 5) as the reactive agent.[54] Turjanmaa et al. fractionated a number of proteins from latex gloves and isolated allergenic fractions with molecular weights of 2, 5 and 30 kDa.[48] Morales et al. isolated four latex proteins that bound IgE with molecular weights of 10, 14, 35 and 100 kDa.[63] Slater was able to demonstrate specific binding of IgG and IgE to a 14 kDa latex protein.[59] Warpinski et al. found active binding at 30 and 66 kDa and felt this was best explained

TABLE 3. *Commonly Encountered Products Containing Latex*

Baby nipples	Golf grips
Balloons	Headsets
Bandages	Latex cuffs[†]
Belts	Milking machines
Brassieres	Ostomy bags
Catheters	Paint
Chewing gum	Pacifiers
Clothing	Rubber bands
Condoms	Rubber cement
Corsets	Shoewear
Dental cofferdams	Suspenders
Face masks*	Surgical gloves
Foam pillows	Tennis grip
Garden hoses	Teething ring
Gloves	Weatherstripping

* Dust and vapor canister masks as well as anesthesia masks.
   † Used in the delivery of barium enemas.

by a 66 kDa glycoprotein that was a dimer of the smaller antigen.[36]

Exquisitely sensitive patients may have to seek alternative work due to severe work-related inhalant allergy and asthma. However, most patients in recent studies have been able to limit exposure and continue their work. Some may require symptomatic treatment intermittently. Health care workers have been urged to carry their own non-latex gloves for possible emergencies.[63a]

In summary, contrary to what has occurred with many other occupational antigens, latex sensitivity and the incidence of adverse reactions to it are on the rise. The emergence of this trend appears closely related to the dissemination of the human immunodeficiency virus, and the need for protection with the use of latex gloves and condoms. It may become increasingly necessary to develop rubber products that have a very stable inner matrix incapable of releasing latex antigen. In the interim, clinicians must be alert to this new potential for both work and non-work-related allergy. This is especially true in the medical, dental, and janitorial fields, where gloves have become firmly entrenched as a necessary protection.

HYPERSENSITIVITY TO THE REACTIVE DYES, ASSOCIATED AZO COMPOUNDS, AND OTHER UNRELATED DYES

The initial reactive dye for cotton was marketed in 1956 by Imperial Chemical Industries (ICI) and since that time hundreds have appeared on the market. They are widely employed because of their bright colors and capacity to bind to cellulose, protein, and polyamide fibers. The dye moiety contains a chromophobic system (usually an azo or anthracene group), hydrophilic groups to improve water solubility, and reactive groups such as a heterocyclic halogen unit or an aliphatic chain with reactive groups. The reactive groups are capable of forming covalent bonds with hydroxyl and amino groups in the fiber molecule[64] (Fig. 6).

Employment of reactive dyes has been very popular due to excellent colorfastness, despite

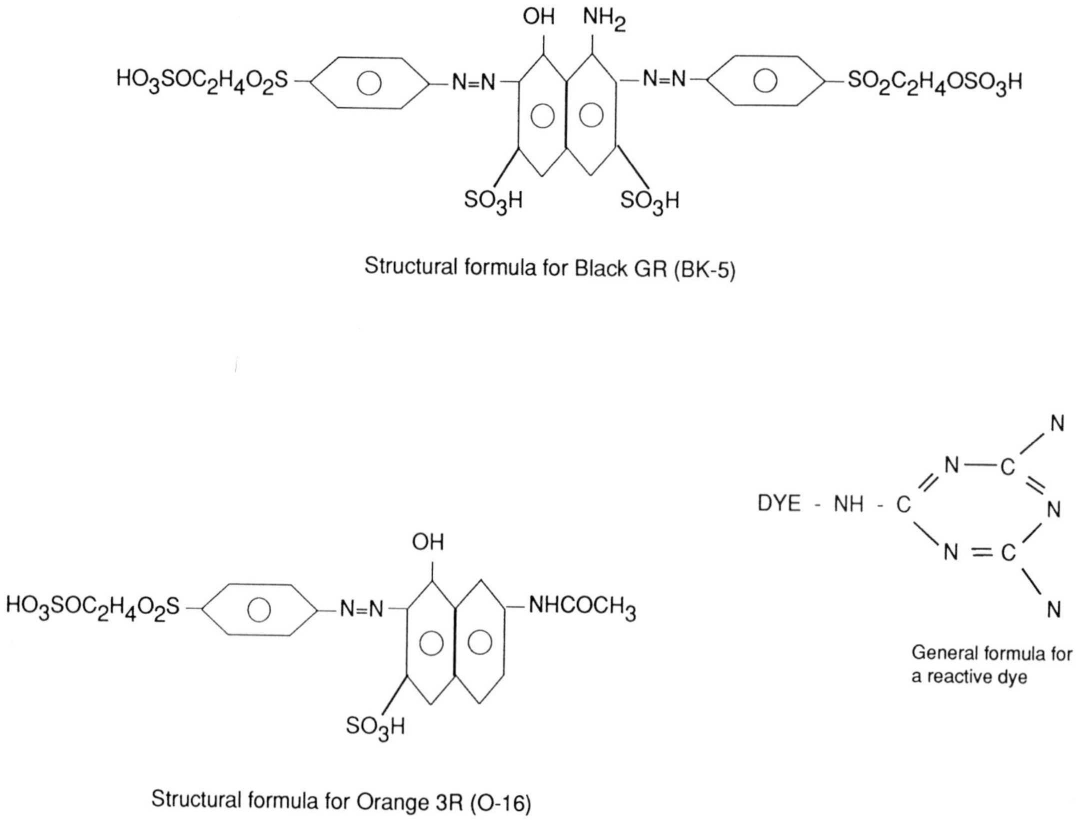

Structural formula for Black GR (BK-5)

Structural formula for Orange 3R (O-16)

General formula for a reactive dye

FIGURE 6.   General structural formula for a reactive dye and specific chemical formulas for two frequently used dyes, i.e., Black GR (BK-5) and Orange 3R (O-16).

repeated bleaching and washing. There is remarkable heterogeneity between these various dyes, but they do share common characteristics of reacting and binding covalently to nucleophilic groups. A number of different reactive groups have been employed in this system. Sulfotoethyl sulfon or dichlorotriazine reactive groups have been used commonly.

Although the number of reported adverse reactions to these reactogenic dyes has been small in number, several reports have associated respiratory or nasal symptoms and exposure to these dyes. Most of these observations have appeared in the last decade.[64-70] It is not known to what extent the reactive group is important to the immunologic response. Direct dyeing of RAST discs has been used to assay dye-specific IgE.[64] However, recent studies have found this technique unreliable.[71]

Luczynska and Topping initially reported good results employing an optimized preparation of conjugates between human serum albumin and dye, which resulted in efficient binding of specific IgE.[67] Wass et al. showed significant levels of specific IgE binding in a patient's sera, whereas sera from 36 exposed workers without symptoms and sera from unexposed subjects with high total IgE were entirely negative.[71] Available data suggest that physical adsorption of the dye may play a major role and that covalent bonds may not be necessary in the in vivo formation of hapten-carrier conjugates.[71]

A Korean group of investigators in Seoul recently studied 309 workers in a reactive dye plant.[72-74] A questionnaire survey revealed that 78 (25.2%) had work-related upper or lower respiratory symptoms. Among these employees, 38 (48.7%) manifested nonspecific bronchial hyperreactivity. Thirteen symptomatic employees with a methacholine PC_{20} less than 5 mg/ml showed immediate (six), dual (six), or solitary delayed (one) responses after inhalation of four types of reactive dyes tested. Twenty-five workers showed immediate skin reactions to Black GR dye, whereas 21 workers manifested reactions to Orange 3R dye (Fig. 6). Fifty-three employees had serum-specific IgE antibodies against Black GR and/or Orange 3R dyes. Specific IgE was detected more frequently in symptomatic employees (30%) and smokers (100%). No association was found between atopy and specific IgE binding. RAST inhibition tests of Black GR revealed significant dose-response inhibitors by Black GR-HSA conjugate and minimal inhibitions by unconjugated Black GR. Orange 3R RAST

inhibition tests revealed significant inhibitions by conjugated forms of Orange 3R and Black GR and some inhibitions by two unconjugated forms of the two dyes, suggesting immunologic cross-reactivity between them. These new data support the contention that the reactive dyes can induce IgE-mediated responses in exposed employees, which lead to the induction of allergic occupational asthma.

Quite apart from what has been described above with the reactive dyes, cochineal is a natural dye extracted from the insect *Dactylopius coccus,* a tropical American species that feeds on certain cacti. The pigment is called carmine. Burge et al. reported two patients with work-related asthma to carmine in 1979.[75] One of the two patients worked at a facility where the dye was being extracted from insects and the other used carmine as a cosmetic colorant (Fig. 4). Both patients had dual asthmatic reactions after carmine inhalation. Oral challenge induced gastrointestinal symptoms in one patient and bronchial asthma in both patients. Skin testing with the extract of *Dactylopius coccus* was positive. Up to this point, there had been no other reports of respiratory symptoms due to carmine, although a contact cheilitis had been reported in 1961.[76]

Methyl blue is a frequently used dye both within the textile industry and as an ink for recording electrocardiography studies. It is a disodium salt of benzenesulfonic acid with a molecular weight of 800 Da. It is highly soluble in water, making it an excellent dye for cotton and silk. It also has antiseptic properties. Several cases of occupational asthma have been reported in hospital technicians as a result of repeated inhalation of ink aerosol near electrocardiographic machines[77-79] (Fig. 7). Dye-specific IgE antibodies have been demonstrated to methyl blue,[77] and both nasal and bronchial provocation studies have confirmed the diagnosis.[77,78]

Azodicarbonamide is a low-molecular-weight amide used in industry as an expanding and blowing agent for resins and rubbers. It is generally a fine yellow powder, and it is said to release a large volume of gas when heated. In the past it was utilized to mature and bleach cereal flours. The initial report of asthma secondary to inhalation of azodicarbonamide powder was in 1971, when Ferris et al. reported 10 cases in a grinding factory,[80] with subsequent additional reports occurring in other parts of the world.[81,82] Almost all cases develop after a latent period of 6 to 12 months. Symptoms are typically of a delayed nature. As in

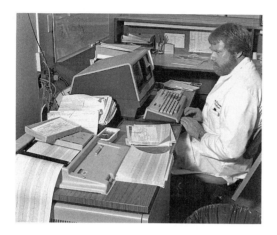

FIGURE 7. Technician generating graphic reproductions of tracings is exposed to methyl blue vapors for significant portions of the work day.

the case with other low-molecular chemicals, no increased incidence of azodicarbonamide-induced asthma has been reported in atopic workers.[83] There have also been a number of observations linking eczematoid dermatitis with azodicarbonamide.[84]

A highly reactive chemical category is comprised of colors resulting from the combination inside the fiber of a diazo compound (or a diazonium salt) and a coupling component. The diazonium salts and coupling components generally have small molecules, permitting easy penetration into the interior of a fiber. Because of the instability of the diazonium salt, the preparation is carried out at low temperatures (0–5°C), and the dye procedure is often referred to as "ice-dyeing." Aside from the dye manufacturing industry, diazonium compounds are also used in the photocopying industry. Armeli reported four cases of occupational asthma after exposure to diazonium chloride.[85] Graham et al. described an individual with delayed, recurrent asthma associated with the use of diazonium chloride in the production of photocopying paper.[86] Recently, Luczynska et al. described sensitization to a diazonium salt intermediate—diazonium tetrafluoroborate (DTFB)—produced during the manufacture of a fluorine polymer precursor.[87] Most workers studied were felt to have suffered mucosal irritation. However, 20% of 43 exposed workers had developed IgE-specific antibodies to DTFB-human serum albumin conjugates. There was a correlation between the presence of IgE-specific antibody and exposure-related respiratory symptoms. In two individuals clinical and immunologic

studies including bronchial provocation testing, and specific IgE measurements confirmed a diagnosis of occupational asthma.

OCCUPATIONAL ASTHMA DUE TO INHALATION OF AMMONIUM PERSULPHATE SALT AND HENNA IN HAIRDRESSERS

A variety of substances have been noted to have the potential to sensitize workers in the hairdressing industry. The persulfate salts are the most notable of these reactive chemicals. In the past, ammonium and potassium persulfate were used in some European countries to improve the appearance of bread by whitening it. It was reported as a frequent cause of contact dermatitis in bakers.[88,89] It was also noted that some bakers had immediate hypersensitivity to ammonium persulfate, probably because it was acting as a direct histamine liberator.[88-92]

There are over a half-million cosmetologists employed in the U.S. It has been estimated that about a third operate their own businesses, sometimes in small underventilated store-front salons, and not infrequently in their own homes. Hairdressers and hairstylists apply bleaches, dyes, and tints to hair using an applicator or brush. They also may shampoo and rinse hair. In carrying out these tasks they are exposed to a number of irritants and allergens[88,89,93] (Fig. 8).

The presence of ammonium persulfate as an accelerator in hair bleaches has been reported to cause anaphylaxis in some individuals.[93] In some cases the mechanism was felt to be a direct histamine liberation, whereas in others an IgE-mediated reaction is felt to be operative. Very early on Brun et al. demonstrated typical wheal-and-flare reactions to epicutaneous testing with ammonium persulfate.[94] These authors described the induction of bronchial asthma and anaphylaxis with skin testing. In addition to acceleration of the bleaching reaction, persulfates also reduce the amount of peroxide that must be used. They also facilitate the attainment of a lighter shade.

The majority of immediate respiratory allergic reactions has been reported in the European literature. The earliest observations were made by Barsotti et al. in Italy.[95] This group studied eczematoid dermatitis and asthmatic reactions in 106 factory workers engaged in the production of hydrogen peroxide. This constituent was produced by the continuous transformation of potassium bisulfate into potassium persulfate in the presence of ammonium persulphate. Of

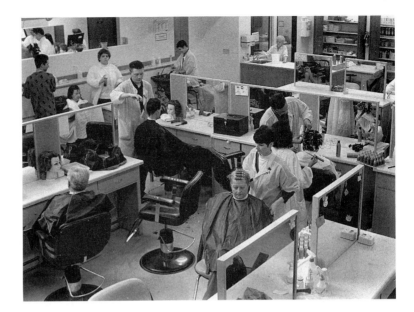

FIGURE 8. Relatively large beauty salon operation with employees performing a variety of operations. Over a half-million cosmetologists are employed in the U.S., and most are exposed to a variety of irritants and allergens.

the 106 workers studied, 34% showed an eczematoid dermatitis and 15% were diagnosed as having an asthmatic bronchitis, both of which were felt to be work-related. Symptoms usually appeared within the first year of work after a brief latent period. Patch tests with ammonium persulphate were positive in 32 of 46 workers, whereas patch testing with potassium persulfate and other constituents was negative. The most important observation made by these workers was the fact that bronchial provocation with aerosols of ammonium persulphate reproduced asthmatic symptoms in a number of workers, suggesting an IgE-mediated process.[95]

Meindl and Meyer reported the development of bronchial asthma and urticaria in hairdressers secondary to persulfates.[96] Pepys et al. studied two female hairdressers with work-related asthma.[97] Skin tests and bronchial provocation were carried out. One was found to be having an immediate asthmatic reaction to fumes originating from a mixture of bleach containing potassium persulphate and hydrogen peroxide. Epicutaneous skin tests as well as patch tests with sodium and potassium persulphate were positive for immediate reactions. The other worker was observed to have a delayed asthmatic reaction with negative skin tests to persulphate preparations, but an immediate cutaneous and asthmatic response to henna extract.[97] Among the dyes used by hairdressers, henna is a reddish brown vegetal dye from the Asian plant *Lawsonia inermis* (the mignonette tree) that is infrequently used. Henna is a catechol derivative and is also referred to as Natural Orange-6 and has the chemical name

2-hydroxy 1,4-naphtha-quinone. It is found in some commercial hair rinses and nail dyes. It has some anti-fungal properties and has been used as a sunscreen in the past.

The most recent observation of persulfate-induced allergy was reported by Pankow et al.[98] These workers reported a young hairdresser who developed rhinoconjunctivitis and bronchial asthma after a relatively long latent period of 2 years. The agent that was incriminated was a hair bleach containing persulfate. Her symptoms were immediate and believed to be IgE-mediated. Epicutaneous skin test and bronchial provocation both resulted in an immediate reaction.

OCCUPATIONAL ASTHMA DUE TO POLYVINYL CHLORIDE RESINS

Polyvinyl chloride (PVC) resins are widely used in industry. PVC suspension resins are granular in nature and usually dust-free. PVC emulsion resins are small particles and are known to contain small amounts of free monomer.[99] Depending on the manufacturing process and the product generated, PVC resins are generally used with admixtures of stabilizers (to reduce degradation), lubricants, plasticizers (to facilitate flexibility), blowing agents, and pigments.[99] One product that remains popular is PVC soft wrap film, which is employed to package meat and other produce in retail food markets (Fig. 9).

Clinical symptoms related to exposure to PVC meatwrapping fumes were first noted in

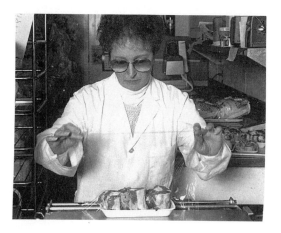

FIGURE 9.   Meatwrapper employing polyvinyl chloride wrap cut with a relatively cold wire. There is essentially no pyrolysis with this technique.

Virginia in 1969, prompting an initial investigation by Polakoff and Vandervort.[100] These studies suggested air contaminants produced by thermal cutting of PVC film caused mucous membrane irritation. In 1973 Sokol et al. published his series of three meatwrappers who developed acute bronchospasm while working.[101] The authors attributed these respiratory symptoms to prolonged exposure to PVC soft wrap film. In 1975 work-simulated bronchial provocation studies carried out by Andrasch et al. indicated that the mucous membrane irritation and bronchospasm in meatwrappers were primarily related to the pyrolytic fumes generated by price-label adhesive.[102-104] Later studies revealed the thermal decomposition products of PVC soft wrap to contain di-2-ethyl-hexyl adipate, hydrogen chloride, and ional and benzyl chloride.[105] Thermal decomposition products of price-label adhesive contained phthalate anhydride along with dicyclohexylphthalate, cyclohexonal, and a quinone derivative.[106] Ultimately it was demonstrated that the major cause of occupational asthma in meatwrappers was phthalate anhydride.[104] The pyrolytic products of PVC film were implicated as a primary irritant and capable of aggravating preexisting disease. However, none of the constituents has ever been shown to act as a sensitizer. With the automation of the wrapping and labeling process in an enclosed, vented machine, meatwrappers' asthma has all but vanished.[107]

Aside from the pyrolytic products of PVC clear wrap film, pulmonary disease has been associated with exposure to vinyl chloride fumes as well as PVC resin dust.[108-113] Abnormalities

in pulmonary function and a spectrum of lower respiratory symptoms have been reported in workers exposed to PVC dust.[112,113] Both pneumoconiosis[108-110] and interstitial lung disease[111] has been reported with vinyl chloride fumes and PVC resin dust.

Recently Lee and associates reported on a case of occupational asthma caused by unheated PVC resin dust.[114] This was confirmed by bronchial provocation, which generated 0.12 mg/M^3 of PVC respirable dust. A delayed asthmatic response was noted about 9 hours after exposure.

REFERENCES

1. Kern RA: Asthma and allergic rhinitis due to sensitization to phthalate anhydride. J Allergy 10:164, 1939.
2. Vaughn WT: The Practice of Allergy. St. Louis, C.V. Mosby, 1939, pp 677.
3. Anon: Asthma induced by epoxy resin systems [editorial]. Br Med J 2:655, 1977.
4. Eckardt RE, Hindin R: The health hazards of plastics. J Occup Med 15:808, 1973.
5. NIOSH: Glycidyl ethers. Current Intelligence Bulletin, Publication 79-104. Cincinnati, OH, U.S. Dept. of Health, Education and Welfare, Public Health Service, National Institute of Occupational Safety and Health, 1978.
6. Lee H, Neville K: Handbook of Epoxy Resins. New York, McGraw-Hill, 1967.
7. Foussereau J, Benezra C, Maibach H: Occupational Contact Dermatitis. Philadelphia, W.B. Saunders Co., 1982, pp 216-235.
8. Dernehl CU: Clinical experiences with exposures to ethylene amines. Ind Med Surg 20:541, 1951.
9. Grandjean E: The danger of dermatoses due to cold-setting ethoxylene resins (epoxide resins). Br J Ind Med 14:1, 1957.
10. Morris GE: Epoxy resins. AMA Arch Derm 76:757, 1957.
11. Fregert S: Epoxy dermatitis from the non-working environment. Br J Derm 105(Suppl 21):63, 1981.
12. Thorgeirsson A, Fregert S: Allergenicity of epoxy resins in the guinea pig. Acta Derm Venereol 57:253, 1978.
13. Fregert S: Contact dermatitis from epoxy resin systems. In Maibach HI, Gellin GA (eds): Occupational and Industrial Dermatology. Chicago, Year Book Medical Publishers, 1982, pp 285-288.
14. NIOSH: A recommended standard for occupational exposure to epichlorohydrin. Cincinnati, OH, U.S. Dept. of Health, Education and Welfare, Public Health Service, National Institute of Occupational Safety and Health, 1977.
15. Epstein E: Allergy to epichlorohydrin masquerading as trichlorhydrin allergy. Contact Dermatitis Newsletter 16:475, 1974.
16. van Joost TH: Occupational sensitization to epichlorhydrin and epoxy resin. Contact Dermatitis 19:278, 1988.
17. Bourne LB, Milner FJM, Alberman KB: Health problems of epoxy resins and amine curing agents. Br J Ind Med 16:81, 1981.
18. Hine CH, Kodama JK, Anderson HH, et al: The toxicology of epoxy resins. Arch Ind Health 17:129, 1958.

19. Pletscher A, Schuppli R, Reifert R: Uber Gesundheids-schaden durch Giessharze. Z Unfallmed Berufskr 47:83, 1954.
20. Tolot F, Colin M, Soubrier R: Asthme et Araldite. Arch Mal Prof 3:163, 1961.
21. Fawcett IW: Asthma caused by fumes from pine rosin and epoxy resin systems. In Frazier CA (ed): Occupational Asthma. New York, Van Nostrand Reinhold, 1980, pp 283–295.
22. Dernehl CU: Hazards to health associated with the use of epoxy resins. J Occup Med 5:17, 1963.
23. Gelfand HH: Respiratory allergy due to chemical compounds encountered in the rubber, lacquer, shellac and beauty culture industries. J Allergy 34:374, 1963.
24. Popa V, Teculescu D, Stanescu D, et al: Bronchial asthma and asthmatic bronchitis determined by simple chemicals. Dis Chest 56:395, 1969.
25. Pepys J, Pickering CAC: Asthma due to inhaled chemical fumes: Amino-ethyl ethanolamine in aluminum soldering flux. Clin Allergy 2:197, 1972.
26. Sterling GM: Asthma due to aluminum soldering flux. Thorax 22:533, 1967.
27. Vallieres M, Cockcroft DW, Taylor DM, et al: Dimethyl ethanolamine-induced asthma. Am Rev Respir Dis 115:867, 1977.
28. Fawcett IW, Newman-Taylor AJ, Pepys J: Asthma due to inhaled chemical agents: Epoxy resin systems containing phthalic acid anhydride, trimellitic acid anhydride and triethylene tetramine. Clin Allergy 7:1, 1977.
29. Lam S, Chan-Yeung M: Ethylenediamine-induced asthma. Am Rev Respir Dis 121:151, 1980.
30. Hagmar L, Bellender J, Bergod B, et al: Piperazine-induced occupational asthma. J Occup Med 24:193, 1982.
31. Pepys J, Hutchcroft B: Bronchial provocation tests in etiologic diagnosis and analysis of asthma. Am Rev Respir Dis 112:829, 1975.
32. Hagmar L, Bellender J, Ranstam T, et al: Piperazine-induced airway symptoms: Exposure-response relationships and selection in an occupational setting. Am J Ind Med 6:347, 1984.
33. Hagmar L, Welinder H: Prevalence of specific IgE antibodies against piperazine in employees of a chemical plant. Int Arch Allergy Appl Immunol 81:12, 1986.
34. Horn CR, Jones RM, Lee D, et al: Late response in exercise-induced asthma. Clin Allergy 14:307, 1984.
35. Matroli S, Foresi A, Corbo GM, et al: Effects of two doses of cromolyn on allergen-induced late asthmatic response and increased responsiveness. J Allergy Clin Immunol 79:747, 1987.
36. Warpinski JR, Folgert J, Cohen M, Bush RK: Allergic reaction to latex: A risk factor for unsuspected anaphylaxis. Allergy Proc 12:95, 1991.
37. Adams RM: Occupational Skin Disease. New York, Grune & Stratton, 1983, p 298.
38. Rodriquez E, Reynolds GW, Thompson JA: Potent contact allergen in the rubber plant guayule (Parthenium argentatum). Science 211:1444, 1981.
39. Baginsky E: Occupational skin disease. San Francisco, CA, State Dept. of Ind. Relations, Division of Labor Statistics and Research, 1982.
40. Fregert S: Occupational dermatitis in a 10-year material. Contact Dermatitis 1:96, 1975.
41. Nutter AF: Contact urticaria to rubber. Br J Dermatol 101:597, 1979.
42. Forstrom L: Contact urticaria from latex surgical gloves. Contact Dermatitis 6:33, 1980.
43. Kopman A, Hunnaksela M: Contact urticaria to rubber. Duodecim 99:221, 1983.
44. Meding B, Fregert S: Contact urticaria from natural latex gloves. Contact Dermatitis 10:52, 1984.
45. Kleinhans D: Contact urticaria to rubber gloves. Contact Dermatitis 10:125, 1984.
46. Frosch PJ, Wohl R, Bahmer FA, et al: Contact urticaria to rubber gloves is IgE-mediated. Contact Dermatitis 14:241, 1986.
47. Grattan CEH, Kennedy CTC: Angioedema during dental treatment. Contact Dermatitis 13:333, 1985.
48. Turjanmaa K, Laurila K, Makinen-Kiljunen S, et al: Rubber contact urticaria. Allergic properties of 19 brands of latex gloves. Contact Dermatitis 19:302, 1988.
49. Turjanmaa K, Reunala T: Contact urticaria from rubber gloves. Dermatol Clin North Am 6:47, 1988.
50. Geimeier WJ, Minor C, Wales B, et al: Immediate systemic allergic reactions to latex rubber. Pediatr Asthma Allergy Immunol 4:65, 1990.
51. Axelsson JG, Johansson SG, Wrangsjo K: IgE-mediated anaphylactoid reactions to rubber. Allergy 42:46, 1987.
52. Carillo T, Cuevas M, Munoz T, et al: Contact urticaria and rhinitis from latex surgical gloves. Contact Dermatitis 15:69, 1986.
53. Spaner D, Dolovich J, Tarlo S, et al: Hypersensitivity to natural latex. J Allergy Clin Immunol 83:1135, 1989.
54. Seaton A, Cherrie B, Turnbull J: Rubber glove asthma. Br Med J 296:531, 1988.
55. Tarlo SM, Wong L, Roos J, et al: Occupational asthma caused by latex in a surgical glove manufacturing plant. J Allergy Clin Immunol 85:626, 1990.
56. Axelsson IGK, Eriksson M, Wrangsjo K: Anaphylaxis and angioedema due to rubber allergy in children. Acta Pediatr Scand 77:314, 1988.
57. Taylor JS, Cassettari J, Wagner W, et al: Contact urticaria and anaphylaxis to latex. J Am Acad Dermatol 21:874, 1989.
58. Segger JS, Mawhinney TP, Yunginger J, et al: Anaphylaxis due to surgical glove powder. J Allergy Clin Immunol 83:267, 1989.
59. Slater JE: Rubber anaphylaxis. N Engl J Med 320:1126, 1989.
60. Jancelowicz Z, Sussman G, Tarlo S, et al: Clinical presentation of five patients allergic to latex. J Allergy Clin Immunol 83:267, 1989.
61. Healy M, Snead E: The risk of latex allergies growing. USA Today D-1, V. 5-29-91.
62. Turjanmaa K: Incidence of immediate allergy to latex gloves in hospital personnel. Contact Dermatitis 17:270, 1987.
63. Morales C, Basomba A, Carreira J, et al: Anaphylaxis produced by rubber glove contact: Case reports and identification of the antigens involved. Clin Exp Allergy 19:425, 1989.
63a. Sussman GL, Tarlo S, Dolovich J: The spectrum of IgE-mediated responses to latex. JAMA 265:2844, 1991.
64. Alanko K, Keskinen H, Bjorksten F, et al: Immediate hypersensitivity to reactive dyes. Clin Allergy 8:25, 1978.
65. Kalas D, Runstukova J: The effect of working with ostazine dyes on the development of bronchospasm and occupational bronchial asthma. Pracovny Lekarskri 32:103, 1980.
66. Stern MA: Occupational asthma from a reactive dye. Ann Allergy 55:264, 1985.
67. Luczynska CM, Topping MD: Specific IgE antibodies to reactive dye-albumin conjugates. J Immunol Methods 95:177, 1986.

68. Hagmar L, Welinder H, Dahlquist I: Immunoglobulin E antibodies against a reactive dye—a case report. Scand J Work Environ Health 12:221, 1986.

69. Docker A, Wattie JM, Topping MD, et al: Clinical and immunological investigations of respiratory disease in workers using reactive dyes. Br J Ind Med 44:534, 1987.

70. Thoren K, Meding B, Nordlinder R, et al: Contact dermatitis and asthma from reactive dyes. Contact Dermatitis 15:186, 1986.

71. Wass U, Nilsson R, Nordlinder R, et al: An optimized assay of specific IgE antibodies to reactive dyes and studies of immunologic responses in exposed workers. J Allergy Clin Immunol 85:642, 1990.

72. Park HS, Kim YJ, Lee MK, Hong CS: Occupational asthma and specific IgE antibodies to reactive dyes. Yonsei Med J 30:298, 1989.

73. Park HS, Lee MK, Kim BO, et al: Clinical and immunologic evaluations of reactive dye-exposed workers. J Allergy Clin Immunol 87:639, 1991.

74. Park HS, Hong CS: The significance of specific IgG and IgG$_4$ antibodies to a reactive dye in exposed workers. Clin Exper Allergy 21:357, 1991.

75. Burge PS, O'Brien IM, Harries MG, et al: Occupational asthma due to inhaled carmine. Clin Allergy 9:185, 1979.

76. Sarkany I, Meara RH, Everall J: Cheilitis due to carmine in lip salve. Trans Ann Report of St. John's Hosp Derm Soc 46:39, 1961 (cited in ref. 60).

77. Keskinen H, Nordman H, Terho EO: ECG ink as a cause of asthma. Allergy 36:275, 1981.

78. Rodenstein D, Stanescu DC: Bronchial asthma following exposure to ECG ink. Ann Allergy 48:351, 1982.

79. Norback D, Larsson E, Gothe CJ: Emission of ink aerosol from ink-jet recorders. Am Ind Hyg J 46:85, 1985.

80. Ferris BG, Peters JM, Burgess WA, et al: Apparent effect of an azodicarbonamide in the lungs. A preliminary report. J Occup Med 19:424, 1977.

81. Slovak AJM: Occupational asthma caused by a plastics blowing agent, azodicarbonamide. Thorax 36:906, 1981.

82. Malo JL, Pineau L, Cartier A: Occupational asthma due to azobisformamide. Clin Allergy 15:261, 1985.

83. Normand J-C, Grange F, Hernandez C, et al: Occupational asthma after exposure to azodicarbonamide: Report of four cases. Br J Ind Med 46:60, 1989.

84. Bonsal JL: Allergic contact dermatitis to azodicarbonamide. Contact Dermatitis 10:42, 1984.

85. Armeli G: Asma bronchiale da sali di diazonio. Med Lav 59:463, 1986.

86. Graham V, Coe MSJ, Davies RJ: Occupational asthma after exposure to a diazonium salt. Thorax 36:950, 1981.

87. Luczynska CM, Hutchcroft BJ, Harrison MA, et al: Occupational asthma and specific IgE to a diazonium salt intermediate used in the polymer industry. J Allergy Clin Immunol 85:1076, 1990.

88. Calnan CD, Shuster S: Reactions to ammonium persulfate. Arch Dermatol 112:1407, 1976.

89. Fisher AA, Doms-Goossens A: Persulphate hair bleach reactions. Arch Dermatol 112:1407, 1976.

90. Young E: Allergic reactions in bakers. Dermatologica 148:39, 1964.

91. Subiza E: Eczema and asthma caused by the combination of flour and ammonium persulfate. Allergologica 1:343, 1951.

92. Grianti V, Bartalini E: Allergy in workmen in mills. Rass Med Ind 22:257, 1953.

93. Brubaker MM: Urticarial reactions to ammonium persulfate. Arch Dermatol 106:413, 1972.

94. Brun R, Jadascohn W, Paillard R: Epicutaneous test with immediate type reaction to ammonium persulfate. Dermatologica 133:89, 1960.

95. Barsotti M, Parmeggiani L, Sassi C: Symptoms of bronchial asthma and eczema in workers assigned to hydrogen peroxide production units. Medicina del Lavoro 42:49, 1951.

96. Meindl VK, Meyer R: Asthma and urticaria in hairdressers caused by bleaching agents containing persulfates. Zentralblatt fur Arbeitsmed. Arbeitschutz 19:75, 1969.

97. Pepys J, Hutchcroft BJ, Breslin ABX: Asthma due to inhaled chemical agents: Persulfate salts and henna in hairdressers. Clin Allergy 6:399, 1976.

98. Pankow W, Hein H, Bittner K, et al: Asthma in hairdressers induced by persulfate. Pneumologie 43:173, 1989.

99. Wheeler RN Jr: Poly (vinyl chloride) processes and products. Environ Health Perspect 41:123, 1981.

100. Polakoff PL, Vandervort R: Health hazard evaluation determination. Reports 52–58. Thermal decomposition products of PVC meatwrapping film. Cincinnati, OH, National Institute of Occupational Safety and Health, 1973.

101. Sokol WN, Aelony Y, Beall GN: Meatwrappers' asthma. A new syndrome? JAMA 226:639, 1973.

102. Andrasch RH, Bardana EJ: Thermo-activated price label intolerance: A cause of meatwrappers' asthma. JAMA 235:937, 1976.

103. Andrasch RH, Bardana EJ, Koster F, et al: Clinical and bronchial provocation studies in patients with meatwrappers' asthma. J Allergy Clin Immunol 58:291, 1976.

104. Bardana EJ, Anderson CJ, Andrasch RH: Meatwrappers' asthma: Clinical and pathogenetic observations. In Frazier CA (ed): Occupational Asthma. New York, Van Nostrand Reinhold, 1980.

105. Vandervort R, Brooks SM: Polyvinyl chloride film thermal decomposition products as an occupational illness. J Occup Med 19:188, 1977.

106. Levy SA, Storey J, Phashko BE: Meat workers' asthma. J Occup Med 20:116, 1978.

107. Bardana EJ, Andrasch RH: Occupational asthma secondary to low molecular weight agents used in the plastic and resin industries. Eur J Respir Dis 64:241, 1983.

108. Szende B, Lapis K, Nemes A, et al: Pneumoconiosis caused by the inhalation of polyvinyl chloride dust. Med Lav 61:433, 1970.

109. Arnaud A, Pommier de Santi P, Garbe L, et al: Polyvinylchloride pneumoconiosis. Thorax 33:19, 1978.

110. Mastrangelo G, Manno M, Marcer G, et al: Polyvinyl chloride pneumoconiosis: Epidemiological study of exposed workers. J Occup Med 21:540, 1979.

111. Cordasco EM, Demeter SL, Kerkay J, et al: Pulmonary manifestations of vinyl and polyvinyl-chloride dust. Thorax 6:828, 1978.

112. Soutar CA, Copeland LH, Thornley PE, et al: Epidemiological study of respiratory disease in workers exposed to PVC dust. Thorax 35:644, 1980.

113. Soutar CA, Gauld S: Clinical studies of workers exposed to PVC dust. Thorax 38:834, 1983.

114. Lee HS, Wang YT, Lee CS, et al: Occupational asthma due to unheated polyvinylchloride resin dust. Br J Ind Med 46:820, 1989.

Chapter 18

OCCUPATIONAL ASTHMA DUE TO INHALATION OF ANTIBIOTICS AND OTHER DRUGS

Anthony Montanaro, MD

Although many drugs can act as potent allergens, a limited number of agents have been described as inducing asthma in an occupational setting. Most at-risk workers are in the pharmaceutical industry, but airborne exposure may affect laboratory and health care workers as well (Table 1). The pharmaceutical manufacturing industry has acted responsibly in minimizing airborne exposure to dusts in the production setting, but a significant risk remains. In addition, many of the drugs that induce asthma can be easily aerosolized in pharmacy and laboratory settings (Fig. 1 and 2). This chapter will review the relevant literature on the drugs that have been reported to be associated with occupational asthma in any setting.

β-LACTAM ANTIBIOTICS

The beta-lactam antibiotics have long been considered the cornerstone of our antibiotic armamentarium. Shortly following their introduction, anaphylactic reactions to these compounds were reported. Interestingly, while asthma had long been recognized as part of an anaphylactic response to systemic administration of these antibiotics, reports of documented industrial asthma did not occur for over 20 years.

In 1974 Pepys and co-workers reported on four workers who developed respiratory complaints after working in an ampicillin production factory for up to 12 years.[1] Three workers developed typical delayed-onset occupational asthma and rhinitis after 2 years of employment, while the fourth developed symptoms of cough and dyspnea suggesting occupational asthma. These patients were investigated by routine skin testing of relevant antibiotic antigens, as well as by bronchial and oral provocation studies. Skin tests were negative to ampicillin, benzyl penicillin, and 6-amino penicillanic acid (6APA). Three of the four patients had delayed and prolonged responses to bronchial provocation. All three patients reacted to commercial and purified ampicillin, while one reacted to purified 6APA and another to benzyl penicillin. This pattern of response indicated that impurities in the antibiotic preparations were unlikely to be the compounds responsible for the decline in FEV_1. Furthermore, oral antibiotic challenges confirmed systemic hyperresponsiveness in two of the three positive reactors.

The potential for airborne exposure to semisynthetic penicillins was highlighted in a study by Moller.[2] In this survey of Danish pharmaceutical workers, a semiquantitative assay using Petri dishes inoculated with test organisms was used to detect airborne concentrations of antibiotic. The factory area was found to be highly contaminated with pivampicillin dust. Forty-five workers developed either dermatitis or respiratory complaints. None of these workers developed occupational asthma, which was confirmed by bronchial provocation. Interestingly, all 45 patients manifested positive delayed skin-testing to one or more patch tests with semisynthetic penicillins. The duration of exposure prior to the

TABLE 1. *Occupational Asthma from Inhaled Antibiotics and Drugs*

Drug	Described At-risk Workers
Beta lactam antibiotics	Pharmaceutical production pharmacists, nurses
Spiramycin	Pharmaceutical production
Tetracycline	Pharmaceutical production
Isonicotinic acid Hydrazide (INH) (Isoniazid^R)	Pharmacists
Chloramine-T	Laboratory workers butcher kitchen production
Piperazine	Chemists
Methyldopa	Chemists
Amprolium hydrochloride	Pharmaceutical production
Salbutamol	Pharmaceutical production
Ipecac	Pharmaceutical production

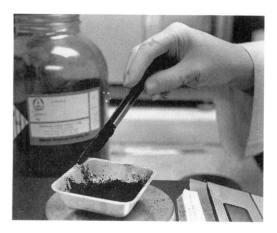

FIGURE 2. Laboratory worker weighing pharamceutical product.

onset of symptoms varied from 1 week to 1 year and tended to be shorter in patients with respiratory complaints as opposed to contact dermatitis. Although these patients were not comprehensively studied from a clinical standpoint, these observations underscore the potential risk for airborne exposure to antibiotic dust in pharmaceutical workers.

Subsequent immunologic studies on workers with beta-lactam antibiotic sensitivity using allergen skin testing, RAST, and basophil histamine release were reported by Moller in 1984.[3] In this study, eight pharmaceutical workers exposed to penicillin while feeding a powder machine were evaluated. Penicillin antigens used included pivampicillin hydrochloride (PA), pivmecillinam hydrochloride (PM), ampicillin (AM), the major penicillin determinate, benzylpenicilloyl-polylysine, as well as a minor determinate mixture (MDM) containing benzylpenicillin and benzylpenicilloate. Immediate scratch tests and RAST studies were negative. Basophil histamine release was positive in five workers, two responding to the MDM alone. The others responded to PA and AM, but not to the MDM. Patch tests were positive in four patients to PA, PM, and AM. This study suggested immediate and delayed immunologic mechanisms in penicillin-induced allergy in workers with airborne exposures, but highlighted the limitations of skin and serologic testing in establishing the diagnosis.

MACROLIDE ANTIBIOTICS

Although spiramycin has had little use in the U.S., it is a member of a macrolide group of antibiotics, which includes erythromycin. Macrolides appear to have a surprisingly low incidence of generalized anaphylaxis associated

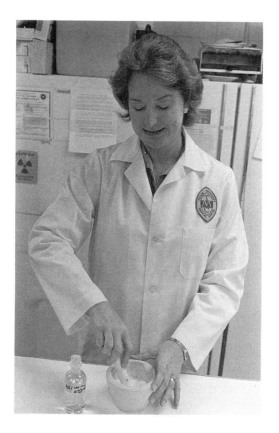

FIGURE 1. Pharmacist preparing medication by grinding into fine dust.

with their use. However, recent observations describing occupational asthma in a pharmaceutical worker exposed to spiramycin[4,5] have been published.

Pepys and Davies first reported spiramycin occupational asthma in 1975.[4] In this case report the authors describe a 35-year-old nonatopic maintenance engineer who had inhalational exposure to spiramycin while employed in a pharmaceutical production plant. The patient developed delayed attacks of nocturnal sneezing, coughing, and breathlessness. Bronchial provocation studies using 20 mg of spiramycin resulted in delayed onset of nasal and respiratory symptoms. Subsequent bronchial challenge with 2 g of spiramycin resulted in significant declines in FEV_1 within 1 to 2 hours of exposure. After removal from his workplace, the worker's symptoms improved, but interestingly they did not clear until his wife, who also worked at the same plant, discontinued her employment.

More recently Malo and Cartier in Montreal investigated 51 employees of a pharmaceutical company processing spiramycin.[5] These workers were exposed to spiramycin processing for brief periods (5–10 days), four to five times/year. Twelve subjects related symptoms suggesting occupational asthma, and 21 subjects reported symptoms of rhinoconjunctivitis following exposure to spiramycin in the past. Forty-eight workers were then studied during a spiramycin production period. Methacholine bronchial provocation testing was undertaken before and during the production periods. Prior to the production period, only nine workers demonstrated hyperresponsiveness to methacholine. During production, six workers had a PC_{20} of 16 mg/ml of methacholine or less, and seven workers experienced a 2.5-fold or greater fall in PC_{20}. The concentration of spiramycin in the production area was measured and found to be 0.54 to 2.33 mg/M^3.

Follow-up bronchial provocation studies to spiramycin were performed on those workers who were determined to be hyperresponsive to methacholine prior to or during production. Three workers had positive challenges with immediate response. Two of these workers were smokers and two were atopics. Skin testing was performed to spiramycin but could not be interpreted due to presumed irritant effect. Although the mechanism, pathophysiology, and risk factors remain unknown, these observations suggest that pharmaceutical workers are at risk for developing occupational asthma due to inhalational spiramycin exposure. As in other occupational asthmatic states, workers with predisposing factors to bronchial hyperresponsiveness, such as atopy and cigarette smoking, may be at increased risk.

TETRACYCLINE

While tetracycline is one of the most widely used antibiotics worldwide, isolated asthmatic responses are rare.[6] Systemic allergic reactions have been well recognized for many years, but occupational asthma following inhalational exposure was not reported until 1977. Mencin and Das have described a pharmaceutical worker who developed typical immediate onset occupational asthma 1 year after beginning work at a production plant.[7] Intradermal skin testing to pure tetracycline resulted in a four-plus dermal reaction and severe dyspnea and wheezing. Subsequent oral provocation to 250 mg and inhalation challenge to 100 mg of tetracycline resulted in declines of greater than 50% in FEV_1.

ISONIAZID (INH)

Isonicotinic acid hydrazide (INH) (Isoniazid) is a small-molecular-weight substance that is used extensively throughout the world as an antimycobacterial drug. Although skin rash, fever, and liver function abnormalities are infrequently observed in patients taking this medication, occupational asthma in pharmacists and pharmaceutical workers had not been described until 1987. Fugiwara and colleagues have described a nonatopic 26-year-old pharmacist who developed work-related rhinitis 1 year after beginning work, and occupational asthma 1 year later.[8] Her job duties had included grinding crystals of INH once/week. Skin tests to INH and INH-human serum albumin (INH-HSA), as well as INH incubated in the patient's serum, yielded positive results. Passive transfer of dermal reactivity was positive in the patient's mother. Bronchial provocation to INH and INH-HSA at a concentration of 10^{-4} g/ml resulted in an approximate 30% decline in FEV_1. The affected worker was observed to develop symptoms of cough within 9 minutes following INH crystal grinding, accompanied by a 50% decline in peak flow.

CHLORAMINE-T

Chloramine-T is a simple chlorinated amide compound. Its potent oxidizing properties, as well as its water solubility, have led to its application as a disinfectant. For decades, it has been used around the world in kitchens, butcher shops, and laboratories. More importantly, this agent has been employed in operating rooms, used as a sterilizing agent for nebulizers by respiratory therapists, and used around patients with chronic lung disease with underlying bronchial hyperreactivity. It also has had laboratory application as a catalyzer for radiolabeling protein with iodine.

The first report of occupational asthma to chloramine-T, by Van Bork from the Netherlands in 1973,[9] was in operating room nurses. Subsequently, others noticed both immediate and delayed bronchial symptoms that correlated with positive immediate skin reactions.[10] More recently Dijkman and colleagues from the Netherlands reported detailed clinical observations, as well as bronchial provocation studies, in five patients who had been exposed to chloramine-T in a variety of occupational settings. All four workers skin-tested to chloramine-T developed both immediate and delayed skin responses to epicutaneous testing. Bronchial provocation studies undertaken in three subjects revealed significant immediate and delayed declines in FEV_1 in one patient and isolated late asthmatic responses 4 to 8 hours after challenge in the remaining two. Interestingly, the late bronchial responses persisted for hours to days in these patients and were accompanied by fever in one subject and leukocytosis in all three. These findings suggested mechanisms in addition to IgE-mediated hypersensitivity as important in the immunopathogenesis of this disorder. Because this material is commercially available as a powder, it affords optimal conditions for inhalational exposures. It should be stressed to workers using this substance that chloramine-T should be dissolved in water away from their breathing zone. Once dissolved, it remains a potent oxidant and potential immunologic sensitizing agent and should not be considered safe. Appropriate industrial hygiene measures must be followed at all times to avoid contact or inhalation injuries and/or sensitization.

In a subsequent publication, Dijkman and co-authors[10] demonstrated specific IgE antibodies by in vitro methods in these same patients. Using solid-phase radioimmunoassay, these authors were able to detect IgE to human serum albumin-bound chloramine-T in the serum of patients with well-documented chloramine-T occupational asthma. Chloramine-T-specific antibodies of IgG subclasses 1, 3 and 4 were not found. Furthermore, these investigators were able to confirm by inhibition studies that the P-toluene sulfonyl group of the chloramine-T molecule was partially responsible for the antigenic determinant. Although there have been very few patients studied in detail, these observations support an IgE-mediated mechanism for some cases of chloramine-T-induced asthma.

Although other aerosolized disinfectants are commonly used in the health care industry, none has been studied as extensively as chloramine-T. Chlorhexidine is a widely used aerosolized disinfectant that has previously been described as a potential skin sensitizing agent.[11] Recently occupational asthma has been reported in two nurses exposed to a chlorhexidine alcohol aerosol.[12] In this report these nurses were noted to have a 13 and 22% immediate decline in FEV_1 following exposure to these agents, accompanied by cough and chest discomfort. Neither individual had a previous history of asthma and in fact both had demonstrated negative histamine bronchial provocation studies. These limited observations failed to discriminate between possible irritant effects of this chemical and the potential for true occupational asthma from sensitization. Because this agent is used so extensively, clinicians should be aware of its potential for causing significant respiratory complaints, but should also be cautious of diagnosing occupational asthma until further clarifying studies are conducted.

PIPERAZINE

Piperazine is a low molecular weight organic chemical substance that is manufactured as a dust. The manufacturing process consists of conversion of piperazine hydrate to piperazine dihydrochloride by hydrochloric acid. Gaseous or particulate piperazine may be liberated into the ambient air at multiple stages of its production or processing. Presumed occupational asthma and rhinitis were first reported by McCullagh in 1968.[13] In 1972 Pepys and co-workers at the Bromptom Hospital in London performed workplace-simulated controlled bronchial provocation studies on two chemists involved with piperazine production who had developed delayed nasal and asthmatic responses 3–4 hours following their occupational exposures.[14] Bronchial provocation to 250 and 500 g of piperazine hydrochloride in 1 kg of lactose powder resulted in significant declines in FEV_1 3 to 4 hours following challenge. Epicutaneous skin testing and nasal provocation to piperazine hydrochloride were negative (see Chapter 17).

PSYLLIUM

Psyllium is a high molecular weight gum, the seed of which is widely used as a "bulking agent" in the treatment of constipation. These laxative preparations contain ground husks and/or seeds of the psyllium plant and are available in a powder form that, when mixed with liquid, creates a hydrophilic mucilloid. Psyllium is a member of the genus *Plantago*, a large group of weeds that also contains the highly allergenic English plantain weed. Patients with clinical evidence of psyllium and English plantain sensitivity have been described with apparent cross-reacting IgE to both allergens.[18] While the potential allergenicity of psyllium seeds had been recognized for decades, the medical consequences of exposure were first detailed in 1970.[19] Despite its widespread production usage, the first cases of occupational asthma were not described until 1975.[20]

In 1975 Busse and colleagues reported on their observations in three atopic psyllium manufacturing workers.[20] In their initial report, they noted positive bronchial provocation studies to psyllium extracts in two of three workers who had reported respiratory complaints in response to inhalation of the psyllium dust generated in the manufacturing of a psyllium-containing laxative. All three patients exhibited positive immediate cutaneous hyperreactivity to psyllium extracts, whereas none of the allergic or nonallergic controls demonstrated any dermal reactivity. Previously Bernton had reported a single patient who had manifest asthmatic responses to inhaled psyllium powder used as a bulk laxative while merely measuring a tablespoon of the powder for personal use.[19] Subsequent to Busse's report in 1975, numerous cases of occupational asthma due to the inhalation of psyllium-containing products by pharmaceutical manufacturing personnel[21] and health care workers have been reported.[22-24]

Despite the relative lack of awareness in the general medical community, hypersensitivity responses to inhaled psyllium are well reported.

One recent survey by Malo and co-workers indicated that 18% of exposed health care workers reported "allergic" symptoms that were temporally associated with psyllium powder exposure.[24] Approximately 12% of the study population demonstrated psyllium-specific IgE antibodies by positive skin tests. Twenty workers who had a history suggestive of occupational asthma or pre-existing asthma, or with positive skin tests to psyllium, underwent specific bronchial provocation studies to psyllium dust. Four of these 20 patients developed bronchospastic responses to the inhaled psyllium. The authors concluded that the prevalence of occupational asthma was 4% in this group of 193 workers who had responded to their survey. These findings, as well as those previously discussed, support the conclusion that occupational or nonoccupational exposure to inhaled psyllium dust may result in IgE-mediated bronchial hyperresponsiveness and severe bronchial asthma. At-risk pharmaceutical and health care workers, as well as patients, should be aware of this hazard and appropriately protected.

IPECACUANHA

Ipecacuanha (ipecac) is a vegetable protein that is derived from the dried rhizome and roots of the plant *Cephaelis ipecacuanha* (see Chapter 1). In the pharmaceutical industry, the substance prepared from the root of this plant is reduced to a fine powder. In small doses, ipecacuanha has been used as an expectorant. In larger doses ipecacuanha is the active ingredient in ipecac formulations, which have been used for decades to induce vomiting and diarrhea. For its antiemetic action, ipecacuanha is usually administered in liquid form, but as an expectorant it can be taken in tablet form. In 1984 Luczynska and colleagues described the results of their investigation of a pharmaceutical manufacturing plant in the United Kingdom involved in the production of ipecacuanha tablets.[25] Their findings indicated that 20 of 42 employees complained of work-related respiratory complaints. Twenty-three percent of these employees were found to be atopic. Twelve of eighteen (67%) with work-related respiratory complaints were found to have dermal reactivity to a skin prick test with 10% ipecacuanha. Details of the specific "allergic symptoms" unfortunately were not presented. No specific bronchial provocation studies were undertaken. Despite the relative lack of detailed information in this study, the findings did indicate the potential hazard of presumed IgE sensitization following inhalational exposure of ipecacuanha dust.

OTHER CHEMICALS/DRUGS

Pharmaceutical and chemical industry workers have been further described as demonstrating bronchial hyperresponsiveness to many other agents. Occupational asthma has been reported in an analytical chemist working in a pharmaceutical lab who inhaled **methyldopa** powder.[15] The patient presented with work-related nasal symptoms and exercise-induced asthmatic symptoms. Controlled bronchial provocation studies to 100 g of methyldopa powder over 30 minutes revealed a 30% fall in FEV_1, 10 hours following exposure.

A chemical worker employed in quality control in the manufacture of a poultry food additive (**pancoxin**) was noted to develop nasal and bronchial symptoms when exposed to the powdered chemical.[16] This additive contains amprolium hydrochloride, which is a simple, low molecular weight, water-soluble thiamine antagonist. Because of its thiamine antagonism, it is effective as a feed additive in preventing coccidiomycosis in poultry. Work-simulated bronchial provocation studies in this worker demonstrated reproduction of nasal and bronchial symptoms accompanied by a 27% decline in FEV_1 20 minutes following exposure. Chemical production workers may be at particular risk with this agent due to their risk of high-level exposure, but poultry workers using feed containing amprolium hydrochloride may have significant inhalational exposures.

Although these production workers appeared to have reacted to "active ingredients" in the manufactured products, other workers have reacted to intermediates in the production of pharmaceutical substances. Pepys and coworkers have reported their detailed observations concerning a pharmaceutical worker involved in the production of the selective beta-2 adrenergic agent **salbutamol**.[17] Controlled bronchial provocation studies demonstrated no response to inhaled salbutamol but significant declines in FEV_1 to a glycyl intermediate. This glycyl compound, Z-(N-benzyl-N-tert-butylamino)-4' hydroxy-3'-hydromethyl-acetophenache diacetate, is an intermediate chemical powder prepared during the manufacturing of salbutamol. Skin-prick tests to salbutamol and

intermediates were negative. Interestingly, inhaled salbutamol was successfully prescribed as a bronchodilator in this patient.

CONCLUSIONS

These observations indicate that inhalational exposure to antibiotics and chemicals in the pharmaceutical and chemical-processing industries are important causes of occupational asthma. Although the number of documented cases in the literature is small, it is likely that these cases represent only the "tip of the iceberg." Physicians and employers must maintain a constant vigilance and awareness of this problem in at-risk workers. These isolated occurrences also highlight the value of detailed studies, including industrial hygiene investigations and controlled bronchial provocation studies. The number of at-risk workers is extremely high, and the potential for inhalation of fine particulates and dusts of chemicals is great.

REFERENCES

1. Davies RS, Hendricks DS, Pepys J: Asthma due to inhaled chemical agents: Ampicillin, benzyl penicillin, 6 amino penicillanic acid and related substances. Clin Allergy 4:227–247, 1974.
2. Moller NE, Nielsen B, Van Wurdenk: Contact dermatitis to semisynthetic penicillins in factory workers. Contact Dermatitis 14:307–311, 1986.
3. Moller NE, Skov PS, Norm S: Allergic and pseudoallergic reactions caused by penicillins, cocca and peppermint additives in factory workers examined by basophil histamine release. Acta Pharm Tox 55:139–144, 1984.
4. Pepys J, Davies RJ: Asthma due to inhaled chemical agents: The macrolide antibiotic spiramycin. Clin Allergy 99:107, 1975.
5. Malo J, Cartier A: Occupational asthma in workers of a pharmaceutical company processing spiramycin. Thorax 43:371–377, 1988.
6. Fawcett IW, Pepys J: Allergy to a tetracycline preparation: A case report. Clin Allergy 6:301–306.
7. Menon NPS, Das AK: Tetracycline asthma: A case report. Clin Allergy 7:285–290, 1977.
8. Asai S, Shimoda T, Hara K, Fujiwara K: Occupational asthma caused by isonicotinic acid hydrazide inhalation. J Allergy Clin Immunol 80:578–582, 1987.
9. Dijkman JH, Piet HY, Kramps JA: Occupational asthma due to inhalation of chloramine-T. Int Arch Allergy Appl Immunol 64:422–427, 1981.
10. Dijkman JH, Piet HY, Kramps JA: Occupational asthma due to inhalation of chloramine-T: Demonstration of specific IgE antibodies. Int Arch Allergy Appl Immunol 64:428–438, 1981.
11. Lyunnggren B, Moller H: Eczematous contact allergy to chlorhexidine. Acta Derm Venereol (Stock) 52:308–310, 1972.

12. Waclawski FR, McAlpine LG, Thomson NC: Occupational asthma in nurses caused by chlorhexidine and aleonal aerosols. Br Med J 298:929-930, 1989.
13. McCullagh SF: Allergenicity of piperazine: A study in environmental allergy. Br J Ind Med 25:319-320, 1968.
14. Pepys J, Pickenng CAC, Loudon HW: Asthma due to inhaled chemical agents: Piperazine dihydrochloride. Clin Allergy 2:189-196, 1972.
15. Harries MG, Neuman Taylor AJ, Wooden J, MacAuslan A: Bronchial asthma due to alpha methyldopa. Br Med J 2:1461, 1979.
16. Greene SA, Freedman S: Asthma due to inhaled chemical agents—amprolium hydrochloride. Clin Allergy 6:105-108, 1976.
17. Fawcett IW, Pepys J, Erooga MA: Asthma due to 'glycol compound' powder: An intermediate in the production of salbutamol. Clin Allergy 6:405-409, 1976.
18. Rosenberg S, Landay R, Klotz SD, Fireman P: Serum IgE antibodies to psyllium in individuals allergic to psyllium and English plantain. Ann Allergy 48:294-298, 1982.
19. Bernton HS: The allergenicity of psyllium seed. Medical Annals of the District of Columbia 39:313-317, 1970.
20. Busse WW, Shoenwetter WF: Asthma from psyllium in laxative manufacture. Ann Intern Med 83:361-362, 1975.
21. Bardy JD, Malo JL, Sequin P, et al: Occupational asthma and IgE sensitization in a pharmaceutical company processing psyllium. Am Rev Respir Dis 135:1033-1038, 1987.
22. Gross R: Acute bronchospasm associated with inhalation of psyllium hydrophilic mucilloid. JAMA 241:1573-1574, 1979.
23. Cartier A, Malo JL, Dolovich J: Occupational asthma in nurses handling psyllium. Clin Allergy 17:1-6, 1987.
24. Malo J-L, Cartier A, L'Archeveque J, et al: Prevalence of occupational asthma and immunologic sensitization to psyllium among health personnel in chronic care hospitals. Am Rev Respir Dis 142:1359-1366, 1990.
25. Luczynska CM, Marshall PE, Scarisbrick PA, Topping MD: Occupational allergy due to inhalation of ipecacuanha dust. Clin Allergy 14:169-175, 1984.

Chapter 19

ASTHMA DUE TO INSECTS

Mark T. O'Hollaren, MD

When one considers insect allergy, it is often in reference to IgE-mediated sensitivity to the stinging insects. However, inhalant sensitivity to airborne insect allergens may be a significant problem, especially in those who work with or are involved with regular exposure to large quantities of insects.

The mite has been identified as an important inhaled aeroallergen; however, technically the mite is not an insect but an arthropod.[1] Nonetheless, mites as potential occupational allergens will also be covered.

Occupational exposures to insects have resulted in some rates of allergic sensitization surpassing 25% of those working with the insects.[2] The allergens may be extremely potent, and inhalant allergy to insects has been reported in the United States, Japan, Australia, Taiwan, Pakistan, the United Kingdom, Germany, France, Sudan, and Egypt.[2,3]

Occupational exposures have provided us with some of the most clear-cut examples of inhaled insect-associated allergic disease. Many of the reported cases of inhalant insect allergy have been from entomologic researchers investigating various insects as pests[2-4] (Fig. 1). Quantification of the actual insect aeroallergens has been impeded by the amorphous nature of airborne insect debris (Fig. 2). Newer immunochemical methods for assaying these particles will improve our ability to monitor and evaluate these aeroallergens[2] (Table 1).

BACKGROUND AND HISTORICAL PERSPECTIVE

In 1713, Ramazzini wrote, "Small fragments of dead silkworms as well as brukes [locust larvae] and caterpillars possess some sort of noxious and corrosive acrimony injurious to the lungs."[5] In the years since Ramazzini's insightful observations, it has become evident that inhaled particles of airborne insect debris may be causative agents in both occupational and domestic asthma. Although this chapter will focus on insects as occupational allergens, they are also important allergens in the domestic setting as well. For example, the U.S. is known to be inhabited by 55 species of cockroaches, five of which can be considered domestic pests.[3] The resulting indoor allergens have been shown to play a role in the pathogenesis and worsening of symptoms in some patients with asthma.[6-13] Cockroaches are constant nuisances to urban dwellers in infested regions due to their rapid spread and resistance to attempts at extermination.[8]

Historically, allergic symptoms secondary to inhaled insect debris have occurred in workers with heavy exposure.[2] In occupational settings these heavy exposures have usually (but not always) occurred in those involved with research or other employment utilizing insects.[3] In addition to those working with insects commercially, gardeners have also been reported to develop asthma secondary to moth exposure.[14] Asthma was reported in the mid-1970s by Perlman et al. in loggers and mill workers who were exposed to high concentrations of the tussock moth.[15] During slack flow along the Nile river in the Sudan, numbers of "green nimitti" midge may be so high that physical distress is caused in those living in the area, and outdoor activity is hindered significantly. Asthma due to allergic sensitization to this insect has been reported in those living along the river in this area.[16]

Earlier studies of inhalant sensitivity to insects often used extracts made from the crude

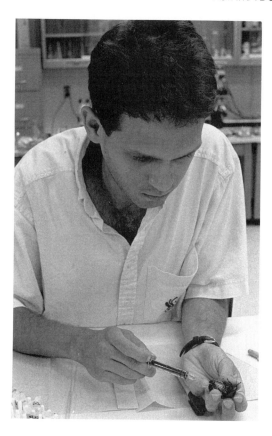

FIGURE 1. Entomological researcher working with cockroaches.

insect material; some of these studies not using the proper concentration resulted in irritant reactions on skin testing. Newer techniques employing the radioallergosorbent test (RAST) assays are helpful in some, but not all, cases of suspected insect allergy. Skin testing still remains extremely important in the diagnosis of inhalant insect allergy.[2]

EPIDEMIOLOGY AND PATHOPHYSIOLOGY

Epidemiology

The varieties and distribution of ambient insects vary significantly from place to place, as well as from year to year, even within a small geographic area.[17] In contrast, occupational exposures to insects may be fairly constant, depending on the nature of the employment or research. There are significant data on occupational exposures to insect aeroallergens.

Allergy to insect aeroallergens appears to occur more commonly in those with an atopic

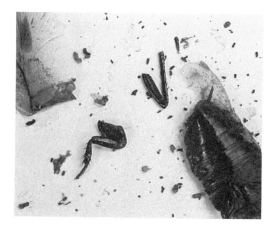

FIGURE 2. Amorphous insect debris from a tray used in a cockroach research facility.

history.[2-4,15,18] Locusts are particularly potent sensitizing antigens. In one study, 26% of 43 locust workers developed lower respiratory symptoms (wheezing or breathlessness) in one facility handling these insects. In addition, one-third of these workers developed rhinitis or urticaria.[4]

The National Institute of Occupational Safety and Health (NIOSH) surveyed 85 Agricultural Research Service facilities in 37 states. They found 25% of workers in these centers had a past or present history suggestive of occupational inhalant allergy. It is noteworthy

TABLE 1. Occupations Where Inhalant Sensitivity to Insects Has Been Reported

Entomologists and insect research workers
Locusts, crickets, fruit flies, house flies, Australian blow-flies, screwworm flies
Grain mill workers, dock loaders, and longshoremen
Beetles, storage mites, grain weevil
Sewer workers
Sewer filter flies
Loggers and lumber mill workers
Tussock moth
Fishermen and bait-handlers
Meal worms, blue-bottle maggots
Poultry workers
Northern fowl mite
Bakers
Storage mites, grain weevil
Small animal handlers
Cat flea
Gardeners
Moths
Amphibian-raising facility workers
Crickets
Honey-packing plant workers
Honey bee body dust
Pet food manufacturing workers
Chironomids

that a third of those working directly with insects reported symptoms of inhalant respiratory allergy.[2,19]

Sensitivity to inhaled cockroach aeroallergen is a significant cause of asthma, which is frequently perennial and may be worse during the winter months.[2,7-13,20] An adult allergy clinic in inner city New Orleans demonstrated that 50% of atopic asthmatics in some areas exhibit positive wheal-and-flare reactions to cockroach antigen.[26] Various species of cockroaches populate different parts of the world, and even in a given community there will be differing species of cockroaches.[21] Cockroach species may vary depending on the type of building, or even the location within a building[21] (see section on Orthoptera).

In some areas of the world, specific IgE to various Lepidoptera species (butterflies, moths and silkworms) may be seen fairly commonly. For example, in Japan, more than 50% of randomly selected asthmatics had reaginic sensitivity to moths and butterflies.[17] Over two-thirds of asthmatic patients in this Japanese study had positive skin tests to silkworm wing, and more than half had positive skin tests to caddis fly wing extract and chironomid (family chironomidae of midges) whole body extract. Only 8.7% of nonasthmatic patients had positive skin test reactions to these reagents. Positive reactions to these insects were seen as commonly as those to house dust. Over 80% of the asthmatic group with positive skin tests were also positive by RAST testing to these antigens.[17] Documented sensitization to Lepidoptera in Japan is as common as sensitization to house dust mite (Dermatophagoides pteronyssinus). Studies have shown no cross-reactivity between house dust mite and Lepidoptera.[1]

Pathophysiology

Inhalant sensitivity to insect aeroallergens appears to be IgE mediated. A number of illustrative studies have demonstrated IgE mediation of these asthmatic reactions.[3,4,14,22,23] Positive skin tests, RAST, and successful transfer of sensitivity with serum via the Prausnitz-Kustner (P-K) reaction was demonstrated in Japanese moth-sensitive asthmatics.[14] These patients were not exposed to moths or butterflies through occupational or hobby interests, and Kino et al. suggest that the majority of these patients were involuntarily sensitized by windborne emanations or those insect allergens present in house dust.[14]

Locust-sensitive asthmatics have had elevated levels of specific IgE and IgG demonstrated by skin tests and RAST analysis.[4] Patients with allergic rhinitis and asthma secondary to cricket exposure have had an IgE mechanism confirmed by skin testing, RAST, leukocyte histamine release, passive transfer studies, and bronchial provocation challenges.[18] An IgE mechanism was also demonstrated for inhaled sensitivity to mealworms in sensitized bait handlers based on allergen skin tests, RAST, and bronchial provocation studies.[22,23] IgE antibodies to sheep blowflies have been demonstrated by skin test and RAST in an entymological worker.[3]

Thirteen cockroach-sensitive perennial asthmatics underwent bronchial provocation challenge studies with cockroach antigen and had significant elevations of circulating plasma histamine levels immediately following antigen challenge, which peaked within 5 minutes after the provocation challenge. Plasma histamine remained elevated until isoproterenol administration reduced the acute bronchospasm.[24] Bronchial provocation with cockroach antigen may elicit an early, late, or dual asthmatic response.[9,11,12,20,24] Inhalation of cockroach antigen causes antigen-specific IgE mediated bronchial asthma and peripheral eosinophilia in specifically sensitized asthmatic subjects.[25]

CHEMISTRY AND ANTIGEN IDENTIFICATION

Various investigators have identified allergenic components in given insects, including excrement of the insect, airborne insect scales or microscopic hairs from the wings, and insect hemoglobin, as well as other body parts or emanations from the insects. Each insect needs to be considered individually and will be discussed in its own section later in this chapter.

For example, the major source of locust allergen, in one study, was found in the peritrophic membrane. This membrane is located in the alimentary tract and is in contact with the fecal material.[2,26] In another report, studies done in bait handlers sensitive to mealworms show cross-reactivity among species, but not between orders.[22,23] Mealworm did not cross react with mite, cockroach, spikeworm, or waxworm extracts.[2,22]

It appears that several parts of the cockroach may contain antigenic material. Cockroach whole bodies and exuviae (cast skins) appear to be important allergens, and whole body extract was found to be more potent than extracts made from egg shells or feces.[2] However, some investigators have demonstrated significant allergenicity of an extract made from cockroach fecal material.[27] Powdered cockroach antigens were advocated by some for use in antigen challenges, but this has since fallen out of favor.[28]

Those patients that may have allergic symptoms working with cats may actually have allergy to cat flea rather than to cat dander, and immunoblotting studies have revealed that there is a diversity of cat-flea allergens.[2] Sodium dodecyl sulfate-polyacrylamide gel electrophoreses (SDS-PAGE) of cat-flea extract followed by incubation of sera with nitrocellulose membrane-bound flea antigen and subsequent exposure to radioactive or enzyme-labeled anti-IgE demonstrated that there are multiple cat flea antigens that may elicit varying IgE responses, depending on the patient.[2]

Moth and butterfly antigen has been shown by RAST inhibition to cross-react almost completely with silkworm wing, but not with mite.[17] Significant allergic activity to chironomid (non-biting midge) larvae has been demonstrated in the hemoglobin molecule.[17] Silkworm moth wing appears to be a more potent sensitizer than other silkworm body parts.[1] Silkworm moth wing (Bombyx mori linne) has been used for allergen testing for moth and/or butterfly.[17] Kino et al. have found that the main allergenic potency in this group of insects is in the wing.[17] They also state that the main antigen for caddis fly is in the hairy wing, and they believe that there appear to be unique antigens present in caddis fly, silkworm wing, and chironomid, because levels of IgE directed against each of these have been shown to fluctuate in any given patient.[17]

In Japan, a bimodal peak (spring/fall) of airborne insect allergens was observed.[17] Perlman et al. prepared moth extracts for skin testing by first defatting crude material with ethyl ether, extracting in buffered saline, and using a 1:25 dilution (W/V) in 50% glycerosaline for scratch testing. If scratch testing was negative or equivocal, they did intradermal testing with a 10-fold dilution. They also found cutaneous sensitivity in those exposed to large amounts of the Douglas fir tussock moth by patch testing with ground crude material applied to the skin directly for 24–48 hours.[15]

CLINICAL PRESENTATION

Historical and Physical Examination Findings

On obtaining the clinical history from a patient suspected of having occupational allergic sensitivity to insects, it is important to elicit the type and duration of exposure, the variety of insect in question, and whether or not the patient has a history of atopic disease. Typical physical examination findings of allergic rhinitis, conjunctivitis, asthma, and contact urticaria have been reported from insect exposure, which may not always be obvious from the patient's occupational description.[2,29,30]

Laboratory and Skin Test Findings

Positive skin tests to silkworm wing in Japanese asthmatics occurred more than two-thirds of the time, with greater than 50% having positive skin tests to chironomid and caddis fly. More than 80% of those with a positive skin test had a positive RAST assay, as defined by greater than twice control levels of binding.[17] It has been shown that the method of preparation of solutions for insect allergen testing may make a significant difference in the percentage of positive skin test reactions, and there have been several acceptable methods described for preparation of allergen testing solutions.[3,14,15] Although positive skin tests do not translate to a symptomatic state, these numbers are helpful in the further elucidation of allergic sensitivity to inhaled insect aeroallergens.

Cricket (family Gryllidae) allergy was identified in two workers in an amphibian-raising plant. A cricket extract was made using ground crickets defatted with diethyl ether. A 1:10 prick test concentration was used, as was a 1:1000 intradermal concentration, because a 1:100 intradermal concentration gave some false positive irritant responses[18] (Fig. 3).

At least one insect, moth, was capable of eliciting a direct cutaneous toxic effect when moth particles were applied using patch tests in nonexposed, nonatopic workers.[15] Skin testing to Lepidoptera antigens has been associated with delayed cutaneous reactions (erythema and induration) in some patients.[30,31] Whether this is indicative of a cutaneous irritant response or true delayed hypersensitivity is not clear at this time. The possibility of delayed

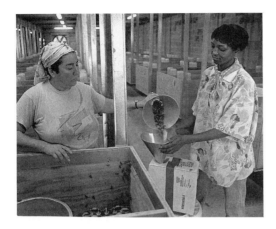

FIGURE 3. Live crickets (*Acheta domestica*—common house cricket) being loaded for shipment as feeder insect and fishing bait for use.

hypersensitivity warrants some consideration in light of a report in which a group of seamen developed contact dermatitis 6–24 hours after being exposed to bedsheets contaminated with crushed moth bodies.[30] Thirty-one of 45 crewmen developed the dermatitis, and all those affected had positive delayed cutaneous reactions to moth skin tests.[30]

Patients living in cockroach-infested dwellings have both a higher incidence of cockroach sensitivity by skin testing, but also a higher total IgE.[6] Twenty to 53% of atopics, and 49–61% of asthmatics have been shown to be sensitive to cockroach antigen by skin testing.[7] The link between positive skin test to cockroach antigen and asthma has been confirmed by bronchial provocation testing, in which six of nine asthmatic patients with positive skin tests to cockroach had positive bronchial provocation tests with that antigen in one study. No patients in this study who had negative skin tests to cockroach antigen demonstrated any fall in FEV_1 after inhalation challenge with that antigen.[7] In another study, 30 of 33 patients with positive skin tests to cockroach had an immediate asthmatic response after bronchial provocation, with a mean 42% fall in FEV_1. Sixteen of those 30 patients also had a late asthmatic response. Asthmatic responses were associated with increased blood histamine values and peripheral eosinophilia.[9] Other investigators have also confirmed the association between positive skin tests to cockroach antigen and positive bronchial provocation tests in patients with asthma.[8,12] Kang et al. demonstrated that those with positive allergen skin tests to cockroach

had a higher total IgE compared to those with negative skin tests; furthermore, those with positive CR skin tests who underwent bronchial provocation challenge had increased peripheral eosinophilia accompanying their fall in FEV_1. Most patients in this study had an immediate asthmatic reaction and half had delayed asthmatic responses.[25] Additional research will clarify the scope of cockroach sensitivity as an occupational allergen in work areas where cockroach infestation is significant.

The sensitivity of RAST assay to demonstrate IgE to insect antigens has been varied. It is clear that RAST sensitivity to cockroach antigen is not particularly reliable when compared with properly performed skin tests, with an approximate 50% false negative rate reported using RAST for cockroach.[7,25,32] It is not clear how reliable the RAST assay is for other insect allergens, although it has been somewhat reliable for some insects such as moths.[17]

SPECIFIC INSECT GROUPS

Orthoptera

Insects in this order include locusts, cockroaches, crickets, and grasshoppers.[2] Because of the demonstrated problem of cockroach allergy, it has been the most thoroughly studied and will be reviewed in the greatest detail.

Specific IgE by skin test and RAST, as well as specific IgG (by ELISA) have been demonstrated in symptomatic locust workers.[4]

Two employees at an amphibian-raising facility developed allergic rhinitis and bronchial asthma from exposure to crickets. An IgE mechanism was demonstrated using allergen skin tests, RAST, P-K reaction, bronchial provocation studies, and leukocyte histamine release assay[18] (Fig. 4).

Five species of cockroaches are considered domiciliary pests.[20,33] For some segments of society, the cockroach is responsible for producing significant airborne allergen, capable of inducing rhinitis and asthma at home.[6,7] The significance of cockroach-antigen sensitivity in asthmatic populations has been well documented.[2,6,7,9-12]

The amount of exposure to cockroach antigen appears to correlate with the development of allergy to the insect. Disadvantaged socioeconomic populations appear to be at higher risk of developing cockroach-associated

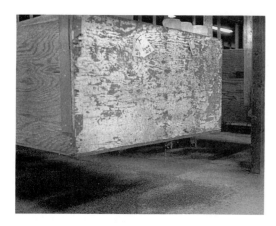

FIGURE 4.   Cricket dander and debris under a cricket cage in one of the largest cricket farms in the U.S.

asthma, as determined by domestic immuno-chemical air sampling data measuring for cockroach antigen in multiple cities.[34] Actual cockroach counts by patients, in one study, roughly correlated with RAST scores to cock-roach antigen in apartment dwellers, and pos-itive skin tests to cockroach antigen were more commonly seen in patients living in cock-roach-infested dwellings compared with those not living in buildings infested with these insects.[6]

Cockroaches may inhabit the kitchens of hotels, hospitals, homes, bakery shops, corn-mills, storehouses, and similar places.[33] They cause considerable problems, because they may devour foodstuffs, leather, paper, and textiles, and may pollute the indoor environment with their excrement and body emanations; in ad-dition they may be vectors of disease.[33]

The German cockroach is the principal indoor cockroach in the United States; how-ever, the Oriental cockroach is the most prev-alent in the United Kingdom.[21] Not only does the type of building influence which type of cockroach may be present, but the location within a building appears to be important as well.[21] For example, the proportion of Oriental to German cockroaches in the U.K. is much higher in homes than in restaurants, hospi-tals, or shops.[21] The German cockroaches favor kitchens; whereas the Oriental cock-roach favors the less humid basement, ducts, and boiler rooms.[21]

Skin testing using cockroach extract is the gold standard in diagnosing cockroach allergy. RAST, basophil histamine release, and total IgE all poorly predict subsequent bronchial provocation results, and the RAST has an approximate 50% false negative rate.[7,24,25] In terms of therapy, allergen immunotherapy was compared to a control group using cock-roach antigen in sensitive individuals and was shown to decrease symptom scores and medication requirements, to increase specific IgG levels, and to decrease basophil histamine release in response to cockroach antigen.[20] Further studies are needed for elucidation of the role of allergen immunotherapy to cock-roach antigen.

Coleoptera

The order Coleoptera has over 250,000 spe-cies, and includes beetles, mealworms, grain weevils, and Mexican bean weevils.[2,35] This order is characterized by six legs and three body segments.[35] Occupational asthma result-ing from beetle exposure appears to have been first reported in a museum curator who used beetle larvae to help digest flesh from zoologi-cal specimens.[36] Species including *Sitophilus oryza,* the "rice weevil," and *S. granarius,* the grain weevil, attack undamaged grain and may presage invasion by other insects, fungi, and bacteria.[35] *S. granarius,* has been the member of this family most commonly impli-cated in allergic respiratory disease, including allergic alveolitis.[35,37] In addition, flour beetles of the genus *Tribolium,* a genus of small grain-infesting beetles, may initiate hypersen-sitivity responses in man.[38,39]

Stevenson reported occupational asthma from bee moth larvae or waxworms *(Galleria mellonella)* in a bait handler in 1967.[23] An entomological researcher has developed aller-gic respiratory symptoms due to sensitization to the lesser mealworm, a grain beetle *(Alphi-tobius diaperinus)*; skin tests, RAST, immuno-blotting, and leukocyte histamine release assays confirmed an allergic mechanism.[40] Bait handlers working with mealworms, the larvae of the *Tenibrio molitor* beetle, have developed occupational asthma and rhinitis, as well as urticaria on contact with mealworms (Fig. 5). The cases were documented with allergen prick tests, bronchial provocation tests, and RAST assays.[41] RAST inhibition studies did not show cross-reactivity with mite, cockroach, or three other species of the Diptera and Lepi-doptera orders.[41]

Occupational asthma due to sensitization to the Mexican bean weevil *(Zabrotes subfas-ciatus)* has been described in bean sorters.[42] For a full discussion on asthma due to the

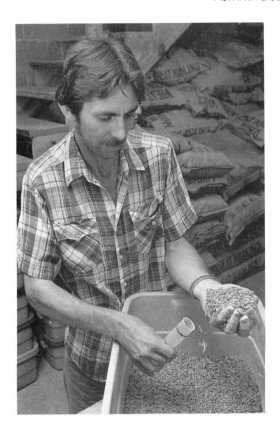

FIGURE 5.   Live mealworms being measured for shipment (species *Tenebrio molitor*).

grain weevil, as well as asthma due to insects and mites in grain millers and bakers, see the chapter on baker's asthma.

Lepidoptera

This order includes moths, silkworms, and butterflies.[2] Because of the nature of these insects, occupational sensitization appears to be fairly uncommon, although there are approximately 75 species of moths that are known to infest stored grain and cereal products.[35,43] The high rate at which these flying insects reproduce ensures their rapid and efficient spread through stored cereals.[35] They can thus be a potential problem for millers and others who store quantities of grain or other milled products.[35]

A commercial fish-bait worker developed occupational asthma while working with bee moths (*Galleria mellonella* [waxworm]).[31] As noted previously, the tussock moth *(Oryia pseudotsugata)* caused both cutaneous and respiratory symptoms in loggers and mill

workers in the Pacific Northwest, especially in those working in infested forests.[15] Perlman noted significant difficulties in attempting to quantify particles of microscopic insect debris in air and dust samples.[44] However, newer immunochemical assays are dramatically improving our capacity to sample these antigens in the air.[2]

Moths and butterflies have wings that are covered on both surfaces with scales of differing shapes (40–80 microns in area per scale).[17] In contrast, caddis flies (order Trichoptera) have their wings covered with thousands of microscopic hairs (80–100 μm in length).[17] These scales and hairs are easily dislodged in flight or rubbed off with gentle contact, and may become airborne or a constituent of house dust.[14]

Moths often appear in the late afternoon and evening and are attracted to lights that may lead to their flying indoors; their scales and other body parts may eventually become a part of house dust.[14] Butterflies are active on a diurnal basis, especially around flowers and vegetables.[14] In Japan, butterflies are present from April through October, with peak numbers in the spring and fall months.[17] Morphologic studies done by Balyeat as early as 1932 demonstrated a count of butterfly scales that was higher than that of grass pollen in June and July.[45]

Immunochemical air sampling by Wynn et al. in southeastern Minnesota showed measurable airborne levels of moth, with particle sizes in the size range of 0.1 to 4.1 μm.[46] Utilizing RAST inhibition assay, there was some cross-reactivity with other insects, but not with pollens or molds.[46]

In Japan, inhalant allergic sensitivity to moth and butterfly is found as commonly as sensitivity to mite, without evidence of cross-reactivity to mite.[1] Kino et al. have shown that > 50% of randomly selected asthmatics had reaginic sensitivity by skin testing to moth and butterfly, with 8% of controls reacting.[17] About two-thirds of those with positive skin tests to moth extract have evidence of specific serum IgE to moth extract by RAST assay.[1] RAST inhibition studies demonstrated cross-reactivity with silkworm moth wing but not with mite.[17] Successful P-K tests have been completed in four patients with moth sensitivity.[14] Silkworm moth wing appears to be a more potent sensitizer, in Japanese asthmatics, than other moth body parts.[1] Allergic sensitization has also been reported to the common clothes moth *(Tineola bisselliella).*[2]

Diptera

This order includes midges, chironomids, lake flies, blow flies, screwworm flies, mushroom flies, sewer flies, fruit flies, house flies, and mosquitoes.

Mosquitoes are one of the most important insect pests of man, transmitting many varied diseases including malaria, yellow fever, and encephalitis.[47] There are 78 species of mosquitoe in the southern U.S. alone, and 67 of those species may be found in Florida.[47] Each species bites at a particular time of the day or night.[17] There are 17 different enzymes in mosquitoe saliva, including anticoagulants and enzymes to prevent platelet aggregation.[47] Although inhalant sensitivity to mosquitoes may exist, it has not been recognized as a significant problem. Asthma has been reported from the bite of a mosquitoe in a 40-year-old female.[47] She had a strong positive skin test reaction to mosquitoe extract and was successfully desensitized.[47]

The American screwworm fly caused significant allergic symptoms, including nasal and eye symptoms, wheezing, shortness of breath, and cough, in those working in planes dropping thousands of sterile flies in an attempt to control the population of these insects. The pilots also had allergic reactions and near-disasters occurred in flight as a result.[3] Occupational asthma has been described in a previously nonatopic individual working with Australian sheep blowflies after approximately 20 months of employment.[3]

A study done in a Sudanese community close to the Nile river showed that inhabitants that were exposed to large numbers of the "green nimitti" midge *(Cladotanytarsus lewisi)* were found to have an increased incidence of asthma and rhinitis compared to a nearby community without the midge infestation.[48] These midges may be present in such large numbers as to cause physical discomfort and limit outdoor activity. Swarms of midges would "make the sky dark," causing the villagers to veil their faces.[16,48] Rates of allergic rhinitis were four times higher, and rates of asthma were 50% higher in the midge-infested communities compared to the control town less than a 20-minute drive away.[48] Crude midge extracts produced positive wheal-and-flare reactions when used to skin test Sudanese asthmatics, and anti-*C. lewisi* IgE has been used to passively sensitize human lung fragments, with subsequent release of allergic mediators.[16] Interestingly, allergenicity of the hemoglobin molecule of the non-biting midge (chironomid) has been demonstrated.[17]

Allergic symptoms have been reported after exposure to insect contaminants of fish and other pet foods. Exposure to the chironomids and their hemoglobins may be a cause of occupational respiratory allergy in pet food manufacturing workers.[2,37,49]

Allergic rhinitis due to exposure to the common house fly *(Musca domestica)* has been reported in a researcher working with these insects. Positive skin tests and RAST were found using house fly extract.[2] Asthma due to exposure to maggots of the common house fly, as well as the "blue bottle" maggots *(Calliphora sp.)*, has been described in fishermen using them for bait, with late-phase asthmatic responses documented after blue bottle maggot exposure.[2]

Asthma due to fruit fly *(Drosophila melanogaster)* exposure has been described in those involved in research utilizing these insects.[2] Sewage filter flies *(Psychoda alternata sp.)* have caused occupational asthma in sensitized sewage workers in both Africa and the United States[2,50] (Fig. 6).

Hymenoptera

Ostrom et al. reported a honey plant employee who experienced severe asthma during the honey packing process. Skin tests to common outdoor aeroallergens were negative, but skin tests, RAST, and bronchial provocation tests with honeybee whole body extract were positive. Eluates from high-volume air-sample filters located inside the honey processing plant gave positive skin tests, RAST, and

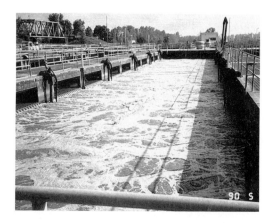

FIGURE 6. Sewage treatment facility. Occupational asthma due to exposure to sewer filter flies has been seen in sewage treatment workers.

bronchial provocation tests. The data supported an IgE-mediated, seasonal occupational sensitivity to honey bee body dust.[51] Beekeepers with an atopic history (although not allergic to bee stings) have been reported to have rhinitis and asthma worsened by bee body dust and have higher levels of specific IgE to honey bee whole body extract compared with non-atopic beekeepers.[52]

Other Insect Orders

Fleas (order Siphonaptera) have been shown to be a non-cross-reacting antigen by RAST and immunoblotting in some patients who experience allergic symptoms around cats. Nearly half of patients with suspected cat allergy also have IgE to cat flea, and up to 9% of patients with allergic symptoms to cats in one study had specific IgE demonstrated to flea without IgE to cat. The clinical significance of this has yet to be determined.[2]

Large amounts of caddis flies (order Trichoptera) have been documented to cause allergic conjunctivitis, rhinitis, and asthma along the Niagra River in Ontario,[53] and sensitivity to caddis fly and May fly has been reported on Lake Erie.[2] Seasonal asthma has been reported in one patient who had his walls and patio infested with box elder bugs (order Hemiptera), and his symptoms cleared once the bugs had been exterminated.[2]

Mites

Mites (order Acarina) have a body with two segments and eight legs, belonging to the subclass Acari, one of several subclasses of the class Arachnida. Storage mites are a small, wingless, translucent species that breed rapidly and require high humidity to reproduce.[35] Although house dust mites such as *Dermatophygoides pteronyssinus* and *D. farinae* are well known to be important indoor aeroallergens, Warren et al. suggest that the storage mite *Lepidoglyphus destructor* may be as important an allergen source in cases of grain dust allergy as *Dermatophygoides* species are in patients who are allergic to house dust.[54] In a survey of mites found in bulk grain stored in Wales and England, Griffiths et al. found that 90% of the grain examined was infested to some degree with storage mites.[55] The most common species found in their study was *Lepidoglyphus* (formerly *Glycyphagus*)

destructor.[55] Cusack et al. have also found a high degree of mite infestation in a wide range of stored products in Ireland. Of the 70 species of mites identified, six species were the most commonly found: *Acarus siro, A. immobilis, cheyletiella eruditus, L. destructor, Tyrophagus longior,* and *T. putrescentiae.*[56] Wraith et al.[57] studied 210 patients whose occupation or living conditions seemed likely to expose them to mite allergens. The patients had bronchial asthma or rhinitis and were skin tested to *D. pteronyssinus* and four storage mites: *A. siro, Glycyphagus domesticus, L. destructor,* and *T. putrescentiae.* The authors concluded that storage mites may present a significant occupational hazard to those who handle material infested with mites, such as farmers.[57] Green and Woolcock found that asthmatics in a New Guinea population had positive skin tests to the storage mite *T. putrescentiae* as commonly as asthmatics in Sydney, Australia had positive skin tests to the common house dust mite *D. pteronyssinus.*[58]

Poultry farmers and those processing poultry may become sensitized to the northern fowl mite *Ornithonyssus sylviarum.*[59] Lutsky et al. studied 16 poultry workers with workplace-associated asthma and rhinitis, 27 atopic individuals with similar symptoms but no occupational exposure to poultry, and 12 asymptomatic nonatopic poultry-exposed controls. Ten of the 16 atopic poultry workers had immediate skin-test reactivity, compared with 2 of 27 non-poultry-exposed controls. Skin-test positivity to the northern fowl mite antigen was distinct from positivity to *D. farinae.* RAST testing also showed specific IgE to the northern fowl mite in 60% of patients with positive skin tests, and bronchial provocation testing done in a patient with positive skin tests and asthmatic symptoms demonstrated an immediate 25% fall in FEV_1 upon challenge.[59]

SUMMARY AND TREATMENT RECOMMENDATIONS

Occupational sensitization to inhaled insect allergens has been described with a large number of insects. Those involved with occupational exposure to large numbers of a particular insect are at increased risk for developing work-related asthma, especially if they have an atopic history, although an atopic history is not a prerequisite for development of inhaled insect allergy. Most of the occupational asthma from insects appears to be IgE-mediated, as demonstrated by skin testing, RAST, P-K results, leukocyte histamine release assays, and bronchial provocation testing.

Immunotherapy has been successfully employed in the treatment of allergic sensitivity to cockroach aeroallergens[20] and has also been useful in a Japanese case study of allergy to inhaled moth particles,[1] but this clearly needs additional study.

It is not clear how long the "typical" period of time is for sensitization to occur after occupational exposure to insects. This most likely depends on the predisposition of the individual, as well as the duration and intensity of the exposure. The recommended treatment for occupational allergy to insects is removal from the antigen source. The role of allergen immunotherapy in this setting is still not clear.

Cautious consideration should be undertaken by those with a strong atopic history who are contemplating employment or research involving heavy and/or prolonged exposure to airborne insect debris. Adequate respiratory protection and ventilation should be provided with such exposure to attempt to avoid sensitization.

REFERENCES

1. Kino T, Oshima S: Allergy to insects in Japan. J Allergy Clin Immunol 64:131–138, 1979.
2. Matthews KP: Inhalant insect-derived allergens. Immunol Allergy Clin North Am 9:2, 1989.
3. Kaufman GL, Baldo BA, Tovey ER, et al: Inhalant allergy following occupational exposures to blowflies. Clin Allergy 16:65–71, 1986.
4. Burge PS, Edge G, O'Brien IM, et al: Occupational asthma in a research centre breeding locusts. Clin Allergy 10:355–363, 1980.
5. Ramazzini B (1713): Workers who handle flax, hemp and silk. In De Morbus Artificum (Diseases of Workers. Tr. Wilmer Cave Wright). Chicago, University of Chicago Press, 1940, pp 257–261.
6. Kang B, Jones J, Johnson J, et al: Analysis of indoor environment and atopic allergy in urban populations with bronchial asthma. Ann Allergy 62:30–34, 1989.
7. Lan JL, Lee DT, Wu CH, et al: Cockroach hypersensitivity: Preliminary study of allergic cockroach asthma in Taiwan. J Allergy Clin Immunol 82:736–740, 1988.
8. Kang B, Sulit N: A comparative study of prevalence of skin hypersensitivity to cockroach and house dust antigens. Ann Allergy 41:333–336, 1978.
9. Kang B, Chang JL, Homburger H, et al: Cockroach cause of allergic asthma. Its specificity and immunologic profile. J Allergy Clin Immunol 63:80, 1979.
10. Shulaner FA: Sensitivity to the cockroach in three groups of allergic children. Pediatrics 45:465, 1970.
11. Mendoza J, Snyder FD: Cockroach sensitivity in children with bronchial asthma. Ann Allergy 28:159, 1970.
12. Bernton HS, McMahan TF, Brown H: Cockroach asthma. Br J Dis Chest 58:49, 1972.
13. Bernton HS, Brown H: Cockroach allergy. II. The relation of infestation to sensitization. South Med J 60:852, 1967.
14. Kino T, Oshima S: Allergy to insects in Japan. I. The reaginic sensitivity to moth and butterfly in patients with bronchial asthma. J Allergy Clin Immunol 61:10–16, 1978.
15. Perlman F, Press E, Googins JA, et al: Tussockosis: Reactions to Douglas fir tussock moth. Ann Allergy 36:302–307, 1976.
16. Cranston PS, Gad El, Rab MO, et al: Immediate-type skin reactivity to extracts of the "green nimitti" midge, (Cladotanytarsus lewisi), and other chironomids in asthmatic subjects in the Sudan and Egypt. Ann Trop Med Parasitol 77:527–533, 1983.
17. Kino T, Chihara J, Fukuda K, et al: Allergy to insects in Japan. J Allergy Clin Immunol 79:857, 1987.
18. Bangantose AH, Mathews KP, Homburger HA, Saaveard-Delgado AP: Inhalant allergy due to crickets. J Allergy Immunol 65:71–74, 1980.
19. Work-related allergies in insect raising facilities. MMWR 33:448, 1984.
20. Kang BC, Johnson J, Morgan C, et al: The role of immunotherapy in cockroach asthma. J Asthma 25:205–218, 1988.
21. Cornwell PB: Can cockroaches cause asthma? [letter] Br Med J 30:1159, 1977.
22. Bernstein DI, Gallagher JA, Bernstein IL: Mealworm asthma: Clinical and immunologic studies. J Allergy Clin Immunol 72:475–480, 1983.
23. Stevenson DD, Matthews KP: Occupational asthma following inhalation of moth particles. J Allergy 39:274, 1967.
24. Chang JL, Ryo UY, Kang B: Changes in free histamine in peripheral circulation following cockroach-antigen challenge in asthmatics. Mt Sinai J Med 51:197–202, 1984.
25. Kang B, Vellody D, Homburger H, et al: Cockroach cause of allergic asthma. J Allergy Clin Immunol 63:80–86, 1979.
26. Stankus RP, Lehrer SB: Common seasonal and environmental allergens. Postgrad Med 82:213–221, 1987.
27. Bernton HS, Brown H: Insect allergy: The allergenicity of the excrement of the cockroach. Ann Allergy 28:543–547, 1970.
28. Hosen H: Bronchial challenge studies with cockroach antigen in asthmatic children (letter). Ann Allergy 32:176, 1974.
29. Monk BE: Contact urticaria to locusts. Br J Dermatol 118:707–708, 1988.
30. Hill WR, Rubenstein AD, Kovacs J: Dermatitis resulting from contact with moths (genus Hylesia). JAMA 138:737, 1948.
31. Stevenson DD, Mathews KP: Occupational asthma following inhalation of moth particles. J Allergy 39:274–283, 1967.
32. Homburger RN: A cautious view of the use of RAST in clinical allergy. Immunol Allergy Pract 3:10, 1981.
33. Zschunke E: Contact urticaria dermatitis and asthma from cockroaches. Contact Dermatitis 4:313–314, 1978.
34. Goldstein IF, Reed CE, Swanson MC, et al: Aeroallergens in New York inner city dwellings of asthmatics. Experientia (Suppl 51):133, 1987.
35. Baldo BA, Sutton R, Wrigley CW: Grass allergens, with particular reference to cereals. Prog Allergy 30:1–66, 1982.

36. Sheldon JM, Johnston JH: Hypersensitivity to beetle *(Coleoptera)*. J Allergy 12:493, 1941.

37. Baur X, Dewain M, Fruhmann G, et al: Hypersensitivity to chironomids (non-biting midges): Localization of the antigenic determinants within certain polypeptide sequences of hemoglobins/erythrocruorins of *Chironomus thummi thummi* (Diptera). J Allergy Clin Immunol 69:66, 1982.

38. Bernton HS, Brown H: Insects as potential sources of ingestant allergens. Ann Allergy 25:381-387, 1967.

39. Popa V, George SA, Gavanescu O: Occupational and nonoccupational respiratory allergy in bakers. Acta Allerg 25:159-177, 1970.

40. Schroeckenstein D, Meier-Davis S, Buch RK, et al: Occupational sensitivity to *Alphitobius diaperinus* (lesser mealworm). J Allergy Clin Immunol 79:246, 1987.

41. Baldo BA, Krilis S, Taylor KM: IgE-mediated acute asthma following inhalation of a powdered marine sponge. Clin Allergy 12:179-186, 1982.

42. Wittich FW: Allergic rhinitis and asthma due to sensitization of the Mexican bean weevil *(Zabrotes sugfasciatus)*. J Allergy 12:42-45, 1940.

43. Hinton HE, Corbet AS: Common Insect Pests of Stored Food Products, 5th ed. London, British Museum, (Economic Ser., No. 15) 1972.

44. Perlman F: Insects as inhalant allergens: Considerations of aerobiology, biochemistry, preparation of material, and clinical observations. J Allergy 29:302-328, 1958.

45. Balyeat RM, Stewen TR, Taft CE: Comparative pollen, mold, butterfly, and moth emanation content of the air. J Allergy 3:227, 1932.

46. Wynn SR, Swanson MC, Reed CE, et al: Immunochemical quantitation, size distribution and crossreactivity of Lepidoptera (moth) aeroallergens in southeastern Minnesota. J Allergy Clin Immunol 82:47, 1988.

47. Gluck JC, Pacin MP: Asthma from mosquito bites: A case report. Ann Allergy 56:492-493, 1986.

48. Kay AB, MacLean CMU, Wilkinson AH, et al: The prevalence of asthma and rhinitis in a Sudanese community seasonally exposed to a potent airborne allergen (the "green nimitti" midge, *Cladotanytarsus lewisi*). J Allergy Clin Immunol 71:345-352, 1983.

49. Rudolph R, Blohm B, Kunkel G, et al: Futtermittelallergien bei tierhaltern. Hautarzt 32(Suppl 5):143, 1981.

50. Ordman B: Sewage filter flies *(Psychoda)* as a cause of bronchial asthma. S African Med J 20:32-35, 1946.

51. Ostrom NK, Swanson MC, Agarwal MK, Yunginger JW: Occupational allergy to honeybee-body dust in a honey-processing plant. J Allergy Clin Immunol 77:736-740, 1986.

52. Yunginger JW, Jones RT, Leiferman KM, et al: Immunological and biochemical studies in beekeepers and their family members. J Allergy Clin Immunol 61:93, 1978.

53. Osgood H: Allergy to caddis fly (Trichoptera). II. Clinical aspects. J Allergy 28:292, 1957.

54. Warren CPW, Sinha RN, Strevens VH: Allergic reactions to the grain mite *Lepidoglyphus destructor*. J Allergy Clin Immunol 63:149, 1979.

55. Griffiths DA, Wilkon DR, Southgate BJ, et al: A survey of mites in bulk grain stored on farms in England and Wales. Ann Appl Biol 82:180-185, 1976.

56. Cusack PD, Evans GO, Brennan PA: A survey of mites of stored grain and grain products in the republic of Ireland. Sci Proc R Dubl Soc Serv B 3:273-329, 1975.

57. Wraith DG, Cunnington AM, Seymour WM: The role and allergenic importance of storage mites in house dust and other environments. Clin Allergy 9:545-561, 1979.

58. Green WF, Woolcock AJ: *Tyrophagus putrescentiae:* An allergenically important mite. Clin Allergy 8:135-144, 1978.

59. Lutsky I, Teichtahl H, Bar-Sela S: Occupational asthma due to poultry mites. J Allergy Clin Immunol 73:56-60, 1984.

Chapter 20

OCCUPATIONAL ASTHMA AND RELATED CONDITIONS IN ANIMAL WORKERS

Emil J. Bardana, Jr., MD

Hypersensitivity reactions to animal dander, saliva, serum, and urinary protein are extremely common among the population. Animals can be encountered at home, at the workplace, in school, or pursuant to one's avocation. Considering that over 60% of the country's 85 million households have dogs and/or cats, distinguishing occupational from nonoccupational health problems can present a unique challenge. Workers who have regular contact with animals represent a heterogeneous group with significant socioeconomic and educational diversity. Table 1 summarizes the major job descriptions with significant animal exposure. The potential group at risk is substantial. It has been estimated that in the United States alone, more than 35,000 workers and scientists are regularly exposed to laboratory animals in connection with the commercial production of laboratory animals, animal care activities, and animal research programs[1] (Table 1). A survey taken in 1978 indicated that 20 million animals were being acquired by major institutions on a yearly basis, and 93% of them were rodents.[2] This chapter will outline some of the epidemiologic considerations of animal-related allergy and discuss the likely clinical presentations and diagnostic approaches available to the clinician.

HISTORICAL PERSPECTIVES

Aside from the observations made by Ramazzini in silk workers and tanners, one of the earliest contemporary reports dealing with animal dander-induced bronchial asthma was made by Henry Salter in 1864.[3] Salter was himself an asthmatic who observed that "one of the most curious incidents in the clinical history of asthma related to its production by certain animal and vegetable emanations." The first edition of his treatise indicated only two animals whose "emanations" could induce asthma, i.e., cats and rabbits. In later editions he maintained that horses, wild beasts, guinea pigs, cattle, dogs, and rabbits could also induce asthmatic paroxysms. Subsequent to Salter's seminal observations, innumerable studies have confirmed that a variety of animal antigens can cause a spectrum of hypersensitivity states in man.

Most of the early allergy textbooks and review articles dealing with animal allergy focused on rats, dogs, rabbits, and other pets.[4-6] The work-related aspects of animal-induced asthma became increasingly known through a variety of case reports. Rackemann was among the first to observe respiratory allergies to murine allergens in laboratory workers.[7] Later publications confirmed murine-related hypersensitivity in a variety of work settings.[8-10] Other laboratory animal species were also incriminated and included the rat,[11,12] guinea pig,[13,14] hamster,[15] and the rabbit.[12,14] The first significant series of work-related animal allergy cases appeared in 1961 and summarized sensitivity reactions in 10 workers at the Karolinska Hospital.[16] In the mid-1970s, Lincoln et al. published their observations concerning 17 animal workers at the Oak Ridge National Laboratory.[17] In Europe, Bohn and Braun followed 19 individuals with dander-induced allergy over a 4-year period.[18]

TABLE 1.   *Occupations in Which Regular Exposure to Animals May Be Found*

Academics	Pharmacologists
Animal breeders	Physician researchers
Animal handlers	Scientists
Biomedical scientists	Stable hands
Circus workers	Students
Cooks	Tanners
Entymologists	Taxidermists
Farmers	Technicians
Grooms	Veterinarians
Jockeys	Zookeepers
Livestock workers	

EPIDEMIOLOGY

It has been said that if conditions are favorable, virtually any mammalian species may cause an allergic response in man.[19] Approximately 100 million domestic animals reside in the U.S., the most common being cats and dogs. The prevalence rate for atopy has been reported at approximately 30% in the general population.[20] In a population of 300 consecutive patients seen at an allergy clinic, 82 individuals (27%) were aware of symptoms following exposure to cats, dogs, or both.[21] In most populations, cat allergy appears to be the most common type of animal allergy. Among a stratified, random sample of 320 white adults in Baltimore skin tested with cat and dog extracts, 13% were positive to cat and 7% to dog antigens.[22]

In 1972 Lutsky and Neuman surveyed 1,293 workers at 39 U.S. research facilities.[23] The majority were employed at medical and veterinary schools, with fewer located at research institutes, pharmaceutical plants, and commercial animal-breeding facilities. They noted that 191 of the 1,293 employees having direct contact with laboratory animals had manifestations of sensitivity to animal antigens, i.e., an incidence of nearly 15%. The species most frequently incriminated as a cause of symptoms were the rat, mouse, and rabbit, in descending order. At about the same time that Lincoln,[17] Bohn and Braun,[18] and Litsky and Neuman[23] published their observations, the British Society of Allergy and Clinical Immunology conducted a survey, which was published in 1976.[24] This catalyzed the formation of an alliance of several investigators into a study group under the auspices of the U.K. Health and Safety Executive.

Up until the 1980s, most of the epidemiologic data dealing with animal allergy consisted of results of cross-sectional prevalence studies. One variety of study sampled exposed individuals at multiple institutions using questionnaires to accumulate raw, subjective data.[23,25] Another group of studies focused on animal-induced allergy in very defined populations, usually at a single institution with careful clinical and immunologic evaluation.[17,26-29] The former observations provided a broad overview of the problem, whereas the latter studies assimilated important clinical and serological fact. The outcome of the collaborative studies led to the realization that exposure to animal allergens could induce common and occasionally serious work-related disease. Symptoms can become quite debilitating and often precipitate change in job or career. Prevalence rates have been consistently higher in the U.K., i.e., 23 to 30%,[25,27,28] than in the U.S. where they range 11 to 15%.[17,23,26] It is not clear what accounts for this difference. It may related to differences in how animals are housed and the ventilation systems servicing the facilities.

A contemporary, cross-sectional study was carried out among animal laboratories of the National Institutes of Health to ascertain the prevalence of laboratory animal allergy.[30] Among the 549 exposed workers, 131 (24%) gave a history of one or more allergy symptoms associated with animal exposure. The investigators felt that a history of atopic disease was not sufficiently sensitive to be employed as a precursor of future laboratory animal allergy. A prior history of atopy was present in only 51% of those with sensitivity to animal allergens. Factors found to be significantly associated with the development of sensitivity to laboratory animals included a history of atopy and, in particular, of allergy to domestic animals. Also important were the number and varieties of animal exposures both at work and in the home.

Studies have shown that the majority of cases of laboratory-animal-induced allergy develop over the initial 36 months of exposure. The majority develop symptoms between 6 and 36 months of exposure.[31] The most common manifestation is allergic rhinoconjunctivitis, which may be associated with palatal itching. It has been estimated that between 25 and 50% of these rhinitis cases go on to develop bronchial asthma. Atopic individuals are much more likely to develop animal allergy, and, once developed, are much more likely to develop bronchial asthma.[17,23,26-28,31,32]

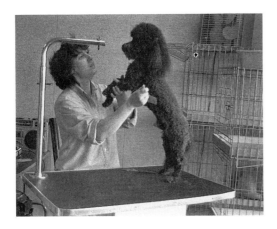

FIGURE 1.   Pet shop employee grooming a dog. Often this type of activity is carried out in the back of a facility with poor ventilation.

TABLE 2.   *Classification of Frequently Encountered Animals and Their Purified Antigens**

Family	Genus	Common Name	Purified Antigen	Mol. Wt.
Muridae	*Mus*	Mouse	Mus m I‡	22,000
	Rattus	Rat	Rat n I‡	20,500
			Rat n II‡	17,000
Cavioidae	*Caviidae*	Guinea pig		
Cricetidae	*Mesocricetus*	Hamster		
	Gerbillus	Gerbil		
Chinchillidae	*Chinchilla*	Chinchilla		
Leporidae	*Oryctolagus*	Rabbit		
Canidae	*Cannus*	Dog	Can ƒ I§	
Felidae	*Felix*	Cat	Fel d I†	18,000
Mustelidae	*Mustela*	Mink		
Didelphyidae	*Didelphis*	Opposum		
Cercopithecoidae		Rhesus monkey		
Callitrichidae		Marmoset, tamarin		
Equidae	*Equus*	Horse	Equ c I†	19,000
			Equ c II†	51,000
Suidae	*Sus*	Pig		
Bovidae	*Bos*	Cow	Bos d I†	24,000
			Bos d II	20,000
			Bos d III	22,000
	Capra	Goat		
	Ovis	Sheep		

*Modified from ref. 34; †dander-derived; ‡urine-derived; §saliva-derived.

ANIMAL ANTIGENS

Small animals present the major source of IgE-mediated sensitization in susceptible workers. This was especially notable in studies of veterinarians[33] (Fig. 1). All animals release protein material into their environment that can potentially sensitize exposed individuals. Like other allergens derived from molds and pollens, animal-derived proteins are complex and only certain moieties have the capacity to sensitize. In a few instances the major allergens have been identified and purified, which has facilitated improved diagnosis and treatment outcomes. Among animals that are preferred as either pets or laboratory animals, Schumacher has identified 13 species belonging to 11 different families and five different orders of mammalia that can cause work-related problems.[34] This has been expanded by adding three families of the common larger species (Table 2).

For many years, epithelial scales on the hair and fur of animals were felt to constitute the most common inhalant allergens in both pet and laboratory animals. However, saliva was implicated as a source of active antigens in the cat, dog and rabbit by Spain et al. in 1942.[35] More recently similar antigens have been identified in rat saliva.[36] Salivary antigens are transferred to the pelt by licking and can be released into the environment when dry or transferred by petting or contact with carpeting or furniture.

In 1977, Newman-Taylor, Longbottom, and Pepys published their observations in five asthmatic laboratory workers.[37] The five workers reported that they developed wheal and flare skin reactions when animals urinated on and then ran across the skin. They wondered whether the skin reaction represented an inadvertent epicutaneous skin test. Their studies demonstrated that mouse and rat urinary proteins represented strong and clinically relevant antigens, both by epicutaneous testing and bronchial provocation.[37] Subsequent to these observations, other studies in a variety of species have identified reactive urinary antigens in mice, rats, guinea pigs, dogs, cats, and rabbits.[36-46]

Mammals have been demonstrated to have substantial amounts of physiologic proteinuria.[47] Perhaps the most significant amounts of urinary protein are found in the male mouse (200–400 mg/kg/day) and male rats (10–35 mg/kg/day).[48,49] Since the gerbil excretes only a few drops of urine daily, it is not felt to pose any allergic potential.[34] Mouse urine contains a complex group of proteins that are relatively heat stable and that have a MW of 17,000 daltons. This protein complex has been identified in dust samples by immunodiffusion. These observations have been verified by quantitative air sampling studies as well.[49,50] Subtle antigenic differences exist among different inbred strains of mice, which may account for strain-specific sensitivity in some laboratory workers.[40] Mouse pelt contains two distinct protein moieties, one of which is probably identical to the urinary protein complex,[51] and the other, which has a molecular weight of between 62,000 and 67,000 daltons. It cross-reacts with mouse serum albumin.[37,41]

Rat urine also contains a significant amount of protein that has been isolated from dust samples taken from the walls and HVAC systems of animal facilities.[54-57] In contrast to homogeneous murine urinary protein, rat protein is quite diverse and is related to several serum constituents.[54,57] Of the two important allergens in rat urine, one is a prealbumin with a molecular weight of 17,000 daltons, and the other is an alpha-2-euglobulin with a molecular weight of 15,000 daltons.

Guinea pig urine also contains two major allergenic moieties. One is a low molecular weight moiety with characteristics of prealbumin. The other has a molecular weight of approximately 60,000 and was thought to represent guinea pig serum albumin. However, the latter does not completely inhibit its binding in a radioassay system.[58] Allergens derived from the guinea pig pelt have characteristics similar to a prealbumin moiety and demonstrate the capacity to partially inhibit binding to guinea pig urine antigens.[58,59] All these allergens have been recovered from animal room air ventilation filters.[60,61]

Allergenic proteins derived from the pelts of rabbits have a molecular weight between 18,000 and 38,000 daltons.[59] Clearly, this moiety has the capacity to sensitize exposed individuals. Some investigators have expressed the opinion that though more is known about the rat and mouse allergens, the guinea pig and rabbit allergens are much more effective sensitizers.[28,30,62]

The allergens involved in cat sensitivity have been extensively studied over the past several years. One of the first studies directed at finding a source of cat allergens was performed by Spain.[35] This study demonstrated no unique allergens in cat pelt that were not also present in saliva. Later investigations using crossed immunoelectrophoresis demonstrated that cat saliva contained all the detectable major allergens present in cat pelt.[63] Immunochemical studies comparing serum, saliva, urine, and dander as potential sources of cat allergen showed that dander and saliva contained the highest levels, with smaller amounts in urine and serum.[64,65] Allergenic reactivity as measured by skin test titrations, modified radioallergosorbent (RAST) tests, and crossed radioimmunoelectrophoresis of cat-derived extracts strongly correlated with the presence of Fel d I purified allergen[64-66] (Table 2). Fel d I has been shown to be an acidic glycoprotein, having an isoelectric point of 3.85 and a prealbumin mobility in 7% acrylamide gel.[67] It has a molecular weight of approximately 18,000 daltons, and it exists primarily as a dimer in physiologic solution. Cat saliva, which has long been known to induce contact urticaria in highly sensitive individuals, is the origin of Fel d I.[68] Transfer to the pelt is believed to occur by virtue of the habitual grooming (licking) of the fur.[69] It has also been demonstrated in the mucous components of salivary glands of the skin[68] but is not found in serum. Recent observations by Charpin et al. suggest that the skin of the cat is also a major source of Fel d I antigen. In the skin, Fel d I appears to be produced by sebaceous and basal squamous epithelial cells and stored on the surface of the epidermis and hair.[69a] A second, less potent, allergen has been found to have a molecular weight of 68,000 daltons, display a mobility similar to cat albumin, and is found in the serum, saliva, and pelt.[65] The level of airborne Fel d I correlates with airway constriction in cat-asthmatic patients and is directly proportional to the dose of cat extract inducing a positive bronchial challenge in the same subject.[70] Cat urine also contains an additional protein moiety distinct from Fel d I and cat serum albumin.[45] The physiologic function of Fel d I remains an enigma.

Allergens derived from dog are believed to be less allergenic than those derived from the cat. Until recently, canine-derived extracts lacked the biochemical standardization described for cat extracts.[71] Because of demonstrated variability in commercial preparations of dog extracts,[72] a recent effort was begun to develop an international standard for dog pelt extract.[73] Initial studies using dander extracts identified two major allergenic components, a dog serum albumin and a serum protein in the gamma globulin regions.[74,75] Subsequent studies established additional antigens, with the major allergenic component being dog serum albumin along with a nonserum protein.[76-78] Serum and urine are also believed to contain sensitizing proteins, although these have not been well characterized.[35] The importance of dog albumin as a clinically relevant aeroallergen remains controversial. A number of studies using skin testing and RAST have shown that less than 20% of dog-sensitive individuals exhibit a positive response to dog serum albumin.[79] Contrary to often expressed lay opinion, no single breed of dog has been found to be more or less allergenic than others, although a number of studies have demonstrated breed-specific allergens.[79,80] Recent observations by de Groot et al. indicate that a newly identified 25 kd moiety, referred to as Can ʃ I, is a major allergen in dog saliva (Table 2).[80a] Additional studies will be required to investigate the size of particles containing dog allergens that become airborne and to establish threshold levels above which atopic subjects become sensitized.

Allergy to horses does not constitute as much a problem as it did early in this century when horses were used as a major form of transport. As well, horse hair is less extensively used in furniture, mattresses, mattings, padding, and felts, which accounted for considerable work-related disease in the past. Nevertheless, significant exposures continue to occur in agricultural workers, mounted law enforcement units, and race track and stable attendants, as well as those who ride as a hobby (Fig. 2). It has been reported that from 8 to 19% of allergic patients react to horse allergens by intracutaneous testing, though clinical symptoms are relatively infrequent.[71,81] A number of immunochemical studies have shown the presence of both horse serum albumin and other unique allergens in horse dandruff.[82] Two of these allergens have been isolated and partially characterized as Equ C I and Equ C II[83] (Table 2).

Occupational asthma and rhinitis from cattle, hogs, sheep and goats have also been reported. Studies of cow dandruff by the RAST technique have demonstrated several fractions reacting with IgE antibodies similar to those in horse dander[84] (Table 2). Recently a laboratory technician was reported to develop occupational asthma from inhalation of crystalline bovine serum albumin powder.[84a] Donham and associates found no significant effect of intense farm animal exposure on pulmonary function, although the hog producers had a significantly higher level of respiratory symptoms if they worked in hog confinement buildings rather than in open, nonconfined facilities.[85] Matson et al. found that symptoms in hog farmers were not related to IgE or IgG allergic mechanisms.[86]

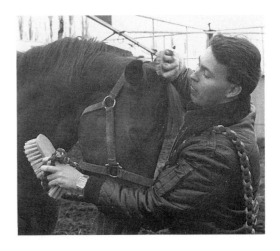

FIGURE 2.   Stablehand grooming a thoroughbred horse at the Portland Meadows Racetrack stable.

Many garments are produced from animal epidermal sources, e.g., furs, cashmere, mohair, alpaca, and vicuna. However, these materials are rarely associated with allergy. Sheep's wool has been found to yield positive skin tests to extracts.[87] However, the physical characteristics of wool suggest that most skin-induced problems are irritant rather than allergy caused. It has also been noted that some sources of wool are contaminated with human dander or housedust allergen, or both.[88]

Although studies are quite limited, shared antigenicity has been demonstrated to exist between mammalian-derived extracts. Cross-reacting allergens between cat and dog dander extracts have been clearly established.[35,89] Skin-testing has shown a significant trend toward multiple reactions to antigens from mammalian species.[90] Furthermore, crossed immunoelectrophoresis gives evidence for partial identity of antigens from several mammalian species.[76,91]

Other species of animals have been reported to cause respiratory allergy. One that is commonly used in a variety of biology classroom settings is the frog. Both IgE-mediated and contact dermatitis has been reported to antigens in bullfrog secretions.[92] Others have observed the induction of occupational asthma due to inhalation of venom expelled from frog skin glands.[93]

Other small animal species known to cause respiratory allergic symptoms as well as IgE-specific antibody are gerbils[94] and tamarin monkeys.[95] Although the dander is allergenic in both species, data on the immunochemical identification of allergens are not available.

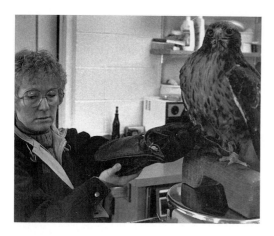

FIGURE 3.   Veterinarian weighing a bird at the Portland Zoo.

Birds are another source of animal-induced hypersensitivity disease. The first reports of allergic alveolitis due to avian antigens were published in 1960.[96,97] Later a similar condition was noted in pigeon breeders.[98,99] Almost all species of birds have been incriminated[100] (Fig. 3). IgG-precipitating antibody has been demonstrated against extracts of feathers, feather dust (bloom), droppings, and serum. Most subjects with this condition have a history of recurrent exposure to dry bird droppings, with subsequent onset of fever, aches, cough, and dyspnea associated with a leukocytosis. Pulmonary function reveals a restrictive pattern, with reduced diffusion capacity. Many individuals with this disease demonstrate both immediate and Arthus reactivity to antigens involved. The antigens have been well characterized in pigeon breeders' disease and include pigeon bloom[101] along with pigeon droppings.[100,102] The major antigenic component is pigeon IgA and IgG, with trace amounts of serum albumin. Pigeon bloom has a very complex nature consisting of pigeon IgA and at least three unique antigens not found in pigeon serum.[103]

CLINICAL PRESENTATION

The occurrence of work-related animal allergy is greater in individuals with a positive personal and family history of atopy. However, it alone cannot be used as a predictor of animal allergy, i.e., in one large study, atopy was present in only 51% of those with proven animal allergy.[30] Atopic status may influence the initial response to an inhalant allergen

but has little effect on the quantity of antibody produced. Platts-Mills et al. reported a significant correlation between positive skin tests to rat urine and reported symptoms (asthma and/or rhinitis), on exposure to rats.[104] Of 179 exposed workers, 17% reported symptoms. Atopy was present in 22% of these workers. A positive skin test alone was present in 40% of workers. Preexisting atopy had a significant influence on the development of asthma, but little on the development of other symptoms. However, atopic status proved to be neither a sensitive nor a specific indicator of which animal handlers would develop asthma. Of 71 with skin test atopy, only 17 developed asthma (24% positive predictive value). Of 108 without atopy, 14 (13%) developed either asthma or rhinitis.[104]

Symptoms of animal allergy usually appear within minutes of exposure to the allergen,[105] and most patients who develop animal allergy will develop multiple symptoms. In one large study of animal allergic individuals, all had manifestations of allergic rhinoconjunctivitis, whereas 71% developed bronchial asthma.[106] It has been said that asthma is a much more common outcome from the development of animal protein sensitivity than as a result of pollen or mold sensitivity.[19] Urticaria and angioedema may be seen following topical exposure, such as from handling or licking. Rare cases of anaphylaxis have occurred secondary to a bite or scratch in which a significant exposure to the allergenic protein occurs. Contact allergic dermatitis has been observed in veterinary surgeons who develop a contact dermatitis to horse amniotic fluid during deliveries.[107]

A few cases of allergic alveolitis (hypersensitivity pneumonitis) have been reported upon exposure to dried, airborne animal proteins. The most common animal source for extrinsic allergic alveolitis is bird antigen.[97-103] However, other animals have also been incriminated. Extrinsic allergic alveolitis has been reported in bench researchers secondary to rat serum protein sensitivity.[108] Allergic alveolitis has also been noted in a gerbil keeper.[109]

DIAGNOSIS OF ANIMAL ALLERGY

The diagnosis of occupational animal allergy has a number of pitfalls that are much less prevalent in other forms of work-related disease. The sheer frequency of contact with animals poses special problems in identifying the cause of the patient's symptoms. Allergies are among the nation's most common and costly health problems, afflicting at least 35 million Americans. Conservative estimates indicate that about 9 million Americans suffer from asthma with or without associated allergic rhinitis, and another 15 million have allergic rhinoconjunctivitis alone.[110] Of these allergic individuals, it has been estimated that nearly 25% are sensitive to dogs or cats.[87] With 100 million domestic animals residing in the U.S.[71] approximately 60% of the country's 85 million households have one or more domestic animals.[111] Therefore, the clinician must first make a diagnosis of animal allergy and, more importantly, must then decide its likely causation among a variety of exposures.

The major diagnostic tool of any clinician is the medical history. In the case of animal allergy, the history must cover a variety of key issues, including the presence of atopy, the totality of animal exposures over the lifetime of the patient (school, work, home, and leisure/avocation activities), and the origin and severity of symptoms, particularly in relation to the putative animal exposures. The history-taking should establish all sources of potential exposure, including frequent sites of visitation, prior animals in a newly purchased home, or the possibility of a second or side job related to the primary job. The author has had numerous cases in which an individual involved in a retail pet store also had strong interests in a second job raising similar domestic pets at home. A thorough review of medical records will provide an insight into severity of symptoms and potential significance of other environmental aeroallergens or irritants. Physical examination is useful during a symptomatic state to record the extent of physical signs in the entire respiratory tract, as well as on the skin. Sequential pulmonary function studies after a period away from work can often be extremely helpful in establishing a diagnosis.

Skin testing and a variety of in vitro studies demonstrating IgG and/or IgE antibodies to the suspected animal protein allergen can be helpful in establishing diagnosis.[17,104-106,112] However, it should be remembered that such studies only assist in the demonstration of antibodies. The latter clearly support prior exposure to the allergen, but not the presence of a symptomatic state. Rarely, bronchial provocation may be required to firmly establish the diagnosis.

ASSESSING THE ANIMAL ENVIRONMENT

The presence of animals in any indoor setting presents potential health problems to any worker or inhabitant. The same is true, to a lesser extent, in confined spaces outdoors as well. Assessing an indoor environment can present very significant problems. Understanding the extent of animal exposures can be difficult, because the risks can be inapparent, falsified, or overlooked entirely. As well, a variety of associated potential irritants and allergens can frequently be disregarded, e.g., pesticides, veterinary pharmaceuticals, and animal feed and feed contaminants.[113] Several key points have been stressed in preparing to assess any animal quarter. First, it is far better to conduct the assessment by a personal visit as opposed to questionnaire. Secondly, a comprehensive evaluation usually requires direct air sampling with analysis by microscopy, culture, and/or immunochemical methodology. Table 3 outlines the important points that should be addressed in assessing an animal facility (Fig. 4).[113]

A number of reports have confirmed the value of methods in which collections of dust are suitably extracted and the allergen content of the resulting eluates determined.[114-117] A descending elution technique has proven useful,[114] and simple in-line extraction of small circular filters has also worked.[115] To measure allergen in the extracts produced, inhibition studies of primary binding assays such as RAST and ELISA have been developed.[114,115] These systems are still in a phase of development and will improve with further experimentation. A recent study employing both the production and removal rates of animal-derived allergens has demonstrated a

TABLE 3. *Principal Issues That Should Be Addressed in Evaluating an Animal Facility*

The number, species, and sexes of animals present

Nature of cages or pens and their bedding

Frequency of bedding change and its disposal

Type of feed utilized and the nature of its storage

Sanitary practices in the facility, i.e., cleansing of floor and wall surfaces

Nature of the HVAC system and associated filters

Frequency of HVAC maintenance

Characteristics of air quality in the facility, i.e., temperature, humidity, exchange rate

Other sources of potential contamination, e.g., mold growth, pesticide, animal feed, etc.

Adapted and modified from ref. 113.

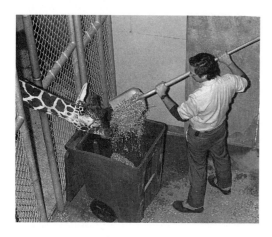

FIGURE 4.   Zookeeper feeding a giraffe in a pen at the Portland Zoo. The environment was exceptionally clean with excellent ventilation.

unique method of quantifying allergen, by measuring the actions taken to reduce levels in an animal facility. This methodology has wide application to a variety of indoor allergens.[118]

PRINCIPLES OF CLINICAL MANAGEMENT

In general, avoidance is the optimal solution to the problem of animal allergy. However, it seems that the socioeconomic impact on affected individuals is greater in this area than many other areas of occupational respiratory disease. One can only imagine the repercussions on a postdoctoral candidate who has developed a unique murine model of disease, or perhaps a veterinarian who has a great deal of emotional and economic investment in his life's work. It is not surprising to note that 72% of individuals diagnosed as having significant animal occupational allergy opted to remain at their work.[23] They relied principally on the use of respiratory protection, industrial hygiene measures, and medications.[119] The success of drug therapy largely depends on the sensitivity of the patient and the continuing extent of occupational exposure. Unless exposure can be extensively reduced, patients with severe allergy will continue to experience symptoms even when receiving adequate medications.

In general, immunotherapy is not recommended for the treatment of most patients with occupational allergy to animals. If they are very sensitive, continued exposure to the species with parallel administration of standardized or partially standardized animal allergens can produce potentially dangerous, life-threatening reactions. This becomes totally impractical in workers with multiple animal allergies or when standardized extracts are not yet available. In the latter case, extracts may contain a variety of foreign proteins, e.g., serum albumin, which could induce a serum sickness-like reaction in the recipient.[105] One must balance these considerations with the growing evidence of immunotherapy efficacy in animal allergy.[58,120-123] Four of these studies demonstrated a reduction in allergen-specific bronchial sensitivity; the fifth study evaluated conjunctival sensitivity, noting an allergen-specific reduction of responses to the challenge in treated individuals. Most importantly, a significant effect on both early and late responses to antigen challenge was demonstrated in one study.[122]

Ideally, coping with animal allergies could be effectively carried out by significantly reducing allergen generation at its source, improving ventilation to remove it despite continued generation or filtering allergens out of the air with personal or area filtration. Although standard animal care procedures already specify a high ventilation rate of 15 changes of air/hour, these are often unachievable in most parts of the country, and even if achieved, would fail to significantly reduce allergen load. In one recent study, it was shown that in a room with 300 rats, an air exchange rate of 172 changes/hour was required to achieve reasonable control.[118] The costs associated with this type of air exchange would be unmanageable. They represent a 1,000-fold greater air-exchange rate than found in a typical energy-efficient American home.

REFERENCES

1. Anon: Institute of Laboratory Animal Resources. Animal Facilities Survey. Lab Anim Care 20:795, 1970.
2. Held JR: Allergy to animals: A laboratory animal science perspective. N Engl Reg Allergy Proc 8:179, 1987.
3. Salter JH: On Asthma: Its Pathology and Treatment. Philadelphia, Blanchard & Lea, 1864, p 90.
4. Freeman J: Toxic idiopathies: Relationship between hay and other pollen ferns, animal asthma, food idiosyncracies, bronchial and spasmodic asthma, etc. Lancet ii:229, 1920.
5. Duke WW: Allergy (asthma, hayfever, urticaria and allied manifestations of reaction). St. Louis, C.V. Mosby, 1925, pp 120–122.
6. Balyeat RM: Allergic Diseases and Their Diagnosis and Treatment. Philadelphia, F.A. Davis, 1930, pp 110–127.

7. Rackemann FM: Asthma. Med Clin North Am 1:65, 1923.

8. Sorrell AH, Gottesman J: Mouse allergy—a case report. Ann Allergy 15:662, 1957.

9. Arbesman CE, Beede RB, Rose NR: Sensitivity to animals: A case report with immunologic studies. J Allergy 29:130, 1958.

10. Czecholinski K, Veltman G: Occupational sensitization of airways by hair and dust of animals (German). Berufsdermatosen 23:87, 1975.

11. Gilday FJ: Bronchial asthma due to rat hair. Delaware Med J 28:110, 1956.

12. Ishiyama H, Kato K, Furuya K, et al: Animal dander allergy found in a laboratory of a cosmetic company (Japanese). Jap J Allergol 23:7, 1974.

13. Braun W: Allergie gegen mecrschweinchen. Allergie Asthma 6:176, 1960.

14. Kobayashi A, Toyoda T, Nakazawa T: Bronchial asthma caused by hair and dander from guinea pig and rabbits. (Japanese). Jap J Allergol 21:244, 1972.

15. Wilson JA: Hamster-hair hypersensitivity in adults of low atopic status. Br Med J 4:341, 1971.

16. Rajka G: Ten cases of occupational hypersensitivity to laboratorry animals. Acta Allergol 16:168, 1961.

17. Lincoln TA, Bolton NE, Garrett AS Jr: Occupational allergy to animal dander and sera. J Occup Med 16:465, 1974.

18. Bohn W, Braun W: Occupational laboratory-animal hair respiratory sensitization. Arbeitsmedizin-Sozial-medizin-Arbeitshygiene (German) 7:94, 1972.

19. Slavin RG: Clinical aspects of allergies to animals: Overview and definition. N Engl Reg Allergy Proc 8:163, 1987.

20. Barbee RA, Lebowitz MD, Thompson HC, et al: Immediate skin-test reactivity in a general population sample. Ann Intern Med 84:129, 1976.

21. Ohman JL: Allergy in man caused by exposure to mammals. J Am Vet Med Assoc 172:1403, 1978.

22. Freidhoff LR, Meyers DA, Marsh DG: A genetic-epidemiologic study of human immune responsiveness to allergens in an industrial population. II. The associations among skin sensitivity, total serum IgE, age and sex in a stratified random sample. J Allergy Clin Immunol 73:490, 1984.

23. Lutsky I, Neuman I: Laboratory animal and dander allergy. I. An occupational disease. Ann Allergy 35:201, 1975.

24. Taylor G, Davies GE, Altounyan REC, et al: Allergic reactons to laboratory animals. Nature 260:80, 1976.

25. Davies GE, McArdle LA: Allergy to laboratory animals: A survey by questionnaire. Int Arch Allergy Appl Immunol 64:302, 1981.

26. Gross NJ: Allergy to laboratory animals: Epidemiologic, clinical and physiologic aspects and a trial of cromolyn in its management. J Allergy Clin Immunol 66:158, 1980.

27. Cockcroft A, Edwards J, McCarthy P, et al: Allergy in laboratory animal workers. Lancet i:827, 1981.

28. Slovak AJ, Hill RN: Laboratory animal allergy: A clinical survey of an exposed population. Br J Med 28:38, 1981.

29. Orr R; quoted by Dwedney JM: Allergy-induced by exposure to animals. J Roy Soc Med 74:928, 1981.

30. Bland SM, Levine MS, Wilson D, et al: Occupational allergy to laboratory animals: An epidemiologic study. J Occup Med 28:1151, 1986.

31. Slovak AJM: Achieved objectives in laboratory animal allergy research: Their significance for policy and practice. N Engl Reg Allergy Proc 8:189, 1987.

32. Davies GE, Thompson AV, Niewola Z, et al: Allergy to laboratory animals: A retrospective, and a perspective study. Br J Ind Med 40:442, 1983.

33. Will LA, Nassif EG, Engen RL, et al: Allergy and pulmonary impairment in Iowa veterinarians. N Engl Reg Allergy Proc 8:173, 1987.

34. Schumacher MJ: Clinically relevant allergens from laboratory and domestic small animals. N Engl Reg Allergy Proc 8:225, 1987.

35. Spain WC, Gillson RE, Strauss MB: Comparative immunologic studies with salivary and epithelial extracts of the dog and cat and rabbit. J Allergy 13:563, 1942.

36. Viander M, Valovirta E, Vanto T, et al: Cross-reactivity of cat and dog allergen extracts. RAST inhibition studies with special reference to the allergenic activity in saliva and urine. Int Arch Allergy Appl Immunol 71:252, 1983.

37. Newman-Taylor AJ, Longbottom JL, Pepys J: Respiratory allergy to urine proteins of rats and mice. Lancet ii:847, 1977.

38. Schumacher MJ: Characterization of allergens from urine and pelts of laboratory mice. Mol Immunol 17:1087, 1980.

39. Lorusso JR, Ohman JL, Picarella D, et al: Immunologic properties of mouse urinary allergen. J Allergy Clin Immunol 75:147, 1985.

40. Schumacher MJ, Tait BD, Holmes MC: Allergy to murine antigens in a biological research institute. J Allergy Clin Immunol 68:310, 1981.

41. Siraganian RP, Sandberg AL: Characterization of mouse allergens. J Allergy Clin Immunol 63:435, 1978.

42. Beeson MF, Dewdney JM, Edwards RG, et al: Prevalence and diagnosis of laboratory animal allergy. Clin Allergy 13:433, 1983.

43. Berrens L, Van Dijk AG, Bollebakker-Baars A, et al: RAST with animal dander, urine, saliva and serum. Ann Allergy 51:543, 1983.

44. Swanson MC, Agarwal MK, Yunginger JW, et al: Guinea pig derived allergens: Characterization, clini-coimmunologic studies and atmospheric immuno-chemical quantitation. J Allergy Clin Immunol 71:95, 1983.

45. Hoffman DR: Dog and cat allergens: Urinary proteins or dander proteins. Ann Allergy 45:205, 1980.

46. McElhinney ME, Findlay SR, Leiterman NM, et al: Cat urinary allergens. J Allergy Clin Immunol 69:144, 1982.

47. Mitruka BM, Rawnsley HM: Clinical, Biochemical and Hematological Reference Values in Normal Experimental Animals and Normal Humans, 2nd ed. New York, Masson, 1981.

48. Finlayson JS, Morris HP: Molecular size of rat urinary protein. Proc Soc Exp Biol Med 119:663, 1965.

49. Twiggs JT, Agarwal MK, Dahlberg MJE, et al: Immunochemical measurement of airborne mouse allergens in a laboratory animal facility. J Allergy Clin Immunol 69:522, 1982.

50. Swanson MC, Agarwal MK, Reed CE: An immunochemical approach to indoor aeroallergen quantitation with a new volumetric air sampler: Studies with mite, roach, cat, mouse and guinea pig antigens. J Allergy Clin Immunol 76:724, 1985.

51. Ohman JL, Moffat S, Lorusso JR: Properties and standardization of a major mouse allergen. J Allergy Clin Immunol 73:191, 1984.

52. Platts-Mills TAE, Longbottom JL, Wilkins SR: Airborne allergens associated with asthma: Particle sizes carrying dust mite and allergens measured with a cascade impactor. J Allergy Clin Immunol 77:850, 1986.

53. Davies GE, Thompson AV, Rackham M: Estimation of airborne rat-derived antigens by ELISA. J Immunoassay 4:113, 1983.
54. Walls AF, Longbottom JL: Quantitative immunoelectrophoretic analysis of rat allergen extracts. I. Antigenic characterization of fur, urine, saliva, and other rat-derived materials. Allergy 38:419, 1983.
55. Longbottom JL: Purification and characterization of allergens from the urines of mice and rats. In Oehling A, Mathav E, Glazer I, Arbesman C (eds): Advances in Allergology and Clinical Immunology. Oxford, Pergamon, 1980, p 483.
56. Walls AF, Longbottom JL: Quantitative immunoelectrophoretic analysis of rat allergen extracts. II. Fur, urne, and saliva studied by crossed radio-immunoelectrophoresis. Allergy 38:501, 1983.
57. Walls AF, Longbottom JL: Comparison of rat fur, urine, saliva and other rat allergen extracts by skin testing, RAST and RAST inhibition. J Allergy Clin Immunol 75:242, 1985.
58. Swanson MC, Agarwal MK, Yunginger JW, et al: Guinea pig-derived allergens: Clinico-immunologic studies, characterization, airborne quantitation and size distribution. Am Rev Respir Dis 129:844, 1984.
59. Ohman JL, Lowell FC, Bloch KJ: Allergens of mammalian origin. II. Characterization of allergens extracted from rat, mouse, guinea pig, and rabbit pelts. J Allergy Clin Immunol 55:16, 1975.
60. Walls AF, Newman-Taylor AJ, Longbottom JL: Allergy to guinea pigs. I. Allergenic activities of extracts derived from pelt, saliva, urine and other sources. Clin Allergy 15:241, 1985.
61. Walls AF, Newman-Taylor AJ, Longbottom JL: Allergy to guinea pigs. II. Identification of specific allergens in guinea pig dust by crossed radioimmunoelectrophoresis and investigation of the possible origin. Clin Allergy 15:535, 1985.
62. Rudolph R, Meier-Duis H, Kunkel G, et al: Uber die bedentung von tierhaarallergien bei erkrankungen deroberen luftwege. Deutsch Med Wachenschr 100:2557, 1975.
63. Anderson MC, Baer H: Allergenically active components of cat allergen extracts. J Immunol 127:972, 1981.
64. Anderson MC, Baer H, Ohman JL: A comparative study of the allergens of cat urine, serum, saliva and pelt. J Allergy Clin Immunol 76:563, 1985.
65. Lowenstein H, Lind P, Weeke B: Identification and clinical significance of allergenic molecules of cat origin. Allergy 40:430, 1985.
66. Ohman JL, Lowell FC, Bloch KJ, et al: Allergens of mammalian origin. V. Properties of extracts derived from the domestic cat. Clin Allergy 6:419, 1976.
67. Leitermann K, Ohman JL: Cat allergen. 1. Biochemical, antigenic and allergenic properties. J Allergy Clin Immunol 74:147, 1984.
68. Bartholome K, Kissler W, Baer H, et al: The origin of cat allergen 1. J Allergy Clin Immunol 73:160, 1984.
69. Ohman JL, Baer H, Anderson MC, et al: Surface washes of living cats: An improved method of obtaining clinically relevant allergen. J Allergy Clin Immunol 72:288, 1983.
69a. Charpin C, Mata P, Charpin D, et al: Fel d I allergen distribution in cat fur and skin. J Allergy Clin Immunol 88:77, 1991.
70. Van Metre TE, Marsh DG, Adkinson NF, et al: Dose of cat (Felix domesticus) allergen I (Fel d I) that induces asthma. J Allergy Clin Immunol 78:62, 1986.

71. Knysak D: Animal aeroallergens. Immunol Allergy Clin North Am 9:357, 1989.
72. Vanto T, Viander M, Koivikko A: Skin prick test in the diagnosis of dog dander allergy: A comparison of different extracts with clinical history, provocation tests, and RAST. Clin Allergy 10:121, 1980.
73. Nedergaard-Larsen J, Ford A, Gjesing B, et al: The collaborative study of the international standard of dog, Canis domesticus, hair/dander extract. J Allergy Clin Immunol 82:318, 1988.
74. Varga JM, Ceska M: Characterization of allergen extracts by polyacrylamide gel isoelectrofocusing and radioimmunosorbent allergy assay. Int Arch Allergy Appl Immunol 42:438, 1972.
75. Yman L, Brande R, Ponterius G: Serum albumin—an important allergen in dog epithelia extracts. Int Arch Allergy Appl Immunol 44:358, 1973.
76. Blands J, Lowenstein H, Weeke B: Characterization of extract of dog hair and dandruff from six different dog breeds by quantitative immunoelectrophoresis. Identification of allergens by crossed radioimmunoelectrophoresis (CRIE). Acta Allergo 32:147, 1977.
77. McLean AG, Glovsky MM, Hoffman DR, et al: Identification of allergens in dog dander extracts. I. Clinical and immunological aspects of allergenicity activity. Ann Allergy 45:199, 1980.
78. Einarsson R, Uhlin T, Erlman P: Isolation and characterization of a dog dander allergen in poodle dandruff extract. J Allergy Clin Immunol 73:191, 1984.
79. Lindgren S, Belin L, Dreborg S, et al: Breed-specific dog-dandruff allergens. J Allergy Clin Immunol 82:196, 1988.
80. Hooker SB: Qualitative differences among canine danders. Ann Allergy 2:281, 1944.
80a. de Groot H, Goei KGH, van Swieten P, et al: Affinity purification of a major and a minor allergen from dog extract: Serologic activity of affinity-purified Can f I and of Can f I-depleted extract. J Allergy Immunol 87:1056, 1991.
81. Rynes SE: A critical analysis of animal dander reactions. J Allergy 8:470, 1937.
82. Markussen B, Lowenstein H, Weeke B: Allergen extract of horse hair and dandruff. Quantitative immunoelectrophoretic characterization of the antigens. Int Arch Allergy Appl Immunol 51:25, 1976.
83. Lowenstein H, Markussen B, Weeke B: Isolation and partial characterization of three major allergens of horse hair and dandruff. Int Arch Allergy Appl Immunol 51:48, 1976.
84. Prahl P, Bucher D, Plesner T, et al: Isolation and partial characterization of three major allergens in an extract of cow hair and dander. Int Arch Allergy Appl Immunol 67:293, 1982.
84a. Joliat TL, Weber RW: Occupational asthma and rhinoconjunctivitis from inhalation of crystalline bovine serum albumen powder. Ann Allergy 66:301, 1991.
85. Donham KJ, Zavala DC, Merchant JA: Respiratory symptoms and lung function among workers in swine confinement buildings: A cross-sectional epidemiological study. Arch Environ Health 39:96, 1984.
86. Matson SC, Swanson MC, Reed CE, et al: IgE and IgG-immune mechanisms do not mediate occupation-related respiratory or systemic symptoms in hog farmers. J Allergy Clin Immunol 72:299, 1983.
87. Fontana VJ, Wittig H, Hoh LE Jr: Observations on the specificity of the skin test: The incidence of positive skin tests in allergic and non-allergic children. J Allergy 34:348, 1963.

88. Berrens L: Structural studies of house dust allergens. Clin Exp Immunol 6:71, 1970.
89. Lowenstein H: Immunological partial identity between animal allergens. Allergy 40:64, 1985.
90. Holley JW, Willen K: The factor analysis method of studying intracutaneous skin reactions. Acta Allergol 24:284, 1969.
91. Lowenstein H, Markussen B, Weeke B: Identification of allergens in extract of horse hair and dandruff by means of crossed radioimmunoelectrophoresis. Int Arch Allergy Appl Immunol 51:38, 1976.
92. Nakazawa T, Inazawa M, Feki R, et al: A new occupational allergy due to frogs. Ann Allergy 51:392, 1983.
93. Armentia A, Martin-Santos J, Subiza J, et al: Occupational asthma due to frogs. Ann Allergy 60:209, 1988.
94. McGivern D, Longbottom J, Davies D: Allergy to gerbils. Clin Allergy 15:163, 1985.
95. Petry RW, Voss MJ, Kroutil LA, et al: Monkey dander asthma. J Allergy Clin Immunol 75:268, 1985.
96. Plessner MM: Une maladie des trieurs de plumes: la fievre de canard. Arch Mal Prof 21:67, 1960.
97. Pearsall HR, Morgan EH, Tesluk H, et al: Parakeet dander pneumonitis. Acute psitticokerato-pneumoconiosis. Report of a case. Bull Mason Clinic 14:127, 1960.
98. Reed CE, Sosman A, Barbee RA: Pigeon-breeder's lung. JAMA 193:261, 1965.
99. Barboriar JJ, Sosman AJ, Reed CE: Serological studies in pigeon breeder's disease. J Lab Clin Med 65:600, 1965.
100. Hargreave FE, Pepys J, Longbottom JL, et al: Bird breeder's (fancier's) lung. Lancet i:44, 1966.
101. Banham SW, McKenzie H, McSharry C, et al: Antibody against a pigeon bloom extract: A further antigen in pigeon fancier's lung. Clin Allergy 12:173, 1982.
102. Tebo TH, Moore VL, Fink JN: Antigens in pigeon breeder's disease: The use of pigeon dropping antigens in detecting antibody activity. Clin Allergy 7:103, 1977.
103. Longbottom JL: Pigeon breeder's disease: Quantitative immunoelectrophoretic studies of pigeon bloom antigen. Clin Exper Allergy 19:619, 1989.
104. Platts-Mills TA, Longbottom JL, Edwards J, et al: Occupational asthma and rhinitis to laboratory rats: Serum IgG and IgE antibodies to the rat urinary allergen. J Allergy Clin Immunol 79:505, 1987.
105. Siraganian RP: Allergy to animals: Principals of clinical management. N Engl Reg Allergy Proc 8:181, 1987.
106. Lutsky I: Occupational asthma in laboratory animal workers. In Frazier CA (ed): Occupational Asthma. New York, Van Nostrand Reinhold, 1980, pp 193–208.
107. Prohl P, Roed-Peterson J: Type 4 allergy from cows in veterinary surgeons. Contact Dermatitis 5:33, 1979.
108. Carroll KB, Pepys J, Longbottom JL, et al: Extrinsic allergic alveolitis due to rat serum proteins. Clin Allergy 5:443, 1975.
109. Korenblat P, Slavin RG, Winzenburger PA, et al: Gerbil keepers lung—a new form of hypersensitivity pneumonitis. Ann Allergy 38:437, 1977.
110. Young P: Asthma and allergies; an optimistic future. U.S. Dept. of Health and Human Services. NIH Publication No. 80-388, March 1980, pp 15 and 16.
111. Beck AM, Meyers NM: The pet owner experience. N Engl Reg Allergy Proc 8:185, 1987.
112. Price JA, Longbottom JL: IgG antibodies in relation to exposure to laboratory-animal antigens. J Allergy Clin Immunol 84:520, 1989.
113. Solomon WR: Assessing the animal associated environment. N Engl Reg Allergy Proc 8:169, 1987.
114. Agarwal MK, Yunginger JW, Swanson MC, et al: An immunochemical method to measure atmospheric allergens. J Allergy Clin Immunol 68:194, 1981.
115. Solomon WR, Burge HA, Mvilenberg ML, et al: Allergen carriage by atmospheric aerosol. 1. Ragweed pollen determinants in smaller micronic fractions. J Allergy Clin Immunol 72:443, 1983.
116. Tovey ER, Chapman MD, Weels CW, et al: The distribution of dust mite antigen in the houses of patients with asthma. Am Rev Respir Dis 124:630, 1981.
117. Findlay S, Stosky E, Leitermann K, et al: Airborne cat-associated antigens. J Allergy Clin Immunol 71:160, 1983.
118. Swanson MC, Campbell AR, O'Hollaren MT, et al: Role of ventilation, air filtration and allergen production role in determining concentrations of rat allergens in the air of animal quarters. Am Rev Respir Dis 141:1578, 1990.
119. Neuman I, Lutsky I: Laboratory animal dander allergy. II. Clinical studies and the potential protective effect of DSCG. Ann Allergy 36:23, 1976.
120. Taylor WW, Ohman JL, Lowell FC: Immunotherapy in cat-induced asthma: Double blind trial with evaluation of bronchial responses to cat allergen and histamine. J Allergy Clin Immunol 61:283, 1978.
121. Sundin B, Lilja G, Graff-Lonnevig V, et al: Immunotherapy with partially purified and standardized animal dander extracts. J Allergy Clin Immunol 77:478, 1986.
122. Rohatgi N, Dunn K, Chai HL: Cat-or-dog-induced immediate and late asthmatic responses before and after immunotherapy. J Allergy Clin Immunol 77:850, 1986.
123. Ohman JL, Findlay SR, Leitermann KM: Immunotherapy in cat-induced asthma. Double blind trial with evaluation of in vivo and in vitro responses. J Allergy Clin Immunol 74:230, 1984.

Chapter 21

BUILDING-RELATED ILLNESS

Emil J. Bardana, Jr., MD

A variety of clinical syndromes have been associated with inferior air quality in tight buildings.[1-3] Individuals encounter a broad range of air pollutants as they travel through a succession of microenvironments over the course of their daily activities. Studies in both the United States and Europe indicate that people spend over 90% of their time indoors.[2] Indoor environments dominate the exposure spectrum, and the potential health consequences are entirely dependent on the number and concentrations of pollution sources, as well as the duration of exposure. Pollutants in an office setting arise from a variety of sources, including emissions from building materials, furnishings, office equipment and activities, and human metabolism, as well as from outside pollution. Contamination of indoor air is occasionally amplified by tight building designs that allow for less than adequate mechanical ventilation. This chapter will review the causes and clinical syndromes encountered in building-related illness.

HISTORICAL PERSPECTIVE

Though humans have constructed buildings to protect themselves from the elements, it is clear that buildings do not protect their inhabitants from pollution. An important outcome of any human activity within buildings is the release of chemicals into their environment. This has been a problem for centuries. Benjamin Franklin wrote "no common air from without is so unwholesome as the air within a closed room that has been often breathed and not changed." Sterling and Kobayashi have reviewed studies on pollution in enclosed living and working spaces and have concluded that the burden of toxic vapors and dusts inside a dwelling may exceed the burden of pollution outdoors.[4]

Environmental medicine had its earliest origins in the writings of Hippocrates, who urged fellow healers to consider their patients' environments before making diagnoses.[5] The Romans found ingenious ways to heat their buildings with minimal pollution. They conceived of a primitive furnace, referred to as a Roman hypocaust, that heated air that was sequestered in spaces between the walls and floors.[6]

In the 17th century, Bernardino Ramazzini published a celebrated monograph, *De Morbis Artificum* (Diseases of Workers), that eventually earned him the title of "Father of Occupational Medicine."[7] He described many conditions related to particular work environments, noting their associated afflictions came as a result of inhaling noxious gases and dusts. Although the majority of his treatise related to outdoor medical crafts, he also observed that scholars had problems with their indoor work environment. He reported that their knees would stiffen up from too much sitting and that they were plagued with eyestrain from working far into the night using candlelight. I am certain that the burning candles also contributed to their exposure to a variety of respiratory irritants.

In 1770, Lavoisier carried out his benchmark studies on the relationship between oxygen and respiration. This gave scientists a solid basis for explaining the requirement for adequate ventilation. The importance of having fresh air indoors was acclaimed by physicians of the 18th century who linked the deaths of English sailors to the crowded, unventilated steerage cabins they lived in on their vessels.

The earliest recommendations on the removal of stale, polluted air were published by Tredgold in 1836. He recommended a minimum air exchange rate of 4 ft^3/min.[8] A clever mechanism for drawing clean outside air into a building and circulating it throughout and later dispelling it was introduced by Drysdale and Hayward in their designs of some environmentally unique Liverpool homes.[9] They used the concept of the "stack effect," with a furnace under a long chimney that drew air upward through the home.

By the end of the 19th century, the need for fresh air was so well established that the American Society of Heating, Refrigerating, and Air Conditioning Engineers (ASHRAE) began advocating a minimum indoor ventilation rate of 30 ft^3/min for all indoor spaces. This recommendation was not changed until 1946, when it was revised downward to 10 ft^3/min. During the first half of our century, the working conditions of the industrial age were vastly improved. Nevertheless, as our century draws to a close, we are in the midst of another economic revolution, which is most evident from the shift of many workers into large commercial buildings to perform services or process information.

In 1982 at a World Health Organization meeting in West Germany, a new work-related entity termed "sick-building syndrome" was initially coined. The complaints of the afflicted inhabitants of certain buildings included dryness of the skin and membranes, mental fatigue, headaches, airway infections, and itching. Most suspected buildings are of a commercial nature and have in common the fact that they are heavily populated, carpeted, and either infrequently or poorly cleaned.[10]

In an attempt to conserve energy during the oil embargo of 1973, ASHRAE further reduced the minimum recommended indoor exchange rate to 5 ft^3/min. However, it was rapidly discovered that at these low air-exchange rates indoor air quality can be adversely affected by accumulation of chemical and physical contaminants.

TERMINOLOGY

Although indoor air pollution has been a well-known problem in industry, the environmental issues relating to large commercial buildings and their occupants are a relatively new phenomenon in medicine.[11,12] The terminology that has arisen in this area has become

TABLE 1. *Definition of Terms Frequently Employed in Office Building-related Health Problems*

Problem building
An office building in which workers' complaints of ill health are more common than might be reasonably expected.

Building-related illness
An office building in which one or more workers develop an accepted, well-defined illness for which a specific cause is found. The cause is clearly related to the building.

Sick-building syndrome
An office building in which an ill-defined illness develops in one or more workers. The illness demonstrates great variability among the workers and no causative agent is apparent.

Tight-building syndrome
Generally used to designate an engineering or architectural flaw as the cause for either a building-related illness or a sick-building syndrome.

Crisis building
Sick building where repeated industrial hygiene surveys have failed to localize a cause for ill-defined symptoms, which precipitates a crisis of concern among the involved employees. Such buildings are frequently evacuated.

somewhat confusing. The author's definitions of commonly used terms are summarized in Table 1, although it should quickly be noted that there is still some disagreement as to the use of these various terms.

In a very generic sense, the term "problem building" can be used to connote any commercial building in which health problems among its occupants are more common than might reasonably be expected. "Building-related illness" is a term applied to a situation in a commercial building where one or more occupants develop a generally accepted, well-defined clinical syndrome for which a specific cause related to the building is found. Though these situations tend to be well defined, they represent only a small fraction of the total number of affected buildings.[3] Examples include hypersensitivity pneumonitis, humidifier fever, and building-related asthma. "Sick-building syndrome" refers to an incident in a building where occupants develop an ill-defined syndrome with great variability among the affected workers, and for which no causative agent is apparent. Symptoms have typically included eye and mucous membrane irritation, cough, chest tightness, fatigue, headache, and malaise.[3,11,12] At times building occupants in this category are said to have developed "multiple chemical sensitivities" or other types of "environmental illness."[13] Depending on the care provider seen, the associated diagnosis of chronic fatigue syndrome and/or chronic candida hypersensitivity may also be invoked. Recently, Terr noted that the majority of 27 office workers and teachers with nonspecific complaints attributed to their workplace had developed their symptoms prior to starting work in the subject building.[14] Trasher and his associates have attempted to link building-related illness to levels of antibody directed against albumin conjugates of formaldehyde, toluene diisocyanate, and trimellitic anhydride.[15] Their data were not conclusive, and their hypotheses were generally not accepted by others in the scientific community.[16-19] The whole area of clinical ecology has been critically reviewed and found to have little or no evidence for scientific validity[20-23] (see Chapter 22).

Some investigators have reserved the term "tight-building syndrome" to apply to problem buildings found to have specific engineering or architectural deficiencies. Hence, this term carries a definite engineering implication that usually relates to the central ventilation system.[24-26]

The term "crisis building" has been employed in instances when repeated studies of a problem building have failed to uncover a source or cause for widespread symptoms.[26] In turn, this precipitates a crisis of concern in the involved occupants, which frequently leads to evacuation, extensive additional testing and renovation, and, at times, litigation.

PREVALENCE AND EPIDEMIOLOGY

In considering the prevalence of buildings associated with symptoms in their occupants, it goes without saying that there should be no obvious nonoccupational explanation for the complaints.[3,27] Most affected buildings are large governmental or commercial office buildings. In 1983 there were 3.9 million commercial buildings defined as nonindustrial and nonresidential structures in the U.S.[28] These units were said to have a total floor space of 52 billion square feet, an average of 13,300 square feet per building. It is apparent that their use mainly determines the nature of the microenvironment in the building. Over one-quarter of all commercial buildings in the U.S. are for mercantile or service applications. Other uses, in decreasing order of number of buildings, include office use, assembly, warehousing, food sales and service, vacant,

residential, educational, lodging, and health care.[2] Most commercial buildings house a single establishment. Government-occupied buildings represent about 9% of all U.S. commercial buildings.

The basic premise of epidemiology is that disease does not occur randomly in the population. Rather, it occurs in patterns that are determined by the characteristics of the causative agent, the affected individual, and the environment.[29] To date, most of the information on building-related illness is derived from health hazard evaluations conducted by federal and state agencies, rather than from formal epidemiologic studies. From 1978 to 1981 only 5% of evaluations of health hazards conducted by the National Institute for Occupational Safety and Health (NIOSH) were because of complaints from workers in nonindustrial settings.[25] Over the following 18 months, that figure increased to 13% of NIOSH's health hazard evaluations.[25] As of January 1986, NIOSH had investigated a total of 356 buildings, with more than 90% of those studies occurring in the first six years of the 1980s. Through December 1990 the figure stood at 783 investigations.* Over three-quarters of the NIOSH evaluations involved government and commercial office buildings.[3,6]

The experience in the United Kingdom has been reported in a series of observations by Finnegan and co-workers at the Leicester Royal Infirmary.[27] The initial study of symptom prevalence was conducted in workers from nine office buildings, three with natural ventilation and six with mechanical ventilation. Seven of the nine buildings were not known to have complaints and the remaining two were known to have problems. Symptoms were self-reported by questionnaire. Annoyance and irritational symptoms were much more common in the mechanically ventilated buildings. Selection bias could not explain the observations, because seven of the buildings were selected without any knowledge of the occupants or their symptoms. These investigators also compared two groups of office workers housed on different floors of the same building, but with identical mechanical ventilation. One group of workers was from the private sector, whereas the other was public service employees. The results suggested that the major determinant

---

*Communication with Hazard Evaluations and Technical Assistance Branch, Division of Surveillance, Health Evaluation and Field Studies, NIOSH, Cincinnati, Ohio, July 24, 1991.

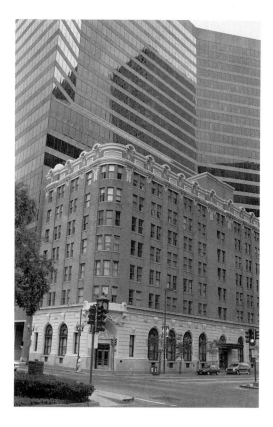

FIGURE 1. View of several commercial buildings in downtown Portland, Oregon with an older structure in the forefront where fresh air is acquired by opening windows, and a modern skyscraper behind where all fresh air is provided by a HVAC system.

in building-related illness is the physical environment rather than the type of work being done.[27,30]

In a subsequent study, workers were surveyed in two buildings, one naturally and the other mechanically ventilated.[31] The prevalence of nonspecific irritational symptoms was significantly higher in workers from the mechanically ventilated building (Fig. 1). However, measurements of temperature, humidity, air velocity, ion concentration, CO, O_3 and CH_2O did not differ between the two buildings. A more recent preliminary report from these authors would indicate that nonspecific building-associated symptoms in 27 buildings are more prevalent in workers of mechanically ventilated buildings when compared to controls.[32] The entire subject of building-related illness was reviewed by these investigators in 1986.[33]

Several groups of Scandinavian investigators have also contributed to our fund of knowledge in the area of indoor air quality. The Danish Indoor Climate Study Group evaluated 3,757

office workers and the environments in 14 Danish town halls with affiliated structures.[34] The lowest prevalence of symptoms were found in the oldest buildings. However, there were no significant differences in frequency of headache, fatigue, malaise, and mucous membrane irritation between mechanically and naturally ventilated buildings. Of interest was the fact that women office workers had a higher rate of work-related symptoms across all job categories. Contrary to many prior observations, the presence of nonspecific building-related symptoms was not well correlated to ambient carbon dioxide levels.[34]

In a more recent publication, the same group of investigators studied the influence of personal characteristics, job-related factors, and psychosocial factors in the genesis of the sick-building syndrome. They showed significant correlation between sex, job category, work functions, and psychosocial factors and work-related mucosal irritation and work-related general symptoms (Table 2). However, these observations did not account for the differences in prevalence of symptoms between different buildings.[35]

In a less focused group of studies sponsored by the Swedish Council for Building Research,

TABLE 2. *Non-building Related Factors Which Have Been Found to Correlate with a Higher Prevalence of Sick-Building Syndrome**

Personal characteristics
- Women have substantially higher symptom prevalence than men
- Allergic rhinoconjunctivitis
- History of migraine headache

Lifestyle and residential factors
- Tobacco abuse
- Contact lenses
- Apartment living
- Living with small children
- Indoor climate problems in private residence

Job category
- Clerk categories
- Social workers

Type of work
- Handling carbon and carbonless paper
- Photocopying
- Work at video display terminal

Psychosocial factors
- Organization of daily work
- Varied work
- Satisfaction with superior
- Work speed
- Excessive workload
- Little influence on organization of work

*From refs. 34 and 35.

the problems of indoor air quality were discussed from multiple perspectives.[36] This collection of studies emphasized formaldehyde off-gassing as one of the major contributors in building-related problems. However, these observations have been supplanted by more contemporary research on the formaldehyde issue (see Chapter 14).

Findings from health hazard evaluations and the cross-sectional epidemiologic studies that are available implicate ventilation as a major contributor to building-related illness,[29,37] although the data base is far from complete.[38] It would appear that in many cases the inadequate ventilation directly reflects faulty design or operation. The effects of building-related indoor air quality problems may be felt by both employers and employees. For the latter there are increased risks of health problems; for the former, there is the probability of reduced employee productivity. Although there are no reliable overall figures for the incidence of building-related illness in the U.S., a committee of the World Health Organization has suggested that up to 30% of new and remodeled buildings may experience indoor air quality problems.[12,39]

CLINICAL SYNDROMES

Just as there are similarities among buildings associated with health complaints, there are a number of well defined syndromes implicated in building-related illnesses (Table 3). In each category of disease, the symptoms observed are dependent on the physical and immunologic properties of the offending agent, as well as the intensity and duration of exposure. In addition, a variety of host factors (Table 2) play a critical role in modifying the clinical presentation observed.

Hypersensitivity Pneumonitis (Allergic Alveolitis) and Humidifier Fever

These conditions represent the best-documented manifestations of building-related illnesses.[40-57] Though they constitute a significant fraction of building-related illness, they represent only a very small share of the numerous etiologic agents incriminated in problem buildings. Both conditions are felt to represent an alveolar and bronchiolar inflammatory reaction secondary to an immune interaction between inhaled organic particles,

TABLE 3. *Spectrum of Clinical Disease Variants in Office Building-related Health Problem*

Building-related illnesses
- Hypersensitivity pneumonitis
- Humidifier fever
- Building-related asthma or allergic rhinitis
- Infectious syndromes
  Legionnaires' disease
  Pontiac fever
  Q fever
- Building-related dermatitis and ocular symptoms
- Intoxication syndromes

Sick building syndrome
- Annoyance and irritational symptoms
- Mass psychogenic illness

circulating antibodies, and sensitized lymphocytes. Although alluded to as early as 1713 by Ramazzini,[7] and described as "farmer's lung" in 1932 by Campbell,[58] many aspects of this inflammatory syndrome continue to remain undefined. One of the most perplexing features of these conditions is the fact that overt disease develops in less than 10% of similarly exposed individuals.[59]

Sixteen outbreaks involving single or multiple cases of either hypersensitivity pneumonitis or humidifier fever resulted in 281 cases of illness. These were reviewed in detail by Kreiss and Hodgson.[60] A number of additional reports have been published since their review, bringing the total to well over 300 cases.[61-68] It must be noted that one of the more recent reports is based upon epidemiologic data alone, and a single causal agent was not identified.[68]

Etiologic agents have represented a wide variety of fungal, bacterial, and protozoal species, including the most frequently incriminated, actinomycetes. Attack rates have varied quite widely among building occupants. The usual source of building dissemination is the heating, ventilation, and air conditioning (HVAC) system. A variety of components have been identified as malfunctioning with resultant growth and dissemination of fungal antigens. These include damaged duct systems, air washers, fan coil units, sump tanks, recirculation vacuum pumps, heater-cooler units, baffle plates, plenums, etc. (Fig. 2). Microbial slime can develop in poorly drained condensation pans serving as cooling coil units (Fig. 3). As the build-up dries, it aerosolizes and contaminates the air supply system. A condition similar to this was uncovered in the General Services Administration building's air conditioner drain pans. The faulty system

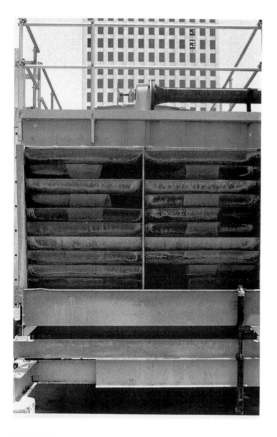

FIGURE 2. Air intake baffle plates of a modern urban structure showing a significant collection of debris on the surface.

was generating more than 83,000 fungal spores/M^3 of air, comparable to levels one might encounter in a chicken coop.[69]

Hypersensitivity Pneumonitis. The clinical presentation of hypersensitivity pneumonitis can be quite variable, even within similarly exposed workers in the same buildings.[45,48,56,57]

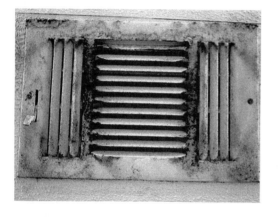

FIGURE 3. A rusted air ventilation duct secondary to moisture build-up with secondary fungal overgrowth.

This may relate to a variety of host factors, particularly major histocompatibility haplotypes and their association with disease expression. As well, subtle differences in antigen concentration can affect exposure, e.g., working in a separately ventilated area, proximity to an open window, etc. Intermittent exposures of high concentrations of antigen may result in acute allergic alveolitis, or alternatively can produce milder bouts of dyspnea and cough, resembling a flu-like illness, i.e., myalgias, fever, headache, chills, cough, fatigue, wheezing, chest tightness or congestion, and dyspnea. Symptoms of acute disease generally begin 4–6 hours after exposure to the causative agent. The observation that repeated flares of disease occur with each return to the source is essential to the diagnosis. Findings of low-grade fever, bibasilar crepitant rales, and a moderate leukocytosis are expected findings. Eosinophilia is not a usual finding. Pulmonary function studies during an acute episode will reveal a restrictive pattern with a reduced diffusion capacity. Many of these acute symptoms and signs may be suppressed with low-level, chronic exposure. However, irreversible pulmonary fibrosis may occur before a diagnosis is made. Chest x-ray may show variable degrees of pulmonary fibrotic changes with reduced lung volumes.

Humidifier Fever. Humidifier fever is probably a distinct pathologic entity, though clearly related to hypersensitivity pneumonitis. The initial attempts to define the clinical and immunologic characteristics of humidifier fever occured at a Medical Research Council Symposium in 1977.[70] Descriptions of the entity have been evolving over the past decade.[71] A rather typical spectrum of this disease was published by Ganier et al.;[44] 26 of 50 office occupants in Tennessee were affected. They experienced episodic flu-like symptoms of fever, chills, headaches, chest tightness, and dyspnea, which came on Monday night after starting the work week. Symptoms subsided over a 12-hour period and would recur each Monday. A similar pattern of symptoms has been described in cotton workers disease, metal fume fever, Pontiac fever, and grain fever. This suggests that the symptoms are a nonspecific pulmonary response that can be evoked by one of a number of mechanisms. Affected employees all worked in an area served by a single HVAC unit. Multiple organisms were detected in the humidifier reservoir, and after the humidifier was removed, no further episodes of the "Monday miseries" occurred. No single causative organism was identified, although an amoeba was suspected. This condition appears to be more common in the winter, and there is a curious negative association with cigarette smoking.[63]

An asthmatic component has been identified as a prominent clinical sign in a few cases.[63] Recently, Anderson et al. described two summer outbreaks in a microprocessor facility and a printing establishment, in which wheezing was a prominent symptom in one facility and not the other.[64] Causative organisms can be similar to those cited for hypersensitivity pneumonitis, but frequently a spectrum of bacteria, fungi, and protozoa is isolated. Serum from exposed occupants generally demonstrates multiple precipitins, whether or not the subjects are symptomatic. Spirometric measurements during an acute episode show a restrictive defect that generally improves over 48-72 hours as the syndrome regresses. Features that are said to set humidifier fever apart from hypersensitivity pneumonitis include: (1) typical "Monday miseries," which clear despite repeated exposure; (2) negative association with tobacco abuse; (3) occasional tendency to have asthmatic symptoms; (4) minimal radiographic findings compared to hypersensitivity pneumonitis; and (5) higher attack rates than are generally encountered with hypersensitivity pneumonitis.

Allergic Rhinoconjunctivitis (Bronchial Asthma)

Allergic rhinoconjunctivitis or bronchial asthma can be aggravated by any indoor pollutants and allergens present in the office environment. However, it is unlikely that these airborne contaminants can precipitate de novo disease. Within the office environment the most important allergens are those derived from pyroglyphid mites (*Dermatophagoides pteronyssinus* and *D. farinae*), which contribute the principal sensitizing immunogens to domestic housedust. As well, numerous fungi and insect antigens could contribute to the indoor contamination. It is well known that the concentrations of both mites and fungi increase proportionately with the relative humidity. The problem can be compounded when these allergens gain access to the HVAC system. Burge et al. reported a number of cases of "humidifier asthma" in 35 employee occupants caused by a contaminated humidifier system.[65] An accompanying editorial indicated the relative surprise that this had not been reported previously. Bronchial hyperreactivity has been associated with hypersensitivity pneumonitis, and many of the antigens involved in its causation have also been implicated in the causation of bronchial asthma. Perhaps the best known association of these conditions is with the spectrum of allergic and hypersensitivity aspergillosis, which has been well known for many years.

A number of fungi have been incriminated in the precipitation of allergic asthma, including *Alternaria, Cladosporium, Aspergillus, Mucor* and *Rhizopus*.[72] Fungi generally flourish at relative humidities in excess of 75%. The latter would be an uncommon circumstance in most modern office buildings. However, faulty repair or inadequate maintenance can result in accumulation of water, e.g., damp carpeting from a rushed cleaning process, leaks in the roof or into ductwork, liquid spills, etc.[1,73] Over-watered decorative plants can be an additional source of fungal growth. Insulated windows can promote condensation along the edge of the frames, with resulting mold growth.[74] Repair and remodeling work has been associated with 20-fold increases in indoor fungal counts.[75]

In addition to allergens, many individuals with asthma can be adversely affected by building-related irritants and odors. Among the most notorious irritants for an asthmatic is involuntary smoking[1,2,11,34,35,76-80a] (Fig. 4). Many asthmatics are also adversely affected by a variety of odors. This observation was initially made by Sir John Floyer in his treatise on asthma in 1698.[81] Although frequently

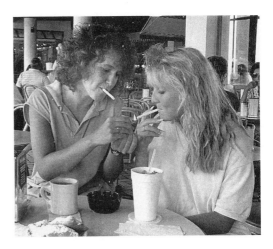

FIGURE 4. Cigarette smoking is frequently restricted to a part of the cafeteria. Unfortunately, all employees must eat in the same area, and usually the same HVAC system serves the whole building.

elicited in the medical history, there are very few comprehensive studies on the effect of malodors on the asthmatic.[82,83] Perhaps the best recent study is one reported by Shim and Williams, who surveyed 60 asthmatics and found that 57 reported aggravation of underlying asthma by odors.[84] Of interest was the observation that the FEV_1 fell 18–58% below baseline during an unblinded 10-minute exposure to cologne in four patients. Though still inconclusive, this area requires further study along with other commonly encountered office odors, e.g., commercial cleaners, photocopy ink, carbonless paper, insecticides, etc.

Building-related Infectious Syndromes

It has been noted that large commercial office buildings may act as excellent incubators for respiratory infections. As well, the recirculation of air within a HVAC system provides an excellent means for transmission of airborne pathogens. There are numerous reports documenting epidemics of airborne infections in buildings with either poor ventilation or poorly maintained air conditioners.[85-88] The incidence of upper respiratory infections and associated absenteeism may be significantly reduced in buildings that are well humidified.[89-91] Low relative humidity may result in the development of rhinitis sicca and a reduction in the capacity to resist viral infectivity.[92,93] In discussing building-related illnesses, it is often quite difficult to draw a distinction between the expected spread of infection and that which is secondary to some deficiency in design or maintenance of the system. The principal infections incriminated in problem buildings include Legionnaire's disease, Pontiac fever, and Q fever.

Legionnaire's Disease. *Legionella pneumophilia* is a gram negative bacterium that was first identified as a cause of death in a man who developed polymyalgia, fever, a nonproductive cough, and chest pain while attending an American Legion convention at the Philadelphia Bellevue Stratford Hotel in 1976.[94] By the fall of 1976, the death toll in that epidemic was 29 of 182 identified cases. The disease was not limited to those attending the convention. Some individuals developed pneumonia after walking down the street outside the hotel, i.e., "Broad Street pneumonia."[94] Later it was realized that *L. pneumophilia* was the same organism originally isolated in a 1947 respiratory infection and retrospectively

implicated in a number of unexplained illnesses by serologic testing.[95]

Some 23 species of *Legionella* have been identified to date. Although all are potential pathogens, about 10 species have been linked to clinical illness. Most cases are associated with serotype I of the species *L. pneumophilia*. It is generally felt that Legionnaire's disease is underreported and probably causes 10% of hospital and nursing home pneumonia. More recent observations suggest that *L. pneumophilia* is responsible for up to 200,000 cases and 40,000 deaths each year.[94-99] Two major forms of legionellosis exist: a pneumonic form (Legionnaire's disease) characterized by a rapidly progressive respiratory illness typical of bacterial pneumonia, with a relatively low attack rate varying between 1–7% and with a case fatality rate of about 15%. It has an incubation rate of 5 to 6 days.

Pontiac Fever. The nonpneumonic form of legionellosis is referred to as Pontiac fever.[100] It was initially described as a building-related epidemic characterized by a 2- to 5-day, mild, flu-like illness with low-grade fever, headache, myalgia, and malaise. Its name is derived from a health care facility in Pontiac, Michigan, where it infected at least 144 individuals in 1968. It has a much higher attack rate than Legionnaire's disease, i.e., about 95%, but it is a less severe disorder, being generally self-limited with a course of about 5 days. It has a shorter incubation period of 36 hours.

Legionella is a ubiquitous organism in the environment and can be isolated from most any location. Its most common reservoir is water, which also seems to amplify the potency of the organism. Airborne transmission has been linked to bacteria-filled droplets. This occurs for both Legionnaire's disease and Pontiac fever. Muder et al. have provided some evidence that transmission may occur via ingestion or aspiration of oropharyngeal isolates.[101] Development of Legionnaire's disease appears to be increased in males, individuals over the age of 50, cigarette smokers, those with a heavy consumption of alcohol, and individuals with preexisting pulmonary disease (bronchitis/emphysema), diabetes, cancer, or other types of disordered immunity[102] Renovation or new construction also appears to increase prevalence. It has been suggested that Pontiac fever represents a humidifier-like disease caused by amoebae that have been infected with *L. pneumophilia*.[103] There is a striking similarity in the epidemiology of humidifier fever and Pontiac fever.

Q Fever. During the past decade there have been a number of building-related outbreaks of Q fever. This infection is caused by airborne transmissions of *Rickettsia burnetii*. Influenza-like symptoms are the most common presentation, but pneumonitis, hepatitis, and endocarditis may occur.[104,105] The most common reservoir is an infected laboratory animal in a research laboratory complex. In addition to Q fever, a number of other infections have been transmitted within HVAC systems, including tuberculosis, measles, rubella, chickenpox, and the common cold.[106,107]

Building-related Dermatitis and Ocular Disease

A variety of noninfectious skin eruptions directly attributable to office buildings have been reported. Building-related dermatitis generally occurs as an outbreak of nonspecific rash and pruritus affecting several employees in an office setting.[3,60,108-113] Eye irritation manifested by itchiness, grittiness, tearing, and erythema is a frequent associated finding.[114] A variety of factors have been incriminated in the causation of these ocular, mucous membrane, and skin symptoms (Table 4).

Mechanical irritation and resultant evanescent rashes and pruritus are most frequently attributed to fibrous glass or mineral wool particles.[108] These particles are most often released secondary to water damage of ventilation duct linings. Fibers break off the water-damaged fibrous material, and then are released through ducts. An evanescent pruritus and nonspecific dermatitis ensue, principally over the skin-exposed areas. Personnel wearing contact lenses may be at special risk. Corneal lacerations can be seen if fibers access the space between the contact lens and the cornea. This is frequently encountered, because office workers may remove the lenses to clean them. Soft lenses may suffer significant irreparable damage secondary to fibrous particles. Verification of the problem can be obtained by microscopic inspection of a Scotch tape sample from a horizontal surface. Collection beneath an exhaust vent is usually the most rewarding.

Photodermatitis has been attributed to monochromatic light from video display terminals. This appears to be more common in females.[113,115-117] Dermatitis is usually localized to the face, neck, and hands. Eye symptoms of redness, itching, or smarting are a frequently associated problem.[115]

TABLE 4. *Factors Involved in the Causation of Skin, Mucous Membrane and Ocular Symptoms*

Mechanical irritation
  Release of fibrous glass or mineral wool particles
Photodermatitis
  Monochromatic light from video display terminals
Low humidity and temperature dermatosis
  Xerosis and mild eczema
  Pyodermas
Dermatitis secondary to office materials
  Carbonless copy paper
    Allergic contact dermatitis
    Contact irritation
    Contact urticaria
  Formaldehyde
    Allergic contact dermatitis
    Contact irritation
    Contact urticaria
  Miscellaneous
    Ozone
    Mixtures of volatile organic compounds
    Fine angular particles of the hygroscopic polymer
Psychogenic

Skin and ocular problems can be associated with low humidity in the workplace. Temperature and relative humidity play a vital role in the comfort of any occupant. Engineers design buildings and HVAC systems to maintain temperatures between 73° and 78° F, with relative humidities between 30 and 60%. Air velocity should be below 0.23 ml. Relative humidity is the ratio of actual vapor pressure of water to the saturated vapor pressure of water at the same temperature and expressed as a percentage. Low relative humidity implies a scarcity of water in the air, and the human skin can become an unwilling source during the work day. Drying of the superficial skin layers usually results in pruritus. The skin can appear relatively normal or show minimal dryness and scaling. Urticaria can occasionally ensue secondary to the scratching of dry pruritic skin.[112,118] This may progress to a low-grade eczema. The condition tends to favor areas of skin with low sebaceous gland activity and generally affects women more than men.

The combination of high relative humidity and high temperatures facilitates a different spectrum of skin disorders, which is generally encountered during the humid, summer months of the southeastern United States. A higher than usual incidence of miliaria rubra and pyodermas has been encountered in this setting.[119]

Many skin disorders have been related to several common office constituents. Perhaps the most often cited product producing skin disease is carbonless paper. A wide variety of carbonless papers are produced throughout the world. Carbonless paper is coated with chemical-containing microcapsules designed to transmit an image from writing or mechanical pressure. Nonimpact printing papers produce images by a heat process. Dermatitis has been linked to one of a multiple of chemical constituents in the paper, depending on the manufacturer. Among the chemicals that can be encountered in these products are a variety of acrylic components, formaldehyde, isocyanates, starch, biocides, and an assortment of inks used in printing on the paper.[109-111] Most prior outbreaks of office dermatitis related to carbonless paper also are connected to significant eye irritation.[111] Respiratory symptoms have also been encountered.[111]

A variety of miscellaneous chemicals have been incriminated in the induction of office dermatitis. This is more frequent in areas where the office is in continuity with a manufacturing area, e.g., production of silicon chips, soft contact lenses, etc. Contact with fine, angular particles of polymer or other byproducts may produce a dermatitis similar to those encountered with fibrous glass or mineral wool.[120] Pruritus has also been encountered in instances of mass psychogenic illness.[121]

Building-related Intoxication Syndromes

The application of a pesticide has frequently triggered fear and, occasionally, a spectrum of

TABLE 5. *Frequency of Symptoms Encountered in the Sick-Building Syndrome*

Parameter	Rate of Frequency
Headache	100
Eye irritation/tearing	90
Fatigue/drowsiness	85
Perception of odors	80
Nasal/sinus congestion	75
Skin irritation	70
Sore throat	65
Dizziness	60
Nausea	50
Sneezing	40
Chest tightness	40
Unusual taste	35
Palpitations	25
Contact lens problems	25
Epistaxis	15
Reduced power of concentration	10

nonspecific symptoms in affected office workers related to residual odor. In the author's experience, responsible pesticide applications are rarely associated with verifiable clinical disease. However, there are isolated reports of unusual incidents involving accidental exposure to a variety of toxic chemicals.

In Butler, Pennsylvania, a small town near Pittsburgh, five office workers in a mail order parts facility developed acute symptoms of organophosphate intoxication. Investigation incriminated chlorpyrifos as the source of the problems. The pesticide was drawn through the air-intake vent as it was injected into small holes accidentally drilled into the walls of the vent from the outside.[122] Similarly, symptoms of carbon monoxide poisoning have been encountered as a result of poorly planned ventilation air intakes being located proximal to parking garages or downwind from large boiler stacks.[123,124] As well, a mild intoxication secondary to moderate concentrations of gasoline fumes has been reported secondary to a breech in an underground storage tank.[125]

SICK-BUILDING SYNDROME

As stated, sick-building syndrome is a term reserved for an office building in which an ill-defined illness develops in one or more workers. Generally, the illness is manifested by a variety of nonspecific symptoms of different intensity and a causative agent is rarely found. Symptoms range from easily demonstrable watering and irritation of the eyes with nasal congestion, to less distinct lethargy, headache, and dry throat (Table 5). Symptoms are usually transient and worsen with each work day. Dramatic improvement is noted in bona fide cases when away from the incriminated work area for several days. Previous descriptions of this condition characterized complaints as either annoyances or mucous membrane irritational syndromes.[19,20,123] Because this symptom complex resembles many common ailments, including viral coryzas and allergic rhinoconjunctivitis, most employers are reluctant to interpret it seriously. For this and other reasons some investigators suggest that buildings where this type of complaint is found should be referred to as "problem buildings." They argue that this generic term avoids the inference that either the building or its occupants are sick.[26]

Even within the medical community there is debate as to whether many of these symptoms are real or perceived. As is often the case with any self-reported illness, especially when it relates to workers' compensation, many factors influence reports of ill health. A number of authors have suggested the use of the term "tight building syndrome" to further segregate those engineering issues related to a sealed or tight-building envelope.[26] It has been said that the tight-building syndrome is as frequently precipitated by complex spectrum of psychosocial issues as it is with toxic substances in the workplace. In this respect it is important to keep in mind that psychological, social, and organizational factors may be acting as either causative or modifying factors in the induction of sick-building syndrome (Table 2). Peer group reaction and the nature of the work environment, as well as the performance of dull, repetitive tasks, all influence symptom prevalence.

Many complaints within the sphere of sick-building syndrome relate to an obvious annoyance factor that is associated with a heightened sense of olfactory awareness. The capacity to cope with a nonirritating, but yet undesirable odor, may relate to genetic factors or acquired factors that blunt olfactory capacity. Congenital familial dysautonomia and Turner's syndrome are both associated with an increased detection and recognition threshold, whereas hypothyroidism, sinusitis, polyposis, and many rhinoplastic procedures result in anosmia, hyposmia, or parosmia.[126] Cigarette smoking, inhalation of cocaine, and chronic use of nasal decongestants all lead to variable hyposmia. Nasal hyperirritability is commonly associated with head cold and symptomatic allergic pollenosis (hay fever).

The cause of sick-building syndrome is frequently never determined. This in fact occurs in about half of all investigations into the nature of problem buildings.[29] In 1980, the Board of Toxicology and Environmental Health Hazards of the National Academy of Sciences appointed a committee on indoor pollutants, which produced a voluminous report.[1] The report fixes the major responsibility for pollution hazards and associated illness in buildings on worker activity, rather than structural or ventilatory defects. Tobacco smoking was especially singled out, perhaps to the exclusion of many other key factors. There is little question that tobacco smoke is an important source of many irritating substances (Table 6). Since the 1950s there has been an extraordinary accumulation of data that implicate tobacco abuse as a preventable

TABLE 6. Composition and Distribution of Constituents of the Vapor and Particulate Phase of Tobacco Smoke

Constituent	Amount in Mainstream Smoke*	
Vapor Phase		
Carbon monoxide	10-23	mg
Carbon dioxide	20-40	mg
Benzene	12-48	ug
Toluene	100-200	ug
Formaldehyde	70-100	ug
Acrolein	60-100	ug
Acetone	100-200	ug
Hydrogen cyanide	400-500	ug
Ammonia	50-130	ug
Nitrogen oxides	8-10	ug
Methyl chloride	150-600	ug
Dimethylamine	12-29	ug
Particulate Phase		
Particulate matter	15-40	mg
Nicotine	1-2.5	mg
Phenol	60-140	ug
Benzo(a)pyrene	20-40	ng
Cadmium	100	ng
Nickel	20-80	ng
Polonium	0.04-0.1	pCi

*Modified from Committee on Passive Smoking: Environmental Tobacco Smoke: Measuring Exposures and Assessing Health Effects. National Research Council, National Academy Press, 1986, p 30.

cause of mortality and morbidity.[127,128] However, the health effects of involuntary smoke have only been the subject of intense study over the past decade. Two recent reports have noted that recirculation of air does not lead to complaints in nonsmokers, and that smoke-related pollutants are not elevated in such buildings[129,130] In this respect, a review of a series of studies by NIOSH found no difference in the concentrations of pollutants between buildings where smoking was permitted and where it was not.[25] The NIOSH experience incriminated tobacco smoke in only 2% of buildings that were studied.[25] Similar observations were made in the United Kingdom and Denmark.[34,35,131,132]

A variety of other compounds have been incriminated as a cause of sick-building syndrome. Several studies have incriminated volatile organic compounds. Volatile organic compounds were measured at indoor levels that were two to 10 times that found outdoors.[2,37,39,133] Extraordinary indoor levels have been noted infrequently.[134,135] A variety of sources have been identified for these compounds, including maintenance products, building materials, and combustion processes, chief among which is tobacco-smoking (Table 6) (Fig. 2). Volatile organic compounds can be broken down into four major classes of chemicals, i.e., aliphatic hydrocarbons, alkylated aromatic hydrocarbons (including benzene), halogenated hydrocarbons, and oxygenated hydrocarbons (including alcohols, aldehydes, ketones, etc.).[136] Most of these compounds can cause mucous membrane, skin, and ocular irritation at high enough concentrations. However, controlled clinical studies are needed to provide clearer insight into their likely role as irritants at the levels they are generally encountered.[137]

Mass Hysteria, Hyperventilation, and Psychogenic Illness

A variety of psychologic and social factors may play a major role in the development of sick-building syndrome. Most cases of sick-building syndrome do not yield any specific chemical or microbial cause.[25,121,138-140] There are instances in which a health care professional may unknowingly precipitate unwarranted concerns in one or more workers, which then results in a chain reaction.[141] If the building occupants have strong beliefs about environmental injury or chemical sensitivity and are further frustrated or ignored by the medical establishment, they may seek consultation with nontraditional care providers. Maladaptive patients who believe they have no other choices find the premises of clinical ecology comforting and useful. Once they are labeled with "multiple chemical sensitivity," they often make this the focal point of their lives[142] (see Chapter 22).

Industrial outbreaks of mass psychogenic illness have occurred in industries where the work is repetitive and uninteresting; where there is a rigid authoritarian administration, lack of social support, and unusual work stress, e.g., demand overload; and where there is lack of windows, poor lighting, shift work, isolationism, overtime, and other factors.[141] There are many modifiers that need to be addressed, including family and marital stresses, job insecurity, behavioral style, and prior psychiatric illness. It is possible that nontoxic levels of aversive pollutants may adversely affect a worker's level of general arousal, perceived threat, and overall anxiety.

An example of this phenomenon was reported at the Commerce Building, a state office facility in Salem, Oregon.[143] Over a period of 72 hours, 93 out of 150 employees became ill and manifested nonspecific symptoms of sick-building syndrome. In addition, there were

six reports of fainting and five workers complained of convulsions. The workers most affected worked in the basement and had been recently asked to convert a major office system from card catalog to a computerized system. In addition, they were expected to keep up all their usual work routine. State officials evacuated the building. After exhaustive evaluations, the air was found to be a bit dry (relative humidity 34%) and the basement had been filled with environmental tobacco smoke when the "outbreak" began, though the entire building was found to be extremely well ventilated. Moreover, medical evaluations produced no measurable evidence of ill health in any of the workers. Most of those with syncope and convulsions were found to be suffering with typical panic-fear reactions with resultant hyperventilation syndrome.[143] In evaluating individuals in this setting, health professionals should not lose sight of the global manifestations of hyperventilation syndrome.[144]

The diagnosis of mass psychogenic illness should not be made without careful consideration of all other organic factors. Whenever possible the clinician should employ strict criteria before arriving at this conclusion.[145]

Causes of Sick-Building Syndrome

In attempting to define the origins of this problem, many investigators have been unable to define any causative agent(s).[140,143] Through January 1986, health hazard evaluation teams from NIOSH had completed 356 investigations of problem buildings.[25] Through December 1990 the figure stood at 783 investigations.* The Medical Services Branch, Indoor Air Quality Investigations of Canada had completed 94 investigations through early 1983.[146] The majority of these investigations in both countries ascribed the problem to inadequate ventilation.[3] Indoor air contaminants were found in about 15% of U.S. cases. Types of environmental stressors included chemical and particulate contaminants (malodors, formaldehyde, tobacco smoke, volatile organic compounds, etc.), thermal discomfort, microbiological contaminants, and nonthermal humidity problems.[147,148] Miscellaneous factors included lighting, electromagnetic radiation, noise, and vibration.

Physical causes have been divided into two broad categories, dealing either with design

---

*See footnote, page 239.

TABLE 7. Major Physical Causes of Sick-Building Syndrome

Problem Category	Specific Cause	Frequency of Occurrence (%)*
Design	*System Problems*	
	Inadequate outdoor air	60–75
	Inadequate air distribution to building spaces (supply/return)	50–75
	Equipment Problems	
	Inadequate filtration of supply air	55–65
	Inadequate drain lines and drain pans	60–65
	Contaminated ductwork on duct linings	35–40
	Malfunctioning humidifiers	15–20
Operations		
	Inappropriate control strategies	90
	Inadequate maintenance	75
	Thermal and contaminant load changes	60

* Derived from Refs. 144 and 145 and modified from ref. 146, with permission.

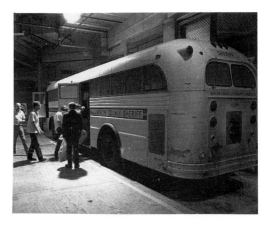

FIGURE 5. The author went to the Justice Building in Portland to evaluate complaints of building-related symptoms in workers on the 12th floor. The problem was related to carbon monoxide and other pollutants which rose in the elevator shaft as prisoners were loaded into an idling prison bus parked inside the building.

problems or operational difficulties.[147,148] These are outlined in Table 7. A detailed discussion of these engineering problems is beyond the scope of this chapter and has been recently reviewed by Woods.[148,149]

Evaluation of Building-Associated Illness

The treating physician will often be the initial contact with regard to evaluating a problem building. The medical history is often the key piece of information suggesting this type of problem. Thus far, thousands of investigations have been completed by NIOSH, state agencies, CDC, and comparable agencies in Canada over the past decade. What has emerged from these studies is the understanding that the usual industrial hygiene techniques that are helpful in the industrial settings are not adequate to resolve the challenges of problem buildings. Extensive air sampling in several building investigations has frequently failed to detect pollutants exceeding or even approaching any threshold limit value, OSHA permissible exposure limits, or NIOSH recommended standard.[24] Only rarely have investigators demonstrated contaminants indoors that exceeded their presence in outdoor air.[37]

There are instances of building-associated illness that can be addressed directly by a

health care provider in a very cost-effective manner (Fig. 5). Problems relating to adequacy of fresh air, smoking policies, temperature, and relative humidity can be discussed with the building manager or HVAC system operator and resolved in a constructive fashion. Clearly, it is to the employer's interest that the issue be resolved as quickly as possible without precipitating a workers' compensation issue. This achieves two goals: (1) maintains the highest worker productivity and (2) avoids a probable rate increase in workers' compensation coverage.

If the problem is deemed too complex and when many workers are involved, a comprehensive evaluation will generally be necessary. Very few physicians are equipped to conduct such an evaluation on their own. They will often require the collaborative assistance of a university research group or commercial investigative team to conduct a thorough evaluation. The author suggests collaboration with an industrial hygienist and/or a National Environmental Balancing Bureau–certified engineer (Fig. 6). NIOSH has developed a guidance document for the investigation of indoor air quality complaints.[150] The guide suggests an initial walk-through assessment in which the building and complaints are characterized, followed by environmental monitoring. This whole approach has been reviewed in some detail by Quinlan and her associates.[151]

Without a suspected work contaminant or apparent defect in the ventilatory rate, most experts recommend the measurement of several

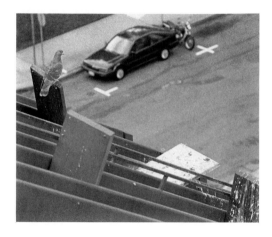

FIGURE 6. An industrial hygienist working with the author uncovered an air intake system contaminated with pigeon droppings, which in turn served as a breeding area for fungal growth.

index pollutants. The contaminants most likely to yield information are carbon dioxide, total hydrocarbons, and volatile organic compounds (VOCs). If allergic symptoms to an office-related allergen are suspected, sample collection from the office carpeting or ventilation system may yield valuable clues, e.g., molds, housedust mite, and bioaerosols, etc.[152]

The most important aspect of investigating any presenting occupant is a willingness to be a careful listener and initiate a serious investigation. A complete history and physical should be carried out. Emphasis should be placed on preexisting medical conditions. An attempt should be made to assimilate all prior medical records for a thorough review (see Chapters 22 and 24). In obtaining a medical history, inquiry should be made as to how many individuals occupy this building and the number of co-workers with similar complaints. It is also of interest to note if only certain groups of workers have the majority of complaints, and whether the issue initially was raised by one or a cluster of individuals. It is important to establish whether a single physician identified all the active cases. It is important to record whether symptoms abate over weekends or on vacations. Absence and sick leave records might also provide clues to similar behavior in the past. Inquiry should be made as to all prior employers and the existence of any preceding workers' compensation matters. In conducting the examination, the physician should record all objective findings. Omission of a mild conjunctivitis, rhinitis, rash, etc. may impede other reviewers in coming to a correct conclusion.

In conducting the examination, any objective parameters that can be quantified can be very helpful. To this end, pre- and post-work provocation with measurement of upper and/or lower airway resistance could prove very helpful. Other studies, including peripheral or nasal/bronchial eosinophilia, dermal reactivity to epicutaneous allergen challenge, and a search for precipitating antibody to fungal constituents can all be helpful in documenting causation. Because there appears to be a significant psychosocial component of building-associated illness, the clinician must make every effort to develop an unassailable objective data base.

CONCLUSION

Concern over the quality of indoor air has become a major issue in many of our modern office buildings. The issues of building-related illness has been reviewed with a view of defining terms and the nature of the adverse health conditions that are encountered. Establishing a cause-and-effect relationship between any indoor air quality parameter and disease is the major challenge facing the health care provider faced with this issue. It becomes evident that the investigation of the occupant and building is a complex matter and requires collaborative efforts between clinicians, industrial hygienists, and building engineers, among others.

REFERENCES

1. National Academy of Sciences: Indoor Pollutants. Washington, D.C., National Academy Press, 1981.
2. Environmental Protection Agency: Report to Congress on Indoor Air Quality. Vol. 11, Assessment and Control of Indoor Air Pollution. EPA/400/1-89/001c, August, 1989.
3. Bardana EJ, Montanaro A, O'Hollaren MT: Building-related illness. Clin Rev Allergy 6:61, 1988.
4. Sterling TD, Kobayashi DM: Exposure to pollutants in enclosed living spaces. Environ Res 3:1, 1977.
5. Chadwick J, Mann WN: The Medical Works of Hippocrates. Oxford, Blackwell Scientific Publications, 1982, p 90.
6. Sterling TD: The politics of indoor pollution; an architectural, engineering and epidemiological overview. Immunol Allergy Pract 9:212, 1987.
7. Ramazzini B: Diseases of Workers (De Morbis Artificum, 1713, tr. by Wright WC). Chicago, University of Chicago Press, 1940.
8. Tredgold T: The Principles of Warming and Ventilation: Public Buildings. London, Taylor, 1836.
9. Bonham R: The Architecture of the Well-tempered Environment. Chicago, University of Chicago Press, 1969.

10. Gravesen S, Larsen L, Gyntelberg F, et al: Demonstration of microorganisms and dust in schools and offices: An observational study of non-industrial buildings. Allergy 41:520, 1986.

11. Samet JM, Marbury MC, Spengler JD: Health effects and sources of indoor air pollution, Part II. Am Rev Respir Dis 137:221, 1988.

12. Lyles WB, Greve KW, Bauer RM, et al: Sick building syndrome. South Med J 84:65, 1991.

13. Cone JE, Harrison R, Reiter R: Patients with multiple chemical sensitivities: Clinical diagnostic subsets among an occupational health clinic population. Occup Med State Art Rev 2:721, 1987.

14. Terr A: Clinical ecology in the workplace. J Occup Med 31:257, 1989.

15. Trasher JD, Broughton AD, Micevich P: Antibodies and immune profiles of individuals occupationally exposed to formaldehyde. Six case reports. Am J Ind Med 14:478, 1988.

16. Hodgson MJ: Clinical diagnosis and management of building-related illness and the sick-building syndrome. Occup Med State Art Rev 4:593, 1989.

17. Greenberg GN, Stave G: Formaldehyde case reports. Am J Ind Med 16:329, 1989.

18. Beavers JD: Formaldehyde exposure reports. Am J Ind Med 16:331, 1989.

19. Bardana EJ, Montanaro A: Formaldehyde: An analysis of its respiratory, skin and immunologic effects. Ann Allergy (in press).

20. Bardana EJ, Montanaro A: "Chemically sensitive" patients: Avoiding the pitfalls. J Respir Dis 10:32, 1989.

21. Cowart VS: Health fraud's toll: Lost hopes, billions spent. JAMA 259:3229, 1988.

22. American College of Physicians: Position paper: Clinical ecology. Ann Intern Med 111:168, 1989.

23. Kahn E, Letz G: Clinical ecology: Environmental medicine or unsubstantiated theory? Ann Intern Med 111:104, 1989.

24. Hicks JB: Tight building syndrome: When work makes you sick. Occup Health Safety 54:51, 1984.

25. Melius J, Wallingford K, Keenlyside R, et al: Indoor air quality—the NIOSH experience. Ann Am Conf Gov Ind Hyg 10:3, 1984.

26. Baker DB: Social and organizational factors in office building-associated illness. Occup Med State Art Rev 4:607, 1989.

27. Finnegan MJ, Pickering CAC, Burge PS: The sick building syndrome: Prevalence studies. Br Med J 289:1573, 1984.

28. Department of Energy (DOE): Nonresidential Buildings Energy Consumption Survey: Characteristics of Commercial Buildings, 1983. Washington, D.C., Energy Information Administration DOE/EIA-0246(83), 1985.

29. Baker DB: Epidemiologic investigation of office environmental problems. Ann Am Conf Gov Ind Hyg 10:37, 1984.

30. Robertson AS, Burge PS: Occup Health March:78-81, 1986.

31. Robertson AS, Burge PS, Hedge A, et al: Comparison of health problems related to work and environmental measurements in two office buildings with different ventilation systems. Br Med J 291:373, 1985.

32. Harrison J, Pickering AC, Finnegan MJ, et al: The sick building syndrome: Further prevalence studies and investigations of possible causes. In Seifert B, Esdorn H, Fischer M, et al (eds): Indoor Air '87. Proceedings of the 4th International Conference on Indoor Air Quality and Climate. Berlin, Inst. for Water, Soil, and Air Hygiene, 1987, pp 487–491.

33. Finnegan MJ, Pickering CAC: Building-related illness. Clin Allergy 16:389, 1986.

34. Skor P, Valbjorn O: Danish indoor climate study group. The "sick" building syndrome in the office environment. The Danish Town Hall Study. Environ Int 13:339, 1987.

35. Skor P, Valbjorn O, Pedersen BV: Influence of personal characteristics, job-related factors and psychoscial factors on the sick building syndrome. Scand J Work Environ Health 15:286, 1989.

36. Berglund B, Lindrall T, Sundell J: Indoor Air. Vol. 3, Sensory and Hyperreactivity Reactions to Sick Buildings. Swedish Council for Building Research. Stockholm, Liber Tryck AB, 1984.

37. Turiel I, Hollowell CD, Miksch RR, et al: The effects of reduced ventilation on indoor air quality in an office building. Atmos Environ 17:51, 1983.

38. Lippmann M, Lioy PJ: Critical issues in air pollution epidemiology. Environ Health Perspect 62:243, 1985.

39. Environmental Protection Agency: Report to Congress on Indoor Air Quality. Vol. I, Federal Programs Addressing Indoor Air Quality. Washington, D.C., EPA/400/1-89/001B, August 1989.

40. Baxter PJ: An outbreak of allergic-type symptoms among staff of an elementary school: A hazard of moldy air filters? Atlanta, Centers for Disease Control, Special Studies Branch, Center for Environmental Health, 1982.

41. Arnow PM, Fink JN, Schlueter DP, et al: Early detection of hypersensitivity pneumonitis in office workers. Am J Med 64:236, 1978.

42. Bernstein RS, Sorenson WG, Garabrant D, et al: Exposures to respirable, airborne penicillium from a contaminated ventilation system: Clinical, environmental, and epidemiological aspects. Am Ind Hyg J 44:161, 1983.

43. Pickering CAC, Moore WKS, Lacey J, et al: Investigation of a respiratory disease associated with an air conditioning system. Clin Allergy 6:109, 1976.

44. Ganier M, Lieberman P, Fink JN, et al: Humidifier lung—an outbreak in office workers. Chest 77:183, 1980.

45. Friend JAR, Gaddie J, Palmer KNV, et al: Extrinsic allergic alveolitis and contaminated cooling-water in a factory machine. Lancet ii:297, 1977.

46. Edwards JH: Microbial and immunological investigations and remedial action after an outbreak of humidifier fever. Br J Ind Med 37:55, 1980.

47. Pestalozzi VC: Febrile gruppener krankungenin einer modell schreinerei durch inhalation von mil schimmelpitzen kontaminiertem befeuchterwasser (Befeuchterfieber). Schwiez Med Wochenschr 89:710, 1959.

48. Banaszak EF, Thiede WH, Fink JN: Hypersensitivity pneumonitis due to contamination of an air conditioner. N Engl J Med 283:271, 1970.

49. Edwards JH, Griffiths AJ, Mullins J: Protozoa as sources of antigen in "humidifier fever." Nature (Lond) 264:438, 1976.

50. Ashton I, Axford AT, Bevan C, et al: Lung function of office workers exposed to humidifier fever antigen. Br J Ind Med 38:34, 1981.

51. Rylander R, Haglind P, Lundholm M, et al: Humidifier fever and endotoxin exposure. Clin Allergy 8:511, 1978.

52. Scully JJ, Galdabini JJ, McNeely BU, et al: Humidifier fever. Eur J Respir Dis 63(Suppl 123):104, 1982.

53. Parrott NF, Blyth W: Another causal factor in the production of humidifier fever. J Soc Occup Med 30:63, 1980.

54. Cockcroft A, Edwards J, Bevan C, et al: An investigation of operating theatre staff exposed to humidifier fever antigens. Br J Ind Med 38:144, 1981.
55. Morey PR, Hodgson MJ: Union Building Fever. Interim Report to the Director, Division of Respiratory Disease Studies, Technical Assistance Request, 82-031. Morgantown, WV, NIOSH, Feb. 28, 1982.
56. Johnson CL, Bernstein IL, Gallagher JS, et al: Familial hypersensitivity pneumonitis induced by *Bacillus subtilis*. Am Rev Respir Dis 122:339, 1980.
57. Miller MM, Patterson R, Fink JN, et al: Chronic hypersensitivity lung disease with recurrent episodes of hypersensitivity pneumonitis due to a contaminated central humidifier. Clin Allergy 6:451, 1976.
58. Campbell JM: Acute symptoms following work with hay. Br Med J 2:1143, 1932.
59. Hendrick DJ, Faux JA, Marshall R: Budgerigar fancier's lung: The commonest variety of allergic alveolitis in Britain. Br Med J 2:81, 1987.
60. Kreiss K, Hodgson MJ: Building-associated epidemics. In Walsh PJ, Dudney CS, Coppenhaver E (eds): Indoor Air Quality. Boca Raton, FL, CRC Press, 1984, pp 87–106.
61. Fergusson RJ, Milne LJR, Crompton GH: Penicillium allergic alveolitis: Faulty installation of central heating. Thorax 39:294, 1984.
62. Robertson AS, Burge PS, Wieland A: Extrinsic allergic alveolitis due to antigen from a humidifier at 15° C. Thorax (Aust) 40:229, 1985.
63. Finnigan MJ, Pickering CAC, Davies PS, et al: Development of precipitating antibodies in workers exposed to humidifier fever antigen. Thorax 39:691, 1984.
64. Anderson K, Wah AD, Sinclair D, et al: Climate intermittent humidification and humidifier fever. Br J Ind Med 46:671, 1989.
65. Burge PS, Finnigan M, Horsfield N, et al: Occupational asthma in a factory with a contaminated humidifier. Thorax 40:248, 1985.
66. Liebert CA, Hood MA, Deck FH, et al: Isolation and characterization of a new cytophago species implicated in a work-related lung disease. Appl Environ Microbiol 48:936, 1984.
67. Hodgson MJ, Morey PR, Attfield M, et al: Pulmonary disease associated with cafeteria flooding. Arch Environ Health 40:96, 1985.
68. Hodgson MJ, Morey PR, Simon JS, et al: An outbreak of recurrent acute and chronic hypersensitivity pneumonitis in office workers. Am J Epidemiol 125:631, 1987.
69. Bronson G: Some like it comfortable. Forbes, June 30, 1986, p 116. and the Washington Post (Health Section), September 16, 1986.
70. Edwards JH, Harbord P, Skidmore JW, et al: Humidifier fever. Thorax 32:653, 1977.
71. Hendrick DJ: Contaminated humidifiers and the lung. Thorax 40:244, 1985.
72. Gravesen S: Fungi as a cause of allergic disease. Allergy 34:135, 1979.
73. Burge HA, Boise JR, Solomon WR, et al: Fungi in libraries: An aerometric survey. Mycopathologica 64:67, 1978.
74. Kapyla ML: Frame fungi on insulated windows. Allergy 40:558, 1985.
75. Maunsell K: Airborne fungal spores before and after raising dust. Int Arch Allergy Appl Immunol 5:373, 1954.
76. Samet JM, Marbury MC, Spengler JD: Respiratory effects of indoor air pollution. J Allergy Clin Immunol 79:685, 1987.
77. Rogier C, Dabis F, Teissier JF, et al: What role do smoking and air conditioning play in the occurrence of otorhinolaryngological and upper respiratory symptoms in the personnel of a hospital center. Rev Epidemiol Sante Publique 37:255, 1989.
78. Environmental Protection Agency: The Inside Story: A Guide to Indoor Air Quality. Washington, D.C., EPA 400-1-88-004, Sept. 1988.
79. Environmental Protection Agency: Environmental Tobacco Smoke (No. 5). Washington, D.C., Office of Air and Radiation (ANR-445) June, 1989.
80. Hodgson MJ: Environmental tobacco smoke and sick building syndrome. Occup Med State Art Rev 4:735, 1989.
80a. Hein HO, Suadicani P, Skov P, et al: Indoor dust exposure: An unnoticed aspect of involuntary smoking. Arch Environ Health 46:98, 1991.
81. Floyer J: A Treatise of the Asthma. London, 1698 (as quoted by Sakula A, Thorax 39:249, 1984).
82. Brown EA, Colombo NH: The asthmogenic effect of odors, smells and fumes. Ann Allergy 12:14, 1954.
83. Herbert M, Glick R, Black H: Olfactory precipitants of bronchial asthma. J Psychosom Res 11:195, 1967.
84. Shim C, Williams MH Jr: Effect of odors in asthma. Am J Med 80:18, 1986.
85. Pennington JH, Lumley J, O'Grady F: The growth of *Pseudomonas pyocyanea* in Garthur condenser humidifiers: An experimental study. Anesthesia 211, 1966.
86. Grieble HG, Colton FR, Bird TJ, et al: Fine-particle humidifiers: Source of *Pseudomonas aeruginosa* infections in a respiratory disease unit. N Engl J Med 282:531, 1970.
87. Rosenzweig AL: Contaminated humidifiers. N Engl J Med 283:1056, 1970.
88. Scott CC, Jacobson I: *Pseudomonas* in ventilators. Lancet i:239, 1970.
89. Knight V: Viruses as agents of airborne contamination. Ann NY Acad Sci 353:147, 1980.
90. Hemmes JH, Winkler KC, Kool SM: Virus survival as a seasonal factor in influenza and poliomyelitis. Nature 188:430, 1960.
91. Green GH: The effect of indoor relative humidity on colds. ASHRAE Trans 85:747, 1979.
92. Lubart J: The common cold and humidity imbalance. NY State J Med 62:817, 1962.
93. Zeterberg JM: A review of respiratory virology and the spread of virulent and possibly antigenic viruses via air conditioning systems. Ann Allergy 31:228, 1973.
94. Fraser DW, Tasi TF, Orenstein W, et al: Legionnaires' disease: Description of an epidemic of pneumonia. N Engl J Med 297:1189, 1977.
95. Smith HM: Legionnaires' disease: A troubling anniversary. MD Magazine August:79–89, 1986.
96. Muder RR, Yu VL, McClure JK, et al: Nosocomial Legionnaires' disease uncovered in a prospective pneumonia study: Implications for underdiagnosis. JAMA 249:3184, 1983.
97. Muder RR, Yu VL, Zuravleff JJ: Pneumonia due to the Pittsburgh pneumonia agent: New clinical perspective with a review of the literature. Medicine (Baltimore) 62:120, 1983.
98. Lunau F: Controlling Legionnaires' disease. Occup Health March:86–88, 1986.
99. Meyer RD: Legionella infections: A review of five years of research. Rev Infect Dis 5:258, 1983.

100. Glick TH, Gregg MB, Berman B, et al: Pontiac fever— an epidemic of unknown etiology in a health department. I. Clinical and epidemiologic aspects. Am J Epidemiol 107:149, 1978.

101. Muder RR, Yu VL, Woo AH: Mode of transmission of Legionella pneumophilia: A critical review. Arch Intern Med 146:1607, 1986.

102. England AC, Fraser DW, Plikaytis BD, et al: Sporadic legionellosis in the U.S.: The first thousand cases. Ann Intern Med 94:164, 1981.

103. Rowbotham TJ: Pontiac fever, amebae and legionellae. Lancet i:40, 1981.

104. Hornibrook JW, Nelson KR: An institutional outbreak of pneumonitis. Public Health Rep 55:1936, 1940.

105. Schachter J, Sung M, Meyer KF: Potential danger of Q fever in a university hospital environment. J Infect Dis 123:301, 1971.

106. Burge HA: Indoor air and infectious disease. Occup Med State Art Rev 4:713, 1989.

107. Brundage JF, Scott RM, Lednar WM, et al: Building-associated risk of febrile acute respiratory diseases in Army trainees. JAMA 259:2108, 1988.

108. Sterling TD, Sterling E, Dimich-Ward H: Building illness in the white-collar workplace. Int J Health Serv 13:277, 1983.

109. Marks JG, Trautlein JJ, Zwillich CW, et al: Contact urticaria and airway obstruction from carbonless copy paper. JAMA 252:1038, 1984.

110. Marks JG: Allergic contact dermatitis from carbonless copy paper. JAMA 245:2331, 1981.

111. Calnan CD: Carbon and carbonless copy paper. Acta Dermatol Venereol 85:27, 1979.

112. Rycroft RJG: Low-humidity occupational dermatoses. Dermatol Clin 2:553, 1984.

113. Nilsen A: Facial rash in visual display unit operators. Contact Dermatitis 8:25, 1982.

114. Franck C: Eye symptoms and signs in buildings with indoor climate problems (office eye syndrome). Acta Ophthalmol 64:306, 1986.

115. Knave BC, Wibom RI, Voss M, et al: Work with video display terminals among office employees. 1. Subjective symptoms and discomfort. Scand J Work Environ Health 11:457, 1985.

116. Feldman LR, Eaglestein WH, Johnson RB: Terminal illness. J Am Acad Dermatol 12:336, 1985.

117. Murray WE, Moss CE, Parr WH, et al: Potential health hazards of video display terminals. Cincinnati, OH, Public Health Service, National Institute of Occupational Safety and Health, 1981 (NIOSH Report 81-129).

118. Rycroft RJG, Smith WDL: Low humidity occupational dermatoses. Contact Dermatitis 6:488, 1980.

119. Sams WM: Humidity, its relation to problems of dermatology. South Med J 44:140, 1951.

120. White IR, Rycroft RJG: Low humidity occupational dermatoses—an epidemic. Contact Dermatitis 8:287, 1982.

121. Maguire A: Psychic possession among industrial workers. Lancet i:376, 1978.

122. Hodgson MJ, Block GD, Parkinson DK: Organophosphate poisoning in office workers. J Occup Med 28:434, 1986.

123. Bardana EJ: Office epidemics. The Sciences (NY Acad Sci) 26:38, 1986.

124. Flachsbart PG, Ott WR: A rapid method for surveying CO concentrations in high-rise buildings. Environ Int 12:255, 1986.

125. Anon: Employee illness from underground gas and oil contamination. MMWR 31:451, 1982.

126. Scott AE: Clinical characteristics of taste and smell disorders. Ear Nose Throat J 68:297, 1989.

127. Committee on Passive Smoking: Environmental tobacco smoke: Measuring exposures and assessing health effects. National Research Council. Washington, D.C., National Academy Press, 1986.

128. U.S. Dept. Health, Education and Welfare; Public Health Service: Smoking and Health. A Report of the Surgeon General. Washington, D.C., U.S. Government Printing Office, 1979, DHEW (PHS) 79-50066.

129. Sterling TD, Collett CW, Mueller B, et al: The effect of instituting smoking regulations in an office building on indoor contaminant levels. In Proceedings of IAQ 87: Practical Control of Indoor Air Quality. Atlanta, ASHRAE, 1987, pp 66-70.

130. Sterling TD, Mueller B: Concentrations of nicotine, RSP, CO and CO_2 in non-smoking areas of offices ventilated by air recirculated from smoking designated areas. Am Ind Hyg Assoc J 49:423, 1988.

131. Cain WS, Leaderer BP, Isseroff R, et al: Ventilation requirements in buildings—control of occupancy odor and tobacco smoke. Atmospheric Environ 17: 1183, 1983.

132. Burge S, Hedge A, Wilson S, et al: Sick building syndrome: A study of 4373 office workers. Ann Occup Hyg 31:493, 1987.

133. Wallace LA: The total exposure assessment methodology (TEAM) study: Summary and analysis, Vol I. Washington, D.C., U.S. Environmental Protection Agency, Office of Research and Development, 1987.

134. Sheldon LS, Handy RW, Harwell TD, et al: Indoor air quality in public buildings, Vol. I. Washington, D.C., U.S. Environmental Protection Agency Report, EPA/ 600/6-88/009a, 1988.

135. Sheldon LS, Zelon H, Sickles J, et al: Indoor air quality in public buildings, Vol. II. Washington, D.C., U.S. Environmental Protection Agency Report, EPA/ 600/6-88/099b, 1988.

136. Girman JR: Volatile organic compounds and building bake-out. Occup Med State Art Rev 4:695, 1989.

137. Norback D, Torgen M, Edling C: Volatile organic compounds, respirable dust and personal factors related to prevalence and incidence of sick building syndrome in primary schools. Br J Ind Med 47:733, 1990.

138. Levine RJ, Sexton DJ, Romm FJ, et al: Outbreaks of psychosomatic illness at a rural elementary school. Lancet ii:1500, 1974.

139. Morse DL: Epidemic respiratory tract irritation. Atlanta, Centers for Disease Control, Center for Environmental Health, Special Studies Branch (Florida), December 8, 1978.

140. Whorton MD, Larson SR, Gordon NJ, et al: Investigation and work-up of tight building syndrome. J Occup Med 29:142, 1987.

141. Colligan MJ, Murphy LR: Mass psychogenic illness in organizations: An overview. J Occup Psychol 52: 77, 1979.

142. Brodsky CM: "Allergic to everything"—a medical subculture. Psychosomatics 24:731, 1983.

143. Heumann M, Campbell DT, Wright L: Report on an illness outbreak at the Commerce Building in Salem, Oregon, July 30, 31 and August 1, 1984. Oregon State Health Department (unpublished).

144. Magarian GJ: Hyperventilation syndromes: Infrequently recognized common expressions of anxiety and stress. Medicine 61:219, 1982.

145. Colligan MJ, Smith MJ: A methodological approach for evaluating outbreaks of mass psychogenic illness in industry. J Occup Med 20:401, 1978.

146. Kirkbride J: Sick building syndrome: Causes and effects. Ottawa, Canada, Health and Welfare, 1985.
147. Robertson G: Sources, nature and symptomatology of indoor air pollutants. In Berglund B, Lindvall T (eds): Proceedings of Healthy Buildings, 88, Vol. 3. Stockholm, Swedish Council for Building Research, 1988, pp 507–516.
148. Woods JE: Recent developments for heating, cooling and ventilating buildings: Trends for assuring healthy buildings. In Berglund B, Lindvall T (eds): Proceedings of Healthy Buildings, 88, Vol. 3. Stockholm, Swedish Council for Building Research, 1988, pp 99–107.
149. Woods JE: Cost avoidance and productivity in owning and operating buildings. Occup Med State Art Rev 4:753, 1989.
150. NIOSH—Health Hazard Evaluation Program: NIOSH Hazard Evaluations and Technical Assistance Branch. Cincinnati, OH, NIOSH, 45226.
151. Quinlan P, Macher JM, Alevantis LE, Cone JE: Protocol for the comprehensive evaluation of building-associated illness. Occup Med State Art Rev 4:771, 1989.
152. Burge H: Bioaerosols: Prevalence and health effects in the indoor environment. J Allergy Clin Immunol 86:687, 1990.

Chapter 22

THE CHEMICALLY SENSITIVE PATIENT

Anthony Montanaro, MD
Emil J. Bardana, Jr., MD

Chemical sensitivity is increasingly perceived as an occupational disease. The diagnosis of "chemical sensitivity" has largely been popularized by practitioners who do not routinely deal with occupational health issues. Nontraditional practitioners describing themselves as clinical ecologists or others who are "ecologically oriented" have championed diagnoses such as "cerebral allergy," "environmental illness," "20th century disease," and "candida hypersensitivity" as being associated with chemical sensitivity. The rapid proliferation of complex chemicals in the workplace has further confounded issues related to this diagnosis. Worker awareness of the potential toxicities of these chemicals has heightened the interest in this field.

Our contention is that the diagnosis of chemical sensitivity offers very little to the physician or worker. It is clearly not a specific diagnosis and in its broadest context may imply a wide range of potential adverse health effects. Although it is true that some workers may develop hypersensitivity responses to one or more chemicals in the workplace, these hypersensitivity responses should be specifically characterized by the physician so that appropriate treatment can be undertaken. Since the diagnosis of "chemical sensitivity" or "multiple chemical sensitivity" carries no specific pathogenetic implication, there can be no meaningful treatment or prevention that can be undertaken without further elucidating the nature of these reactions.

In this chapter we will attempt to outline what we feel to be a very pragmatic approach to this problem. Whereas we accept the notion that many individuals may react adversely to a diverse range of chemicals, we do not feel that "multiple chemical sensitivity" is a meaningful diagnosis. This diagnosis has been described by Cullen.[1] He defines this condition as an acquired disorder characterized by recurrent symptoms referable to multiple organ systems occurring in response to demonstrable exposure to many chemically unrelated compounds at doses far below those established in the general population to cause harmful effects. In stating this, no single widely accepted test of physiologic functioning can be shown to correlate with symptoms. Nevertheless, this entire area continues to receive national attention in a variety of forums and has recently been spotlighted in a text authored by Ashford and Miller.[2]

Because many practitioners who employ this diagnosis are adherents of doctrines taught by clinical ecology, it is critical for the health care provider to recognize that these issues have received critical review by a diverse group of organizations. The clinical ecology ideation has been rejected on scientific grounds by the American Academy of Allergy and Immunology (1986),[3] the California Medical Association (1986),[4] the American College of Physicians (1989),[5] and the American Academy of Occupational Medicine (1990).[6] In addition to these organizational reviews and position papers, numerous clinical studies of patients labeled with the diagnosis of multiple chemical sensitivity have concluded that there is inadequate support for the beliefs and practices of clinical ecology.[7-10] Nor can the practice of clinical ecology be considered harmless. In many cases severe and costly constraints are placed upon the patients, including extreme environmental

255

control, relocation, and unconventional therapy such as megadoses of vitamins, neutralizing sublingual drops, dietary manipulation, cleansing colonic enemas, etc. Occasionally, timely and appropriate treatment of an underlying psychiatric illness is avoided.[8-10]

Many physicians, when faced with a patient with perceived chemical sensitivity, are uncertain of how to cope with the issues involved. Much of this stems from their lack of training and expertise in areas of occupational medicine and toxicology. They tend to dismiss such patients or treat them without proper tolerance, commitment, and creativity. It is precisely this attitude that reinforces symptom-reporting by the patient and encourages him or her to seek nontraditional approaches, with resultant implications for their underlying health problems.[11]

What follows in this chapter is an outline of experiences we encountered in evaluating many of these patients in our practice. A practical cost-effective approach is presented that may be useful in clinical practice. We believe that such an approach can only be successful if medical toxicologic, environmental, and psychosocial factors are carefully considered in a comprehensive evaluation.[12,13]

CLASSIFICATION OF SYMPTOMS PERCEIVED AS CHEMICAL SENSITIVITY

When considering symptoms of chemical sensitivity, a spectrum of possible health effects should be considered. The classification of potential reactions should include annoyance reactions, mucous membrane irritation, immunologic sensitivity, and intoxication syndromes[14] (Table 1). **Annoyance reactions** occur in many individuals who possess a heightened sense of olfactory awareness. The ability to tolerate a variety of nonirritating, but yet undesirable, odors, is dependent on a variety of genetic and acquired factors that may affect olfaction. These factors may include allergic or nonallergic rhinitis, infectious paranasal sinusitis, nasal and sinus polyposis, tobacco use, and the nasal use of over-the-counter prescription and illicit drugs, among others.

Irritational syndromes are the result of extensive exposure to irritating chemicals. These exposures are more likely to penetrate the mucous layer into the periciliary regions. Such reactions may primarily affect olfactory and trigeminal irritant nerve receptors, causing transient burning of the eyes, nasal passages,

TABLE 1. Common Examples of Chemicals Causing Adverse Health Effects

Annoyance symptoms	
Perfumes	Household cleaners
Colognes	Cooking odors
Detergents	Flower fragrances
Newspaper print	Low concentrations of
Exhaust fumes	tobacco smoke
Wave sets	Clothing stores
Body odor	
Irritational syndromes	
High concentrations of	Paint fumes
tobacco smoke	Volcanic ash
Pollution/smoke	Garden sprays
Field and slash burning	Ozone
Formaldehyde	Sulfur dioxide
Toluene/xylene	Nitrogen dioxide
Anhydrous ammonia	Chlorine gas
Immune hypersensitivity	
Acid anhydrides	Latex
Toluene diisocyanate	Ammonium persulfate
Colophony	Chloramine-T
Amine epoxy resins	Piperazine
Reactive dyes	Ipecacuanha
Beta-lactam antibiotics	Platinum salts
Intoxication syndromes	
Vinyl chloride	Carbon monoxide
Organophosphorus	Organic sulfur-containing
compounds	compounds
Cyanide, nitriles	Phenols and related
Aromatic hydrocarbons	compounds
Mercury	Acrylamide
Lead	

and throat. It is important to note that irritational syndromes may occur by stimulating nerve endings without the production of pathologic changes in the affected mucous membranes, e.g., inflammation. Formaldehyde is an example of a low molecular weight chemical capable of causing mucous membrane irritation (see Chapter 14).[15]

There are relatively few chemicals that are capable of inducing **immune hypersensitivity.** In most cases these low molecular weight substances require formation of a chemical-human serum albumin conjugate, with resultant chemical conjugate-specific antibody formation. Acid anhydrides (see Chapter 13) and isocyanates (see Chapter 12) are prominent examples of highly reactive, low molecular weight chemicals that may induce immunologic hyperreactivity and respiratory disease in specific occupational settings.[16-20]

Finally, under circumstances of prolonged and excessive chemical exposures, **intoxication syndromes** may occur. Almost any chemical can cause intoxication if the concentration is high enough and the exposure long enough.[21,22] Intoxication syndromes may result in a significant disease in multiple organs and may result in death. It is important to note that, as opposed to annoyance and irritational syndromes, the sequelae of immunologic hyperresponsiveness and intoxication syndromes may be permanent.[22] The outcomes of these reactions are dependent on the nature and extent of the exposures.

CLINICAL PRESENTATION

The diagnostic and therapeutic approach to individuals with perceived chemical sensitivity will vary, depending on the specific clinical presentation. The most common complaints in our experience are associated with exposure to ambient pollution.[23-25] Individuals may be exposed to a complex mixture of volatile and particulate substances in both indoor and outdoor environments. Pollution of the ambient air can occur as a result of natural phenomena, e.g., volcanoes, dust storms, forest fires, etc. More often than not, pollution is man-made and follows industrial generation of exhaust fumes, fossil fuel combustion, or petroleum refining. Important outdoor pollutants include carbon monoxide, nitrogen oxides, sulfur oxides, hydrocarbons, ozone, and respirable particulates. Common indoor air pollutants include many of the outdoor pollutant chemicals, as well as those more commonly associated with the use of household chemicals, aerosolized personal hygiene products, and most importantly, cigarette smoke. A number of important indoor allergens must also be considered as potential sources of allergy, which might account for perceived chemical sensitivity.

There is a substantial body of evidence linking specific air pollutants to increased respiratory illness and decreased pulmonary function, particularly in children.[25-28] Atopic individuals, particularly those with allergic asthma, appear to be at increased risk of demonstrating hypersensitivity to inhaled sulfur dioxide.[29-32] In addition to bronchospasm, urticaria, and gastrointestinal symptoms, vasculitic-like symptoms have been associated with inhalational exposures to sulfur dioxide.[33] Long-term exposure to nitrogen dioxide in some settings has been associated with the increased prevalence of respiratory illness.[34-36]

Despite our major efforts to control outdoor pollution, it has become increasingly apparent that individuals have their most significant exposure to airborne pollutants in the indoor environment. The typical employed adult male and female spend about 20 hours indoors at home or at work, with another hour in transit.[25] Of the time spent indoors, the greatest percentage of time for most individuals is in their home or in nonindustrial settings. Unfortunately these settings have been largely ignored by air quality control agencies. Pollutants found indoors are similar to those found outdoors and in many instances are derived from outdoor sources. One of the most prominent sources of indoor air pollution is tobacco smoke, which is comprised of a complex mixture of gases and particulates containing a wide range of chemical constituents.[14,15,37] Indoor tobacco smoking substantially increases the ambient levels of carbon monoxide, formaldehyde, nitrogen dioxide, acrolein, polycyclic aromatic hydrocarbons, hydrogen cyanide, respirable particulates, and many other substances. Other potentially toxic chemical indoor pollutants may include styrene, xylene, benzene, toluene, methylene chloride, 1,1-1-trichloroethane, chloroform, carbon tetrachloride, and a variety of other volatile organic compounds that are emitted from building products, furniture, cleaning fluids, pesticides, and paints.[38,39] Although increased recognition of the potential toxicity of these substances has led to a greater focus on the indoor environment, a great deal more study is required to achieve clear data on health effects. We have made marginally more progress in the study of woodburning stoves and potential adverse effects of formaldehyde. These topics are reviewed individually because they have achieved such importance in the medical community.

The use of **woodstoves** and fireplace inserts has greatly increased over the past decade. Homeowners have increasingly used wood as a heat source because of economic savings compared to increasing oil and natural gas prices. In addition, many individuals feel that woodburning stoves provide a "clean and natural" source of heat. The National Research Council Committee report suggested that this trend has been more substantial in the northeastern and northwestern United States.[40]

Although woodstoves and fireplace inserts are vented to the outdoor environment and ideally effectively transfer smoke to the outdoor environment, there are many circumstances that allow smoke to re-enter the home. In investigations of indoor air quality, it is our experience that many owners of woodstoves and fireplace inserts have improperly installed their units, with an inadequately fitted stovepipe or improper stack height.[41] In addition, it is common that doors to these units are left open, allowing for potential leakage of smoke into rooms that have negative air pressure. The emissions from wood-burning stoves have been studied by Duncan[42] and others[43,44] and include significant quantities of respirable particulates, sulfur oxides, nitrous oxides, hydrocarbons, carbon monoxide, formaldehyde, acid aldehydes, phenols, and acetic acids (Table 2). It is clear from a review of the nature of these substances that residents of homes with woodburning stoves expose themselves to potential respiratory irritants.

Study of comparable indoor and outdoor concentrations of particles have frequently found the indoor concentrations to be much higher than those found outdoors. While a specific discussion on the toxicologic effects of individual pollutants is beyond the scope of this discussion, it is quite clear that many of the substances emitted by woodburning stoves contain a wide array of potential respiratory irritants as well as carcinogenic compounds. Because combustion of drier wood may be more complete, resulting in less generation of products of incomplete combustion, owners of woodburning stoves and fireplaces should be advised to use dry cured wood. Even the best-made, most modern stoves have been shown to emit considerable respirable particulates into the outdoor air and should be considered a source of significant indoor and outdoor air pollution.[45]

Formaldehyde is a simple organic compound (HCHO) that has significant medical and industrial applications. It is used extensively in the production of textiles and building materials and has been identified as a significant indoor and outdoor air pollutant in many settings. With the advent of the energy crisis in the early 1970s, many buildings were retrofitted with urea formaldehyde foam insulation. Subsequent investigation suggested that buildings and homes that contain this material may emit significantly elevated levels of formadehyde, which could result in harmful health effects. Over the prior decade there has been a great deal of new literature generated on the health effects of formaldehyde. We will briefly review only those issues that specifically relate to chemical sensitivity and refer the reader to Chapter 14 for more details on formaldehyde as an allergen.

The adverse health effects of formaldehyde have been well documented. Exposure to lower levels of formaldehyde (i.e., 0.03 to 0.3 ppm) may result in annoyance complaints associated with heightened sense of olfactory awareness.[14,15] In addition, exposure to higher levels of formaldehyde, which have been estimated to range between 0.3 and 3 ppm, may result in irritation of eyes, nasal passages and throat.[15,46] While dermal sensitivity may result following dermal exposure to formaldehyde,[47] there are no consistent or convincing data that respiratory sensitization occurs.[15] Formaldehyde in high concentrations may be neurotoxic; several epidemiologic studies have attempted to relate subjective complaints of fatigue, forgetfulness, headache, inability to concentrate, or inability to sleep with environmental exposures to formaldehyde.[48] However, careful case-controlled studies have failed to show significant differences in nonspecific symptoms such as these in residents of homes with urea formaldehyde foam insulation as compared to controls.[49] It is our opinion, having reviewed this extensive literature, that with most formaldehyde exposures in the range of 0.3 ppm and 3.0 ppm that significant neurotoxicity would be quite unlikely.[15]

In summary, formaldehyde may be one of the most ubiquitous chemicals in our indoor and outdoor environment. While there is a substantial body of literature supporting potential toxic and immunologic consequences of exposure, the great majority of routine formaldehyde exposures result in annoyance or irritant reactions that are entirely reversible in nature. Health care providers should be aware of potential sources of formaldehyde exposure and their biologic significance.

TABLE 2.   *Woodburning Stove Contaminants**

Emission	Emission Range
	lb/cord†
Particulates	3–93
SO$_x$	0.5–1.5
NO$_x$	0.7–2.6
Hydrocarbons	1–146
Carbon monoxide	300–1,220
Polyclic organic materials	0.6–1.22
Formaldehyde	0.3–1.0
Acetaldehyde	0.1–0.3
Phenols	0.3–8
Acetic acid	5–48

* Adapted with permission from Pierson et al., ref. 41.
† The factor used to convert 1 lb per ton was 1.65 lb per cord.

PATIENT EVALUATION

When initially evaluating a patient with suspected chemical sensitivity, it is imperative to consider the common medical and psychologic conditions that may present as perceived toxicity or hypersensitivity to environmental exposures (Table 3). As a means of introduction, we present three clinical case studies that typify the basic patient profile of perceived "chemical sensitivity" seen in our practice:

Case 1. Building-related Illness

A 40-year-old white female telephone operator was referred to us for evaluation of "building-related illness" and possible occupational asthma. She had been transferred 2 months earlier to the Willamette valley from coastal Oregon, where she had apparently been completely healthy.

Within 3 days of her transfer to her new workplace, she began to experience nonproductive cough and chest tightness. In addition to her cough, she also complained of nasal and ocular congestion with palatal itching

TABLE 3. *Medical Conditions Commonly Presenting as Toxicity or Hypersensitivity to Environmental Exposures**

Infectious diseases
    Acute/chronic sinusitis
    Pharyngitis
    Tonsillitis
    Bronchitis
    Mononucleosis

Allergic/inflammatory states
    Allergic rhinoconjunctivitis
    Bronchial asthma
    Atopic dermatitis
    Contact dermatitis
    Hypersensitivity pneumonitis

Nonallergic respiratory diseases
    Chronic serous otitis media
    Chronic eustachian tube dysfunction
    Nasal polyposis
    Vocal cord polyps/tumors
    Vasomotor rhinitis
    Gastroesophageal reflux
    Rhinitis medicamentosa

Metabolic/toxic conditions
    Hypothyroidism/hyperthyroidism
    Diabetes mellitus
    Drug use
    Rheumatic disorders

* Reproduced in modified form from Bardana and Montanaro, ref. 12, with permission.

and profuse rhinorrhea. All of these symptoms reportedly improved within hours of leaving the workplace.

Following presentation to our office, it was clear that the patient appeared to have signs and symptoms of atopic disease. Her physical examination revealed changes of allergic rhinitis and conjunctivitis, with typical findings of conjunctival injection and with pale, swollen inferior nasal turbinates. This examination failed to reveal signs of bronchial obstruction, but spirometry showed an FEV_1 of 68% of predicted. Epicutaneous skin testing at the time of her original evaluation revealed marked dermal reactivity to grass, trees, and weed pollens, as well as to *Dermatophagoides pteronyssinus* and multiple molds.

A workplace evaluation resulted in a number of significant findings. The patient's new workplace had been undergoing extensive remodeling. Examination of the ceiling tiles noted prominent water staining. Inspection of the heating and air conditioning units uncovered standing water and obvious mold growth in the air intake system. Specific fungal sampling of the ambient air in the office subsequently resulted in prominent growth of *Cladosporium*. Further industrial hygiene evaluation noted a temperature of 72° and a relative humidity of 32% with a carbon dioxide level of greater than 1500 ppm. While the office appeared to be well heated with reasonable relative humidity, the carbon dioxide level substantiated the subjective appraisal of most workers in the environment as being "stuffy."

Simple and inexpensive interventions proved to be therapeutic in this case. A cleaning of the heating, ventilation, and air conditioning systems with an increase in exchange rate of fresh outdoor air resulted in dramatic and prompt improvement in the patient's work-related symptoms. While this patient clearly had underlying allergic rhinoconjunctivitis, as well as possible intermittent bronchospasm that may have been rendered more symptomatic in her workplace, she has been able to return to the workplace on a full-time basis without symptoms by being maintained successfully with a low dose of intranasal corticosteroids.

Case 2. Multiple Chemical Sensitivities

A 32-year-old female sign painter presented to our office for further evaluation of apparent paint and solvent sensitivity. She had been previously healthy and had worked for the state of Oregon at the same position for approximately 3 years. Over the 6 weeks prior to her evaluation, she had noted prominent headache, cough, chest discomfort, mood swings, irritability, and difficulty concentrating on and completing fine motor movements.

Her initial evaluation had been undertaken by her primary care physician, who noted no abnormalities on physical examination or on screening laboratory tests. Office spirometry as well as workplace peakflow monitoring were entirely normal. She had subsequently been referred by her primary care physician for neuropsychologic testing, which revealed "findings consistent with solvent encephalopathy." At the time of her evaluation in our office, a careful history suggested the diagnosis of endogenous depression. She presented with a history of frequent crying spells, chronic fatigue, nonrestorative sleep, anorexia, and weight loss. Her social history indicated that her second husband had left her after 18 months of marriage. A routine urine drug screen was positive for both marijuana and cocaine. A final diagnosis of situational depression and drug abuse was established, which clearly explained her symptoms.

Case 3. Environmentally Induced Immunologic Abnormalities

A 50-year-old printer was referred to our office by his internist for evaluation of potential immunodeficiency caused by "multiple chemical sensitivities" from his workplace. For the 2 years prior to his evaluation he had complained of increasing rhinorrhea, ocular signs, nasal congestion, sneezing, cough, chest pain, and exertional dyspnea. It had been suggested to him by a family member that his workplace exposures had led to a global deficit in his immune system, resulting in newly acquired sensitivities to a number of foods and environmental agents.

He was then evaluated by a practitioner of clinical ecology. Cytotoxic testing revealed the presence of multiple food sensitivities. Immune complex assays were said to confirm the presence of food sensitivities. Extensive B- and T-cell phenotypic testing, which had been done in the practitioner's office, were interpreted as "typical chemically-induced immune dysfunction."

The results of these tests and the patient's belief that he was being "poisoned" by his workplace prompted a complaint to the State

Accident Prevention Division. A subsequent inspection of the workplace detected a number of instances of unsafe storage and inadequate ventilation of volatile organic solvents, paints, and inks. However, dual cartridge charcoal filter respiratory protective devices had been made available to the workers and had been appropriately fitted and employed whenever workers had been exposed to solvents or paints.

Following his initial evaluation by the clinical ecologist, the patient discontinued his job and filed a claim for total and complete disability. Following denial of this claim, he sought legal counsel from an attorney, who then appealed this denial. This appeal subsequently led to the request for an independent medical evaluation in our office.

Our evaluation conducted approximately 4 months after the patient left his workplace included a thorough review of the medical records, a comprehensive history and physical examination, office spirometry, and flexible fiberoptic nasopharyngoscopy. The patient's history suggested that he had problems with irritant and vasomotor rhinitis that dated back at least 10 years. Physical examination revealed mild erythema and edema of the nasal turbinates but was otherwise normal. Repeat B- and T-cell phenotypic studies were entirely normal. A diagnosis of vasomotor rhinitis symptomatically aggravated by organic solvents and paints was made. There did not appear to be any evidence to confirm suspicions of occupational asthma. We determined his condition to be medically stationary with no long-term impairment or disability. The patient's appeal was subsequently denied. The patient is now a plaintiff in a product liability case against the manufacturers of the organic solvents and respiratory protective devices. We feel that this case represents an astonishing waste of medical and legal manpower, and that it is likely that it may have been predicated on a baseless belief system established by one of the health care workers who initially evaluated the individual.[50]

These cases highlight many of the difficulties that health care providers encounter when evaluating patients suspected of having chemical sensitivities.

MAKING THE CORRECT DIAGNOSIS

As can be discerned from the three case histories provided above, the issue of chemical sensitivity frequently emerges in the setting of workers' compensation or in product liability litigation. On the basis of what we have learned in evaluating patients presenting with chemical sensitivities, a pragmatic approach has been developed that attempts to avoid the common pitfalls and addresses the alternative disorders that frequently masquerade as sensitivity.

Three major pitfalls arise in the evaluation of possible attribution of chemical sensitivity to a particular industrial agent or household product. The three areas that we recognize as possible traps include: (1) failure to recognize an explanatory preexisting medical disorder; (2) oversight of an underlying condition masquerading as chemical sensitivity; and (3) inappropriate patient advocacy.

For any investigation of an environmental illness, a comprehensive medical history and physical examination are fundamental to achieving a correct diagnosis. In taking a medical history the evaluator should elucidate all preexisting disease. The patient may be confused or unable to recall prior diagnoses. However, prior health care providers should be meticulously documented so that all prior medical records can be obtained for review. In our experience, prior records frequently provide insight into health conditions or habits that explain the current symptoms. An important corollary of the medical history and examination is a complete differential diagnosis. Without systematic consideration and exclusion of a variety of equally plausible alternatives, inappropriate diagnoses may be made. The differential diagnostic approach should consider common conditions that may present as chemical sensitivity. We have arbitrarily divided these alternative diagnoses into four clinical classes of disease (Table 3).

DIFFERENTIAL DIAGNOSIS

Infectious Diseases. Chronic and/or acute paranasal sinusitis is clearly the most common infectious disease that we encounter in our patients who present with presumed respiratory chemical sensitivities. Chronic drainage frequently promotes problems that give the appearance of pharyngitis, laryngitis, or bronchitis. We have also observed patients with bona fide tonsillitis, pharyngitis, and bronchopneumonitis presenting as "sensitivity" to a pollutant. Acute and chronic forms of infectious mononucleosis must also be considered.

We feel that these infectious diseases many times cause complaints that are mistakenly interpreted by the patient or physician as manifestations of chemical sensitivities. It is entirely conceivable that these infectious diseases may in fact predispose an individual to have heightened sensible olfactory awareness, and thus experience annoyance or, in fact, have heightened reactivity to irritants in the environment.

Allergic Conditions. The presence of an underlying allergic seasonal disease may in fact predispose the individual to a perception of heightened reactivity. It is common, for example, for individuals with atopic dermatitis to experience prominent irritant effects of nonspecific exposures, such as frequent washing and drying of hands. Allergic rhinoconjunctivitis, which affects 15–20% of the general population, may also render an individual more sensitive to nasally inhaled irritants. It is very clear that allergic individuals with underlying bronchial hyperreactivity have nonspecific bronchial hyperresponsiveness to many environmental irritants. Atopic individuals may also have underlying bronchial asthma as part of a spectrum of allergic disease. Finally, the health care provider must be aware of conditions such as hypersensitivity pneumonitis, which may present with cough, dyspnea, and chest pain and which can lead the patient or physician to suspect a toxic or a chemical response. Although in fact cases of chemically induced hypersensitivity pneumonitis have been described,[51-54] most cases occur as a response to organic causes, e.g., mold, bird droppings, etc.[55]

Nonallergic Diseases of the Upper and Lower Airways. These diseases may result in signs or symptoms that can be interpreted as chemical sensitivity or toxicity. We have found individuals, for instance, with chronic serous otitis media, chronic eustachian tube dysfunction, nasal or vocal cord polyps, tumor, and vasomotor rhinitis who have presented with an exacerbation of these underlying disorders following exposure to chemicals. Gastroesophageal reflux is an exceedingly common cause of hoarseness or sore throat. One of the most frequent iatrogenic conditions that appears to predispose individuals to heightened symptoms is rhinitis medicamentosa. This occurs in settings where individuals are abusing over-the-counter topical nasal vasoconstrictors, with resultant rebound congestion, or in some cases of nasal inhalation of illicit recreational drugs.

Metabolic or Toxic Disorders. These disorders may present as presumed chemical toxicity in some patients. It is important to keep in mind that metabolic disorders are many times insidious and protean in their presentation. Endocrinopathies such as hypothyroidism, hyperthyroidism, and diabetes mellitus are commonly encountered conditions. It is critical to consider that many metabolic processes are affected by the use of prescription and nonprescription medications. In this regard, we have found that obtaining a detailed history of prescription medication and recreational drug use may provide clues to the patient's underlying disorders. Rheumatic conditions that may uncommonly present as chemical sensitivity include Sjogren's syndrome, systemic lupus erythematosus, Churg-Strauss syndrome, and Wegener's granulomatosis.[56]

PATIENTS PRESENTING WITH PSYCHOLOGIC DISORDERS WHO HAVE PERCEIVED CHEMICAL SENSITIVITIES

It has been our experience, as well as others who have reported in the literature,[8-10,57,58] that many individuals with perceived chemical sensitivity have serious underlying psychologic conditions. In our experience these conditions are far from "occult." As in the case described, many of these patients have overt manifestations of mood disorders that highly suggest the presence of unipolar or bipolar depression. A recent study using a diagnostic interview schedule found that 15 of 23 (65%) of subjects previously diagnosed as having "environmental illness" met criteria for current or past mood disorders, anxiety, or somatiform disorders, compared to 13 of 46 (28%) of age, sex, community-matched controls.[10] It is very common and well established that patients labeled with "environmental illness" or "multiple chemical sensitivity" in fact may have one or more commonly recognized psychiatric disorders. These disorders in many instances clearly explain their entire presentation.

The Litigious Patient

Unfortunately, all health care providers involved with occupational disease occasionally encounter the litigious patient. Although the past history and manner of presentation may suggest that an individual is seeking "secondary gain," it is essential that the practitioner

undertake a comprehensive evaluation in all cases and never presume that an individual is only pursuing secondary gain. We have encountered many "apparently" litigious patients who in fact have very valid claims. In such patients we have uncovered significant medical or psychologic conditions that need aggressive treatment.

DIAGNOSTIC PROCEDURES

On the basis of our experience with patients with presumed "chemical sensitivity," we have developed what we feel to be a pragmatic approach that emphasizes the use of high yield, low cost procedures (Table 4).[12,13]

High-yield, Low-cost Procedures

Aside from the carefully obtained medical history and review of the medical records discussed above, it may be helpful to acquire

TABLE 4. *Comprehensive List of Diagnostic Measures Ranked According to Yield and Cost*

High yield/low cost
  History and physical examination
  Review all medical records
  Review Material Safety Data Sheets
  Routine laboratory studies
  Nasal smear and cytology
  Chest x-ray
  Screening computed tomography scanning of sinuses
  Schirmer's test
  Nasopharyngoscopy
  Selected skin testing
  Pulmonary function studies
  Methacholine challenge
  Pre- and post-work exposure spirometry

High yield/significant cost
  Workplace/domicile industrial hygiene evaluation
  Toxicology sreeens for illicit drugs
  Immunodeficiency screens
  Psychometric testing
  Exercise stress test
  Psychiatric/neuropsychiatric evaluation
  Determination of diffusion capacity

Low yield/high cost
  Radioallergosorbent testing (RAST)
  Epstein-Barr virus serology
  Autoimmune serology profiles
  Food allergy testing
  Airborne mold/bacterial determination
  Controlled chamber challenge
  Toxicology screen for pesticides

* Reprinted in a modified form from Bardana and Montanaro, ref. 12, with permission.

Material Safety Data Sheets (MSDSs) or product information pamphlets on all suspected exposures. Material Safety Data Sheets are required by the Hazard Communication Standard to be on file in the workplace that uses potentially hazardous substances. Given the great number of toxic substances in industry that can be found in the workplace, it is difficult for the clinician to have a working knowledge of all of these common substances. We have found it particularly helpful to have an understanding of the health effects of commonly encountered chemicals. There are a number of publications available that provide helpful information on commonly encountered chemicals.[59-61] For those who wish a more comprehensive reference, we have found *Patty's Industrial Hygiene and Toxicology* to be invaluable.[62]

The physical examination of course must be the initial step in the evaluation of approaching any patient with chemical sensitivity. A careful examination of the upper respiratory tract may reveal signs of chronic infection or allergy. Skin findings compatible with atopic dermatitis such as flexural eczema may explain the patient's hyperresponsiveness to cutaneous irritants. As part of the physical examination, a careful neurologic examination is essential. For example, we have detected neurologic conditions of multiple sclerosis and cerebellar degeneration in patients who were thought to be exhibiting signs of neurotoxicity to workplace chemicals. Because the differential diagnosis of chemical sensitivity can be so extensive, the physician must be compulsive in performing a complete physical examination.

Laboratory testing does not need to be extremely extensive or expensive. We routinely order a chemistry panel and a complete blood count with differential and platelet count. A Westergren erythrocyte sedimentation rate can sometimes be helpful in detecting underlying inflammation or infectious disease. These studies can be accomplished at a very low cost and in our opinion should be obtained on every patient. Because thyroid disease may be insidious and multifaceted, it is often useful to include measures of thyroid function in the routine screening of the chemically sensitive patient.

Respiratory complaints are the most frequent and often the most prominent presentation in a patient with perceived chemical sensitivity, and further evaluation of the respiratory tract is very useful. A nasal smear is likely to be the least expensive office procedure for determining the cause of chronic nasal complaints. The presence of more than 25% eosinophils on a nasal smear may support the diagnosis of allergic disease, whereas predominance of polymorphonuclear cells may suggest a diagnosis of an infectious process. Although a single Waters x-ray of the sinuses may reveal obvious changes of the maxillary paranasal sinuses, we have found that computed tomographic *screening* of the sinuses is much more useful. Fortunately, in our community this is available for approximately $110/study, which is approximately the same cost as a complete x-ray series of the sinuses. We have also found that by using fiberoptic flexible nasopharyngoscopy as a routine study, abnormalities of the nasal membrane, paranasal sinuses, and larynx can be simply and inexpensively evaluated. We have found this technique to be particularly useful in establishing the diagnosis of occult paranasal sinus disease.

Allergy skin testing can be useful in isolated conditions. Many individuals with underlying atopy clearly are predisposed to multiple irritant and allergic symptoms of the upper and lower respiratory tract. Allergy skin tests can be undertaken with epicutaneous or intracutaneous methodology quite inexpensively, with both negative and positive results providing useful information. Although skin testing is generally preferable to radioallergosorbent testing (RAST), the RAST test offers a scientifically acceptable methodology that is convenient and noninvasive, but clearly more expensive. In a litigious setting where only one evaluation is possible, this may be the most expedient choice.

When symptoms suggest the presence of significant pulmonary disease, office spirometry is exceedingly valuable. Office spirometry may enable the clinician to objectively evaluate patients with prominent respiratory complaints. A normal spirometry result may in fact lead the physician to investigate more extensively the upper respiratory tract as a cause of intermittent cough. In individuals with normal spirometric findings, we find that methacholine challenge can be a valuable adjunct. These challenges with their benefits and drawbacks are reviewed more extensively in Chapters 3, 4 and 24.

If office spirometry and physical examination do not confirm an obvious respiratory diagnosis, peak-flow monitoring at home or in the workplace is quite useful in patients with presumed chemical sensitivity. This is likely to be the most cost-effective modality for use in accumulating objective data to substantiate workplace or home-related respiratory complaints. While peakflow monitoring is clearly effort-dependent, it may allow you to associate specific patient symptoms with some objective data, which may lead to further appropriate workplace or home evaluations. It should not be relied upon as the sole modality to establish the diagnosis (see Chapter 3).

HIGH-YIELD BUT HIGHER COST PROCEDURES

When a definitive diagnosis of the patient's condition has not been established using the previously described protocol, further high-yield studies may be indicated. Industrial hygiene evaluations invariably provide valuable information in identifying possible causations for presumed chemical sensitivity. Most insurance carriers either employ or retain industrial hygienists who can help the physician in this regard. A physician may simply request a workplace evaluation, but in most cases it is helpful to specify which aspect of the evaluation is important. The industrial hygienist, for instance, may be able to obtain simple measures of carbon dioxide as an indicator of adequacy of ventilation. Concentrations of total respirable particulates may suggest the extent of particulate exposure. In addition to working closely with a skilled industrial hygienist, a workplace evaluation by the physician can provide further insights. We have encountered settings where we identified sites of fungal, bacterial, or dust mite proliferation that have explained adverse health effects. In many instances these conditions can be dramatically altered.

Since neuropsychiatric symptoms are quite prominent among patients with suspected chemical sensitivities, neuropsychiatric evaluations can be quite helpful. In any person whose neuropsychiatric complaints suggest illicit drug use, toxicology screens may uncover many unsuspected findings. Many patients who emphatically deny illicit or recreational drug use have been found on their evaluation to have measurable levels of marijuana, alcohol, and cocaine.

Psychometric testing may be useful as a means of obtaining quantitative information, which may help to differentiate organic from nonorganic causes of neuropsychiatric complaints. On many occasions psychometric

testing has established a diagnosis of clinical depression, somatization disorders, or hysteria. Psychiatric referral is many times appropriate in these instances.

As previously mentioned, many patients have been informed of or perceive that they have abnormalities of "immune dysfunction." This belief may be based on inappropriate testing using well-established methodologies such as phenotypic analysis of B- and T-cell subsets. These tests are frequently obtained as part of an evaluation that has included non-validated measures such as sublingual provocation and cytotoxic testing. It is clear from data obtained by Terr and others that the immunologic abnormalities documented in these patients are in almost all cases unsubstantiated.[63]

MEDICAL-LEGAL CONSIDERATIONS

Chemical sensitivity frequently presents in the setting of a workers' compensation claim or product liability litigation. Many times the patient's initial concerns regarding chemical sensitivity have been validated by a busy primary care physician who has no expertise in the area of environmental or occupational medicine.

In considering the attribution of any symptom complex to any specific etiology, the clinician must be certain that a preexisting condition does not account for the patient's complaints. We recognize that the restrictions of a busy primary care practice are such that it is impossible to review a large file of medical records that might suggest a preexisting disorder. Often these records are not available at the time the primary physician is asked to make an assessment. Nonetheless, all physicians must be aware that if these previous records are not evaluated, or if the patient has not undergone a comprehensive evaluation, that they should avoid validating a diagnosis of "chemical sensitivity." Often a failure to consider an alternative explanation for symptoms attributed to chemical sensitivity leads to an inappropriate acceptance of chemical exposures as the explanation for symptoms. Usually this is based solely on the patient's perception. This "cause and effect trap" occurs frequently, because there is a natural tendency to automatically attribute causation to any exposure with which there is a recognized risk. For example, an asthmatic painter exposed to isocyanate-containing paint must have isocyanate-induced bronchial asthma.

Although the primary care physician must act as the patient's advocate, there is no imperative to reach an unsubstantiated diagnosis. A physician should always be conservative in establishing a diagnosis of chemically induced disease. Once this diagnosis is offered, the physician may find it impossible to retract it. Frequently, fear of disloyalty or legal retribution further confounds the problem. We feel it is very appropriate for physicians to utilize the term "possible" or "presumptive" toxicity or work-related disorder until more extensive and definitive evaluation can be undertaken. In this manner, the patient can be removed from further exposure while definitive evaluation proceeds.

The treatment of established chemical sensitivity should be focused on avoidance and education. If the exposure occurs at the workplace, modification of a manufacturing process, improved ventilation, or the use of proper respiratory protection frequently provides definitive therapy. If true sensitivity does exist, the patient will almost always be required to move to an entirely different work location. Clearly, there will be workers who require job retraining. Immunologic respiratory sensitivity has implications for long-term pulmonary effects that need to be conveyed to the patient. If exposures occur in a home or office setting, changes may be required in the equipment delivering fresh outdoor air. It is important to allow the patient to participate in designing programs of home or work modification. Finally, we have found that while many patients with perceived chemical sensitivity may present in an antagonistic fashion, that the problem can many times be resolved amicably. However, the latter usually requires a great deal of patience, time, and commitment on the part of the physician.

REFERENCES

1. Cullen MR: The worker with multiple chemical sensitivities: An overview. Occup Med State Art Rev 2:655, 1987.
2. Ashford N, Miller CS: Chemical Exposures: Low Levels and High Stakes. New York, Van Nostrand Reinhold, 1991.
3. Executive Committee of the American Academy of Allergy and Immunology: Chemical Ecology. J Allergy Clin Immunol 78:289, 1986.
4. California Medical Association Scientific Board Task Force on Clinical Ecology: Clinical Ecology: A Critical Appraisal. West J Med 144:239, 1986.
5. American College of Physicians: Position paper on clinical ecology. Ann Intern Med 111:68, 1989.
6. Dreger M (ed): American College of Occupational Medicine Report. September, 1990.
7. Terr AI: Environmental illness: A clinical review of 50 cases. Arch Intern Med 146:145, 1986.
8. Brodsky CM: "Allergic to Everything": A medical subculture. Psychosomatics 24:731, 1983.
9. Stewart DE, Raskin J: Psychiatric assessment of patients with 20th century disease ("total allergy syndrome"). Can Med Assoc J 133:1001, 1985.
10. Black DW, Rathe A, Goldstein RB: Environmental illness: A controlled study of 26 subjects with "20th century disease." JAMA 264:3166, 1990.
11. Brodsky CM, Green MA, Ogrod ES: Environmental illness: Does it exist? Patient Care Nov. 15:41-45, 1989.
12. Bardana EJ, Montanaro A: "Chemically sensitive" patients: Avoiding the pitfalls. J Respir Dis 10:32, 1989.
13. Bardana EJ, Montanaro A: Chemical sensitivity. In Lichtenstein LM, Fauci AS (eds): Current Therapy in Allergy, Immunology and Rheumatology, 4th ed. St. Louis, Mosby-Year Book, 1991.
14. Bardana EJ, Montanaro A, O'Hollaren MT: Building-related illness. Clin Rev Allergy 6:61, 1988.
15. Bardana EJ, Montanaro A: Formaldehyde: An analysis of its respiratory, skin and immunologic effects. Ann Allergy 66:441-452, 1991.
16. Bardana EJ, Andrasch RM: Occupational asthma due to low molecular weight antigens. Eur J Respir Dis 64:241, 1983.
17. Davies RJ, Butcher BT, Salvaggio JE: Occupational asthma caused by low molecular weight chemical agents. J Allergy Clin Immunol 60:93, 1977.
18. Fawcett IW, Newman-Taylor AJ, Pepys J: Asthma due to inhaled chemical agents-epoxy resin systems containing phthalic acid anhydride, trimellitic acid anhydride and triethylene tetramine. Clin Allergy 7:1, 1977.
19. Zeiss RC, Patterson R, Pruzansky JJ, et al: Trimellitic anhydride-induced airway syndromes. J Allergy Clin Immunol 60:96, 1977.
20. Banks DE, Butcher BT, Salvaggio JE: Isocyanate-induced respiratory disease. Ann Allergy 57:389, 1986.
21. McCarthy TB, Jones RD: Industrial gassing poisonings due to trichlorethylene, perchlorethylene and 1-1-1-trichloroethane. Br J Ind Med 40:450, 1983.
22. Wagoner JK: Toxicity of vinyl chloride and poly (vinyl chloride): A critical review. Environ Health Perspect 52:61, 1983.
23. Urone P: The primary air pollutants—gaseous. Their occurrence, sources and effects. In Stern AC (ed): Air Pollution. Vol. I, Air Pollutants, Their Transformation and Transport. New York, Academic Press, 1976, pp 24-71.
24. Juriel I: Indoor Air Quality and Human Health. Stanford, CA, Stanford University Press, 1985.
25. Samet JM, Marbury MC, Spengler JD: Health effects and sources of indoor air pollution, Parts I and II. Am Rev Respir Dis 136:1486, 1987 and 137:221, 1988.
26. Weiss ST, Tager IB, Speizer FE: Passive smoking: Its relationship to respiratory symptoms, pulmonary function and non-specific bronchial responsiveness. Chest 84:651, 1983.
27. Tager IB, Weiss ST, Munoz A, et al: Longitudinal study of the effects of maternal smoking on pulmonary function in children. N Engl J Med 309:699, 1983.
28. White JR, Froeb HF: Small-airways dysfunction in nonsmokers chronically exposed to tobacco smoke. N Engl J Med 302:720, 1980.

29. Koenig JQ, Pierson WE, Horikem FR: Broncho-constrictor responses to sulfur dioxide or sulfur dioxide plus sodium chloride droplets in allergic non-asthmatic adolescents. J Allergy Clin Immunol 69:339, 1982.
30. Sheppard D, Wong WS, Uehara CF, et al: Lower threshold and greater bronchomotor responsiveness of asthmatic subjects to SO_2. Am Rev Respir Dis 122:873, 1980.
31. Sheppard D, Saisho A, Nadel J, et al: Exercise increases SO_2-induced bronchoconstriction in asthmatic subjects. Am Rev Respir Dis 123:486, 1981.
32. Spengler JE, Dockery DW, Turner WA, et al: Long-term measurements of respirable sulfates and particles inside and outside homes. Atmos Environ 15:23, 1981.
33. Simon RA, Stevenson DD: Adverse reactions to sulfites. In Middleton E, Reed CE, Ellis EF, et al (eds): Allergy—Principles and Practice, 3rd ed. St. Louis, C.V. Mosby, 1988, pp 1555–1568.
34. Jakab GJ: Nitrogen dioxide-induced susceptibility to acute respiratory illness: A perspective. Bull NY Acad Med 56:847, 1980.
35. Ehrlich R, Henry MC: Chronic toxicity of nitrogen dioxide. I. Effect on resistance to bacterial pneumonia. Arch Environ Health 17:860, 1968.
36. Graham JA. Miller FJ: Interference with lung defenses by nitrogen dioxide exposure. In Gammage RB, Kaye SV (eds): Indoor Air and Human Health. Chelsea, MI, Lewis Publishers, 1985, pp 279–294.
37. Committee on Passive Smoking: Environmental Tobacco Smoke: Measuring Exposures and Assessing Health Effects. National Research Council. Washington, D.C., National Academy Press, 1986.
38. Wallace L, Pellizzari E, Hartwell T: Analysis of exhaled breath of 355 urban residents for VOCs. Proceedings of the 3rd International conference on Indoor Air Quality and Climate, Vol. 5. Stockholm, Sweden, August 20–24, 1984, pp 15–20.
39. Sterling DA: Volatile organic compounds in indoor air: An oveview of sources, concentrations and health effects. In Gammage RB, Kaye SV (eds): Indoor Air and Human Health. Chelsea, MI, Lewis Publishers, 1985, pp 387–402.
40. National Research Council: Indoor Pollutants. Washington, D.C., National Academy Press, 1981.
41. Pierson WE, Koenig JQ, Bardana EJ: Potential adverse health effects of wood smoke. West J Med 151:339, 1989.
42. Duncan JR, Monkin KM, Schmlerbach MP: Air quality impact potential from residential woodburning stoves. Paper presented at the 73rd annual meeting of the Air Pollution Control Association, Montreal, Quebec, June 1980.
43. Sexton K, Kai-Shenl, Treitman RD, et al: Characterization of indoor air quality in woodburning residences. Environ Int 12:265, 1986.
44. Butcher SS, Ellenbecker MJ: Particulate emission factors for small wood and coal stoves. J Air Pollution Control Assoc 32:380, 1982.
45. Spengler JD, Duffy CP, Letz R, et al: Nitrogen dioxide inside and outside 137 homes and implications for ambient air quality standards and health effects research. Env Sci Tech 17:164, 1983.
46. Morgan KIT, Patterson DL, Gross EA: Frog palate mucociliary apparatus: Structure, function and response to formaldehyde gas. Fundam Appl Toxicol 4:58, 1984.
47. Epstein E, Maibach HC: Formaldehyde allergy. Arch Dermatol 94:186, 1966.
48. Kilburn KH, Warchaw R, Boylen CJ, et al: Pulmonary and neurobehavioral effects of formaldehyde exposure. Arch Environ Health 40:254, 1985.
49. Bracken JJ, Lisa DJ, Morgan WKC: Exposure to formaldehyde: Relationship to respiratory symptoms and functions. Can J Public Health 76:312, 1985.
50. Cowart VS: Health fraud's tool: Lost hopes, misspent billions. JAMA 259:3229, 1988.
51. Schlueter DP, Banazak EF, Fink JN, et al: Occupational asthma due to tetrachlorophthalic anhydride. J Occup Med 20:183, 1978.
52. Fink JN, Schlueter DP: Bathtub refinishers lung: An unusual response to toluene diisocyanate. Am Rev Respir Dis 118:955, 1978.
53. Malo JL, Zeiss CR: Occupational hypersensitivity pneumonitis after exposure to diphenylmethane diisocyanate. Am Rev Respir Dis 125:113, 1985.
54. Lewis LD: Procarbazine-associated alveolitis. Thorax 39:206, 1984.
55. Fink JN: Hypersensitivity pneumonitis. In Middleton E, Reed CE, Ellis EF, et al (eds): Allergy—Principles and Practice, 3rd ed. St. Louis, C.V. Mosby, 1988, pp 1237–1252.
56. Campbell SM, Montanaro A, Bardana EJ: Head and neck manifestations of autoimmune disorders. Am J Otolaryngol 4:187, 1983.
57. Selner JC, Staudenmayer H: The practical approach to the evaluation of suspected environmental exposures: Chemical intolerance. Ann Allergy 55:655, 1985.
58. Staudenmayer H, Selner JC: Neuropsychophysiology during relaxation in generalized, universal allergic reactivity to the environment: A comparative study. J Psychosomatic Res 34:259–270, 1990.
59. Scott RM: Chemical hazards in the workplace. Chelsea, MI, Lewis Publishers, 1989.
60. Chemical Safety Data Sheets. Vol. 1, Sovlents; Vol. 2, Metals and Their Compounds. Cambridge, Engl, Royal Society of Chemistry, Thomas Graham House, 1989.
61. Finkel AJ: Hamilton and Hardy's Industrial Toxicology, 4th ed. Littleton, MA, PSG Publishing, 1983.
62. Patty's Industrial Hygiene and Toxicology, 3rd rev ed. New York, John Wiley, 1982.
63. Terr AI: Clinical ecology in the workplace. J Occup Med 31:257, 1989.

Chapter 23

THE PATHOGENESIS AND NATURAL HISTORY OF OCCUPATIONALLY INDUCED AIRWAY OBSTRUCTION

Emil J. Bardana, Jr., MD
Anthony Montanaro, MD

Occupational asthma represents only a small segment of the spectrum of occupational lung disorders. Since its earliest descriptions in grain handlers in the 18th century, an enormous body of literature has emerged that has significantly expanded our understanding of work-related bronchial asthma. Its import has been further accentuated because of its interface with our system of jurisprudence. Despite tremendous advances, it is still difficult to understand precisely how much any given set of occupational exposures contributes to the development of adult-onset bronchial asthma.

Approximately 35 million Americans suffer with some form of allergic disorder, and about 9 million are said to have bronchial asthma.[1] It has further been estimated that occupational exposures are responsible for 2% of all U.S. cases of bronchial asthma,[2,3] although the prevalence may approach 15% or more in some parts of the world.[4-6]

A multitude of agents have been incriminated as potential causes of occupational asthma. In 1980, their number was reported to exceed 200,[7] and this number will likely increase with time and the expansion of new polymer systems, adhesives, medicinals, and other chemicals.[8] Whereas the number of at risk workers is enormous, the number of well-documented cases of occupational asthma is relatively small. And although documented cases are relatively infrequent, occupational asthma remains one of the more commonly diagnosed conditions and continues to be responsible for considerable morbidity worldwide.[9,10] Reported cases almost certainly represent the "tip of the iceberg."

PREVALENCE

Because there is some debate about how occupational asthma should be defined, it continues to be difficult, if not impossible, to obtain precise information about the overall prevalence of work-related asthma. There has been a tendency to arrive at dependable information by evaluating specific industries. Examples include Hunter et al.'s survey of platinum refinery workers, in which 46% were found to have asthma,[11] and the initial observations of work-related asthma in the detergent industry after introduction of proteolytic enzymes in the 1960s.[12,13] Neither of these prevalence rates is consistent with exposure risks that are present within these industries at this time. Another deficiency of these types of industry-specific data may reside in the dissimilarity of workplaces. For instance, reports of occupational asthma affecting 7 to 9% of unselected bakers[14,15] is more consistent with bakeries in Europe than in the United States, where we are more likely to encounter large production plants rather than the small, family-run establishments. Industry-specific information cannot be reliably extrapolated to comparable industries worldwide. As well, many of these data were derived in a period when there were fewer restrictions on employers and essentially no incentives to provide

TABLE 1.   *Preexisting Conditions That Can Contribute or Aggravate Respiratory Impairment in Patients with Occupational Asthma*

Developmental
Bronchopulmonary sequestration
Congenital bronchial cysts
Congenital cystic bronchiectasis

Congenital
Immunologic deficiency syndromes
Kartagener's syndrome
Alpha-1 antitrypsin deficiency
Cystic fibrosis

Infections
Tuberculosis
Childhood bronchiolitis
Viral pneumonia

Diseases of the airways
Childhood or adult bronchial asthma
Chronic bronchitis
Emphysema
Bullous disease of the lungs
Bronchiectasis

Diseases of uncertain origin
Collagen vascular disorders
Sarcoidosis
Ankylosing spondylitis
Idiopathic pulmonary fibrosis
Bronchiolitis obliterans
Aspirin idiosyncrasy syndrome

safe work environments. Federal and state agencies, as well as insurers providing coverage for workers' compensation, have emerged as major regulators in the last several decades, putting considerable pressure on employers to safeguard employees.

DEFINITION

Bronchial asthma has always generated controversy when attempts were made to define it.[2,16-21] It is a disease that can be approached from several different perspectives. The clinician defines it as a reversible, obstructive airway disorder. The physiologist views it as a disorder of increased bronchial hyperreactivity. The pathologist considers it as an inflammatory disease of the airways and would rather rename the disorder to "desquamative eosinophilic bronchitis."

TABLE 2.   *Concomitant or Underlying Upper Respiratory Conditions That May Contribute to or Aggravate Asthmatic Symptoms*

Allergic rhinoconjunctivitis
Rhinitis medicamentosa
Nasal polyposis
Infectious sinusitis

Occupational asthma has been defined as a condition characterized by reversible obstruction of the airways, with its origin in the inhalation of ambient dusts, vapors, gases, or fumes that are either manufactured or employed by the worker, or incidentally present at the workplace.[3] The condition may occur in association with chronic bronchitis and varying degrees of chronic irreversible obstructive airway disease.[16-18] Occupational asthma may also develop in a predisposed individual with preexisting bronchial asthma, e.g., via immune or nonimmune sensitization to a specific industrial antigen.[19,20] De novo occupational asthma must be distinguished from either a transient symptomatic expression or more permanent aggravation of a preexisting nonoccupational asthmatic state.

It is important to consider patients with work-related inhalational syndromes in the context of their entire medical history. Any preexistent lung disorder should be considered as potential contributors to the ultimate respiratory impairment (Table 1). As well, a variety of genetically determined disorders have the capacity to induce or contribute to respiratory disease. Examples include the genetic predisposition to develop early emphysema with alpha-1-antitrypsin deficiency, paranasal sinusitis and bronchiectasis associated with Kartagener's syndrome, and the increased frequency of bronchitis, pneumonitis, and occasionally bronchiectasis with congenital or acquired humoral immunodeficiency states. A number of other diseases can be associated with pulmonary sequelae, e.g., collagen-vascular disorders, adverse drug reactions, sarcoidosis, etc. (Table 1). Additionally, a number of upper respiratory conditions may accentuate or aggravate asthmatic symptoms (Table 2).

As indicated above, there is still some controversy with some aspects of the definition for occupational asthma. For example, in Great Britain the Industrial Injuries Advisory Council defines occupational asthma as "asthma which develops after a variable period of symptomless exposures to a sensitizing agent at work."[21] The Council has implicated only seven groups of industrial agents, including platinum salts, isocyanates, epoxy resins, colophony fumes, proteolytic enzymes, laboratory animals and insects, and grain (or flour) dust. This definition is too restrictive and potentially could eliminate affected workers.

Smith has recently raised a number of medical-legal issues regarding the definition of occupational asthma.[22] He correctly noted that the repercussions of how to define and diagnose occupational asthma frequently assume greater importance in the litigation arena relative to workers' compensation statutes and third-party product liability lawsuits. He suggests a number of criteria for establishing the diagnosis of occupational asthma, including: (1) the presence of asthma characterized by variable airway obstruction that is persistent and not just related to a chemical spill or viral illness; (2) association with an established asthmogenic agent in the workplace; (3) exposure for a sufficient time for hyperreactivity to develop; (4) physiologic demonstration of airway obstruction to the suspected asthmogenic agent at work or by simulated work provocation; (5) development of asthma with low concentrations (subirritant doses) of the suspected asthmogenic agent, i.e., far below the TLV set for the irritant effect of that agent; and (6) symptomatic improvement that occurs when the patient is removed from the suspected agent, with the demonstrated return of symptoms upon re-exposure.[22] Although the last criterion is not always true, it is our strong belief based upon the available data that the manifestations of de novo, work-related airway obstruction should either remit or significantly improve in all patients who are diagnosed and removed from the offending agent in a timely manner.

PREDISPOSING FACTORS

Epidemiologic studies have looked for personal as well as social and medical factors that are associated with the development of occupational asthma. There is limited knowledge in this area, but some factors have been explored in some detail (Table 3).

Atopy. Individuals with a personal and family history of allergic rhinoconjunctivitis (hayfever), bronchial asthma, urticaria/angioedema, and atopic eczema are more likely to be sensitized to certain industrial agents than those who are not so predisposed.[8,16,23] Atopy clearly predisposes to asthmatic states resulting from IgE production to one or more work antigens. This is particularly true with respect to industries where high-molecular-weight compounds are the incriminated agents, e.g., animal handlers, grain and flour handlers, seafood processors, agricultural research workers, etc.[24] In general, this is not true in industries where low-molecular-weight antigens are the principal agents inducing disease.[20,25]

TABLE 3. *Predisposing Factors in the Development of Occupational Asthma*

1. **Atopy**

   Increased likelihood of developing sensitivity to high-molecular-weight antigens in industry or environment.

   There is synergy between smoking and atopy.

   Greater likelihood of developing adult-onset asthma.

2. **Smoking**

   Associated with significant inflammation of the tracheobronchial system.

   Associated with varying stages of chronic obstructive pulmonary disease.

   Higher incidence of respiratory tract infections.

   Increased incidence of bronchial hyperreactivity.

   Presence of increased levels of total serum IgE and a higher prevalence of sensitization to certain antigens.

   Increased bronchial permeability to allergens and perhaps a greater access to submucosal immuno-competent cells.

3. **Recreational drug use**

   Marijuana is capable of causing similar inflammatory changes in bronchial system as tobacco.

   There is synergism of all adverse effects in tobacco smokers who also use marijuana.

   Smoking freebase cocaine is associated with hypersensitivity pneumonitis, bronchial asthma, obliterative bronchiolitis, and pulmonary edema, among other disorders.

4. **Respiratory infections**

   Viral infections frequently precipitate the initial asthmatic episode in adults and are frequently associated with exacerbations.

   Viral infections may cause damage to irritant receptors and result in a decreased threshold of reactivity.

   Viral-specific IgE antibodies could result in release of vasoactive amines from mast cells.

   Viral infections could depress cellular immunity.

   Certain bacterial infections may depress beta-adrenergic activity and act as adjuvants.

5. **Nonspecific bronchial hyperreactivity**

   Probably genetically transmitted.

   Major characteristic of bronchial asthma.

   Almost universally present in patients with documented occupational asthma.

   Rare instances of its absence are known.

   Unknown whether bronchial hyperreactivity is the result of work exposures or a predisposing factor to the development of occupational asthma.

6. **Miscellaneous**

   Aspirin idiosyncracy syndrome

   Beta adrenergic blockers

   Angiotensin converting enzyme inhibitors

   Gastroesophageal reflux

   Exercise

   Stress and anxiety

   Offensive or irritating odors

Bronchial asthma has at least two genetic influences on its development. One relates to the capacity of an individual to develop allergic disease or atopy; the other relates more specifically to the development of bronchial hyperresponsiveness independent of atopy.[26] Cumulative incidence figures for asthma ranging as high as 20% support the contention that the genetic possibility for the development of asthma must be very common.[26] In this respect, care must be taken to distinguish de novo, work-related asthma from a simple reappearance of childhood asthma or the initial appearance of adult-onset asthma associated with the first encounter of a very prominent environmental (non-work) allergen or in the wake of a viral infection.

Smoking.   Approximately 50 million Americans still smoke cigarettes. Several groups of investigators have considered smoking both a predisposing and an aggravating factor in the development of occupational asthma.[27-30] There is little doubt that chronic tobacco abuse is associated with significant inflammation of the tracheobronchial system[31] and frequently with the development of obstructive pulmonary disease.[32] There is no relationship between smoking and the de novo development of bronchial asthma. However, there appears to be a clear relationship between chronic tobacco abuse and a higher incidence of respiratory tract infections. In one of the larger prospective studies in a group of healthy individuals, smoking was associated with a 46% greater risk of upper respiratory tract infection.[33] There is also a relationship between respiratory infection with viruses and the development of bronchial hyperreactivity and/or bronchial asthma.[34-38] Cigarette smoking has also been linked with an increased incidence of bronchial response to methacholine and histamine.[39-42]

A number of studies have also suggested an increased association between cigarette smoking and the development of sensitization to occupational agents. Burrows and his associates observed higher mean levels of total serum IgE in smokers than in nonsmokers.[43] Howe et al. noted an increased sensitization to tetrachlorophthalic anhydride (TCPA) in smokers.[44] The latter observations were recently expanded by noting 20 of 24 workers with specific IgE antibodies to TCPA-HSA conjugate were current cigarette smokers.[45] This group also reported a positive interaction between the presence of an atopic state and smoking. Similar associations between chronic tobacco abuse and sensitization have been reported in Sweden in pharmaceutical workers exposed to ispaghul and in coffee workers.[46] An increased incidence of occupational asthma was noted in cigarette-smoking enzyme-detergent workers[47] and crab processors.[48] One possible explanation for these observations is the fact that smoking is known to increase lung permeability in man[49] and experimental animals,[50] leading several groups of investigators to speculate that smoking may potentiate allergen access to submucosal immunocompetent cells.[8,51,52] On the other hand, Chan-Yeung noted no such association in 185 patients with western red cedar asthma diagnosed by inhalation provocation.[53] Seventy percent of these occupational asthmatics were never smokers and only 5% were present smokers.

Recreational Drug Use.   Marijuana smoking on a regular basis, i.e., one cigarette daily, is thought to be practiced by 20 million individuals in the U.S.[54] It appears that consumption of a few marijuana cigarettes has the potential to cause the same degree of epithelial damage and bronchitis as a larger number of tobacco cigarettes, because of the manner in which the substance is inhaled and the quantity particles retained.[55] Studies in both animal models and healthy young adults indicate that marijuana smoke can: (1) induce airway irritation with increased numbers of inflammatory cells; (2) impair host defenses of the lung by limiting their ability to protect against infections and other noxious insults; and (3) produce significant changes in lung function similar to the functional manifestations of early chronic obstructive airway disease.[54-56] It has also been shown that the combined use of marijuana and tobacco may be more harmful than the use of either substance alone.[56]

The current popularity of smoking the alkaloidal form of cocaine ("crack" or "freebase") has also been associated with a spectrum of pulmonary complications that should be considered in any claimant suspected of illicit drug abuse. The pulmonary sequelae of smoking freebase cocaine include hypersensitivity pneumonitis, obliterative bronchiolitis, bronchial asthma, and pulmonary edema, among other disorders.[57]

Infection.   Clinicians have long suspected that viral infections frequently precipitate asthmatic episodes in patients with established asthma, and that they may mark the beginning of symptoms that recur in the future, mainly with subsequent viral infections.[58] In this respect, many patients evaluated for suspected work-related asthma frequently recall symptoms of a viral infection shortly before their asthmatic symptoms began.[16,27,28] Prospective studies have shown that over 40% of asthmatic episodes in children occur in the setting of viral respiratory infections.[59] This relationship also occurs in adults, but to a lesser degree than in children.[34] By contrast, bacterial infections of the respiratory tract do not appear to exacerbate bronchial asthma.[58] The one exception to the latter is pyogenic infections of the paranasal sinuses in which the relationship to worsening underlying asthma is quite strong.[35,60]

Respiratory viral infections are capable of producing a variety of changes having a direct effect on the facilitation of an underlying asthmatic state, including: (1) epithelial damage and inflammation of nerve endings, resulting in a decreased threshold of reactivity[61,62]; (2) viral-specific IgE antibodies that may precipitate the release of vasoactive amines from mast cells[63,64]; (3) viral agents that could themselves affect the stability of mast cells and their products[65,66]; and (4) promotion of defective cellular immune responses secondary to viral infection.[67,68] It is also conceivable that certain of these sequelae could result from bacterial infections, especially if they were severe and recurrent as might be expected with certain immunodeficiency disorders. Certain bacteria such as pertussis have been shown to depress beta-adrenergic activity as well as act as an adjuvant in a sensitization process.[69]

Nonspecific Bronchial Hyperreactivity. Perhaps the major problem in making the initial diagnosis of occupational asthma is the assurance that the condition does not represent a preexisting illness. The same question arises when reviewing medical reports of occupational asthma, because the vast majority of these reports are retrospective or anecdotal in nature. Unfortunately, many patients have a very poor understanding of childhood and young adult illnesses when interviewed, judging from information in available medical records. Additionally, there may be an element of overt deception for the purposes of secondary gain, i.e., a willful omission in one or more aspects of the medical, family, or social history. Perhaps the most striking example of the latter in the author's experience, for whatever reason, is the deliberate underestimation of tobacco abuse (as compared with prior citations in the medical records).

It is believed that the predisposition to the acquisition of bronchial hyperreactivity is genetically transmitted.[70] It has been linked to the determinants of atopy, in that subjects with allergic rhinoconjunctivitis (hayfever) have greater bronchial reactivity than non-atopic individuals.[71-74] Townley and his associates have conducted a number of studies suggesting an increased association between atopy and agents resulting in bronchial hyper-reactivity.[75]

Bronchial hyperreactivity is regarded as a major characteristic of bronchial asthma.[70] It can be defined as an exaggerated airway narrowing in response to a wide variety of stimuli.[70] It is almost universally present in untreated patients with symptomatic occupational asthma. Rare instances of its absence have been noted.[76] It is unknown whether this is a result of occupational exposures or a predisposing factor to the development of occupational asthma.[8] In this respect, it is of interest to note that in a group of 2,363 children from ages 8 to 11 studied by Salome et al., about 18% had bronchial hyperreactivity.[77] However, 37% of these children with bronchial hyperreactivity had neither symptoms nor a previous diagnosis of bronchial asthma.[77] This observation and others like it beg the need for large-scale prospective studies of workers in high-risk industries, measuring for the presence of bronchial hyperreactivity. Unfortunately, the only long-term prospective study of this kind ever undertaken failed to assess workers for this abnormality before any exposure had occurred.[78]

Patients with work-related asthma must be screened for both nonoccupational and occupational factors that can cause bronchial hyper-reactivity. These include a myriad of stimuli that have been documented to cause late-phase responses.[79] The major factors include viral upper respiratory infections, which, as noted above, are the most frequent cause of asthmatic flares,[31] inhalation of antigen,[80] exposure to significant concentrations of oxidizing irritants (e.g., ozone,[81, 81a] NO_2,[82] and SO_2[83]), and exposure to certain occupational agents such as toluene diisocyanate.[18,25] Elements of all these factors might easily be present in a single patient.

Miscellaneous.   A number of other factors are associated with the triggering or aggravation of preexisting asthma. Some of these may truly represent predisposing features and for the most part are incompletely understood. A subset of individuals with bronchial asthma may have upper respiratory sequelae and an idiosyncratic response to aspirin and non-steroidal anti-inflammatory drugs.[84] Aspirin idiosyncrasy is often overlooked and in our experience has been misinterpreted as a work-related phenomenon.

Prescription drugs used for unrelated conditions may also have an adverse effect on the course of asthma or occasionally be the triggering event for its initial appearance. Beta adrenergic blocking agents are increasingly used in many areas of medicine. They probably represent the most common group of medications that can potentially precipitate or worsen preexisting asthma. Not infrequently a new work exposure may be implicated as the cause for a flare in asthma in the absence of a complete history. Angiotensin-converting enzyme inhibitors have become recognized as a common cause of cough, which may be mistaken as an asthmatic condition.[85]

Other factors such as exercise, exposure to cold air, stress, and gastroesophageal reflux can also provoke airway obstruction in asthmatic patients. A large spectrum of ubiquitous odors have been implicated in triggering asthma.[86] Perfume and cologne were two of the most frequent sources of offensive odors implicated by asthmatic patients.[86] Finally, in addition to the myriad of nonspecific irritants that workers are exposed to in the workplace, exposure to many commonly encountered environmental pollutants may act as irritants and aggravate asthmatic symptoms.

PATHOGENETIC MECHANISMS

Some time ago Gandevia noted that in most instances occupational asthma is not a single, simple, or homogeneous entity, even when a single, specific causal factor can be identified in the workplace.[87] Induction of work-related asthma by any industrial agent is dependent on the type, source, and concentration of occupational exposure, work conditions, industrial hygiene factors, climatic influences, and individual characteristics of host response. This is fundamentally why acute, high-level exposures to some respiratory irritants lead to acute inflammatory occupational asthma in some instances, but chronic low-level exposures to the same agent may induce an immunologic or pharmacologically derived occupational asthma in another instance (Fig. 1).

THE LATE-PHASE RESPONSE

Although many older definitions of bronchial asthma characterize it as a bronchospastic disease, there is substantial evidence indicating that prominent inflammatory changes underly this bronchospasm.[88,89] The introduction of bronchoalveolar lavage has afforded studies indicating the presence of significant numbers of eosinophils in patients with mild bronchial asthma.[90] The critical question that cannot be answered completely at this time is whether airway inflammation is the sole cause of airway hyperresponsiveness. There appears to be good evidence linking bronchial hyperreactivity to inflammation in the airways. This is particularly true in most cases of occupational asthma.[91] However, there appear to be factors in addition to bronchial inflammation that operate in the maintenance of airway hyperreactivity. There are good data that show that asymptomatic patients with previously documented western red cedar asthma have no evidence of airway inflammation in BAL fluid in the face of moderate degrees of airway hyperresponsiveness, as determined by methacholine challenge.[8,91] The importance of intact bronchial epithelium has been noted by several groups of investigators recently.[90] Fabbri and associates have emphasized their observations relating to a steroid responsive and unresponsive component of airway hyperresponsiveness.[92] These investigators feel the steroid responsive component is related to inflammation and the unresponsive component is related to unknown factors.

A variety of pulmonary reactions may develop following bronchial challenge in a sensitized individual. These include isolated immediate, isolated late, or dual reactions, with incidences ranging from 9 to 53%, 7 to 50% and 18 to 84%, respectively.[79,93,96] Isolated immediate reactions occur within minutes following antigen challenge and are characterized by a bronchospastic reaction leading to airway obstruction. They generally resolve within 30 to 60 minutes.[79,95] Isolated late reactions start some 3 to 4 hours following exposure and peak by 4 to 8 hours. This reaction is characterized by bronchial inflammation and increased airway hyperresponsiveness.[97] It generally resolves by 12 to 24 hours.[79] The dual response is generally characterized by a more intense and prolonged obstructive reaction.

A wide variety of triggers have been observed to cause late-phase asthmatic reactions, including environmental allergens as well as many occupational antigens.[79] The clinical features of dual or biphasic responses were initially used by Pepys to develop immunopathogenetic hypotheses to explain disease

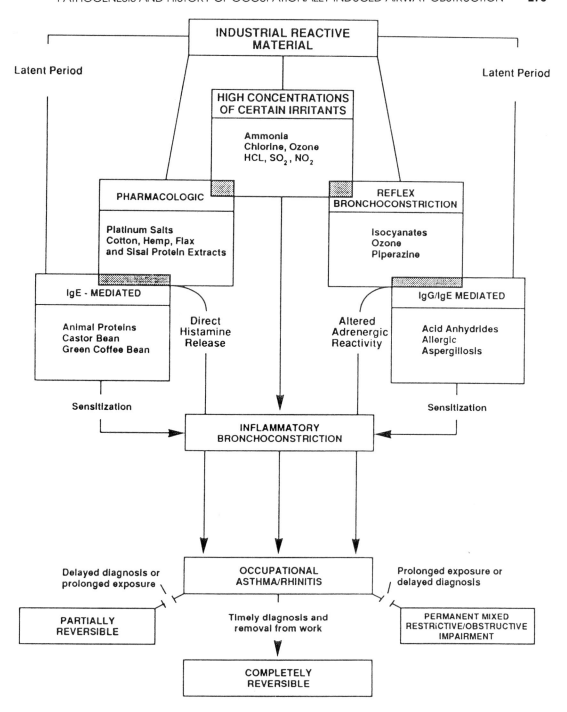

FIGURE 1. Schematic conceptualization of the many possible pathogenetic mechanisms of occupational asthma. (Modified from Ref. 16, with permission.)

processes, i.e., the type I and type III mechanisms of allergic bronchopulmonary aspergillosis (ABPA).[98,99] While perhaps true for ABPA, this formulation did not hold up with respect to other antigens and disease processes. Perhaps most important was the observation

that exercise challenge could produce dual asthmatic reactions in selected patients,[100] though recent observations suggest that the delayed component may also reflect diurnal variability in pulmonary function.[101] Others have shown that ultrasonically nebulized distilled

TABLE 4. *Asthmogenic Triggers Can Be Divided into Bronchospastic or Inflammatory Triggers**

Bronchospastic Triggers (Symptomatic)	Inflammatory Triggers (Causative)
Pharmacologic, e.g., beta blockers, angiotensin inhibitors, and cotton bract	Allergens, e.g., pollens, housedust mite, mold, etc.
Exercise[†]	Viral infections
Cold air	Many low molecular weight chemicals
Hyperventilation	High concentrations of respiratory irritants, e.g., anhydrous ammonia, chlorine, etc.
Emotional stress	Oxidizing pollutants such as ozone, NO_2, or SO_2
Usual concentration of environmental irritants, e.g., cigarette smoke, perfumes, and cologne	

*Adapted from Ref. 97, with permission.
[†] May induce an inflammatory component in selected patients.

water has been reported to produce immediate and late bronchial reactions.[102] It appears that both the immediate and late-phase reactions are primarily IgE-mediated, but that the late-phase response results from a complex amplification of the initial response.

In conceptualizing the development of bronchial asthma, either de novo or as a result of irritating encounters, Cockcroft divided potential triggers into those that would induce a symptomatic expression of asthma, i.e., bronchospastic, and those that could cause or alter the basic nature of asthma, i.e., inflammatory (Table 4). It is believed that the immediate response is modulated by pulmonary mast cells and their mediators, including histamine, LTC_4, and LTD_4. The late-phase response results when chemotactic factors promote the ingress of eosinophils that generate further LTC_4 and LTD_4 and release platelet activating factor and major basic protein. The latter could damage air epithelium, limiting its ability to produce relaxing factors and exposing irritant receptors to further stimuli, perpetuating and worsening airway responsiveness.

MECHANISMS OF DAMAGE

Gandevia initially classified occupational asthma according to pathophysiologic mechanisms.[87] He initially proposed four basic mechanisms including acute inflammation, reflex mechanisms, pharmacologic bronchoconstriction, and immunologic bronchoconstriction. We have assimilated this very useful classification and expanded the immunologic category to include both IgE- and IgG-mediated subsets[16] (Fig. 1).

Inflammatory Bronchoconstriction

This mechanism was initially described by Gandevia in workers exposed to high concentrations of irritant or noxious gases or fumes (Fig. 1). This was generally related to a pyrolytic process or overt combustion.[87] A number of other investigators made similar observations with a variety of toxic materials. The airway obstruction usually develops quite rapidly, secondary to a chemically induced bronchitis or bronchopneumonia. There is no latent period required. The process induces maximal symptoms and signs within the period of a week and gradually regresses over the next several months.[103-105] Pathologic studies of tissue in patients who failed to survive showed changes consistent with chemical bronchitis associated with hemorrhagic pulmonary edema.[106] Many survivors manifested evidence of chronic bronchial asthma or chronic airway hyperresponsiveness, depending on the corrosive properties of the agent involved and the duration of exposure.

Reactive Airways Dysfunction Syndrome

In 1981 Brooks and Lockey coined the diagnostic grouping "reactive airways dysfunction syndrome" (RADS) to describe 13 workers exposed to high concentrations of respiratory irritants with features consistent with inflammatory bronchoconstriction.[107] In a later description of 10 patients, which included the original six index cases, they noted these individuals presented with asthma-like symptoms after high-dose exposure to respiratory irritants.[108] Five of the initial six cases manifested bronchial hyperreactivity as determined by methacholine-challenge testing. Bronchial biopsies were carried out on two of these cases who were said to show evidence of bronchial epithelial desquamation and mucous cell hyperplasia. The authors postulated that the cause of persistent bronchial hyperreactivity was related to the extensive chemically induced inflammatory response.[108] Unfortunately, eight of ten patients had confounding variables related to previous cigarette smoking or atopic disease that may have independently accounted for their bronchial hyperreactivity, aside from the putative high-dose exposure. Interestingly, although the exposures in these cases were irritant in nature, only three of the ten patients had immediate symptoms. Seven of the ten patients went on to have chronic or persistent respiratory symptoms requiring continuous use of bronchodilators. Although these retrospective observations raise the provocative question as to the role of irritants in evoking bronchial hyperreactivity, they fail to clearly discriminate between atopy, smoking, possible viral infection, and a single noxious exposure to a chemical for an uncertain time and concentration.

It remains unclear whether RADS is sufficiently unique to distinguish it from the previously described condition of inflammatory bronchoconstriction.[87] Some authors would argue that RADS is not occupational asthma, because the condition is not exacerbated by reexposure to low levels of the same chemical.[109] It is true that certain toxic chemicals may induce transiently inflamed, irritable, and hyperreactive airways in otherwise normal individuals. Some would prefer to call this an occupational chemical bronchitis rather than occupational asthma. There is also the definitional problem that arises between work-related asthma, which is felt to be an "occupational disease," and RADS, which many consider an "occupational injury."[110] In this respect, the authors of this chapter feel that RADS may in some cases be a misleading designation. Furthermore, it is clear that all cases of occupational asthma do not necessarily imply "sensitization" and that acute inflammatory asthma of industrial origin is very likely to be of a transient nature in the great majority of cases.

Pharmacologic Bronchoconstriction

The second mechanism discussed by Gandevia was related to a direct pharmacologic effect[87] (Fig. 1). The best example of this mechanism is the Monday morning illness commonly observed in many cotton textile workers and referred to as byssinosis[111] (see Chapter 7). The syndrome is seen with inhalation of dusts of cotton, flax, hemp, and jute. The clinical syndrome was initially described by Ramazzini in 1713. The workers most often affected are those engaged in the preparation of cotton, flax, or soft-hemp fibers for spinning. However, workers in later phases of the process, including weavers, may also develop the syndrome. Byssinosis starts as a transitory acute response to dust exposure and is characterized by symptoms of chest tightness, cough, wheezing, and dyspnea, particularly pronounced at the beginning of the work week. The longer the absence from work the more pronounced the symptoms.[111] There remains some considerable controversy regarding the nature of any chronic disease with byssinosis—so-called "brown lung disease."[112] The precise mechanisms of byssinosis are still unclear, but the acute bronchoconstriction is thought to be related to histamine content in the bract as well as a release of histamine from pulmonary mast cells.[112,113] In addition, cotton bract dust is known to be contaminated with endotoxin. Rylander et al. reported that acute bronchoconstriction in cardroom workers correlated better with the quantity of gram-negative bacteria contaminating bale cotton than the bacteria-free dust[114] (see Chapter 7). Another example of a direct pharmacologic effect is the pulmonary toxicity reported with organophosphate insecticide. Acute bronchial asthma has been described in farm workers spraying crops with organophosphate insecticides. In this condition the anticholinergic effect precipitates airflow obstruction on a pharmacologic basis.[115]

Reflex Bronchoconstriction

Certain chemicals and inert agents are felt to have the capacity to cause reflex bronchospasm by disrupting the delicate balance of adrenergic control involved in maintaining bronchial tone (Fig. 1). This is felt to be mediated via the irritant receptors in the bronchial wall.[116,117] The reaction tends to be acute in nature and does not require a latent period. Examples of this type of mechanism are seen with inhalation of ozone, SO_2, and NO_2.[81-83] This type of reaction is commonly seen in patients with preexistent bronchial asthma. Permanent residual effects are not generally a feature of this mechanism. Davies et al. have shown that isocyanates can act as pharmacologic inhibitors, reducing the ability of beta-adrenergic receptors to produce cyclic AMP levels in sufficient quantities necessary to maintain bronchial tone.[118] Monomeric isocyanates at high concentrations can also stimulate cyclic

AMP production, suggesting that they act as partial agonists.

Immunologic Bronchoconstriction

Immunologic mechanisms are operative in the large majority of cases of occupational asthma. We have chosen to divide this mechanism into reactions that appear to be purely IgE in nature and those that have both IgE and IgG participation (Fig. 1).[16] Classically, most examples of this type of antigen fall into the category of organic high-molecular-weight antigens.[24] Usually the allergens involved are proteins or glycoproteins with the capacity to elicit IgE and occasionally IgG antibodies to certain ligands. A latent period is required for sensitization to take place. Examples include allergens encountered from exposure to animal products, insects, plants, and biological enzymes. As indicated above, immunologic bronchial reactivity invariably leads to late-phase reactions, and sequential allergen exposure is associated with amplification in airway reactivity.[119] In most instances of allergic asthma, epicutaneous or intracutaneous skin tests with appropriate antigens elicit a typical wheal-and-flare reaction. Specific IgE antibodies can also be demonstrated in serum by using radio-allergosorbent tests. Atopic subjects are more frequently affected than nonatopic individuals.

Another form of sensitization results from the development of IgG antibody to certain inhaled antigens. This leads to the development of hypersensitivity lung disorders, which can be occupational in nature but clearly are not of an asthmatic nature. Clinically one sees cough, dyspnea, rales, pulmonary infiltrates, and a restrictive lung disease with reduced diffusion capacity. Examples include farmer's lung disease, pigeon breeder's lung, mushroom worker's lung, etc.[120]

There are also a number of occupational asthmatic syndromes that result from mixtures of IgE and IgG immune responses. A latent period is required for sensitization to occur. There appears to be a predilection to affect atopic individuals to a greater extent, although there are exceptions to this rule. Perhaps the best example of this variant is allergic bronchopulmonary aspergillosis, when it occurs in the framework of an occupational exposure, e.g., malt worker's lung.[121] In another arena, Zeiss and co-workers reported on a spectrum of occupational asthmatic states caused by trimellitic anhydride.[29] One subset termed

"phthalate flu syndrome" characteristically manifested IgE or IgG phthalate-specific antibodies associated with myalgia, arthralgia, headache, and fatigue. Similar reeactions have been noted with other phthalates[28] (see Chapter 13).

Despite what is known about the pathogenesis of occupational asthma, there are many occupational agents that are associated with the induction of work-related asthma but for which the precise mechanism is still poorly understood. Plicatic acid is the chemical compound thought to be responsible for western red cedar asthma. Yet, it has never been measured in the actual work environment and the mechanism by which it causes the asthma has never been fully elucidated. It clearly has been shown to have irritant, immunizing, and pharmacologic properties, i.e., activation of the classic complement pathway (see Chapter 8).[8] However, none of these mechanisms explains why only a small percent of workers are affected. It is very likely that a specific industrial reactant can induce asthma by more than a single mechanism, and further, that more than a single mechanism may be operative in any given patient. This merely reinforces the previous observations of Gandevia[87] and Farr,[122,123] who have emphasized the heterogeneity of asthma.

PROGNOSIS IN OCCUPATIONAL ASTHMA

As can be determined from the discussion relating to the definition of bronchial asthma, there still remains some controversy as to what should be appropriately called occupational asthma and the minimum criteria for its absolute diagnosis.[52,124] In attempting to define the natural history of occupational asthma, one must currently rely on the diverse clinical criteria employed by different investigators studying entirely different patient populations in unique industrial settings. With rare exceptions, these studies are all retrospective in nature, and there are no assurances that a significant percentage of these cases did not have preexistent mild, unrecognized asthma. Similarly, there is no assurance that some of these cases did not have asymptomatic bronchial hyperreactivity.[42]

Chan-Yeung et al. published their support for the concept of chronic occupational asthma persisting after discontinuation of the offending work exposures.[125] While these authors and others have estimated that chronic occupational asthma may occur commonly, we believe that before one can make meaningful statements about the chronicity of occupational asthma, it will be necessary to develop information relating to a cohort of workers who were screened *prior* to any potential adverse work exposure. This would have to include data on prior history of asthma or lung disease, and more importantly, whether they might have asymptomatic bronchial hyperreactivity. At this point in time, there are no controlled, prospective studies addressing these issues, i.e., a well-screened population about to enter a high-risk industry where both preexposure pulmonary function studies and methacholine challenge testing has been carried out. As well, there are no prospective studies that longitudinally follow such a group of workers, identify the onset of work-related asthma, remove the worker from further exposure, and then determine the features of the asthma and bronchial hyperreactivity over an extended period of time. Without such longitudinal studies, one can only speculate about the issue of prognosis.

In reviewing some of the frequently cited papers supporting the higher frequency of chronic symptoms in occupational asthma, they all suffer common weaknesses. In 1975 Adams reported persistent respiratory symptoms in 46 patients with toluene diisocyanate asthma.[126] He studied 565 men in two toluene diisocyanate plants, none of whom had preexposure pulmonary function or methacholine challenge. The 46 men removed from further exposure were identified because of "symptoms." None had documented challenge-proven isocyanate asthma. Adams compared the 46 symptomatic men to 46 control men with similar smoking habits. It is of interest that 40 of the "symptomatic" group continued to have symptoms along with 28 of the "normal controls." Given the lack of preemployment health data and the presence of these confounding variables, it would be exceedingly difficult to ascribe causation to the chronic complaints. Moller et al. reported that 7 of 12 patients with toluene diisocyanate asthma continued to have persistent symptoms after removal from further exposure nearly 2 years following cessation of exposure.[127] This study is also retrospective and purports to investigate 12 individuals with "suspected" toluene diisocyanate asthma. The latter was verified by bronchial challenge with subirritant levels of isocyanate in only seven individuals. Four of the seven individuals had

been exposed to spills of toluene diisocyanate. The heterogeneity of the population makes it difficult to extrapolate the meaning of these observations in the broad context of occupational asthma. The retrospective study by Paggiaro et al. reports chronic symptoms in 27 of 47 furniture workers believed to have toluene diisocyanate asthma, but who continued to work and experience exposure to isocyanate.[128] Only 17 or 27 asthmatics had demonstrable bronchial hyperreactivity by bethanechol challenge.

The only prospective study ever carried out in the toluene diisocyanate industry was done by the Tulane group between 1973 and 1978 in a toluene diisocyanate plant before production began.[78,129] Clinically important sensitivity to toluene diisocyanate developed in 4.3% of the study population. This was proven by inhalation challenge to a maximum concentration of toluene diisocyanate of 0.02 ppm. Fully 75% of the reactors became asymptomatic within 7 months of the initial exposure to toluene diisocyanate. There was universal improvement in symptoms in all identified asthmatics removed from the offending agent.

In attempting to define factors affecting prognosis, Chan-Yeung et al. considered a multitude of potential factors.[130] They observed that those with persistent asthma had a significantly longer duration of symptoms before diagnosis, poorer lung function for a variety of reasons, and a severer degree of bronchial hyperreactivity at the time of diagnosis. Similar observations were made by Hudson et al. in 1985,[131] as well as in a 1989 follow-up study.[132] The latter study suggests that their observations are restricted because of the retrospective nature of the design.[131,132] Our own experience indicates that while symptoms and functional changes may persist on removal from the workplace, most patients should experience a symptomatic improvement. This is especially true when the diagnosis is established in a timely fashion and the patient promptly removed from the offending agent. This favorable outcome is facilitated when there is an absence of prior pulmonary disease and atopy, and relatively normal pulmonary function at the time of diagnosis. In this respect, it should be noted that 17 of 25 patients reported by Allard et al. who failed to improve upon removal from work were atopic. It is possible their failure to improve simply reflects a preexisting nonoccupational asthmatic state.[132]

REFERENCES

1. Young P: Asthma and allergies: An optimistic future. Washington, D.C., U.S. Dept. of Health and Human Services. NIH Publ. 80-388, March, 1980.
2. Salvaggio J, et al: Task force on asthma and other allergic diseases. Washington, D.C., U.S. Dept. of Health and Welfare, NIAID Task Force Report, Publication No. 79-389, 1979, p 330.
3. Brooks SM: Bronchial asthma of occupational origin. Scand J Work Environ Health 3:53, 1977.
4. Kobayayashi S: Occupational asthma due to inhalation of pharmacological dusts and other chemical agents with some reference to other occupational asthmas in Japan. In Yamamura Y, Frick OL, Horiuchi Y, et al (eds): Allergology. Proceedings of the Eighth International Congress of Allergology, Tokyo, 1973. New York, Elsevier, 1973, p 124.
5. Introna I: L'asme bronchiale allergica come malattia professionale. Minerva Med 86:176, 1966.
6. Cotes JE: Epidemiology and prevention of occupational asthma [editorial]. Br J Ind Med 44:73, 1987.
7. Newman Taylor AJ: Occupational asthma. Thorax 35:241, 1980.
8. Chan-Yeung M, Lam S: Occupational asthma. Am Rev Respir Dis 133:686, 1986.
9. Ad Hoc Committee on Occupational Asthma of the Standards Committee of the CTS: Occupational Asthma. Can Med Assoc J 140:1029, 1989.
10. Parkes WR: Occupational asthma (including byssinosis). In Parkes WR: Occupational Lung Disorders, 2nd ed. London, Butterworths, 1982, pp 415–453.
11. Hunter D, Milton R, Perry KMA: Asthma caused by complex salts of platinum. Br J Ind Med 2:92, 1945.
12. Newhouse ML, Tagg B, Pocock SJ, et al: An epidemiological study of workers producing enzyme washing powders. Lancet i:689, 1970.
13. Mitchell CA, Gandevia B: Respiratory symptoms and skin reactivity in workers exposed to proteolytic enzymes in the detergent industry. Am Rev Respir Dis 104:1, 1971.
14. Bjorkstein F: Immunological methods in the identification of occupational asthma. Eur J Respir Dis 63 (Suppl 123):21, 1982.
15. Thiel H, Ulmer WT: Baker's asthma: Development and possibility for treatment. Chest 78:400, 1989.
16. Anderson CJ, Bardana EJ: Work-induced asthma: I. Clinical features, evaluation and pathogenesis. Immunol Allergy Pract 1:54, 1979.
17. Morgan WKG: Industrial bronchitis. Br J Ind Med 35:285, 1978.
18. Salvaggio JE: Occupational asthma: Overview and mechanisms. J Allergy Clin Immunol 64:646, 1979.
19. Pepys J: Occupational asthma: Review of present clinical and immunologic status. J Allergy Clin Immunol 66:179, 1980.
20. Bardana EJ, Andrasch RH: Occupational asthma secondary to low molecular weight agents used in the plastic and resin industries. Eur J Respir Dis 64:241, 1983.
21. Report by the Industrial Disease Committee of the Industrial Injuries Advisory Council in Occupational Asthma. Dept. of Health and Social Security. London, HMSO, 1981, pp 7–19.
22. Smith DD: Medical-legal definition of occupational asthma. Chest 98:1007, 1990.
23. Seaton A: Occupational asthma. In Morgan WKC, Seaton A (eds): Occupational Lung Diseases, 2nd ed. Philadelphia, W.B. Saunders, 1984, pp 498–501.
24. Novey HS, Bernstein IL, Mihalas LS, et al: Guidelines for the clinical evaluation of occupational asthma due to high molecular weight antigens. J Allergy Clin Immunol 85(Part 2):829, 1989.
25. Butcher BT, Bernstein IL, Schwartz HJ: Guidelines for the clinical evaluation of occupational asthma due to small molecular weight chemicals. J Allergy Clin Immunol 85(Part 2):835, 1989.
26. Smith JM: Epidemiology and natural history of asthma, allergic rhinitis, and atopic dermatitis (eczema). In Middleton E, Reed CE, Eclis EF, et al (eds): Allergy: Principles and Practice, 3rd ed. St. Louis, C.V. Mosby, 1988, p 899.
27. Andrasch RH, Bardana EJ, Koster F, et al: Clinical and bronchial provocation studies in patients with meatwrappers' asthma. J Allergy Clin Immunol 58:291, 1976.
28. Bardana EJ, Anderson CJ, Andrasch RH: Meatwrappers' asthma: Clinical and pathogenetic observations. In Frazier CA (ed): Occupational Asthma. New York, Van Nostrand Reinhold, 1980.
29. Zeiss CR, Patterson R, Pruzansky JJ, et al: Trimellitic anhydride-induced airway syndromes: Clinical and immunologic studies. J Allergy Clin Immunol 60:96, 1977.
30. Gandevia B: Pulmonary reactions to organic chemicals: Clinical history, physical examination and x-ray changes. Ann NY Acad Sci 221:10, 1974.
31. U.S. Public Health Service: The Health Consequences of Smoking: A Report of the Surgeon General. Rockville, MD, Dept. Health and Human Services, Pub. No. DHHS [PHS]82-50179, 1982.
32. Doll R, Peto R: Mortality in relation to smoking: 20 years' observations in male British doctors. Br Med J 2:1525, 1976.
33. Blake GH, Abell TD, Stanley WG: Cigarette smoking and upper respiratory infection among recruits in basic combat training. Ann Intern Med 109:198, 1988.
34. Minor TE, Dick EC, Baker JW, et al: Rhinovirus and influenza A infections as precipitants of asthma. Am Rev Respir Dis 113:149, 1976.
35. Slavin RG, Cannon RE, Friedman WH, et al: Sinusitis and bronchial asthma. J Allergy Clin Immunol 66:250, 1980.
36. Pullan CR, Hey EN: Wheezing, asthma and pulmonary dysfunction 10 years after infection with respiratory syncytial virus in infancy. Br Med J 284:1665, 1982.
37. Empey DW, Laitinen LA, Jacobs L, et al: Mechanisms of bronchial hyperreactivity in normal subjects after upper respiratory tract infection. Am Rev Respir Dis 113:131, 1976.
38. Halperin SA, Eggleston PA, Beaseley P, et al: Exacerbations of asthma in adults during experimental rhinovirus infection. Am Rev Respir Dis 132:967, 1985.
39. Cerveri I, Bruschi C, Zoia M, et al: Distribution of bronchial nonspecific reactivity in the general population. Chest 93:26, 1988.
40. Cerveri I, Bruschi C, Zoia MC, et al: Smoking habit and bronchial reactivity in normal subjects. A population-based study. Am Rev Respir Dis 140:191, 1989.
41. Mullen JBM, Wiggs BR, Wright JL, et al: Nonspecific airway reactivity in cigarette smokers. Relationship to airway pathology and baseline lung function. Am Rev Respir Dis 133:120, 1986.
42. Kennedy SM, Burrows B, Vedal S, et al: Methacholine responsiveness among working populations: Relationship to smoking and airway caliber. Am Rev Respir Dis 142:1377, 1990.

43. Burrows B, Halonen M, Barbee RA, et al: The relationship of serum immunoglobulin E to cigarette smoking. Am Rev Respir Dis 124:523, 1981.

44. Howe W, Venables KM, Topping MD, et al: Tetrachlorophthalic anhydride asthma: Evidence for specific IgE antibody. J Allergy Clin Immunol 71:5, 1983.

45. Venables KM, Topping MD, Howe W, et al: Interaction of smoking and atopy in the production of specific IgE antibodies against a hapten protein conjugate. Br Med J (in press).

46. Zetterstrom O, Osterman K, Machado L, et al: Another smoking hazard: Revised serum IgE concentration and increased risk of occupational allergy. Br Med J 283:1215, 1981.

47. Greenberg M, Milne JF, Watt AA: A survey of workers exposed to dusts containing derivatives of Bacillus subtilis. Br Med J 2:629, 1970.

48. Cartier A, Malo J-L, Forest F, et al: Occupational asthma in snow crab-processing workers. J Allergy Clin Immunol 74:261, 1984.

49. Jones JG, Minty BD, Royston JP: Carboxyhemaglobin and pulmonary epithelial permeability in man. Thorax 38:129, 1983.

50. Hulbert WC, Walker DC, Jackson A, et al: Airway permeability to horseradish peroxidase in guinea pigs: The repair phase after injury by cigarette smoke. Am Rev Respir Dis 123:320, 1981.

51. Anon: Smoking, occupation and allergic lung disease [editorial]. Lancet ii:965, 1985.

52. Venables KM: Epidemiology and the prevention of occupational asthma [editorial]. Br J Ind Med 44:73, 1987.

53. Chan-Yeung M: Immunologic and non-immunologic mechanisms in asthma due to western red cedar (Thuja plicata). J Allergy Clin Immunol 70:32, 1982.

54. Gong H Jr, Fligiel S, Tashkin DP, et al: Tracheobronchial changes in habitual heavy smokers of marijuana with and without tobacco. Am Rev Respir Dis 136:142, 1987.

55. Wu T-C, Tashkin DP, Djahed B, et al: Pulmonary hazards of smoking marijuana as compared with tobacco. N Engl J Med 318:347, 1988.

56. Anon: Marijuana: A second look (position paper). ATS News 11:7, 1985.

57. Ettinger NA, Albin RJ: A review of the respiratory effects of smoking cocaine. Am J Med 87:664, 1989.

58. Busse WW: The effect of viral infections in asthma and allergic disorders. Insights in Allergy 3(4):October 1988. St. Louis, C.V. Mosby, 1988.

59. McIntosh K, Ellis EF, Hoffman LS, et al: The association of viral and bacterial respiratory infections with exacerbations of wheezing in young asthmatic children. J Pediatr 82:578, 1973.

60. Rachelefsky CS, Katz RM, Siegel SC: Chronic sinus disease with associated reactive airway disease in children. Pediatrics 73:526, 1984.

61. Hudgel DW, Langston L, Selner JC, et al: Viral and bacterial infections in adults with chronic asthma. Am Rev Respir Dis 120:393, 1979.

62. Smith CB, Golden CA, Kanner RE, et al: Association of viral and mycoplasma pneumonial infections with acute respiratory illness in patients with chronic obstructive pulmonary disease. Am Rev Respir Dis 121:225, 1980.

63. Bloom JW, Halonen M, Dunn AM, et al: Pneumococcus-specific IgE in cigarette smokers. Clin Allergy 16:25, 1986.

64. Welliver RC, Sun M, Rinaldo D, et al: Predictive value of respiratory syncytial virus-specific IgE responses for recurrent wheezing following bronchiolitis. J Pediatr 109:776, 1986.

65. Busse WW, Swenson CA, Borden EC, et al: Effect of influenza A virus on leukocyte histamine release. J Allergy Clin Immunol 71:382, 1983.

66. Alam R, Kuna P, Rozniecki I, et al: The magnitude of the spontaneous production of histamine releasing factor (HRF) by lymphocytes in vitro correlates with the state of bronchial hyperreactivity in patients with asthma. J Allergy Clin Immunol 79:103, 1987.

67. Welliver RC, Kahl TN, Sun M, et al: Defective regulation of immune responses in respiratory syncytial virus infection. J Immunol 133:1925, 1984.

68. Welliver RC, Sun M, Rinaldo D: Defective regulation of immune responses in croup due to parainfluenza virus. Pediatr Res 19:716, 1985.

69. Frick OL, German DF, Mills J: Development of allergy in children. I. Association with virus infections. J Allergy Clin Immunol 63:228, 1979.

70. Boushey HA, Holtzman MJ, Sheller JR, et al: Bronchial hyperreactivity. Am Rev Respir Dis 121:389, 1980.

71. Townley RG, Dennis M, Iekini JM: Comparative action of acetyl-beta-methacholine, histamine and pollen antigens in subjects with hayfever and patients with bronchial asthma. J Allergy 36:121, 1965.

72. Fish JE, Rosenthal RR, Batra G, et al: Airway responses to methacholine in allergic and non-allergic subjects. Am Rev Respir Dis 113:579, 1976.

73. Cockcroft DW, Killian DN, Mellon JJA, et al: Bronchial reactivity to inhaled histamine: A clinical survey. Clin Allergy 7:235, 1977.

74. Townley RG, Ryo UY, Kolotkin BM, et al: Bronchial sensitivity to methacholine in current and former asthmatic and allergic rhinitis patients and control subjects. J Allergy Clin Immunol 56:429, 1975.

75. Townley RG, McGready S, Bewtra A: The effect of beta-adrenergic blockade on bronchial sensitivity to acetyl-beta-methacholine in normal and allergic rhinitis subjects. J Allergy Clin Immunol 57:358, 1976.

76. Hargreave JE: Occupational asthma without bronchial-hyperresponsiveness. Am Rev Respir Dis 130:513, 1984.

77. Salome CM, Peat JK, Britton WJ, et al: Bronchial responsiveness in two populations of Australian school children. I. Relation to respiratory symptoms and diagnosed asthma. Clin Allergy 17:271, 1987.

78. Diem JE, Jones RN, Weill H, et al: Five-year longitudinal study of workers employed in a new toluene diisocyanate manufacturing plant. Am Rev Respir Dis 126:420, 1982.

79. Lemanske RF Jr: The late phase response: Clinical implications. Adv Intern Med 36:171, 1991.

80. Cockcroft DA, Ruffin RE, Dolovich J, et al: Allergen-induced increase in non-allergic bronchial reactivity. Clin Allergy 7:503, 1977.

81. Euston RE, Murphy SD: Experimental ozone pre-exposure and histamines. Arch Environ Health 15:160, 1967.

81a. Molfino NA, Wright SC, Katz I, et al: Effect of low concentrations of ozone in inhaled allergen responses in asthmatic subjects. Lancet ii:199, 1991.

82. Orehek J, Mussari JP, Gayrard P, et al: Effect of short-term, low level nitrogen dioxide exposure on bronchial sensitivity of asthmatic patients. J Clin Invest 57:301, 1976.

83. Islam MS, Vastag E, Ulmer WT: Sulfur-dioxide-induced bronchial hyperreactivity against acetylcholine. Int Arch Arbeits Med 29:221, 1972.
84. Stevenson DD: Diagnosis, prevention, and treatment of adverse reactions to aspirin and non-steroidal anti-inflammatory drugs. J Allergy Clin Immunol 74:617, 1984.
85. O'Hollaren MT, Porter GA: Angiotensin converting enzyme inhibitors and the allergist. Ann Allergy 64:503, 1990.
86. Shim C, Williams MH: Effect of odors on asthma. Am J Med 80:18, 1986.
87. Gandevia B: Occupational asthma. Part I. Med J Aust 2:332, 1970.
88. Cockcroft DW: Airway hyperresponsiveness and late asthmatic responses. Chest 94:178, 1988.
89. Chung KF: Mediators of bronchial hyperresponsiveness. Clin Exp Allergy 20:453, 1990.
90. Beasley R, Roche WR, Roberts JA, et al: Cellular events in the bronchi in mild asthma and after bronchial provocation. Am Rev Respir Dis 139:806, 1989.
91. Chan-Yeung M, Lam S: Evidence for mucosal inflammation in occupational asthma. Clin Exp Allergy 20:1, 1990.
92. Fabbri LM, Chiesure-Corona P, DalVecchio L, et al: Prednisone inhibits late asthmatic reactions and the associated increase in airway hyperresponsiveness induced by toluene-diisocyanate in sensitized subjects. Am Rev Respir Dis 132:1010, 1985.
93. Robertson DG, Kerigan AT, Hargreave FE, et al: Late asthmatic responses induced by ragweed pollen allergens. J Allergy Clin Immunol 54:244, 1974.
94. Metzger WJ, Nugent K, Richerson HB: Site of airflow obstruction during early and late phase asthmatic responses to allergen provocation. Chest 88:369, 1986.
95. Booij-Noord H, deVries K, Sluiter HJ, et al: Late bronchial obstructive reaction to experimental inhalation of housedust extract. Clin Allergy 2:43, 1972.
96. Lam S, Tan F, Chan H, et al: Relationship between types of asthmatic reaction, non-specific bronchial reactivity and specific IgE antibodies in patients with red cedar asthma. J Allergy Clin Immunol 72:134, 1983.
97. Cockcroft DW: Modulation of airway hyperresponsiveness. Ann Allergy 60:465, 1988.
98. Pepys I: Clinical and therapeutic significance of patterns of allergic reactions of the lungs to extrinsic agents. Am Rev Respir Dis 116:573, 1977.
99. Pepys J: Occupational asthma: Review of present clinical and immunologic status. J Allergy Clin Immunol 66:179, 1980.
100. Bierman CW, Spiro SG, Petheram I: Characterization of the late response in exercise-induced asthma. J Allergy Clin Immunol 74:701, 1984.
101. Rubinstein I, Levison H, Slutsky AS, et al: Immediate and delayed bronchoconstriction after exercise in patients with asthma. N Engl J Med 317:482, 1987.
102. Foresi A, Mattoli S, Corbo GM, et al: Late bronchial response and increase in methacholine hyperresponsiveness after exercise and distilled water challenge in atopic subjects with asthma with dual asthmatic response to allergen inhalation. J Allergy Clin Immunol 78:1130, 1986.
103. Harkonen H, Nordman H, Korhonen O, et al: Long term effects of exposure to SO_2 lung function four years after a pyrite dust explosion. Am Rev Respir Dis 128:890, 1983.
104. Flurry KE, Dines DE, Rodarte JR, et al: Airway obstruction due to inhalation of ammonia. Mayo Clin Proc 58:389, 1983.
105. Hasan FM, Gehshan A, Fulechan FJD: Resolution of pulmonary dysfunction following chlorine exposure. Arch Environ Health 38:76, 1983.
106. Charan ND, Myers CG, Lakshminarayan S, et al: Pulmonary injuries associated with acute sulfur dioxide inhalation. Am Rev Respir Dis 119:555, 1979.
107. Brooks SM, Lockey J: Reactive airways dysfunction syndrome (RADS). A newly defined occupational disease [Abst]. Am Rev Respir Dis 123(suppl):A133, 1981.
108. Brooks SM, Weiss MA, Bernstein IL: Reactive airways dysfunction syndrome (RADS). Persistent airways hyperreactivity after high level irritant exposure. Chest 88:376, 1985.
109. Boulet LP: Increase in airway responsiveness following acute exposure to respiratory irritants. Chest 94:476, 1988.
110. Hendrick D: Occupational asthma—problems of definition. J Occup Med 25:484, 1983.
111. Bouhuys A, Zuskin E: Byssinosis: Occupational lung disease in textile workers. In Frazier CA (ed): Occupational Asthma. New York, Van Nostrand Reinhold, 1980, p 33.
112. Kleinerman J, Bardana EJ, Battigelli MC, et al: Byssinosis: Clinical and research issues. Washington, D.C., National Academy Press, 1982.
113. Edwards J: International conference in byssinosis. Mechanisms of disease induction. Chest 79(Suppl): 38, 1981.
114. Rylander RK, Imbus HR, Suh MW: Bacterial contamination of cotton as an indicator of respiratory effects among cardroom workers. Br J Ind Med 36:299, 1979.
115. Weiner A: Bronchial asthma due to organic phosphate insecticide. Ann Allergy 19:397, 1961.
116. Widdicombe JT, Kent DC, Nadel JA, et al: Mechanisms of bronchoconstriction during inhalation of dust. J Appl Physiol 17:613, 1962.
117. Frank NR, Amdur MO, Worcester J, et al: Effect of acute controlled exposure to SO_2 on respiratory mechanics in healthy male adults. J Appl Physiol 17: 252, 1962.
118. Davies RJ, Butcher BT, O'Neil CE, et al: The in vitro effect of toluene diisocyanate on lymphocyte cyclic adenosine monophosphate production by isoproterenol, prostaglandin and histamine. J Allergy Clin Immunol 60:223, 1977.
119. Cockcroft DW: Mechanism of perennial allergic asthma. Lancet ii:253, 1983.
120. Fink JN: Immunologic lung diseases. Hosp Pract 6:53, 1981.
121. Bardana EJ: The clinical spectrum of aspergillosis. Part II. Classification and description of saprophytic, allergic and invasive variants of human disease. CRC Lab Sci 13:21, 1981.
122. Farr RS: Asthma in adults: The ambulatory patient. Hosp Pract 14:113, 1978.
123. Spector SL, Farr RS: The heterogeneity of asthmatic patients—an individualized approach to diagnosis and treatment. J Allergy Clin Immunol 57: 499, 1976.
124. Porter R, Birch J (eds): Identification of Asthma. Edinburgh, Churchill Livingstone, 1971 (Ciba Foundation Study Group No. 38).
125. Chan-Yeung M, Grzybowski S: Prognosis in occupational asthma [editorial]. Thorax 40:241, 1985.
126. Adams WG: Long-term effects on the health of en engaged in the manufacture of toluene diisocyanate. Br J Ind Med 32:72, 1975.

127. Moller DR, McKay RT, Bernstein IL, et al: Long-term follow-up of workers with TDI asthma [Abst]. Am Rev Respir Dis 129:A159, 1984.

128. Paggiaro PL, Loi AM, Rossi O, et al: Follow-up study of patients with respiratory disease due to toluene diisocyanate (TDI). Clin Allergy 14:463, 1984.

129. Butcher BT, Karr RM, O'Neil CE, et al: Inhalation challenge and pharmacologic studies of toluene diisocyanate (TDI)-sensitive workers. J Allergy Clin Immunol 64:146, 1979.

130. Chan-Yeung M, Lam S, Koerner S: Clinical features and natural history of occupational asthma due to western red cedar (*Thuja plicata*). Am J Med 72:411, 1982.

131. Hudson P, Cartier A, Pineon L, et al: Follow-up of occupational asthma due to various agents. J Allergy Clin Immunol 73:174, 1984.

132. Allard C, Cartier A, Ghezzo H, et al: Occupational asthma due to various agents. Chest 96:1046, 1989.

Chapter 24

EVALUATION OF THE PATIENT
WITH OCCUPATIONAL ASTHMA

Mark T. O'Hollaren, MD
Anthony Montanaro, MD
Emil J. Bardana, Jr., MD

The respiratory tract is the most commonly affected organ system in occupational diseases because it represents the portal of entry for annoying, irritating, sensitizing, and intoxicating agents.[1] A large number of chemicals and organic dusts have been identified as causing occupational asthma in the workplace.[2-4] The prevalence of the condition varies widely. In some parts of the world it has become the most prevalent occupational lung disorder,[5,6] whereas in other geographic areas it remains an unusual work-related condition[7,8] (see Chapter 23). One of the difficulties in arriving at dependable prevalence rates is the lack of a universally accepted definition. We define occupational asthma as a condition characterized by reversible obstruction of the airway, its origin being in the inhalation of ambient dusts, vapors, gases, or fumes that are either manufactured or employed by the worker, or incidentally present at the workplace.[9] The most important characteristic of this condition is an increased airway responsiveness to a known sensitizing or inducing agent.[10] Once symptoms begin, the inhalation of subirritant concentrations of the incriminated agent results in asthmatic symptoms.

Although immunologic mechanisms have been identified in many instances of work-related asthma, they cannot always be identified as the primary pathogenetic mechanism in every case of asthma. More often than not, immunologic mechanisms are operative in work-related asthma owing to high molecular weight antigens.[11,12] In the case of low molecular weight antigens, a specific immune response may be present, but rarely is it identified as the principal or exclusive pathogenetic mechanism.[12-14] In most cases, in addition to specific sensitivity, a nonspecific bronchial hyperresponsiveness is also present.[10]

In evaluating patients with suspected occupational asthma, it is critical to define the parameters of diagnosis that distinguish it from a variety of closely related conditions. In this respect, we have already discussed reactive airways dysfunction syndrome (RADS) in Chapter 23. It remains unclear whether RADS is sufficiently unique to distinguish it from the previously described condition of inflammatory bronchoconstriction.[15] In its recent reelucidation, it has been defined as occurring after a single massive exposure to an irritant gas, vapor, aerosol, fume, or smoke, usually as a result of an accident.[10] It generally begins within minutes or hours of the exposure, and the airway abnormality may persist for months or years. The mechanism is probably similar to the development of an acute chemical bronchitis or pneumonitis. Clearly, classic antibody-mediated immunologic mechanisms are not operative within the time frame related to this condition.

Industrial bronchitis is a disorder characterized by chronic cough and/or sputum production that is likely a response to moderate or low-level exposure to an irritant dust, gas, or fume.[10] This condition has been reviewed in detail in Chapter 6. Considerable clinical heterogeneity exists in the population with chronic bronchitis regarding the presence or severity of concomitant pulmonary syndromes, such as chronic airflow obstruction and bronchial hyperreactivity. This diversity is best explained by differences in individual susceptibility and the wide range of chemical exposures that may result in a common pathologic state.

Bronchiolitis obliterans is a fibrotic, obliterative lesion of the terminal airways resulting from inhalation of irritant gases or fumes, the prototype being inhalation of nitrogen dioxide.[10] Patients with this disorder manifest airway obstruction as well as reduced carbon dioxide diffusion.

Many years ago Gandevia noted that in most instances occupational asthma is not a single, simple, or homogenous entity, even when a single, specific causal factor can be identified in the workplace.[15] It is also probable that a specific industrial reactant can induce asthma by more than a single mechanism. Furthermore, multiple mechanisms may be operative in any given patient.[15,16] In this chapter we will concentrate on features of the evaluation that may help to establish the diagnosis and distinguish work-related asthma from those closely related disorders, or from occupationally induced conditions that represent true aggravation or symptomatic expression of an underlying respiratory condition.

MEDICAL AND OCCUPATIONAL HISTORY

A detailed and comprehensive medical and occupational history remains the cornerstone of establishing the diagnosis of occupational asthma. In our practice we routinely request that each patient complete a questionnaire prior to his or her visit as a supplement to our history (Appendix I). Because of the limited time that may be available, the questionnaire serves as an important tool to amplify the interview process. Patients may spend 2 or 3 hours completing this questionnaire. For this reason we feel it is important to mail the questionnaire to individuals with an explanatory letter indicating the importance of their accurate answers. However, we agree entirely with Malo et al. that an open questionnaire alone is not a satisfactory means of facilitating a diagnosis of occupational asthma.[16a]

Each individual evaluated for the possibility of occupational asthma should be prepared to provide a clear chronological medical history before and after any harmful work exposures.

The questionnaire facilitates obtaining the nonoccupational history by allowing the patient to answer questions related to each major organ system of the body. The functional inquiry can be very helpful in understanding the pre-exposure medical status. This should include a documentation of all prior hospitalizations and surgical procedures from childhood. A complete family medical history is important in the understanding of genetic predispositions inherent in many significant medical conditions, including recurrent infections, emphysema, alcoholism, atopic disease, diabetes, heart disease, etc. It is important to obtain ages of close family members, their ages at the time of death and the causes of death. It goes without saying that the most important issue in the family history is the presence of any familial proclivity to allergic or nonallergic respiratory disease.

The occupational history as outlined in the questionnaire provides an initial framework in the acquisition of current and past employment history. This information should ultimately include length of time on the job, employer, nature of industry, number of hours worked/week, amount of overtime, and the nature of the shift. The latter is important, particularly if it tends to change on a regular basis. This is frequently associated with discontent in the worker. So often, examiners will fail to inquire about the nature and extent of second jobs. The starting and ending point of each employment is an essential component of the history if the evaluator is to ultimately judge the presence of any temporally related symptoms.

During the personal interview process, the facts on the questionnarie are augmented with details regarding the industrial hygiene characteristics of current as well as prior workplaces. The nature of ventilation, availability of exhaust, presence of open doors or windows, chemicals and dusts encountered, and the presence of passive cigarette smoke should be included (Fig. 1). The presence or absence of similar symptoms in co-workers may be quite important. A complete inventory of worker protection devices (or lack thereof) is sought, including face mask, earplugs, goggles, gloves, uniform, steel-tipped shoes, etc. It is important to detail the nature of any protective masks, including their characteristics (cloth versus cardboard, cartridge or air supply respirators). One should inquire as to whether the mask was properly fitted, whether the worker wore a beard (which may affect proper fit), whether

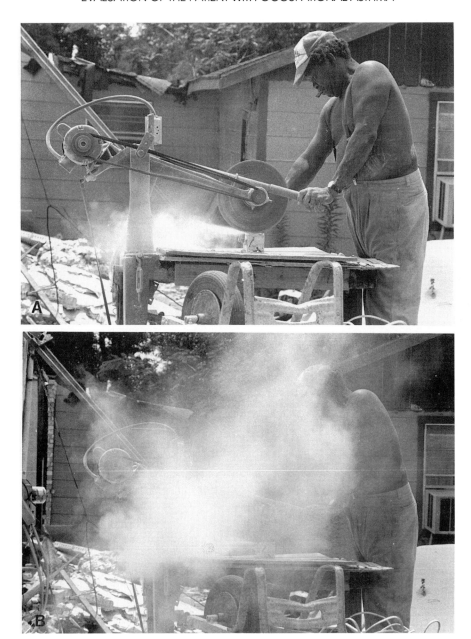

FIGURE 1. **A** and **B**, Yard worker in Mississippi grinding grey brick. Note the absence of worker safety guards. The worker is not using safety goggles and does not wear a respirator despite being enveloped in a cloud of dust. Additionally, he is smoking a cigar while working in these suboptimal conditions.

he changed charcoal cartridges and prefilters, and if so, how often they were changed. Detailed inquiry as to how often respiratory equipment is worn is essential to the work history. With respect to the chemicals handled and processes used, details are generally available from most employers. The availability of Material Safety Data Sheets (MSDS) is mandated by law (Fig. 2).[17] The worker may also

be aware of inspections carried out by state or federal agencies. These should be recorded so details can be obtained. The employer may have data from prior industrial hygiene evaluations of the plant or facility. All these facts facilitate making the correct diagnosis.

Social aspects of the history are also important in acquiring information relating to general factors that predispose to the development

MATERIAL SAFETY DATA SHEET

I PRODUCT IDENTIFICATION		
MANUFACTURER'S NAME	REGULAR TELEPHONE NO EMERGENCY TELEPHONE NO	
ADDRESS		
TRADE NAME		
SYNONYMS		

II HAZARDOUS INGREDIENTS		
MATERIAL OR COMPONENT		HAZARD DATA

III PHYSICAL DATA		
BOILING POINT 760 mmHG		MELTING POINT
SPECIFIC GRAVITY ($H_2O \cdot 1$)		VAPOR PRESSURE
VAPOR DENSITY (AIR $\cdot$ 1)		SOLUBILITY IN H_2O BY WT
% VOLATILES BY VOL		EVAPORATION RATE (BUTYL ACETATE)
APPEARANCE AND ODOR		

FIGURE 2.   Format of Material Safety Data Sheet (MSDS). Daytime and emergency telephone numbers are usually located in the right upper hand corner.

of medical illness. Information relating the geographic region in which the patient has lived may provide better understanding of seasonal symptoms and also facilitate the later location of medical records. Information related to the number of marriages and whether there were special problems with a spouse may provide critical insights into the psychosocial circumstances surrounding the disease and chemical exposures, stress, etc. (e.g., whether a former spouse smoked or was engaged in behavior that would put him or her at high risk for AIDS, or if the spouse might have been physically or sexually abusive, etc.). Insights into these social issues assist in explaining certain stressors and medical conditions that may have arisen at the time. An accurate military history may be helpful in the determination of health status at an early age, i.e., revealing medical and psychological problems. Military medical records may also provide information about service-connected disability, illnesses in the service, nature of medical discharge, etc. Similarly, an educational history provides insight into social behavior, e.g., premature departure from the educational system or occasionally heavy absenteeism from school suggests chronic illness or an early behavior problem.

Social habits also are very important with respect to their influence on long-term health. We inquire carefully into smoking habits, specifically about age of onset, nature of the tobacco substance (cigarette, filtered or non-filtered, cigar or pipe), maximum daily habit and duration, average habit, and date of cessation. Of equal importance in some cases are the smoking habits of parents, spouses, friends, roommates, etc. Although many individuals have never smoked tobacco, we find a large number have used recreational drugs, which can similarly affect respiratory health. We determine use of cannabis and similar drugs. Similarly, we make detailed inquiry about alcohol use or abuse, both in the past and present.

Inquiry is also made regarding regular exercise, sleep habits, hobbies, drug and food allergies, and the nature of the residence. With regard to the worker's residence, specific inquiry is made regarding a description and age of the home; how it is heated, humidified or air conditioned; and the presence of woodstove or insert and its venting characteristics. The number and nature of pets may be important factors that precipitate respiratory symptoms.

When using the health questionnaire as a basis for the history, close attention should be paid to several aspects that may have a significant connection to the potential diagnosis of occupational asthma. While many patients will deny a previous history of childhood asthma, when specifically questioned about childhood "wheezy" bronchitis, or recurrent croup or whooping cough, they will recall significant episodes that may have represented the early onset of reversible obstructive airways disease. In addition, it is important to question patients concerning previous response to upper respiratory tract infections. Many individuals with underlying bronchial hyperresponsiveness will relate a history of persistent cough, wheezing, and shortness of breath that last for weeks to months following an otherwise uncomplicated viral or bacterial upper or lower respiratory tract infection. The worker must be questioned carefully regarding upper respiratory complaints. Frequently, a history of recurrent nasal and ocular complaints can suggest a diagnosis of underlying atopic disease, which the worker may have not previously recognized as a significant "allergic" disease. The presence of persistent facial pain or headache with post-nasal discharge may have been associated with indolent or recurrent sinusitis. In this respect, inquiry should include questions about unusual responses to aspirin or nonsteroidal anti-inflammatory drugs. The presence of nasal polyps and sinusitis might imply the presence of aspirin idiosyncracy syndrome. Similarly, a previous history of childhood or adult skin disorders may be important. Longstanding eczema may indicate a diagnosis of atopic dermatitis in an individual not previously suspected of having a significant atopic predisposition. The gastrointestinal review of systems may be important, because many individuals with peptic disease may present with chest pain or cough from gastroesophageal reflux, which may be either their primary disorder or a significant aggravating factor for asthma.

A neuropsychologic review of systems is quite important. Many patients with alleged occupational disease may have neuropsychiatric disorders that may lead to a somatiform predisposition. A careful history relative to physical or sexual abuse is important.

The temporal relationship of occupational exposures to the presence of symptoms is critical. It is also extremely important to detail with the worker the extent of symptoms during his or her most recent vacation away from the workplace. Documentation regarding the typical latent period that characteristically exists between exposure and development of the symptoms is very important. One must keep in mind that an ever-increasing number of substances known to cause occupational asthma (particularly the low molecular weight substances) may result in symptoms that may be delayed by many hours after exposure. Thus, workers who have only delayed symptoms may characteristically present with cough and shortness of breath 4 to 8 hours following their workplace exposure. Nevertheless, the great majority of patients with acute and/or delayed onset respiratory symptoms will improve following cessation of exposure, which may occur on weekends or during vacations. In this respect, consistency in the history is important. So often there is a clear history of marked improvement away from work until a change in job description, termination of employment, or initiation of a claim, when without explanation the symptoms become permanent and unremitting.

COMPREHENSIVE REVIEW OF MEDICAL RECORDS

We have found that an exhaustive review of the medical records may be rewarding for two major reasons: (1) the acquisition of medical information of which the patient had no awareness; and (2) as an excellent tool to corroborate many important elements of the medical history.

Many patients may not have an appreciation for their underlying airways hyperresponsiveness, but have a significant history of asthmatic responses well documented in their medical record. A review of the medical records with attention to hospital admissions as well as physician and emergency (urgency care) visits following respiratory tract infections can be very rewarding in this respect. Special care should be focused on reviewing events near or at the time the industrial illness began. On numerous occasions we have found a variety of alternative explanations to account for the pulmonary complaints, e.g., acute sinusitis, viral pneumonitis, institution of a beta blocker drug for hypertension, etc. We are constantly surprised by medical records that reveal a previous history of important medical and surgical conditions suggesting contributory nonoccupational disease states.

Secondly, the medical records serve to corroborate facts obtained in the interview and questionnaire process. Special attention should be given to reviewing events at the inception of the occupational disease process. As well, documenting all prior illnesses and medications taken by the patient can be very helpful. Medical record review is also helpful in checking for completeness and accuracy of the family history and social history. For example, it is often true that the patient's estimate of smoking at the time of an active workers' compensation action is frequently underestimated when compared to physician records prior to any action. The same is often true, though perhaps not as pronounced, with respect to alcohol consumption, treatment for alcoholism, and use of recreational drugs.

HAZARDOUS WORKPLACE CHEMICALS

Because it is virtually impossible for any physician to maintain an exhaustive knowledge of the composition and toxicity of hazardous compounds in the workplace, **Material Safety Data Sheets** (MSDS) can be extremely helpful (Fig. 2).[17] The Occupational Safety and Health Administration (OSHA) estimates that there are at least 575,000 hazardous chemical products in the American workplace.[18] OSHA requires that all manufacturers and importers of chemicals prepare MSDS on their products. The MSDS must include the identification of the compound, and its physical hazards as well as the health hazards associated with exposure to the compound.[19] The revised Hazard Communication Standard of 1987 requires that every employer that utilizes or produces hazardous chemicals must keep all MSDS on file.[18] The employer must not only maintain MSDS on file, but must make them readily available to the employee as well as health care providers.

Although a standard has been established, one must realize that this federal regulation is new, and it is not clear at this time how local and federal statutes affect not only the preparation and provision of information, but those who employ its content, i.e., a physician evaluating a patient with occupational asthma. It is important for the physician to realize that in the preparation of the MSDS, the term "health hazard" has been defined as "a chemical for which there is statistically significant evidence based on at least one study conducted in accordance with established scientific principles that acute or chronic health effects may occur in exposed individuals."[18] The availability of reproducible human data is lacking in many instances. It must also be noted that only compounds that have been previously determined to be health hazards are required to have an MSDS. Many constituents are identified as "inert ingredients." These inert ingredients may include active ingredients or carriers and vehicles that may be shown to be potentially toxic in the future. It should be noted that if the specific chemical identity of a product is a trade secret (proprietary), the specific chemical composition of the product may be withheld. If specific chemicals in a proprietary compound are known to represent potential health hazards, they must be listed. However, the inclusion of the chemical as a hazardous material is left up to the discretion of the manufacturer under the previously described standard. While the MSDS frequently lacks sufficient toxicologic data on each chemical in the product, it should serve as a basis for further investigation should there be a specific concern.

If the examining physician has specific questions regarding the chemical composition of a product, the MSDS is required to list both a regular hour and emergency phone number of the manufacturer in the upper right hand corner (Fig. 2).[17] For those physicians who frequently evaluate occupational disease, it may be helpful to have updated sources of health hazard information on frequently used chemicals. The ACGIH publishes a looseleaf volume entitled "Documentation of the Threshold Limit Values and Biological Exposure Indices." This publication contains every chemical for which the organization has established a threshold limit value (TLV), appearing in alphabetical order, and it provides synonyms, chemical formulas, exposure limits, and information related to biologic key effects, with references.[20] Of interest is the fact that updates are provided on a regular basis, with additions and revisions of the text. The United Kingdom has enacted similar legislation, which stimulated a series of publications setting forth standardized information on a variety of compounds. (Volume I—*Solvents;* Volume II—*Metals and Their Compounds;* Volume III—*Corrosives and Irritants*).[21] These fact sheets closely approximate information by U.S. manufacturers and, at times, provide greater detail on certain chemicals. They may be a ready source of information before the employer makes the official MSDS available to the physician.

It becomes apparent that the occupational history with respect to potential reactive chemicals in the workplace is only as good as the worker's knowledge of his or her exposures, or the physician's awareness of which chemicals are likely to be present. In our experience, physicians cannot depend entirely on a precise awareness on the part of the worker. Appendix II presents an alphabetical list of industrial agents (immunogens and irritants) that are likely to be found in a variety of occupations as an aid in the development of an exposure history.

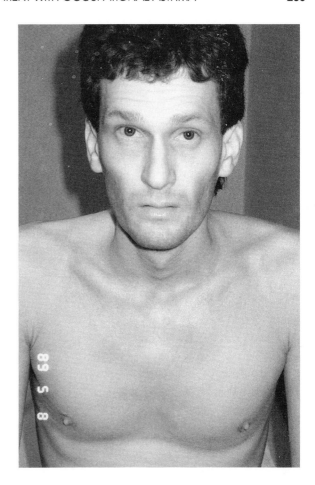

FIGURE 3.   Typical erythematous skin changes and features associated with atopic dermatitis. Note the edema of the infraorbital folds and lichenification due to constant rubbing. These signs can be seen with allergic rhinoconjunctivitis as well.

a comprehensive examination of all organ systems. Though the physical findings from an examination may be very helpful, the key objective findings may have improved in proportion to the time away from the putative workplace exposure.

One should be aware of physical signs that suggest underlying atopy. In the skin, it is useful to note findings such as atopic dermatitis, chronic contact dermatitis, or the presence of Denny's lines (Fig. 3). Systematic examination of the head and neck should be completed, specifically noting the presence or absence of conjunctival injection, serous otitis, and nasal mucosal appearance, as well as character of the nasal secretions (Fig. 4). The presence of pale, boggy nasal mucosa suggests allergic rhinitis, whereas beefy red mucosa is typical for infection, rhinitis medicamentosa, or chronic cigarette smoking.[22] Chronic paranasal

PHYSICAL EXAMINATION OF THE WORKER WITH SUSPECTED OCCUPATIONAL ASTHMA

The physical examination of a worker with suspected occupational asthma should include

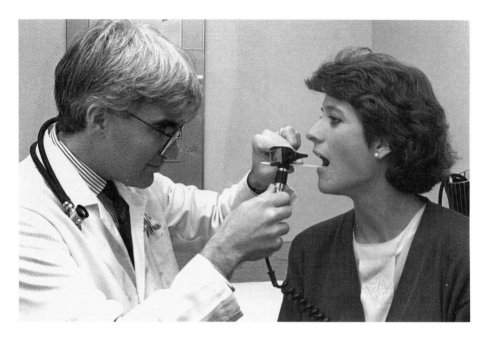

FIGURE 4.   Author (TM) examining the upper airways of a patient with suspected occupational asthma.

sinusitis with or without polyposis may be associated with significant inflammatory nasal disease and postnasal drainage associated with cough, as well as with bronchial hyperreactivity at and away from the workplace.[23,24] Dryness of the eyes, mouth, and nasal passages, with or without associated ulceration and bleeding, may suggest Sjogren's syndrome.[25] Signs of possible collagen vascular disease should also be noted, in particular, nasal septal perforation, nasal and oral ulcerations, enlarged salivary glands, enlarged cervical lymph nodes, etc.[26]

The neck should be examined for the presence of adenopathy, thyroid abnormalities, and vascular bruits suggesting vascular disease. Examination of the thoracic cavity should include any aberration impeding normal respiration, e.g., ankylosing spondylitis, severe spinal deformity, etc. The lungs should be carefully examined using percussion and auscultation, noting the presence of sibilant or sonorous rhonchi, rales, prolonged expiratory phase, etc. Cardiovascular evaluation is done to look for signs of organic heart disease, such as murmurs or gallops suggesting congestive cardiac failure, as a cause of dyspnea. The abdomen should be evaluated for organomegaly, presence of bruits, and masses. The extremities should be studied for signs of fingernail clubbing, cyanosis, or edema. A screening neurological examination should also be performed.

Signs of chronic infection suggest an immunodeficiency disorder. We have evaluated many patients who have presented with complete or partial IgA, IgG, or IgG subclass deficiency, which has rendered them more susceptible to recurrent pyogenic infections of the sinobronchial tree. These infections may render the worker more susceptible to the irritant effects of many volatile organic compounds, which may cause respiratory tract irritation and symptoms masquerading as occupational asthma.[27]

LABORATORY STUDIES IN THE EVALUATION OF SUSPECTED OCCUPATIONAL ASTHMA

The diagnosis of work-related bronchial asthma is often difficult, particularly since the evaluation is most frequently conducted retrospectively. It would be useful to have laboratory studies to aid in confirming the diagnosis. Unfortunately, the usefulness of immunologic testing is limited to those forms of occupational asthma in which an immunologic mechanism has clearly been demonstrated.[28] High molecular weight antigens implicated in the causation of occupational asthma are usually proteins of animal, plant, bacterial, or fungal origin and range between 20 and 50 kilodaltons in size (Table 1). For many of these agents the presence of sensitization can be established either by in vitro or in vivo tests, or by a combination of both.[29] Where IgE-mediation has been clearly demonstrated, conventional allergy skin testing can be very helpful. Allergens amenable to this type of testing include those derived from animal dander, pelts, or urine insect extracts, fungal antigens, and selected pharmaceutical agents.[11,12] Each of these has an in vitro counterpart that can be done when skin testing is not possible or when independent confirmation is sought, i.e., radioallergosorbent testing or enzyme-linked immunoassay. Unfortunately, many investigators have used evidence derived from cutaneous or serologic sensitization as sufficient to conclude that the allergen was responsible for the patient's occupational asthma[30] (see Chapter 14). Clearly this is not the case with any potential work allergen. Lindblad and Farr demonstrated a significant number of passively transferrable skin tests in completely asymptomatic individuals.[31] The presence of an antibody cannot be interpreted as more than evidence for prior exposure to that allergen with a specific response; it cannot be interpreted as equivalent to a "symptomatic state."

Whereas in vivo and in vitro tests for IgE-specific antibodies have a useful role in the evaluation and diagnosis of occupational asthma caused by high molecular weight antigens, similar assays in work-related asthma due to low molecular weight antigens are problematic. Here the overall value of laboratory tests in establishing a diagnosis is limited. In many cases with low molecular weight antigens, the antigen is hapten and must be conjugated with a protein carrier.[32-35] It is presumed that these avid, cross-linking industrial compounds react with human serum albumin, and the resultant neoantigen stimulates the production of specific IgE antibody. However, to our knowledge, these hapten-protein conjugates have never been proven to be the operative mechanism in affected workers. Standardized and well characterized conjugates are now available from the National Institute of Allergy and Infectious Diseases for diisocyanates and the principal acid anhydride compounds.[13]

Although studies have shown a reasonably good correlation between the presumptive clinical diagnosis and serologic data for IgG and IgE in trimellitic anhydride-induced industrial syndromes,[38] serologic data are much less helpful and tend to fluctuate widely from laboratory to laboratory with respect to specific IgE antibodies to monofunctional isocyanates.[39] In the case of symptomatic or bronchoprovocation-positive workers with isocyanate asthma, the

TABLE 1. *Selected High Molecular Weight Allergens Reported to Cause Occupational Asthma*

Origin	Allergens	Occupations
Animal	Avian	Veterinarians
Danders	Bovine	Pet shop owners
Feathers	Cat	Animal handlers
Pelts	Dog	Farmers
Saliva	Hog	Laboratory workers
Urine	Horse	Zoo keepers
	Rabbit	Animal breeders
	Rodent	
Food	Crustaceans	Food processors
	Mollusks	Pharmaceutical
	Castor bean	workers
	Green coffee bean	Seafood processors
	Papain/pepsin	Truckers/haulers
	Egg	Dock workers
	Mushroom	Bait handlers
	Mealwork	Mushroom growers
Fungal	*Aspergillus* sp.	Woodworkers
HVAC	Graphium	Pulp workers
systems	*Aureobasidium*	Sawyers
Sawdust	*pullulans*	Office workers
Tree bark	(pullularia)	Bark strippers
Wood pulp	*Alternaria* sp.	HVAC engineers
Cork	*Penicillium* sp.	Cork workers
Insect/Mite	*Sitophilus granarius*	Grain handlers
	Tyroglyphus granarius	Bakers
	Glycyphagus destructor	Granary workers
	Sewer fly	Silk processors
	Silkworm	Sewer workers
		Entomologists
Plant/Vegetable	Wheat, rye flour	Florists
	Gum acacia	Printers
	Gum arabic	Nursery workers
	Gum tragacanth	Botanists
	Pollens	Bakers
	Plant components	
Pharmaceutical	Antibiotics	Physicians
	Psyllium	Pharmacists
	Ipecacuanha	Nurses
		Pharmaceutical

percent with positive IgE-specific antibody to paratolyl monoisocyanate varied from 0 to 19%, depending on the laboratory conducting the study.[39] IgE-specific antibody to plicatic acid has an even more limited role as a diagnostic tool in western red cedar asthma.[40] Here also, the presence of IgE- or IgG-specific antibodies cannot be interpreted as diagnostic nor can definitive linkage be made with respect to causation.

In addition to IgE-specific antibodies, a number of studies have shown that IgG-specific antibodies against industrial immunogens have a role in the evaluation of patients.[32,36] It has also been suggested that antigen-specific IgG$_4$ may play a pathogenetic role in the development of work-related asthma.[37] Further study will be required to establish a definitive role of these immunologic tests in the diagnosis of occupational asthma.

CHEST RADIOGRAPHS

The role of chest x-rays in the evaluation of the patient with occupational asthma is limited. One must exclude other conditions that may present with similar signs, particularly diffuse wheezing, such as emphysema and obstructions of the trachea and major bronchi. In adults the x-ray findings in bronchial asthma are almost always normal. Findings of overinflation or air trapping are not diagnostic.

PULMONARY FUNCTION TESTS IN THE EVALUATION OF PATIENTS WITH SUSPECTED OCCUPATIONAL ASTHMA

The initial step in the evaluation of work-related pulmonary disease is the careful delineation of the respiratory disorder. Not infrequently we find ourselves evaluating patients with occupational asthma who have never been demonstrated to have reversible airflow obstruction, the cardinal prerequisite feature of asthma.[41] The diagnosis of bronchial asthma may be uncomplicated, but it can be difficult in a setting where cough is the principal manifestation of the illness. In such a case the differential diagnosis is between bronchitis and asthma. Another situation that causes difficulty in the diagnosis of asthma is where the spirometry is completely normal and there is no objective record of reversible obstruction in the past, while the worker was exposed to the putative agent. Finally, the verification of work-related asthma may be difficult where there is a nonoccupational respiratory disorder that causes wheezing and dyspnea.

As has been noted in the previous Chapter 23, the major problem in making an initial diagnosis of work-related asthma is the assurance that the condition does not represent a preexisting illness. Without the availability of a preemployment pulmonary function study or a determination of a premorbid condition underlying nonspecific bronchial hyeprreactivity, one is left with a clinical judgment based upon the medical history and careful medical record review. Nonspecific bronchial hyperreactivity is an exaggerated airway narrowing in response to a wide variety of nonspecific stimuli,[42] and it is almost universally present in untreated patients with symptomatic

occupational asthma. In making a clinical judgment as to the likely presence of work-related asthma, the decision should be tempered by the fact that there is a genetic relationship between atopy and the later development of nonspecific bronchial hyperreactivity.[42,43] Atopy certainly does not preclude a worker from the development of occupational asthma and could become a predisposing factor with respect to high molecular weight agents.[11] On the other hand, the decision should then be weighted more on the objective data depicting a unique sensitivity to an industrial immunogen rather than the presence of nonspecific bronchial hyperreactivity. Although not diagnostic of bronchial asthma, bronchial hyperreactivity is so often found that its absence is taken as evidence that the respiratory illness is not asthma.[28,42] Conversely, the presence of bronchial hyperreactivity cannot be summarily used as proof that bronchial asthma exists. For example, some siblings of asthmatics, parents of asthmatics, and 20% of individuals with allergic rhinitis may have significant degrees of airway reactivity without any asthmatic symptoms.[44,45] Approximately one-third of normal individuals achieve a positive test with methacholine or histamine if a sufficiently high concentration is employed.[44,46,47]

In those instances when bronchial asthma is in doubt, an assessment for nonspecific bronchial hyperreactivity can be helpful. In our institution, we use methacholine as the reagent to determine nonspecific bronchial hyperreactivity. The indications, methodology, and safeguards required in the conduct of this procedure are discussed in Chapter 4 and have been detailed in other comprehensive reviews.[48] This technique is safe and results are rapidly reversible; there is an immediate decline in peak flow or forced expiratory volume in one second (FEV_1) if nonspecific bronchial hyperreactivity is present. The test also provides a dose-dependent means of quantitating the degree of bronchial hyperreactivity, which strongly correlates with the clinical severity of asthma..[48,49] In addition, the degree of nonspecific bronchial hyperreactivity may be important in determining the dose of an agent to be used in specific bronchial provocation.

Although pharmacologic bronchial challenge tests demonstrate nonspecific bronchial hyperreactivity in nearly all cases of occupational asthma, they do not define the specific industrial agent responsible.[50] There is a wide variety of factors that either enhance or inhibit the response to methacholine (Table 2). Upper respiratory tract infections may become associated with increased bronchial responsiveness or typically increase it. Other factors that enhance methacholine responsiveness include recent exposure to the putative industrial agent, or to a nonindustrial allergen for which there is incidental sensitivity, e.g., grass pollen, house dust mite, dog or cat dander, etc.[48] Factors that reduce potential hyperresponsiveness include avoidance of relevant allergens or the causal industrial antigen, as well as the concomitant use of bronchodilator, cromolyn, or aerosolized steroid.

Once it has been shown that bronchial asthma exists, and assuming the historical account demonstrates the likeliness of a temporal relationship, the next step will be to prove a relationship between the asthmatic condition and the industrial agent. With over 200 industrial agents incriminated in the causation of occupational asthma, this can be a difficult clinical task. A helpful clue to recognizing the etiology of a work-related asthma is found in some facilities where several workers in the same area (or involved with the same process) develop de novo asthma. The clinician has available a number of pragmatic approaches that can be employed to better define the likelihood of work-related asthma. The simplest approach employs the actual work activity as the challenge. The method used can vary with the degree of suspicion. Initially, ambulatory monitoring of the peak expiratory flow rate can be used at the beginning and end of a workshift over a 1 to 2-week period. The test is clearly effort-dependent, but a number of methods have been established to improve the validity of results.[41] Peak expiratory flow rates should be recorded every 2 hours, with each recording being the best of three attempts (given there is not greater than 20L/min variability between readings.)[51] A fall of greater than 25% in the peak expiratory flow rate is probably significant.[41] Measurements should be monitored every 2 hours for 1 week at work, followed by measurement again every 2 hours while awake for 10 days off work, then again for 2 weeks while at work.[52] Having a plant nurse monitor each reading improves the accuracy and validity of such measurements.

TABLE 2. *Factors Suspected of Either Enhancing or Suppressing Responses to Industrial Agents on Bronchial Provocation* *

A. Factors with potential enhancing effects

Exposure or Event	Approx Impact Interval[†]	Reference
Tobacco smoking	6–12 hours	61,62
Exposure to atmospheric pollutants, e.g., SO_2, NO_2, O_3	6–12 hours	63–65a
Exercise	6–12 hours	66
Recent exposure to putative work antigen	3–5 days	67,68
Recent symptomatic exposure to seasonal allergens	3–5 days	67,68
Vaccination	2–4 weeks	69,70
Recent viral bronchitis	2–4 weeks	71

B. Factors with potential suppressive effects

Caffeine, cola, chocolate	4–8 hours	59
Aerosol beta agonists	6–8 hours	75
Anticholinergic agents	6–8 hours	76,77
Sustained action beta agonists	10–12 hours	59
Sustained release theophylline	12 hours	75
Cromolyn sodium (sodium cromoglycate)	24 hours	78
Short-acting antihistamines	24–48 hours	79
Aerosolized steroid	5–7 days	72–74
Hydroxyzine, doxipen HCl, astemizole	2–4 weeks	59

* Adapted from Ref. 59 as well as from Table 2, Chapter 4.
[†] Approximate time of significant impact on bronchial responsiveness.

A second method, which is simple and relatively inexpensive, depends on the use of spirometry with actual work activity as the challenge. Spirometry is simple to administer, rapid, inexpensive, safe, and both sensitive and specific when properly applied and interpreted (see Chapter 3) (Fig. 5). Changes in FVC, FEV_1 or FEF_{25-75} may be found in the same subjects studied repeatedly on the same day or on consecutive days.[53] This issue is important in the setting of occupational asthma where repeated spirometry is an essential aspect of subject evaluation. A reasonable figure for the day-to-day variability of the coefficient of variation for the FVC and the FEV_1 in normal nonsmoking subjects is 3%. For the FEF_{25-75}, the coefficient of variation is between 8 and 21% (see Chapter 3). Where one has established firm "baseline parameters" in a subject with normal pulmonary function without an exposure, e.g., twice daily measurements in an office by the same technician

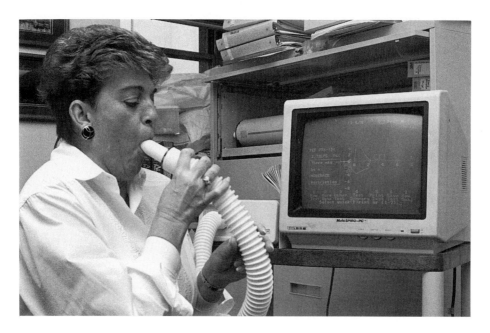

FIGURE 5.   Patient undergoing simple office spirometry as part of a sequential study over the course of a work week.

for a week, then reproducible decrements in FEV_1 over a workshift of greater than 5% should prompt additional studies in incriminating an occupational agent that has induced asthma and that probably should be avoided if verified by specific bronchial challenge. As is often the case, serial measurements are not available, and given only a single-shift examination, Spector has published some minimal changes in pulmonary function data that would be considered significant on bronchial provocation studies[54] (Table 3).

Spirometry is also dependent on patient effort. Principal reasons for poor performance are the presence of disease (e.g., uncontrollable cough), inadequate understanding, or inadequate effort by the patient. A number of parameters suggest that the patient may be providing a submaximal effort. These include: (1) failure to inspire to total lung capacity (TLC); (2) failure to exhale to residual volume (RV); (3) failure to exhale as forcefully as possible; (4) failure to show changes in facial color or expression during a forceful exhalation; and (5) failure to give reproducible expiratory maneuvers. In general the reproducibility of the maximum voluntary ventilation (MVV), a highly effort-dependent test, does not appear to be a reliable index of effort. It is felt that no combination of tests clearly separates good from submaximal efforts better than the FEV_1 reproducibility test.[55-57]

In any event, changes in the measurements of peak expiratory flow rates or spirometry before and after work shifts can only provide the impetus to proceed further in elucidating a potential industrial asthmagenic agent. There are too many nonspecific issues in the work setting to permit use of the peak flow rate or spirometry to incriminate a specific reactant as causative, i.e., the patient may be responding adversely to exercise, cold air, nonspecific irritants including dusts, and environmental tobacco smoke. In order to make a definitive diagnosis, one should carry out bronchial provocation studies with subirritant doses of the suspected industrial agent.

TABLE 3.   *Minimal Percent Change from Baseline Spirometric Data Considered Significant After Bronchial Provocation Challenge*

Parameter	Percent Change from Baseline
Forced vital capacity (FVC)	–10%
Forced expiratory volume (1 second) (FEV_1)	–20%
Maximal mid-expiratory flow rate (FEF_{25-75})	–25%
Peak expiratory flow rate (PEFR)	–25%
Specific airway resistance (SG_{aw})	+35–40%
Functional residual capacity (FRC)	+25%

Modified from Ref. 54 with permission.

BRONCHIAL PROVOCATION STUDIES IN THE EVALUATION OF PATIENTS WITH SUSPECTED OCCUPATIONAL ASTHMA

There are two basic approaches to bronchial provocation with suspected industrial agents. One is of historical interest, because it was the model that later testing would modify. Early studies of bronchial provocation were largely developed by Pepys and his associates.[58] These procedures generally attempted to re-create the workplace and used chemical dusts, wood dusts, vapors from paints, etc. in a small cubicle as the approach to testing. Chemical dusts were mixed with lactose powder to develop different test concentrations. Similar tests could be recreated with flour, wood dusts, and the like. When paints or soldering fumes were suspected, the worker was asked to re-create his workplace by soldering in the pulmonary function laboratory or painting a piece of wood with the suspect catalyzed paint. Despite the imprecision of test concentrations, rather impressive and reproducible data were obtained.[58] This pragmatic approach still has a role in some instances of bronchial provocation, but has largely been supplanted with carefully delineated challenge studies.

Bronchoprovocation tests have become increasingly popular as a method of confirming sensitivity to a non-IgE-mediated sensitizing agent. This relates principally to the low molecular weight chemicals, with which serologic tests are unlikely to assist in establishing cause and effect.[13] Clearly, allergens inducing an exclusive IgE response are also amenable to bronchial provocation, but the availability of both in vivo and in vitro testing, particularly if the allergen is unique to the work environment, makes bronchial provocation less necessary. Because these tests pose some risk to the patient, the patient must be appropriately informed and consent must be obtained for the procedure. These studies must be performed by experienced clinicians in a hospital setting. It may be prudent to admit the patient to hospital where there are adequate emergency facilities.[38,51,59]

Several excellent protocols have been published as a guide for those who are contemplating this procedure.[28,59] Most of these protocols assume the dose of the agent to be tested can be accurately measured at levels below the irritant level. This usually requires the assistance of an industrial hygienist or chemist familiar with the generation and measurement of the agent in air. A physician must be in close proximity during all phases of the testing, principally to assure optimal spirometric effort and to ensure patient safety. Finally, all contraindications to testing must be excluded. The principal contraindications are severe, obstructive lung disease and severe ischemic heart disease. With the former, cessation of bronchodilator therapy may pose serious, unnecessary problems to an individual. The latter may precipitate ischemic symptoms with vigorous and sequential forced expiratory maneuvers.[28,60] There must be a complete knowledge of factors capable of altering the outcome of the bronchial provocation so these can be addressed prospectively (Table 2). Another factor that can affect the bronchial provocation response is emotional trauma. This is especially true in asthmatics with the most hyperreactive airways. Circadian rhythms also have an impact on bronchial response. All asthmatics suffer an increase in histamine reactivity during the night. Hormonal influences have also been reported to affect the outcome of bronchial provocation.[80]

Most inhalation challenge protocols last a minimum of 3 days and with complex testing may last up to 6 days.[38] On the first day the subject worker is evaluated clinically. This includes a complete history, record review, examination, laboratory studies, and complete pulmonary function studies, including a diffusion capacity. A methacholine challenge test should be conducted to acquire information on the presence and severity of underlying nonspecific bronchial hyperreactivity. The latter will largely determine the starting dose of the industrial chemical to be studied.

On the second day the worker is placed in the chamber and undergoes a "mock exposure" for approximately 30 to 60 minutes (Fig. 6). Spirometry is carried out every 15 minutes for 2 hours and thereafter every hour until late afternoon. The patient then continues to undergo bedside spirometry under observation on an hourly schedule until bedtime. Should the patient awaken, bedside spirometry is conducted at that time. If there are any complaints, chest examination is also carried out and recorded with the physiologic measurement. This control day is essential to define the normal circadian variation for the subject.

The third day represents the first true challenge day and the dose of the chemical selected must be based on a clinical judgment, which should consider: (1) baseline pulmonary function; (2) degree of methacholine challenge responsiveness; (3) characterization of the work conditions; (4) historical account of a likely

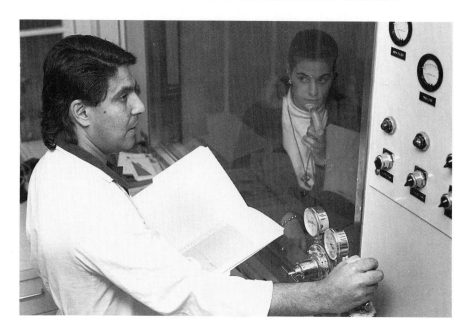

FIGURE 6. Technician administers a "mock challenge" in the Oregon Health Sciences University's provocation chamber. The worker complained of "multiple chemical sensitivity" as a result of her clerical work in an office.

"positive" exposure; and (5) a provocation dose that is clearly below irritant levels. Most investigators use a starting challenge dose that is approximately 50% of the threshold limit value (TLV) for 15 minutes. A challenge test is considered positive when there is a sustained decline in FEV_1 to less than 80% of the baseline value on the day of testing. Though somewhat arbitrary, this is consistent with the agreed-upon criteria used to measure response to pharmacologic bronchoconstrictor agents.[44-51] If the challenge studies on the third day are negative, the challenge done is increased to the TLV level for 1 hour on the fourth day. If this is negative, the challenge dose is increased to the highest level that remains subirritant, i.e., one-and-one-half times the TLV for up to 5 hours. If this is negative, it is concluded that no specific sensitivity to the putative agent exists.[28] This protocol was initially developed at Tulane University. An example of an outcome with toluene diisocyanate is graphically depicted in Figure 5 of Chapter 12.[28,81]

ASSESSMENT OF THE WORKPLACE AND RECOMMENDATIONS

If a patient has occupational asthma, then the treating physician must recommend avoidance of the offending agent, for life-endangering asthma attacks may ensue from continued exposure.[82] One death has been reported in a patient with documented isocyanate-induced asthma who continued to work with a respirator mask, despite the diagnosis of occupational asthma.[82,83] In one study of patients with established occupational asthma due to western red cedar, exposure to cedar continued for an average of 6.5 years after diagnosis. None of the patients recovered their premorbid lung function values. One-half of the patients were able to remain in stable condition on chronic medication use, and one-half continued to deteriorate. Only a twin-cartridge face-mask helped prevent deterioration of pulmonary function.[82,84] As indicated above, when a timely diagnosis is made, prompt removal from the workplace should result in either resolution of all symptoms or a very significant improvement of symptoms.

Patients with occupational asthma should be moved to an area without exposure to the offending agent and retrained if possible. If exposure must continue for whatever reason, then adequate respiratory protection must be provided.[82] An industrial hygienist should be involved in the initial assessment as well as the quantification of the response to remedial measures in that particular workplace[41] (Fig. 7). Air samples collected by accepted techniques should be used. Immunochemical assays are now allowing more detailed investigations of allergens present in the air in small amounts.[85] Immunochemical air sampling technology has also been used to quantify both lab animal aeroallergen production, as well as to document the effectiveness of air filtration apparatus in that setting.[86]

Workplace visitations can result in many practical and effective recommendations. Such recommendations may include personal respiratory protection, modification of ventilation equipment in the workplace, substitution of a different material for the particular job, or isolation (or automation) of the job function so as to minimize the health risk to the worker.[41]

In summary, the evaluation of the patient with suspected occupational asthma includes a thorough history (including an occupational health questionnaire), a complete physical exam, selected allergen skin tests and laboratory tests (when indicated for that antigen), chest radiographs, full spirometric assessment, and, where indicated, assessment of both nonspecific and specific bronchial hyperreactivity.

PITFALLS IN THE DIAGNOSIS OF OCCUPATIONAL ASTHMA

After assimilating all the available medical, social, and industrial hygiene data, the clinician must analyze the information and consider whether the diagnosis of work-related asthma is tenable. The following comments may be of some assistance in this regard.

Variants of Occupational Asthma. The initial hurdle for the evaluating physician lies in the distinction between "pure occupational asthma" and any preexisting respiratory disorders, e.g., bronchiolitis, recurrent pneumonitis, chronic bronchitis, emphysema, or preexisting asthma. With regard to the latter, one must distinguish between: (1) de novo, pure occupational asthma; (2) preexistent asthma which has been *permanently altered* or *worsened* by occupational exposures; (3) preexistent asthma which has become *transiently symptomatic* as a result of work exposures, i.e., no permanent impairment; (4) occupational bronchitis; and (5) no work-related respiratory disease, but the presence of preexisting or

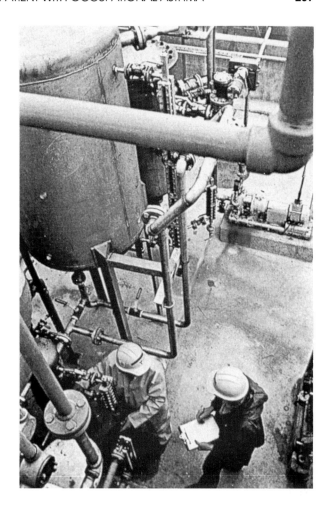

FIGURE 7. Evaluation of a large isocyanate plant by an industrial hygienist reveals areas of prior spills.

nonoccupational respiratory disease, e.g., tobacco-related bronchitis/emphysema.

De Novo Pure Occupational Asthma. Nonoccupational asthma is a relatively common disease affecting between 9 and 12 million Americans. Current estimates suggest that about 2% of all cases of bronchial asthma are of occupational origin.[16] Compared to its non-work-related equivalent, industrial asthma is an uncommon disease. Its prevalence varies widely between industries and their locations. Some 200 agents have been incriminated in the induction of occupational asthma.[2,87] One would anticipate little difficulty in establishing a reasonably certain diagnosis in a nonatopic, lifelong nonsmoker without prior respiratory disease working in a high-risk industry who develops clear-cut asthma after a variable period of documented exposure to a known sensitizing agent. This would become even more evident if the condition regressed after removal from the work exposure. The degree of difficulty rises with the presence of one or more confounding factors, e.g., presence of atopy, chronic cigarette smoking, or preexisting respiratory disease. With the presence of multiple confounding issues, the diagnosis can become extremely difficult. One factor that should provide assistance is the clinical benefit that results with removal from the offending agent. Whether one is dealing with a sensitizer or a significant respiratory irritant, there is little doubt that a timely diagnosis of occupational lung disease with prompt removal of the worker should be accompanied by a definable improvement.[16] Patients with a significant inflammatory asthmatic component may require 1–2 months to demonstrate this improvement. Though variable degrees of chronic work-related bronchial asthma can persist, this is true for only a handful of agents and only if the work exposure has been prolonged or of a large magnitude.[82-84]

Permanent Aggravation of Preexisting Asthma. There are several potent mechanisms by which preexistent asthma can be adversely affected with an occupational exposure. An individual with preexisting allergic, nonallergic, or mixed bronchial asthma may become newly sensitized to a work-related antigen. The sensitization leaves a permanent immunological effect on the worker. An inflammatory-based, late asthmatic response commonly results from such a sensitization. However, despite the continued vulnerability to react adversely upon re-exposure, once the worker is removed from the incriminated agent, the condition should regress entirely. Another mechanism by which preexistent asthma can be permanently worsened is by significant exposure to a highly irritating fume or gas, e.g., chlorine, anhydrous ammonia, hydrochloric acid fumes, etc. To induce a chemical bronchitis/pneumonitis, the exposure must be to high concentrations of a particularly corrosive agent for a significant period of time. Again, an inflammation-mediated late asthmatic response is likely to occur in this situation. Such an exposure frequently results in an irritative, contact dermatitis or burn over exposed parts of the body, as well as inflammation of the mucous membranes of the eyes, nose, and mouth. The resulting acute inflammation of the airways has been referred to as reactive airways dysfunction syndrome (RADS).[88] The condition can be transient or permanent, dependent on the inducing agent,

its concentration, and duration of exposure. The damage to the irritant receptors of the bronchial tree can be such that the underlying bronchial responsiveness is permanently altered (lowered threshold), and the course of the preexisting asthma is permanently altered. Although this condition has been reported in a small number of patients, it is not considered a frequent clinical occurrence. In addition, the authors have pointed out many confounding variables that complicate the interpretation of this data (see Chapter 23).

Occupationally-induced Transient Symptoms. Pre-existent asthma is more frequently worsened by exposure to industrial fumes, gases, or dusts that are considered either minor annoyances or minor mucous membrane irritants.[89] These are considered bronchospastic triggers and are not associated with a late asthmatic response. Examples would include many common industrial exposures, including wood dust and smoke, many solvent and paint fumes, diesel fumes, welding fumes, passive cigarette smoke, and many other agents (see Table 1, Chapter 22). This type of exposure could precipitate a symptomatic asthmatic state, i.e., increased, but transient, cough, sputum production, and wheezing respiration. Definite, but reversible changes in pulmonary function may occur. However, the symptoms would be expected to abate entirely within a few hours of discontinuing the exposure. Such exposures would not be associated with any permanent sequelae. Since bronchial asthma is a significantly reversible condition, incidental contacts with respiratory irritants do not necessarily worsen the basic underlying bronchial condition. They therefore do not produce any lasting respiratory impairment. The same can be said for certain types of stress, cold air exposure, and all forms of exercise (see Table 4, Chapter 23).

Despite the particular mechanism involved in precipitating either de novo occupational asthma or a re-expression of a preceding asthmatic state, one would expect a dramatic relief of symptoms on removal from the source of the "sensitizing" or "irritating" agent. This would be especially true where the diagnosis is established in a timely fashion, i.e., within 3 to 6 months of onset.

Cause and Effect Trap. All too often there is a tendency to automatically attribute causation for any asthmatic condition developing in an individual industrially exposed to a high-risk agent, e.g., asthma developing in a cedar mill worker must be due to western red cedar. Such a diagnosis is frequently made without the benefit of a clear past medical history and, more importantly, a thorough review of any past medical records. In order to properly apply the principles of differential diagnosis, the physician must have an accurate and complete knowledge of all current and past medical problems. Too often upper or lower respiratory tract infection is overlooked as the mechanism of inducing bronchial asthma (see Table 3, Chapter 22). Knowledge of a longstanding allergic diathesis can be critical in arriving at a proper assessment. Smoking history is frequently only partially elucidated, e.g., type of cigarette and maximum habit. Whenever possible the smoking history should be corroborated in prior medical records. There is an unconscious tendency for longstanding smokers with respiratory disease to minimize past smoking history. Concomitant use of cigars and pipe smoking are often important. Information relating to inhalation habits is also important in assessing likely sequelae from tobacco abuse. Individuals may deny tobacco smoking and not mention the protracted inhalational use of marijuana or cocaine unless directly asked. The presence of other active smokers in the household is also important. In patients with preceding asthma, the initiation of beta blocker or nonsteroidal anti-inflammatory drugs has profound effects on the course of bronchial asthma.

Every effort should be made to establish the diagnosis of occupational asthma with certainty before formally labeling the patient with this diagnosis. This may require sequential physiological measurements of lung function before and after a work shift, but in the absence of any confounding factors. Alternatively, work-stimulated or controlled bronchial provocation studies may be needed to secure the diagnosis.[12] When the clinician is uncertain, it is much easier to retreat from a provisional diagnosis than what appeared to be a certain diagnosis made in haste.

Occupational Asthma Does Not Imply Permanent Disability. As indicated above, once the asthmatic is removed from the offending irritant or sensitizing agent, there should be either a marked improvement or total abatement of the condition. The worker should be capable of returning to work providing re-exposure is avoided or minimized. Even in those instances where permanent respiratory impairment is attributed to work exposure, aggressive antiasthmatic therapy and removal from further exposure should result in significant symptomatic relief. In any case, only rare cases of asthma are felt to be totally disabling irrespective of causation.

SUMMARY

Occupational asthma can have one of several presentations that are often difficult to distinguish from nonoccupational conditions. Work-related asthma may arise for the first time secondary to inhalational exposure of an occupational irritant or sensitizer. More often, the worker has preexistent asthma that has been adversely affected by work exposures. Occasionally this can cause permanent impairment by virtue of a unique work-related sensitization, i.e., superimposition of an occupational allergy on a preexisting asthmatic state. Permanent impairment may also result from a significant exposure to a potent, corrosive gas or fume with resultant chemical bronchitis/pneumonitis. More commonly, longstanding asthma is made transiently symptomatic with exposure to an annoying or irritating agent without permanently affecting the status of airway responsiveness. It is important to realize that occupational asthma rarely occurs as a "pure" disease process. Prior to making a definitive diagnosis, the diagnostician is well advised to gather as much medical history and objective physiologic data as is possible. The majority of occupational asthmatic conditions regress completely if the diagnosis is timely and the worker is removed from further adverse exposures. This may be true even when longlasting respiratory impairment has occurred. Finally, it is important to recognize that the diagnosis of occupational asthma does not necessarily imply permanent disability.

REFERENCES

1. Cullen MR, Cherniack MG, Rosenstock L: Medical progress: Occupational medicine. N Engl J Med 322: 594, 1990.
2. Chan-Yeung M, Lam S: State of the art: Occupational asthma. Am Rev Respir Dis 133:686, 1986.
3. Salvaggio JE: Hypersensitivity pneumonitis. J Allergy Clin Immunol 79:558, 1987.
4. Newman Taylor AJ: Occupational asthma. Thorax 35:241, 1980.
5. Kobayashi S: Occupational asthma due to inhalation of pharmacological dusts and other chemical agents with reference to other asthma in Japan. In Yamamura Y, Frick OL, Hariuch Y, et al (eds): Allergology. Amsterdam, Excerpta Medica Foundation, 1974, p 124.
6. Venebles KM: Epidemiology and the prevention of occupational asthma. Br J Ind Med 44:73, 1987.

7. McNutt GM, Schleuter DP, Fink JN: Screening for occupational asthma: A word of caution. J Occup Med 33:19, 1991.

8. Salvaggio J, et al: Task force on asthma and other allergic diseases. U.S. Dept. of Health and Welfare, NIAID Task Force Report. Publication No. 79-389, p 330, 1979.

9. Brooks SM: Bronchial asthma of occupational origin. Scand J Work Environ Health 3:53, 1977.

10. Brooks SM, Kalica AR: NHLBI Workshop Summary: Strategies for elucidating the relationship between occupational exposures and chronic air-flow obstruction. Am Rev Respir Dis 135:268, 1987.

11. Novey HS, Bernstein IL, Mihalas LS, et al: Guidelines for the clinical evaluation of occupational asthma due to high molecular weight (HMW) allergens. J Allergy Clin Immunol 84:829, 1989.

12. Grammer LC, Patterson R, Zeiss CK: Guidelines for the immunologic evaluation of occupational lung disease. J Allergy Clin Immunol 84:805, 1989.

13. Butcher BT, Bernstein IL, Schwartz HJ: Guidelines for the clinical evaluation of occupational asthma due to small molecular weight chemicals. J Allergy Clin Immunol 84:834, 1989.

14. Salvaggio JE: Clinical and immunologic approach to patients with alleged environmental injury. Ann Allergy 66:493, 1991.

15. Gandevia B: Occupational asthma, Part I. Med J Austr 2:332, 1970.

16. Anderson CJ, Bardana EJ: Work-induced asthma. I. Clinical features, evaluation and pathogenesis, and II. Agents implicated in its causation. Immunol Allergy Pract 1:54, 1979 and 1:81, 1979.

16a. Malo JL, Ghezzo H, L'Archeveque J, et al: Is the clinical history a satisfactory means of diagnosing occupational asthma. Am Rev Respir Dis 143:526, 1991.

17. Lerman SE, Kipen HM: Material Safety Data Sheets; Caveat Emptor. Arch Intern Med 150:981, 1990.

18. Occupational Safety and Health Administration: Hazard Communication Standard: Final rule. Federal Register. August 24, 1987; 52:31, 852-31, 886.

19. Occupational Safety and Health Administration: Hazard Communication Standard. Federal Register. November 26, 1983; 48:53:280-53, 315.

20. Anon: Documentation of the Threshold Limit Values and Biological Exposure Indices, 5th ed. Cincinnati, OH, ACGIH, 1986, with supplemental documentation, 1989.

21. Anon: Chemical Safety Data Sheets (Vol I: Solvents; Vol II: Metals and Their Compounds; Vol III: Corrosive and Irritants). Cambridge, UK, The Royal Society of Chemistry, Xerox Ventura Publisher, 1990.

22. O'Hollaren MT, Bardana EJ: Chronic rhinitis: A practical approach to the work-up. J Respir Dis 11:443, 1990.

23. Weille FL: Studies in asthma. The nose and throat in five hundred cases of asthma. N Engl J Med 215:235, 1936.

24. Slavin RG, Cannon RE, Friedman WH, et al: Sinusitis and bronchial asthma. J Allergy Clin Immunol 66:250, 1980.

25. Bardana EJ, Montanaro A: Sjogren's syndrome: A rheumatic disorder with prominent respiratory manifestations. Ann Allergy 64:3, 1990.

26. Campbell SM, Montanaro A, Bardana EJ: Head and neck manifestations of autoimmune disorders. Am J Otolaryngol 4:187, 1983.

27. Stiehm ER, Chin TW, Haas A, et al: Infectious complications of the primary immunodeficiencies. Clin Immunol Immunopath 40:69, 1986.

28. Banks DE, deShazo R: An overview of occupational asthma: Principles of diagnosis and management. Immunol Allergy Pract 7:17, 1985.

29. Adkinson NF: Measurement of total serum immunoglobulin E and allergen specific immunoglobulin E antibody. In Rose NR, Friedman H, Fahey JL (eds): Manual of Clinical Laboratory Immunology. Washington, DC, Am Soc Microbiol 664, 1986.

30. Trasher JD, Boughton A, Micevich P: Antibodies and immune profiles of individuals occupationally exposed to formaldehyde: Six case reports. Am J Ind Med 14:479, 1988.

31. Lindblad JH, Farr RS: The incidence of positive intradermal reactions and the demonstration of skin sensitizing antibody to extracts of ragweed and dust in humans without history of rhinitis or asthma. J Allergy 32:392, 1961.

32. Bernstein DI, Patterson R, Zeiss CR: Clinical and immunologic evaluation of trimellitic anhydride and phthalic anhydride exposed workers using a questionnaire with comparative analysis of enzyme-linked immunosorbent and radioimmunoassay studies. J Allergy Clin Immunol 69:311, 1982.

33. Butcher BT, O'Neil CE, Reed MA, Salvaggio JE: Radioallergosorbent testing of toluene diisocyanate-reactive individuals using P-tolyl monoisocyanate antigen. J Allergy Clin Immunol 66:213, 1980.

34. Cromwell O, Pepys J, Parish WE, et al: Specific IgE antibodies to platinum salts in sensitized workers. Clin Allergy 9:109, 1979.

35. Patterson R, Pateras V, Grammer LC, et al: Human antibodies against formaldehyde-human serum albumin conjugates or human serum albumin in individuals exposed to formaldehyde. Int Arch Allergy Appl Immunol 79:53, 1986.

36. Patterson R, Dykewicz MS, Evans R, et al: IgG antibody against formaldehyde human serum proteins: A comparison with other IgG antibodies against inhalant proteins and reactive chemicals. J Allergy Clin Immunol 84:359, 1989.

37. Nielsen J, Welinder H, Schutz A, et al: Specific serum antibodies against phthalic anhydride in occupationally exposed subject. J Allergy Clin Immunol 82:126, 1988.

38. Zeiss CR, Wolkonsky P, Pruzansky JJ, et al: Clinical and immunologic evaluation of trimellitic anhydride workers in multiple industrial settings. J Allergy Clin Immunol 70:15, 1982.

39. Bernstein IL: Isocyanate-induced pulmonary diseases: A current perspective. J Allergy Clin Immunol 70:24, 1982.

40. Tse KS, Chan H, Chan-Yeung M: Specific IgE antibodies in workers with occupational asthma due to western red cedar. Clin Allergy 12:249, 1982.

41. Smith AB, Castellan RM, Lewis D, et al: Guidelines in the epidemiologic assessment of occupational asthma. J Allergy Clin Immunol 84:794, 1989.

42. Boushey HA, Hoiltzman MJ, Sheller JR, et al: Bronchial hyperreactivity. Am Rev Respir Dis 121:389, 1989.

43. Cockcroft DW, Killian DN, Mellon JJA, et al: Bronchial reactivity to inhaled histamine: A clinical survey. Clin Allergy 7:235, 1977.

44. Townley RG, Bewtra AK, Nair NM, et al: Methacholine inhalation challenge studies. J Allergy Clin Immunol 64:569, 1979.

45. Townley RG, Hopp RJ, Bewtra AK, et al: Airway reactivity in asthmatic families and twins. In Spector SL (ed): Provocative Challenge Procedures: Background and Methodology. New York, Futura, 1989, p 341.

46. Cockcroft DW, Benscheid BA, Murdock KY: Unimodal distribution of bronchial responsiveness of inhaled histamine in a random human population. Chest 83: 751, 1983.

47. Townley RG, Bewtra A, Wilson AF, et al: Segregation analysis of bronchial response to methacholine inhalation challenge in families with and without asthma. J Allergy Clin Immunol 77:101, 1986.
48. O'Byrne PM, Zamel N: Airway challenges with inhaled constrictor mediators. In Spector SL (ed): Provocative Challenge Procedures: Background and Methodology. New York, Futura, 1989, p 277.
49. Townley RG, Ryo UY, Miller-Kolotkin B, et al: Bronchial sensitivity to methacholine in current and former asthmatic and allergic rhinitis patients and control subjects. J Allergy Clin Immunol 56:429, 1975.
50. Lam S, Wong R, Chan-Yeung M: Nonspecific bronchial reactivity in occupational asthma. J Allergy Clin Immunol 63:28, 1979.
51. Cartier A, Bernstein IL, Burge PS, et al: Guidelines for bronchoprovocation on investigation of occupational asthma. J Allergy Clin Immunol 84:823, 1989.
52. Burge PS: Single and serial measurements of lung function in the diagnosis of occupational asthma. Eur J Respir Dis 63:47, 1982.
53. Pennock BE, Rogers RM, McCaffree DR: Changes in measured spirometric indices. Chest 80:97, 1981.
54. Spector SL: Bronchial inhalation challenges with aerosolized bronchoconstrictive substances. In Spector SL (ed): Provocative Challenge Procedures: Bronchial, Oral, Nasal and Exercise. Boca Raton, FL, CRC Press, 1983, p 150.
55. Krowka MJ, Enright PL, Rodarte JR, et al: Effect of effort on measurement of forced expiratory volume in one second. Am Rev Respir Dis 136:829, 1987.
56. Sobol BJ: Effort independence and forced expiratory flow. End of an era? Chest 73:566, 1978.
57. Davis JD, Harkins CJ, Marshall SG: Detection of submaximal effort in spirometry. Respiratory Management 20:55, 1989.
58. Pepys J, Hutchcroft BJ: Bronchial provocation tests in etiologic diagnosis and analysis of asthma. Am Rev Respir Dis 112:829, 1975.
59. Spector SL: Bronchial challenge tests: Practical help in asthma. J Respir Dis 5:106, 1984.
60. Salvaggio JE, Hendrick DJ: The use of bronchial inhalation challenge in the investigation of occupational diseases. In Spector SL (ed): Provocative Challenge Procedures: Background and Methodology. New York, Futura, 1989, p 417.
61. Malo JL, Filiatrault S, Martin RR: Bronchial hyperexcitability to inhaled methacholine in young asymptomatic smokers. Am Rev Respir Dis 121:248, 1980.
62. Mink JT, Gerrard JW, Cockcroft DW, et al: Nonspecific bronchial hyperreactivity in cigarette smokers with normal lung function. Am Rev Respir Dis 121:379, 1980.
63. Islam MS, Vastag E, Ulmer WT: So_2-induced bronchial hyperreactivity against acetylcholine. Int Arch Arbeits Med 29:221, 1972.
64. Orehek J, Massari JP, Gayrard P, et al: Effect of short-term, low level NO_2 exposure on bronchial sensitivity of asthmatic patients. J Clin Invest 57:301, 1976.
65. Golden JA, Nadel JA, Boushey HA: Bronchial hyperirritability in healthy subjects after exposure to ozone. Am Rev Respir Dis 118:287, 1978.
65a. Molfino NA, Wright SC, Katz I, et al: Effect of low concentrations of ozone on inhaled allergen responses in asthmatic subjects. Lancet ii:199, 1991.
66. O'Byrne PM, Ryan G, Morris M, et al: Asthma induced by cold air and its relation to nonspecific bronchial responsiveness to methacholine. Am Rev Respir Dis 125:281, 1982.
67. Cockcroft DW, Ruffin RE, Dolovich J, et al: Allergen-induced increase in non-allergic bronchial reactivity. Clin Allergy 7:503, 1977.
68. Bryant DH, Burns MW: Bronchial histamine reactivity: Its relationship to the reactivity of the bronchi to allergens. Clin Allergy 6:523, 1976.
69. Parker CD, Bilbo RE, Reed CE: Methacholine aerosol as test for bronchial asthma. Arch Intern Med 115:452, 1965.
70. Laitinen CA, Elkin RB, Empey DW, et al: Changes in bronchial reactivity after administration of live attenuated influenza virus. Am Rev Respir Dis 113:194, 1976.
71. Empey DW, Laitinen LA, Jacobs L, et al: Mechanisms of bronchial hyperreactivity in normal subjects after upper respiratory tract infections. Am Rev Respir Dis 113:131, 1976.
72. Kraan J, Koeter GH, van der Mark TW, et al: Dosage and time effects of inhaled budesonide on bronchial hyperreactivity. Am Rev Respir Dis 137:44, 1988.
73. Vathenen AS, Knox AJ, Wisniewski A, et al: Time course of change in bronchial reactivity with an inhaled corticosteroid in asthma. Am Rev Respir Dis 143:1317, 1991.
74. Szefler SJ: Glucocorticoid therapy for asthma: Clinical pharmacology. J Allergy Clin Immunol 88:147, 1991.
75. Cockcroft DN, Killian DN, Mellon JJA, et al: Protective effect of drugs on histamine-induced asthma. Thorax 32:429, 1977.
76. Simonsson BT, Jacobs FM, Nadal JA: Role of the autonomic nervous system and the cough reflex in the increased responsiveness of airways in patients with obstructive airway disease. J Clin Invest 46:1812, 1967.
77. Harnett J, Spector SL: Blocking effect of SCH1000 and isoproterenol on the combination of methacholine and histamine inhalations (abstract). J Allergy Clin Immunol 57:174, 1976.
78. Woenne R, Kattan M, Levison H: Sodium cromoglycate-induced changes in the dose-response curve of inhaled methacholine and histamine in asthmatic children. Am Rev Respir Dis 119:927, 1979.
79. Nathan RA, Segall N, Glover GG, et al: The effects of H_1 and H_2 antihistamines on histamine inhalation challenges in asthmatic patients. Am Rev Respir Dis 120:1251, 1979.
80. Smolensky MH, Reinberg A, Queng JT: The chronobiology and chronopharmacology of allergy. Ann Allergy 47:234, 1981.
81. Banks DE, Butcher BT, Salvaggio JE: Isocyanate-induced respiratory disease. Ann Allergy 57:389, 1986.
82. Chan-Yeung M: Occupational asthma. Chest 98:149(S), 1990.
83. Fabbri LM, Danieli D, Crescioli S, et al: Fatal asthma in a subject sensitized to toluene diisocyanate. Am Rev Respir Dis 137:1494, 1988.
84. Cote J, Kennedy SM, Chan-Yeung M: Outcome of patients with cedar asthma with continuous exposure. Am Rev Respir Dis 139:A388, 1989.
85. Agarwal MK, Yunginger JW, Swanson MC: An immunochemical method to measure atmospheric allergens. J Allergy Clin Immunol 68:194, 1981.
86. Swanson MC, Campbell AR, O'Hollaren MT, et al: Role of ventilation, air filtration, and allergen production rate in determining concentrations of rat allergens in the air of animal quarters. Am Rev Respir Dis 141:1578, 1990.
87. Chan-Yeung M, Malo JL: Occupational asthma. Chest 91:1315, 1987.
88. Brooks SM, Weiss MA, Bernstein IL: Reactive airways dysfunction syndrome. Chest 88:378, 1985.
89. Bardana EJ, Montanaro A, O'Hollaren MT: Building-related illness. Clin Rev Allergy 6:61, 1988.

APPENDIX I

HEALTH QUESTIONNAIRE

Prior to your arrival to see the doctor, we ask your cooperation in the completion of the questionnaire that follows. Base your answers on your own observations and what you feel to be the most accurate and complete response. Though the information requested is rather detailed, it could be a major help in arriving at a more accurate diagnosis or decision related to your condition.

1. GENERAL INFORMATION

NAME _____ DATE _____

ADDRESS _____

CITY _____ PHONE ( ) _____

Please briefly describe your major complaints(s) _____

_____

_____

_____

_____

Do you relate this complaint to anything in your work environment? _____

If yes, please describe: _____

_____

_____

_____

_____

When did this complaint begin? _____

Address of the home you were living in at the time: _____

_____

Which doctors (and their addresses) have you consulted for this or any related health problems?

1) _____   3) _____

_____   _____

_____   _____

2) _____   4) _____

_____   _____

_____   _____

If you have not already done so, please request that your records from any past physician be mailed to our office prior to your appointment.

2. PAST MEDICAL HISTORY

Have you ever had or have you now (please check at left of each item):

Yes (past)	Yes (now)	Never	Don't know	Check Each Item
				1. Whooping cough, frequent croup
				2. Scarlet fever or rheumatic fever
				3. Swollen or painful joints or arthritis
				4. Frequent or severe headache including migraine
				5. Dizziness, fainting spells, seizures
				6. Eye trouble including cataracts, glaucoma
				7. Ear, nose, throat trouble, or nasal polyps
				8. Hearing loss
				9. Chronic or frequent colds
				10. Severe tooth or gum trouble
				11. Sinusitis
				12. Hayfever (sneezing, watery eyes, itchy nose)
				13. Head injury with/without unconsciousness
				14. Skin disease, e.g., hives, eczema or psoriasis
				15. Swelling of eyelids, lips, or body
				16. Tuberculosis
				17. Asthma or asthmatic bronchitis
				18. Pneumonia
				19. Shortness of breath or wheezing
				20. Pain or pressure in chest
				21. Chronic cough or bronchitis
				22. Palpitation or pounding heart
				23. Heart trouble (angina, heart failure)
				24. High or low blood pressure
				25. Anemia or low blood count
				26. Diabetes or thyroid problems
				27. Venereal disease, e.g., gonorrhea, syphilis
				28. Frequent indigestion or ulcer disease
				29. Stomach, liver, or intestinal trouble
				30. Nervous trouble, irritability, anxiety
				31. Recurrent back pain, ruptured disc
				32. Gallbladder trouble or gallstones
				33. Jaundice or hepatitis
				34. Adverse reaction to serum, drug, food
				35. Broken bones or torn ligaments
				36. Tumor, growth, cyst, cancer
				37. Rupture/hernia
				38. Piles or rectal disease
				39. Kidney or bladder infections
				40. Painful or bloody urination
				41. Bed wetting since age 12
				42. Depression or loss of memory
				43. Lack of coordination
				44. Inability to concentrate
				45. Recent gain or loss of weight

Please explain all "yes" answers on the previous page by indicating when the problem began, which physician you saw, and what treatment was given.

Number of the item   Comments

_____

_____

_____

_____

_____

_____

_____

_____

_____

_____

_____

_____

_____

_____

_____

_____

_____

_____

_____

PREVIOUS SURGERY

Operation   Year   Hospital/Surgeon

_____

_____

_____

_____

_____

_____

_____

_____

_____

PREVIOUS HOSPITALIZATION

Reason for Admission   Year   Hospital

_____

_____

_____

_____

_____

_____

_____

_____

_____

3. FAMILY MEDICAL HISTORY

	Age (if living)	Age (at death)	Year (of death)	Please list cause of death and all major illnesses that you are aware of during each family member's life.
Mother				
Father				
Brothers 1.				
2.				
3.				
4.				
5.				
Sisters 1.				
2.				
3.				
4.				
5.				
Children 1.				
2.				
3.				
4.				
5.				

Do any of your blood relatives have problems with these conditions? Please make a check on the left for any "yes" answer and indicate which relative to the right in the space provided.

_____ Tuberculosis _____
_____ Cancer _____
_____ Diabetes _____
_____ Kidney disease _____
_____ Gallbladder _____
_____ Heart problems _____
_____ Allergy (hayfever, hives) _____
_____ Liver disease _____
_____ Stroke _____
_____ Hypertension _____
_____ Nervous or psychiatric disorder _____
_____ Migraine _____
_____ Ulcer _____
_____ Arthritis _____
_____ Skin disorders _____
_____ Bleeding disorder _____
_____ Diarrheal disorder _____
_____ Goiter _____
_____ Glaucoma _____
_____ Alcoholism _____
_____ Drug addiction _____
_____ Eating disorders (anorexia nervosa, bulemia) _____
_____ Deformities _____
_____ Birth defects _____
_____ Thyroid disease _____
_____ Asthma _____
_____ Cystic fibrosis _____
_____ Sinus disease _____
_____ Nasal polyps _____

4. OCCUPATIONAL HISTORY

What is your current or most recent employment?

Employer: _____
Location: _____
Type of industry: _____
Job title: _____
Date of hire: _____
Pre-employment physical exam: _____ Yes   _____ No.
Examining physician: _____
_____
Were you laid off at any time: _____ Yes   _____ No.
If yes, when: _____

Job status:

_____ Full time, hrs/wk   (   )   _____ Part time, (hrs/wk) (   )

_____ Retired, date   (   )   _____ Laid off, date   (   )

_____ Multiple jobs   (#   )   _____ Disabled, date   (   )

_____ Discharged? When? _____

                        Reason _____

_____ Second job? How long? _____

Nature of second job: _____

_____

Shift   _____ Day shift   _____ Graveyard

         _____ Swing shift

         _____ Rotating shifts   _____ Overtime (average hrs/wk)

Briefly describe your work in your current (or most recent) job. Mention any possible hazardous exposures (fumes or dusts) and describe ventilation.

_____

_____

_____

_____

_____

When appropriate have you employed any of the following protective equipment at your current (or most recent job?

Protection	Always	Occasionally	Never
Air supply respirator			
Charcoal filter respirator			
Surgical mask type			
Safety goggles			
Gloves			
Coveralls/apron			
Earplugs			
Hardhat			
Steel tipped shoes			

Please indicate places of employment prior to current or most recent job:

Year From	To	Employer (City)	Type of Industry (Generalize)	Job Description

Were you ever injured at the jobs cited above? If so, please indicate which job and how.

_____

_____

_____

_____

To the best of your knowledge, have you ever been in contact with, or worked at a job handling, any of the following materials? (CIRCLE).

Acetone	Chromates	HDI	Parathion	Rubber
Acids	Cobalt salts	Henna extract	Persulfate salts	Shellac
Acrylic resins	Colophony	Herbicides	Pesticides	Silica
Aerosols	Cutting oils	Hydrazine	Phenol	Solders
Aluminum dust	Detergents	Hog trypsin	Phenolic resins	Solvents
Alkalis	Diamines	Inks	Phthalic anhydride	Spiramycin
Ammonia	Dyes	Insecticides	Pigments	Stains
Antibiotics	Emery	Isocyanates	Piperazine	Storage mites
Arsenic	Enzymes	Latex	Plastic fumes	Toluene
Asbestos	Epoxy resins	Lime	Platinum salts	TDI
Benzene	Ethylene diamine	MDI	Plicatic acid	Thinners
Bleaching agents	Exhaust fumes	Mercury	Polyvinyl chloride	Vanadium
Brake fluids	Fiberglass	Mineral wool	Potassium dichromate	Vinyl chloride
Carbonless paper	Formaldehyde	Nickel salts	Resins	Welding fumes
Cement	Food vapors	Paints	Red cedar	Wood dust
Chlorine	Glue fumes	Papain	Rock dust	Xylene
				Zinc salts

5. SOCIAL HISTORY

A. General

Place of birth:_____ Date of birth:_____

Please list cities you lived in to the present:

City	Dates
_____	_____
_____	_____
_____	_____
_____	_____
_____	_____
_____	_____

Are you married? _____ Date:_____

Prior marriages (indicate number and inclusive dates) and whether divorced (D) or widowed (W).

_____

_____

Spouse's occupation: _____

Have you ever participated in sexual practices that may make you vulnerable to venereal disease, including AIDS? _____ Yes _____ No.

If Yes, please elaborate: _____

_____

_____

Have you ever served in the Armed Forces?

    Branch of service _____

    Date of induction _____

    Date of discharge_____ Honorable? _____

    Top rank and job _____

    Places stationed _____

        _____

        _____

        _____

Have you traveled outside the U.S. in the past 2 years? If yes, where?

_____

_____

Education:

    Grammar school (name) _____

    High school diploma (name) _____

    GED equivalent _____

    College (circle no. of years)   1   2   3   4;   major: _____

    Professional education? _____ Degree: _____

B. Habits

Have you ever smoked cigarettes?   Yes _____   No _____.

If yes, age started _____ Brand _____

Switched brands?/filter/menthol (specify) _____

_____

Maximum habit (packs/day) _____

Decreased smoking (when) _____

How many packs do you currently smoke on a daily basis? _____

When did you stop smoking? _____

Why? _____

Have you ever been told to stop smoking by your doctor? _____

Have you ever smoked cigars?   Yes _____   No _____.   If yes, how many cigars/day? _____

Have you ever smoked a pipe?   Yes _____   No _____.   If yes, how many pipefuls/day? _____

Does anyone in your household smoke?　Yes _____　No _____.

If yes, how many individuals? _____

Do you drink alcohol?　Yes _____　No _____.

Average amount per week (e.g., glasses bottles, oz., etc.)?　　　For how many years?

Beer _____　　　_____

Wine _____　　　_____

Liquor _____　　　_____

Have you ever used alcohol to excess?　　　　　　Yes _____　No _____

Have you ever been treated for alcoholism?　　　　Yes _____　No _____

Have you ever been cited for driving under the influence?　Yes _____　No _____

Have you ever used recreational or pleasure drugs?　Yes _____　No _____

If yes, which drugs and how much (check and indicate time frame and frequency of use).

_____ Marijuana (pot)　　　_____

_____ Cocaine/crack　　　_____

_____ Heroin　　　_____

_____ Amphetamines　　　_____

_____ Sedatives/tranquilizers　　　_____

_____ LSD, mescaline, other hallucinogens _____

_____ I.V. use (mainline)　　　_____

Do you use any nonprescription drugs?　Yes _____　No _____.

If yes, which drugs (e.g., Primatene Mist, vitamins, Afrin Nasal Spray, Dristan Nasal Spray, etc.)?

_____

_____

_____

Do you currently take any prescription medications?　Yes _____　No _____.

If yes, which? (Name them with their dosage and number of doses taken daily.)

_____

_____

_____

Do you exercise regularly?　Yes _____　No _____.　If yes, describe:

_____

_____

_____

Average hours of sleep per night? _____

C. Hobbies (Check)

_____ Aviation	_____ Gardening	_____ Rock collecting
_____ Bird study	_____ Golf	_____ Sailing
_____ Boating	_____ Hiking	_____ Sewing
_____ Bowling	_____ Hunting	_____ Sculpture
_____ Camping	_____ Knitting	_____ Skiing (snow, water)
_____ Car restoration	_____ Macrame	_____ Stamp collecting
_____ Cooking	_____ Movies/TV	_____ Stained glass
_____ Coin collecting	_____ Painting (water,	_____ Welding
_____ Crochet	oil, enamel)	_____ Wood working
_____ Diving (scuba)	_____ Photography	_____ Others: _____
_____ Fishing	_____ Reading	_____

D. Drugs

Do you have any drug allergies?   Yes _____   No _____

Have you every had an allergic or toxic reaction to any of the following kinds of drugs? (Check)

_____ Aspirin	_____ Vitamins	_____ Antihistamines
_____ Nose drops	_____ Sulfa	_____ Cortisone drugs
_____ Laxatives	_____ Penicillin	_____ Codeine
_____ Sedatives	_____ "Mycin" antibiotics	_____ Morphine
_____ Tranquilizers	_____ Hormones	_____ "Caine" drugs

Do you use any aspirin, aspirin-containing drugs, or other anti-inflammatory medications? (See list below.) If yes, which? (Check)

_____ Advil	_____ Clinoril	_____ Fiorinal	_____ Percodan
_____ Alka-Seltzer	_____ Damason-P	_____ Ibuprofen	_____ Robaxisol tablets
_____ Anacin	_____ Darvon Compound	_____ Indocin	_____ Rufin
_____ Anahist	_____ Dolobid	_____ Liquiprin	_____ Soma Compound
_____ APC	_____ Dristan	_____ Meclomin	_____ Supac
_____ Aspergum	_____ Easprin	_____ Medipren	_____ Talwin Compound
_____ Ascriptin	_____ Ecotrin	_____ Midol	_____ Stanback
_____ Axotal	_____ Empirin Compound	_____ Motrin	_____ Tolectin
_____ B-A-C tablets	_____ Encaprin	_____ Nalfon	_____ Trigesic
_____ BC	_____ Equagesic	_____ Naprosyn	_____ 4-Way Cold Tabs
_____ Bromoquinine	_____ Excedrin	_____ Norgesic	_____ Vanquish
_____ Bromo-Seltzer	_____ Feldene	_____ Nuprin	_____ Zorprin
_____ Bufferin	_____ Fiogesic	_____ Pepto-Bismol	

If yes, which drugs and how many tablets per month on average? _____

Have you ever reacted adversely to aspirin? (Explain): _____

_____

E. Foods

Do any foods make your symptoms worse?   Yes _____   No _____   If yes, name them.

_____

_____

_____

What symptoms are produced? _____

_____

_____

Have you been on any special diets? _____

_____

_____

Have you ever reacted to the following foods? (Check)

_____ Avocado dip	_____ Potatoes	_____ Soups
_____ Guacamole	_____ Coleslaw	_____ Wine vinegar
_____ Cider	_____ Shellfish	_____ Wines/wine coolers
_____ Salads (at salad bars)	_____ Fresh mushrooms	_____ Beer

F. Home (Check all applicable answers)

Location of Home	**Type of House**	**Heating System**	
_____ Farm/Country	_____ Frame	_____ Hot air	_____ Electric
_____ Suburban	_____ Stucco	_____ Steam	_____ Gas
_____ City	_____ Brick	_____ Hot water	_____ Oil
_____ Trailer park	_____ Apartment	_____ Space	_____ Propane

What is the age of your home?   _____ yrs.

How long have you lived in the home?   _____ yrs.

Does your home have: (Check or circle all correct answers)

_____ Wood stove?   How many? _____   How well is it (are they) vented? _____

_____ Fireplace insert?   How many? _____

_____ Humidifier?   Describe _____

_____ Air filtration system?

_____ Air conditioner?   Central?_____

_____ Basement?   Finished or not? _____   Is the basement damp or musty? _____

_____ Carpeting?   How extensive? _____   Padded? _____

_____ Recent insulation?   Type? _____

_____ Pets

    Dog   # _____; Indoor/outdoor? Ever sleep in bedroom? _____ Yes   _____ No

    Cat   # _____; Indoor/outdoor? Ever sleep in bedroom? _____ Yes   _____ No

    Birds   # _____; Indoor (canary, parakeet, parrot)/outdoor (pigeons, chickens)?

    Gerbils # _____; Indoor?

_____ Others? _____

_____ Litterbox? How many? _____; Location? _____

_____ Plants? How many? _____

Is your home near a barn? _____

Are you exposed to moldy hay, stables, dairies, horses, cows, or heavy industry? _____

_____

G. Which factors worsen your nasal, sinus, or asthmatic condition? (The factors unchecked will be considered non-offenders.)

_____ Pollens: grass, weeds, trees, hay, flowers

_____ Molds: wet leaves, moldy hay, damp basements

_____ Danders: pet cats, dogs, mice, rats, etc.

_____ Dust: house dust, mattress, pillow, carpet

_____ Foods: fish, berries, peanut, milk

_____ Nasal or chest colds   _____ Exercise or exertion (any kind)

_____ Influenza (flu)   _____ Cold air

_____ Sinus infection   _____ Hot air

_____ Bronchitis   _____ Weather change

_____ Field burning   _____ Deodorant sprays   _____ Newspaper fumes

_____ Air conditioning   _____ Detergent odors   _____ Paint/varnish fumes

_____ Pollution/smog   _____ Wave sets   _____ Food cooking odors

_____ Volcanic ash   _____ Cigarette/cigar smoke   _____ Clothing stores

_____ Cosmetics/perfumes   _____ Toothpaste/mouthwash

_____ Garden sprays   _____ House deodorants

H. Miscellaneous

Have you ever had a rash from exposure to:

_____ Poison ivy, sumac, oak?

_____ Chemicals or contacts at work? _____

_____ Ointments? _____

_____ Cosmetics? _____

_____ Clothing? _____

_____ Metals? _____

Have you ever had an unusual reaction to a bee, hornet, or wasp sting?

If yes, describe: _____

_____

Did you complete this questionnaire yourself?   Yes _____   No _____.

If not, why not? _____

Who assisted you to complete this? _____

_____

Thank you very much for completing this questionnaire.

_____   _____

DATE   SIGNATURE

APPENDIX II

AN ALPHABETICAL LIST OF OCCUPATIONS AND SELECTED IMMUNOGENS AND IRRITANTS THAT MAY BE ENCOUNTERED

Industry or Occupation	Immunogens	Irritants
Abrasive wheel makers (grinders)	Adhesive resins	Emery carborundum
Aircraft or aeronautical	Epoxy resins Phthalates Formaldehyde Latex products Rubber accelerators Acrylic glues Isocyanate paints	Cutting oils Anticorrosives Solvents Chromates Fiberglass Lubricants Thinners
Animal handlers (cattle, horse breeders, veterinarians)	Antibiotics Bacteria Grains Fungi Storage mites Parasites Vermifuges (piperazine and phenothiazine) Cat fleas	Germicides Insecticides Disinfectants Deodorants Detergents Cleaners Food additives Preservatives
Artists (painters and sculptors)	Acrylics Epoxy resins Isocyanates Colophony Pigments Phthalates Exotic woods Azo pigments	Thinners Solvents Plaster of Paris Polishes Dusts
Automotive (assembly, body mechanic)	Latex products Anticorrosive paints Catalyzed paints Isocyanates Chromium Colophony Epoxy resins Formaldehyde Potassium dichromate Nickel	Asbestos Brake fluids Flame retardants Gasoline Antioxidants Solvents Cleansers Hydraulic fluids Alkalis Bonding/metallic dusts
Bakers (pastry makers, confectioners)	Natural fragrances Wheat, rye flour Fungi Storage mite Food dyes Egg wash Malt	Benzoyl peroxide Dust Flavor oils Spices
Battery makers	Cobalt Epoxy sealer Nickel Pitch Plastics	Alkali Fiberglass Solvents Sulfuric acid Zinc chloride

Continued on next page.

Industry or Occupation	Immunogens	Irritants
Bookbinders	Formaldehyde Resin glues Shellac Colophony	Solvents Thinners Inks
Brick masons (cement workers)	Chromates Epoxy resins Cobalt	Cement Lime Pitch Muriatic acid
Bronzers	Lacquers Epoxy resins Varnishes	Acetone Ammonia Benzene Cyanides Hydrochloric acid Methyl alcohol Hydrocarbons Sodium hydroxide Sulfur dioxide
Cable splicers	Epoxy resins Isocyanates Dyes Ammonium chloride Zinc chloride Amino-ethyl ethanolamine	Chlorinated diphenyls Chlorinated naphthalene Zinc oxide Fluroborate
Carpenters (cabinet makers, woodworkers)	Amino resin glues Rosin Colophony Epoxy glues Exotic woods Western red cedar Formaldehyde Chromium Fungi Polyurethane coatings	Acid bleaches Shellac Oils Polishes Solvents Stains Preservatives Fillers Wood dusts
Carpet makers	Reactive dyes Guar gum Formaldehyde Epoxy glues	Solvents Cleaners Textile dusts
Chemical	Chromium Formaldehyde Azo pigments Aniline dyes Paraphenylene-diamine Hydrazine Pharmaceuticals Chloramine-T	Acids Alkalis Cleaners Disinfectants Dusts
Clerks (office workers)	Adhesives Carbonless paper (NCR) Formaldehyde Latex	Duplicating fluids Ink removers Inks Solvents
Dairy workers	Antibiotics Bacteria	Deodorants Detergents

Continued on next page.

Industry or Occupation	Immunogens	Irritants
Diary workers *(Cont.)*	Fungi Storage mites Viruses Potassium dichromate	
Degreasers	None	Alkalis Hydrocarbon solvents Petroleum solvents Trichloroethylene
Dentists	Formaldehyde Antibiotics Chromium, nickel Latex Mercury Epoxy resins Acrylic resins	Disinfectants Soaps Dentin dust Waxes
Dock workers (longshoremen)	Beetles Castor bean pomace Chemicals Fungi Storage mites Bacteria Grains Grain weevil Insects Tropical woods Paints Coffee/tea dust	Fumigants Insecticides Petroleum Tar Sanitary products Anticorrosives
Dry cleaners	Formaldehyde Perchlorethylene Dyes	Acetic acid Ammonia Benzene Carbon tetrachloride Methanol Stoddard solvent Trichloroethylene
Dye makers (dyers)	Azo dyes Formaldehyde Vegetable gums Mercury Acid anhydrides	Benzene Acids Alkalis Cresol Hydroquinone solvents Zinc chloride
Electricians (electronics)	Colophony Epoxy resin and hardeners Polyurethanes Phenolic resins Latex	Solvents Waxes Chlorinated diphenyls Rubber antioxidants Asbestos Varnishes
Entomologists (insect research workers)	Locusts Crickets House flies Australian blowflies Screwworm flies	Pesticides Fungicides Preservatives Disinfectants

Continued on next page.

Industry or Occupation	Immunogens	Irritants
Farmers (agriculture)	Amprolium HCl Antibiotics Bacteria Feeds Fungi Paints Mercurials Liverworts Storage mites Animal protein Garlic	Detergents Disinfectants Fertilizers Fungicides Lubricants Oils Pesticides Solvents Preservatives
Florists (gardeners, horticulturists)	Chrysanthemum Baby's breath Sunflower seed Bacteria Fungi Parasites	Fertilizer Herbicides Phytosanitary products
Food preservers (processors)	Egg Shellfish Coffee dust Sea squirt Garlic dust Cinnamon Honeybee dust Mushrooms Capsaicin Bromelain Pectinase Papain Guar gum Gum acacia Protease	Bleaches Brine Vinegar Waxes Disinfectants
Hairdressers (barbers)	Fungi Ammonium persulfate Latex Formaldehyde Henna	Antiseptics Cosmetics Hairspray Depilatories Dyes Hair conditioners Perfumes Shampoos Wave solutions
Histology technicians	Formaldehyde Epoxy resins Mercury bichloride	Toluene Xylene Waxes Benzol Aniline Alcohol
Jewelers	Chromium Mercury Nickel Colophony Formaldehyde Epoxy resins Platinum salts	Acids Cyanides Rouge

Continued on next page.

Industry or Occupation	Immunogens	Irritants
Joiners (loggers)	Local wood Forestry allergens (frullania, parmelia) Exotic woods Formaldehyde glue Resin glues Potassium dichromate Colophony Tussock moth	Preservatives Creosol Fungicides Pesticides
Laundry workers	Alkalase Enzymes	Bleaches Alkalis Detergents Fungicides Bacteriocides
Machinists (mechanics)	Chromates Latex Rubber accelerators	Antioxidants Cutting oils Germicides Greases Lubricants Rust inhibitors Solvents Gasoline Ethylene glycol
Medical personnel (physicians/nurses)	Chlorhexidine Antibiotics Bacteria Ethylene oxide Fungi Latex Anesthetics Mercurials Formaldehye Piperazine Chloramine-T Ipecacuanha	Antiseptics Detergents Talc Alcohol Disinfectants
Paint makers (painters)	Chromates Epoxy resins Azo dyes Colophony Isocyanates Trimellitic anhydride Formaldehyde Protease Methyldopa	Acetone Acids Alkalis Benzene Strippers Thinners Turpentine Pigments
Pharmaceutical industry	Mercury Antibiotics Furan binder Pancreatic extract Piperazine Latex Psyllium	Antiseptics Disinfectants Detergents

Continued on next page.

Industry or Occupation	Immunogens	Irritants
Plastics and resin makers	Acid anhydrides Polybasic acids Diamines (aliphatic amines) Formaldehyde Azo dyes (see Table 2, Ch. 17) Phenolic resins Polyurethanes Acrylics	Epichlorhydrin Bisphenol A Asbestos Glass fiber Tar
Platers	Chrome Nickel	Acids Organic solvents
Printers	Chromium Cobalt Azo dyes Formaldehyde Gum arabic Gum tragacanth Resin glues	Turpentine Solvents Detergents Roller wash Alkalis Aniline
Railroad workers	Catalyzed paints Epoxy resins Chromates Latex Reactive dyes Fungi	Ethylene glycol Lubricants Cutting fluids Diesel fuel Greases Lacquers Strippers Thinners Solvents
Rubber workers	Accelerators Latex Colophony Activators Formaldehyde Resins Plasticizers	Antioxidants Solvents Acids Adhesive removers Benzol Oils Soaps Solvents Tar Turpentine
Sewer workers	Sewer filter flies Bacteria Fungi	Chlorine Disinfectants Multiple chemicals and odors
Shoemakers	Chromium Formaldehyde Latex Azo dyes Colophony Rubber accelerator Potassium dichromate	Polish Tanning products Insecticides Ammonia Benzene Hexane Naphtha Waxes
Textile industry	Azo dyes Formaldehyde Protease	Sizing chemicals Detergents Bleaches Solvents

Continued on next page.

Industry or Occupation	Immunogens	Irritants
Upholsterers	Formaldehyde Mites Resin glues Lacquer Bacteria	Flame retardants Lacquer solvents Methyl alcohol
Zookeepers	Animal protein Grains Grain weevil Storage mite Fungi Antibiotics Parasites Vermifuges Cereal and insect antigens in animal feed	Germicides Insecticides Disinfectants Deodorants Detergents Cleaners Food additives

INDEX

Page numbers in **boldface type** indicate complete chapters.

Abalone, respiratory hypersensitivity to, 126
Abietic acid, 97
Acacia, occupational asthma associated with, 101
Acarina, allergic reactions to, 221
ACE-inhibitors, and bronchial hyperreactivity, 37
Acetylcholine, inhalation challenge with, 35, 37
Acid anhydrides,
    asthma secondary to, **145-150**, 190, 192
        historical perspective of, 145
    chemistry and physical properties of, 145
    himic anhydride, 149
    immunologic reactivity to, 147
    phthalic anhydride, 145-147
    testing for, 291
    tetrachlorophthalic anhydride, 149
    trimellitic anhydride, 147-149, 276, 291
Acute respiratory distress syndrome, 37, 70
Adenosine, inhalation challenge with, 36
Aerosol generation, delivery, and penetrance, 47-48
Agricola, Georgius, 2
Air pollution, indoor, **237-254**
Air-quality standards, 6-7
Airflow obstruction, chronic, bronchitis and, 67
    criteria for, 23, 26
    small-airway disease and, 68
Airway hyperreactivity, blocking of, 38-39
    response to medications and, 38
    to allergens and bronchoconstrictive substances,
        35-54
Airway inflammation, disorders associated with,
    66-68
Airway obstruction, occupationally induced,
    pathogenesis of, **267-281**
Alcalase, occupational asthma due to, 171-173
Aldehydes, in tobacco smoke, 156
Alder wood dust, asthma in workers exposed to, 92
Aliphatic polyamine hardeners, health effects of, 192-195
Allergen inhalation challenges, 39-44. *See also*
        Bronchial provocation tests
    guidelines for safe, 43-44
    indications for, 39-43
    preparation of patients for, 44
Allergens, airway hyperreactivity to, **35-54**
    immediate- versus late-phase reaction to, 41-43
    reported to cause occupational asthma, 291
Allergic alveolitis, animal-related, 230
    building-related, 241-242
    See also Hypersensitivity pneumonitis
Allergy, as occupational disease, 11-12
Alpha-adrenergic blocking agents, effect on asthmatic
    response, 46
Aluminum exposure, chronic obstructive lung disease
    from, 182
Aluminum soldering flux, asthma due to fumes of, 194
Aluminum workers, occupational (potroom) asthma in,
    181-184
AMA disability classes, work requirements and, 30-31
Amine hydrobromide, asthmatic reactions to, 100
Amine-based epoxy resins. *See* Epoxy resins
Ammonium persulphate, asthma and dermatitis from
    exposure to, 200-201
Amprolium hydrochloride, asthma following exposure
    to, 210

Anhydrides. *See* Acid anhydrides
Animals, antigens of, 227-230
Animal-induced asthma, **225-235**, 314
    animal antigens, 227-230
    assessing animal environment, 231-232
    clinical presentation of, 230
    diagnosis of, 230-231
    epidemiology of, 226
    historical perspective of, 225-226
    immunotherapy and, 232
    management of, 232
    occupations with exposure to, 226
Animal facility, evaluation of, 231-232
Annoyance reactions, 256
Antibiotics, asthma due to inhalation of, **205-211**
        beta-lactam antibiotics, 205-206
        chloramine-T, 208
        macrolide antibiotics, 206-207
        tetracycline, 207
Anticholinergic agents, effect on asthmatic response, 46
Antigen inhalation challenge, 38
ARDS, 37, 70
Asbestos, exposure to,
    and small airways inflammation, 67
    malignancy from, 4-5
    smoking and, 71
Asbestosis, 4-5
Ascidian, occupational asthma from, 127
Ascorbic acid, effect on asthmatic response, 46
Aspergillus flavus, enzyme exposure from, 177
Aspirin idiosyncracy syndrome, 287
Asthma. *See also* Occupational asthma
    definition of, 63
    preexisting, permanent aggravation of, 298
    prevalence of, 56
Asthmatic response, immediate versus late, 41-43
    location of, mechanism and, 41
Atopic dermatitis, 289
Atopy, and development of nonspecific bronchial
        hyperreactivity, 292
    and development of occupational asthma, 269-270
Atropine, effect on asthmatic response, 46
Atypical asthma, 37
Azo compounds, hypersensitivity to, 198-200
Azodicarbonamide-induced asthma, 200

Baby's breath, allergy to, 103
Bait handlers, sensitivity to mealworms in, 215, 218,
    219
Baker's asthma, 3, 12, **107-111**, 314
    clinical presentation of, 109
    diagnosis of, 110-111
    epidemiology and etiology of, 107-108
    historical perspective of, 107
    pathophysiology of, 110
    treatment of, 111
Barley flour, occupational asthma from exposure to, 109
Beauty products industry, asthma in, 193
Bee moth larvae, asthma from, 218, 219
Beekeepers, occupational asthma in, 128, 221
Beer, asthma and, 174
Beetle exposure, asthma resulting from, 218

Beta agonists, effect on asthmatic response, 42, 45
Beta-lactam antibiotics, asthma from, 205–206
Beverage industry workers, bromelain-induced asthma in, 175
Birds, allergy to, 229–230
Bisphenol A, dermatitis from exposure to, 192
Blocking agents, 43
Box elder bugs, allergy to, 221
Bradykinin, producing bronchial provocation with, 36
Brewery, asthma in, 174
Britannicus, 2
Broad Street pneumonia, 244
Bromelain, occupational asthma to, 176
Bronchial asthma, building-related, 243–244
    definition of, 268
Bronchial hyperreactivity, 68, 271, 292
    in western red cedar workers, 94
    nonspecific, 26–28
Bronchial inflammation, mechanisms of airway injury secondary to, 65–66
Bronchial provocation tests, 26–28, **35–54**, 272, 293, 295–296. *See also* Allergen inhalation challenges *and* in text under specific entities
    comparison of, 36–37
    cumulative doses for, 48
    factors affecting responses to, 293
    indications for performing, 37–39
    safety considerations for, 48
Bronchiolitis, 64, 67–68
Bronchiolitis obliterans, 284
    bronchitis and, 70
Bronchitis,
    chronic, airway hyperreactivity in, 68
        and airflow obstruction, 67
        byssinosis and, 80
        causative agents in, 7
        definition of, 63
        determining impairment and disability with, 72–73
        evaluation and treatment of, 72
        mechanisms of airway injury secondary to, 65–66
        occupational causes of, 68–70
        pathology of, 64–66
        prevention of, 73
    occupational, **63–75**, 283–284
    smoking-induced, 63, 64, 67, 69
Bronchoconstrictive agents, comparison of, 36–37
    storage of, 37
Bronchoconstriction,
    immunologic, 276
    pharmacologic, 275
    reflex, 275–276
Bronchogenic carcinoma, 71
Brown lung disease, 275
Budesonide, 39
Building-related illness, **237–254**, 259. *See also* Chemical sensitivity *and* Sick-building syndrome
    evaluation of, 249–250, 259
    historical perspective of, 237–238
    humidifier fever, 242–243, 244
    non-building-related factors and, 240
    prevalence and epidemiology of, 239–241
    psychogenic illness and, 248
    sick-building syndrome, 246–249
    symptoms of, 246
    syndromes implicated in, 241–246
        allergic alveolitis, 241–242
        allergic rhinoconjunctivitis, 243–244
        dermatitis and ocular disease, 245–246
        hypersensitivity pneumonitis, 241–242

Building-related illness *(Cont.)*
    syndromes implicated in *(Cont.)*
        infectious syndromes, 244–245
        intoxication syndromes, 246, 256–257
        Legionnaire's disease, 244
        Pontiac fever, 244
        Q fever, 244–245
    terminology of, 238–239
Bullfrogs, allergy to, 229
Butterflies, asthma from exposure to, 215, 216, 219
Byssinosis, 56, **77–85**, 275
    characteristics of, 77
    chemistry, antigen identification and pathophysiology of, 80–82
    clinical presentation and evaluation of, 82–83
    effect of smoking on, 82
    epidemiology of, 80
    etiologic agents of, 78–80
        coir, 80
        cotton, 78
        flax, 78–79
        hemp, 79
        jute, 79–80
        kapok, 79
        sisal, 79
    historical perspective of, 77
    prevention of, 84
    symptoms, 82

Caddis flies, allergy to, 221
Cadmium pneumonitis, 187
Capsaicin-containing peppers, allergy from, 129
Carbamylcholine, inhalation challenge with, 35
Carbon monoxide, building-related, 246
    diffusing capacity for, 26
Carbonless paper, dermatitis from, 245–246
Cardiac stimulants, piperazine in, 195
Carmine, work-related asthma to, 199
Carpet manufacturers, asthma in, 102, 315
Castor bean dust, asthma due to, 117, 118, 121–124
    occupations associated with, 123
Castor-bean pomace, 121–122
Cat flea, allergy to, 216, 221
Cats, allergic symptoms to, 216, 221, 226, 228
Cattle, allergy to, 229
Cayenne peppers, allergy from, 128–129
Cedar asthma. *See* Western red cedar asthma
Celsus, Aulus Cornelius, 1
Cereal flour-associated asthma, 108–110
Chemical industry workers, occupational asthma in, 208–210, 315
Chemical production, occupational asthma from 145–146
Chemical sensitivity, **255–266**. *See also* Building-related illness
    classification of symptoms perceived as, 256–257
    clinical presentation of, 257
    diagnosis of, 260–264
        procedures for, 262–264
    evaluation of, 259–260, 263–264
    medical conditions commonly presenting as, 259
    medical-legal considerations of, 264–265
    patient evaluation for, 259–260
    psychologic factors in, 262
    symptoms of, 256–257
    treatment of, 265
Chemicals, common, adverse health effects from, 256
    hazardous workplace, 288–289
Chemonucleolysis, allergy to, 174–175

Chest x-ray, for evaluation of occupational asthma, 14, 292
Chili peppers, allergy from, 129
Chironomids, allergy to, 220
Chloramine-T, asthma following exposure to, 208
Chlorhexidine alcohol aerosol, 208
Cholinergic antagonists, effect on asthmatic response, 45
Chromium, occupational asthma from, 186
Chronic obstructive lung disease, 63, 67
from aluminum exposure, 182
Chrysanthemum pollen, occupational asthma to, 103
Chymopapain-induced allergy, 173–175
Chymotrypsin-induced allergy, 172, 177
Cigarette smoking. See Smoking
Cinnamon-induced asthma, 128
Circadian rhythms, and asthma, 47
Clam liver extract, occupational asthma from, 126
Clinical ecology, 255–256
Coal dust exposure, chronic bronchitis from, 69–71
Coal workers' pneumoconiosis, 71
Cobalt-induced asthma, 184–185
Cocaine use, and development of occupational asthma, 270
Cochineal, asthma from exposure to, 199
Cockroaches, asthma from exposure to, 213, 215–218
Code of Federal Regulations, Z-Tables of, 7
Coefficients of variation, 20, 22
Coffee-bean dust,
asthma due to, **117–121**, 127
chemistry and antigen identification, 117–118
clinical presentation and diagnosis of, 120
epidemiology and etiology of, 118–120
historical perspective of, 117
treatment of, 120–121
Coffee-bean sacks, dust contaminant of, 118, 127
Coir, byssinosis from exposure to, 80
Coleoptera, allergic reactions to, 218–219
Colophony, occupational asthma associated with, 97–100
Confidence intervals, for pulmonary function testing, 22–23
Congestive heart failure, and hyperresponsiveness, 47
Contact lenses, and building-related eye irritation, 245
Copper exposure, metal fume fever from, 187
Cork, suberosis from bark dust of, 102
Corticosteroids, effect on asthmatic response, 42, 46
to block hyperreactivity, 38
Cosmetologists, occupational asthma in, 200–201
Cotton dust, antigens in, 81–82
byssinosis from exposure to, 78, 80
Cotton textiles, castor oil for preparation of, 121
Cottonseed allergy, 83
Crack, use of, and the development of occupational asthma, 270
Cricket exposure, asthma secondary to, 215–218
Cromolyn sodium, effect on asthmatic response, 42, 45–46
to block hyperreactivity, 38
Cross-reactivity, among grain antigens, 109–110
Cutting fluids, castor oil for preparation of, 121

Dermatitis, atopic, 289
building-related, 245–246
from exposure to epoxy resin, 191–192
from exposure to formaldehyde, 158–159
Dermatophagoides pteronyssinus, allergic reaction to, 215, 221
Detergent industry, exposure to alcalase in, 171–173
Dialysis-associated formaldehyde infusion, 164

Diamines, asthma associated with, 190, 192–194
Diamond polishers, cobalt exposure in, 184
Diazonium compounds, asthma from exposure to, 200
Diethylenediamine, sensitivity to, 195
Diffusing capacity, for carbon monoxide, 26
Diisocyanates, asthma from, testing for, 291
Dimethyl ethanolamine, asthma associated with, 194
Diptera, allergic reactions to, 220
Disability, 13. See also Pulmonary disability
dyspnea, 31
patient motivation, 31
permanent, 299
reversible disease, 31–32
Disinfectants, asthma following exposure to, 207–208
Documentation of the Threshold Limit Values and Biological Exposure Indices, 289
Dogs, allergy to, 226, 228–229
Doll R, 4
Douglas fir dust, asthma in workers exposed to, 92
Dover's powder, 3
Drug abuse, and the development of occupational asthma, 270
Drugs, inhaled, asthma from, **205–211**
Dyes, asthma from, 145–146, 198–200, 316

Egg-processing workers, asthma in, 125–126
Electrocardiographic machines, exposure to ink aerosol with, 199–200
Electronic workers' asthma, 97–100
Emotional factors, in asthma, 46–47
Emphysema, and small-airways disease, 68
coal mining exposure and, 71
definition of, 63
Endotoxins, as cause of byssinosis, 81–82
Environmental illness. See Building-related illness *or* Chemical sensitivity
Enzyme-induced occupational asthma, 172
Enzymes. See Proteolytic enzymes
Eosinophils, elevated, and evaluation of occupational asthma, 14
Epichlorohydrin, dermatitis from exposure to, 192
Epidemiologic studies of occupational asthma, problems in, 59–61
types of, 57–59
case-control studies, 58
cohort studies, 58–59
cross-sectional studies, 59
descriptive studies, 57–58
experimental studies, 59
Epidemiology, and occupational asthma, **55–62**
history of, 3–4
Epoxy resins, acid anhydrides and, 145
allergens in, 192
amine-based, asthma associated with, **189–196**
chemistry of, 190–191
hardeners and, 145, 190–191, 193
health effects of, 191–196
dermatitis, 191–192
respiratory irritation and sensitivity, 192
historical perspective of, 189–190
industries using, 192
occupational asthma from production of, 146–148
Ethylene diamine-induced asthma, 193–195
Exercise testing, assessing pulmonary disability with, 29, 30, 36
Exposure. See Occupational exposure
Eye irritation, building-related, 245–246
from exposure to formaldehyde, 158

Face masks, protective, 284–285, 296
Fair Labor Standards Acts of 1938, 6
Farmer's lung disease, 276
Farr, William, 4
Federal Coal Mine and Safety Act of 1969, 6
Federal Employee Health Service Act of 1941, 6
Federal Mine Inspection Act of 1941, 6
FEF_{25-75}, 20
    coefficient of variation in, 22–23
    normal values for, 22–23
Fertilizer, use of pomace as, 121
FEV_1, 20
    coefficient of variation in, 22–23
    normal values for, 23
    to measure bronchoconstrictor response, 45
FEV_T, 20
Fiberglass-exposed workers, risk of asthma in, 56
Fire retardants, himic anhydride in production of, 149
Fireplace inserts, indoor pollution from, 257–258
Flax dust exposure, byssinosis from, 77, 78–79
Flea, allergy to, 216, 221
Fleischer WE, asbestos and, 5
Floral industry, occupational asthma in, 103, 317
Flour, allergens in, 108. *See also* Bakers' asthma
Food industry workers, asthma in, **125–130**, 175, 317.
    See also Bakers' asthma
Forced expiratory maneuver, 20
Forced vital capacity, 20–24
    coefficient of variation in, 20–23
    normal values for, 23
    unacceptable performance of, 23
Forest workers, hypersensitivity pneumonitis in, 102
Formaldehyde, as a carcinogen, 165
    as an immunogen, 163–164
    chemical and physical properties of, 153–154
    chemical sensitivity to, 258–259
    concentrations of, 155
    distribution and exposure to, 154–157
    indoor sources of, 156–157
    major species and their application, 154
    neurotoxic reactions to, 164–165
    occupations with exposure to, 157
    pathophysiologic reactions to, 163–165
    physical effects of exposure to, 157–158
        annoyance reactions, 157–158
        dermatologic reactions, 158–159
        ocular and mucous membrane irritation, 158
        respiratory symptoms, 159–163
    product uses of, 157
    smoking as source of, 156
    systemic reactions to, 164
    vehicular emissions and, 155
Formaldehyde asthma, **151–170**
    clinical evaluation of, 165–166
    historical perspective of, 151–153
Formalin, 153
    respiratory disease from exposure to, 159–160
Foundry workers, occupational asthma in, 134–135
Frogs, allergy to, 229
Fruit fly, asthma due to, 220
Fungi, building-related allergy to, 243–244
FVC, 20
    coefficient of variation in, 22–23
    normal values for, 23
FVC maneuver, acceptability, reproducibility and test
    failure in, 23–24

Galen, 2
Gardeners, asthma secondary to moth exposure in, 213

Garlic dust occupational asthma, 127
Gasoline fumes, and building-related illness, 246
Gerbils, allergy to, 229, 230
Goats, allergy to, 229
Grain dust, bakers' asthma from exposure to, **107–111**
Grain dust allergy, 221
Grain dust fever, 110, 114
Grain dust-induced asthma, 112–115
    antigen identification and pathophysiology of, 113–114
    epidemiology and etiology of, 112–113
    evaluation and treatment of, 114–115
Grain handlers' asthma, 112–115
Grass species, bakers' asthma and, 109–110
Graunt, John, 3
Guar gum, occupational asthma associated with,
    101–102
Guinea pig, allergy to, 228
Gum acacia, occupational asthma associated with, 101
Gum arabic, printers' asthma due to, 101

Hairdressers, occupational asthma in, 200–201, 317
Hamilton, Alice, 6
Handicap, meaning of, 29
Hard-metal workers' asthma, 184–185
Hardwood dust, 96–97
Health hazard, definition of, 288
Health questionnaire, 302–313
Heart failure, and hyperresponsiveness, 47
Hemlock dust, asthma in workers exposed to, 92
Hemp dust exposure, byssinosis from, 79
Henna, asthma from exposure to, 201
Hexamethylene-diisocyanate. *See* Isocyanates
Hill AB, 4
Himic anhydride, 149
Hippocrates, 1
Histamine inhalation challenge, 36–38
History, medical, 284–287
    questionnaire for, 302–313
    occupational, 284–287
    of occupational medicine, **1–7**
Hogs, allergy to, 229
Honeybee, occupational asthma to, 128, 221
Horse amniotic fluid, contact dermatitis to, 230
Horses, allergy to, 2, 229
Hot pepper workers, occupational asthma in, 128–129
House dust mites, allergy to, 215, 221
House fly, allergy to, 220
Humidifier fever, building-related, 242–243, 244
Humidity, in workplace, skin and ocular problems
    associated with, 245
Hydrogen peroxide, dermatitis and asthmatic reactions
    during production of, 200–201
Hymenoptera, allergic reactions to, 220–221
Hyperreactive state, 37
Hyperreactivity. *See* Airway hyperreactivity
Hypersensitivity, immune, 256
Hypersensitivity pneumonitis, building-related, 241–242
    diagnosis of, 140
    following exposure to isocyanates, 135–136
    wood dust-induced, 102
Hypertonic saline, inhalation challenge with, 36
Hyperventilation, in sick-building syndrome, 248

Immune hypersensitivity, 256
Immunodeficiency, environmentally induced, 260
Immunogens, by occupation, 314–319
Immunologic bronchoconstriction, 276
Immunologic testing, for occupational asthma, 290–292

Immunotherapy, and bronchial hyperresponsiveness, 39, 43
Impairment, definition of, 28-29, 72-73
  meaning of, 13
  vs. disability, 13
Incidence, 56
Industries, immunogens and irritants present in, 289, 314-319
Inert ingredients, meaning of, 288
Infectious diseases, differential diagnosis of chemical sensitivity and, 261
Inflammatory bronchoconstriction, 274
Inhalation challenge, with nonantigens, 35-36. *See also* Allergen inhalation challenge
  safe procedure for, 43-44
Ink aerosol, asthma from inhalation of, 199-200
Insect allergy, inhalant. 128
Insect-induced asthma, **213-223**
  chemistry and antigen identification in, 215-216
  clinical presentation of, 216-217
  epidemiology of, 214-215
  historical perspective of, 213-214
  pathophysiology of, 215
  to coleoptera, 218-219
  to diptera, 220
  to hymenoptera, 220-221
  to lepidoptera, 219-220
  to orthoptera, 217-218
  occupations with, 214
  treatment of, 221-222
Insulation. *See* Urea-formaldehyde foam insulation
Interstitial lung disease, airflow obstruction in, 25-26
Intoxication syndromes, 246, 256-257
Ipecacuanha, asthma following exposure to, 3, 209
Irritants, by occupation, 314-319
Irritational syndromes, 256
Isocyanate asthma, 100, **131-143**, 277, 296
  diagnosis of, 140
  dose response and, 134
  industrial studies of, 134-135
  natural history and outcome of, 138-139
  pathophysiology of, 136-138
    immunologic hypotheses and, 136-138
    pharmacologic studies and, 138
  prevention of, 140-141
  testing for, 291
Isocyanates, chemistry of, 131-132, 133
  history of, 131
  hypersensitivity pneumonitis following exposure to, 135-136
  industrial hygiene recommendations for, 140-141
  occupations with exposure to, 132
  pulmonary effects of exposure to, 133, 135
  toxicity of, 132-134
Isoniazid, asthma following exposure to, 207

Jute, byssinosis from exposure to, 79-80

Kapok, byssinosis from exposure to, 79
Karaya gum, occupational asthma associated with, 101

Labor Management Relations Act of 1947, 6
Laboratory studies, of occupational asthma, 14, 290-292
Lacquer handlers, exposure to ethylene diamine by, 193-194
Late-phase response, to allergens, 41-43, 272-274
Late respiratory systemic syndrome, 147, 148
Latency period of disease, following exposure, 4-5

Latex, occupational allergy to, 196-198
  products containing, 197
Laundry workers, exposure to alcalase in, 171-173, 318
Laxative preparations, asthma following exposure to, 209
Lead, as work-related disorder, history of, 1
Legionnaire's disease, 244
Lepidoptera, allergic reactions to, 215, 216, 219-220
Leukotrienes, inhalation challenge with, 36
Lidocaine, aerosolized, effect on asthmatic response, 46
Litigious patient, 262
Locusts, asthma from exposure to, 214, 215, 217
Loggers, asthma in, 213, 219
Logistic regression, 56
Lung volumes and capacities, measurement of, 25-26

Macrolide antibiotics, asthma from, 206-207
Maggots, asthma from exposure to, 220
Maple bark strippers' disease, 102
Marijuana use, and development of occupational asthma, 270
Masks, protective, 284-285, 296
  grain handlers and, 114-115
Mass hysteria, in sick-building syndrome, 248
Material Safety Data Sheets, 263, 285-286, 288-289
May flies, sensitivity to, 221
Mealworms, sensitivity to, 215, 218, 219
Meat tenderizers, asthma and, 174
Meatwrapper's asthma, 146, 201-202
Medical history, and evaluation of occupational asthma, 284-287
  questionnaire for, 302-313
Medical records, review of, 288
Medications, influence of, on pulmonary function tests, 45-46
Menstrual cycle, and asthma, 47
Mercury vapor, pneumonitis from, 187
Metabolic disorders, differential diagnosis of chemical sensitivity and, 262
Metal fume fever, 186-187
Metal salts, asthma due to, **179-188**
Metal workers, platinum sensitivity in, 179-181
Metals, asthma due to, **179-188**
Methacholine challenge testing, 26-27, 35-36, 37, 47, 292, 295
Methyl blue, asthma from exposure to, 199-200
Methyldopa powder, asthma following exposure to, 210
Methylene diphenyl-diisocyanate. *See* Isocyanates
Midges, allergy to, 220
Mill workers, asthma in, 213, 219
Mineral dust small-airways disease, 67, 68
Mining, asthma from, 2
Mites, allergy to, 221, 243-244
Monkeys, allergy to, 229
Mortality ratio, standardized, 56
Mosquitoes, allergy to, 220
Moths, asthma from exposure to, 213, 215-217, 219-220
Mouse, allergy to, 227-228
Mucous gland hypertrophy, 63
Mucous membrane irritation, from exposure to formaldehyde, 158
Mushroom worker's lung, 128, 276
Mushrooms, dried, asthma from, 128

Nasal passage irritation, from exposure to formaldehyde, 158
National Institute for Occupational Safety and Health (NIOSH), 6

National Labor Relations Act of 1935, 6
Nedocromil, effect on asthmatic response, 42
Neurologic sequelae, exposure to, 132–133
Neuropsychologic evaluation, of patient with
    occupational disease, 287
Neutrophils, toxic effects of, 66
Nickel, occupational asthma from, 185
Nifedipine, effect on asthmatic response, 46
Nonspecific bronchial hyperreactivity, 292
Nonspecific bronchial reactivity, 26–28
Northern fowl mite, allergy to, 221

Occupational asthma, atopy and, 269
  bronchial hyperreactivity and, 271
  bronchial provocation studies for, 26–28, **34–54**, 272,
      293, 295–296
  cause and effect, 298–299
  chronic, 276–277
  de novo pure, 297–298
  definition of, 13, 60, 268–269, 283
  diagnosis of, 13–14
      pitfalls in the, 297–299
  drug abuse and, 270
  epidemiology and, 55
  evaluation of, 14–16, **283–319**
      assessment of workplace and recommendations,
          11–13, 296–297
      bronchial provocation studies, 14–15, 295
      chest radiographs, 14, 292
      laboratory studies, 14, 290–292
      medical and occupational history, 13–14, 284–287,
          302–313
      physical examination, 14, 289–290
      pulmonary function testing, 14–15, 292–294
      review of medical records, 288
  immunologic mechanisms in, 283
  infection and, 270–271
  laboratory tests for, 14, 290–292
  late-phase response, 272–274
  measurement of, 60
  mechanisms of damage in, 274–276
      immunologic bronchoconstriction, 276
      inflammatory bronchoconstriction, 274
      pharmacologic bronchoconstriction, 275
      reactive airways dysfunction syndrome,
          274–275
      reflex bronchoconstriction, 275–276
  other respiratory conditions and, 268
  pathogenesis and natural history of, **267–281**
  pathogenic mechanisms of, 272–273
  permanent disability from, 299
  physical examination for, 289–290
  physician's report of, 15–16
  pitfalls in diagnosis of, 297–299
  predisposing factors in the development of,
      269–272
  preexisting asthma and, 298
  preexisting conditions and, 268
  prevalence of, 56, 267–268
  prognosis in, 276–277
  pulmonary function testing for, 14–15, 292–294
  role of physician in assessing, 13–16
  smoking and, 270
  studies of, 59–61
  transient symptoms of, 298
  variants of, 297
  workers' compensation and, **9–17**
Occupational bronchitis, **63–75**
  See also Bronchitis

Occupational disease, definition of, 10–11
  workers' compensation for, 10
Occupational exposure, and asthma, 61
  measurement of, 60–61
Occupational history, and evaluation of occupational
    asthma, 284–287, 302–313
Occupational lung disease, role in physician in
    assessing, 13–16
Occupational medicine, development of, 5–6
  history of, **1–7**
Occupational Safety and Health Act of 1970, 6–7
Occupational safety laws, history of, 5
Occupations, immunogens and irritants present in, 289,
    314–319
Ocular disease, building-related, 245–246
Odds, ratio, 56
Odors, aggravation of asthma by, 243–244
Oligomers, dermatitis from exposure to, 191–192
Organophosphate intoxication, building-related, 246
Orthoptera, allergic reactions to, 217–218
Oyster workers, sea squirt-induced asthma in, 127

Pancoxin, asthma following exposure to, 210
Pancreatic extract, exposure to, 177
Papain-induced allergy, 173–175
Paracelsus, 2
Paraformaldehyde, 153–154
Paraphenylenediamine exposure, asthma from, 194
Particleboard, asthma from exposure to urea-
    formaldehyde in, 160–161
PC_{20}, 27, 35
Peak expiratory flow rates, 24–25, 293
Pepper, hot, asthma from, 128–129
Period prevalence, 56
Permanent disability, occupational asthma and, 299
Perkin WH, 4
Persulfate-induced allergy, 200–201
Pesticides, and building-related illness, 246–247
Pet food manufacturing workers, allergy in, 220
Pharmaceutical workers, asthma due to inhalation of
    antibiotics and other drugs by, **205–211**
      bromelain-induced asthma in 175
      guar gum-induced asthma in, 101–102
      papain-induced asthma in, 174
      trypsin-induced asthma in, 176
Pharmacologic bronchoconstriction, 275
Phenothiazine tranquilizers, exposure to piperazine in
    manufacture of, 195
Photocopying paper, diazonium chloride in production
    of, 200
Photodermatitis, from exposure to formaldehyde, 159
Photographic workers, platinum sensitivity in, 179–181
Phthalates, and asthma, 276
Phthalic anhydride, asthma secondary to, 145–147
Physical examination, for occupational asthma, 14,
    289–290
Physician, report of, following assessment for
    occupational asthma, 15–16
  role in assessing occupational lung disease, 13–16
Pigeon breeders' disease, 229–230, 276
Pimaric acid, 97
Pine resin, occupational asthma associated with,
    97–100
Piperazine, asthma following exposure to, 208–209
  cutaneous and respiratory sensitivity to, 195
  use in rubber production, 196
Plant pollens, occupational asthma to, 103
Plant-derived materials, occupational asthma secondary
    to, 103

Plastics industry, exposure to amine-based epoxy resins in, 189–196
  occupational asthma in, 146–147, 318
Platelet activating factor, 42
Platinum salts, asthma due to, 179–181
Plicatic acid, and western red cedar asthma, 88, 90, 92–95, 276
Pliny the Elder, 2
Point prevalence, 56
Pollens, occupational asthma to, 103
Polyamine hardeners, health effects of, 192–195
Polyurethane. *See* Isocyanates
Polyurethane-coated wire, asthma from, 100
Polyvinyl chloride, occupational asthma from, 146, 201–202
Pomace, allergic problems associated with, 121–122
Pontiac fever, 244
Potassium aluminum tetrafluoride, asthma in workers using, 183
Potassium persulfate, asthma and dermatitis from exposure to, 200–201
Potroom asthma, 181–184
  criteria for, 183
Poultry food additives, asthma following exposure to, 210
Poultry workers, allergy in, 221
Prednisone, effect on asthmatic response, 42
Pregnancy, airway responsiveness during, 47
Prevalence, 56
Prevention, of chronic bronchitis, 73
Printers' asthma, 100–102, 318–319
Procedures, diagnostic, cost of, 262–264
Prostaglandins, inhalation challenge with, 36
Protease-exposed workers, 172
Protection devices, 284–285
Proteolytic enzymes,
  occupational asthma due to, **171–177**
    alcalase, 171–173
    bromelain, 175
    papain and chymopapain, 173–175
    trypsin, 176
Psychogenic illness, in sick-building syndrome, 248
Psyllium, asthma following exposure to, 209
Public Contracts Act of 1936, 6
Pulmonary disability, 72
  assessment of, 29
  definition of, 13, 28–29
  evaluation and grading of, 28–29
  grading degree of, 29–31
  permanent, occupational asthma and, 299
  problems in evaluation of, 31–32
  vs. impairment, 13
Pulmonary disease-anemia syndrome, 148
Pulmonary function, criteria for grading impairment of, 16
Pulmonary function testing, **19–34**, 44–45
  acceptability, reproducibility and test failure in, 23–24
  choice of, 44–45
  for disability evaluation, 29
  for evaluation of occupational asthma, 14–15, 16
  normality in, 22–23
  of occupational asthma, 292–294

Q fever, 245

Rabbits, allergy to, 227, 228
Radioallergosorbent test (RAST), *See text* under specific entities.

Radiographic examination, and evaluation of occupational asthma, 14
Ramazzini, Bernardino, 2–3
Rat, allergy to, 227–228, 230
Reactive airways dysfunction syndrome, 39, 274–275, 283, 298
Reactive dyes, hypersensitivity to, 198–200
Recreational drug use, and the development of occupational asthma, 270
Red cedar asthma. *See* Western red cedar asthma
Redwood, allergy from, 102
Reflex bronchoconstriction, 275–276
Rehn L, 4
Reid index of bronchial gland enlargement, 64, 67
Resin, definition of, 189
  epoxy, 189–196
  production of, occupational asthma from, 146–148
  synthetic, 151–153
Respiratory disability. *See* Pulmonary disability
Respiratory impairment, 72–73
Respiratory flow, peak, measurement of, 24–25
Rhinoconjunctivitis, building-related, 243–244
Ricin toxin, in castor beans, 122, 123
Risk factors, for occupational asthma, 56–57
Rubber, synthetic, production of, 196
Rubber industry workers, asthma in, 176, 319
Rubber latex, occupational allergy to, 196–198
Rye flour, occupational asthma from exposure to, 109–110

Salbutamol, asthma following exposure to, 210
Screening tests, 57
Screwworm fly, allergy to, 220
Sea squirt-induced asthma, 127
Seafood processing, asthma due to, 126
Sensitivity, meaning of, 57
Serotonin, inhalation challenge with, 36, 37
Sewer filter flies, 220
Sheep, allergy to, 229
Shellac handlers, exposure to ethylene diamine by, 193–194
Shellfish, allergy to, 126
Skin tests, 40
Sick-building syndrome, 238, 240, 246–249. *See also* Building-related illness
  causes of, 247–249
  non-building-related factors and, 240
  psychologic and social factors in, 248
  symptoms of, 246
  volatile organic compounds and, 247–248
Silica, exposure to, and small-airways inflammation, 67
Silkworm, asthma from exposure to, 215, 216, 219
Sisal dust exposure, byssinosis from, 79
Skin irritation, from exposure to formaldehyde, 158–159
Skin testing, for evaluation of occupational asthma, 40, 44, 291
  for diagnosis of byssinosis, 82–83
Small-airways disease, 64, 67–68
Smelting, asthma from, 2
Smoking, and asbestos exposure, 71
  and building-related illness, 243, 247
  and development of chronic bronchitis, 63, 64, 67, 69
  and development of occupational asthma, 83–84, 269, 270, 287, 299
  and occupational lung disease, 12
  and respiratory infection, 270
  and sensitization to occupational agents, 270
  as source of formaldehyde, 156
  effect on course of byssinosis, 82

Smoking *(Cont.)*
   effect on occupational exposures, 71–72
   involuntary, and building-related illness, 247
      exposure to formaldehyde from, 156
   protective masks and, 115
Snow, John, 4
Soaps, castor oil for preparation of, 121
Social habits, influence on long-term health, 287
Social Security Disability Insurance, 30
Soldering fluxes, occupational asthma from, 97–100
Soybean dust, asthma from, 112
Soybean flour, antigens in, 107–108, 110
Specificity, meaning of, 57
Spice workers, occupational asthma in, 129
Spiramycin, asthma from exposure to, 206–207
Spirometry, 15, 19–21, 292–294, 295
   acceptability, reproducibility and test failure in, 23–24
   coefficients of variation in, 20, 22
   definition of, 19
   examples of spirograms, 21
   for disability evaluation, 29
   normal values for, 22–23
   peak flow measurements in, 24–25
Sponge, marine, occupational asthma from, 126
Stainless steel, occupational asthma from, 186
Standard error of the estimate (SEE), 22–23
Standardized mortality ratio, 56
Steel foundry workers, occupational asthma in, 134–135
Storage mite, allergic reaction to, 221
Suberosis, from bark dust of cork, 102
Sudden infant death syndrome, 197
Sunflower pollen, occupational asthma to, 103

Tamarin, allergy to, 229
Tannin, in cotton dust, byssinosis and, 82
Tea dust, asthma due to, 121
Tetrachlorophthalic anhydride, 149
Tetracycline, asthma following exposure to, 207
Textile dust exposure, byssinosis from, 80
Textile workers, byssinosis in, 275
Theophylline, effect on asthmatic response, 45
Throat irritation, from exposure to formaldehyde, 158
Tight-building syndrome, 237, 238, 247
Time-forced expiratory volume (FEV$_T$), 20
Tobacco leaf exposure, 83–84
Tobacco smoke, aldehydes in, 156
   See also Smoking
   composition of, 247
   distribution of, 247
Toluene-diisocyanate, 100, **131–143**
   See also Isocyanates
   occupational exposure limits to, 141
Toxic disorders, differential diagnosis of chemical sensitivity and, 262
Tragacanth-induced asthma, 101
Triethylene, tetramine, asthma associated with, 195
Triggers, asthmogenic, 274

Trimellitic anhydride, 147–149
   asthma caused by, 276
      testing for, 291
   respiratory syndromes associated with, 147
Troleandomycin, to block hyperreactivity, 38
Trypsin, occupational asthma to, 177
Tungsten carbide workers, cobalt exposure in, 184
Turkey red oil, 121

Uranium hexafluoride, occupational asthma from, 186
Urea-formaldehyde,
   in particleboard, asthma from exposure to, 160–161
   foam insulation, asthma from exposure to, 160–162
Urticaria, from exposure to formaldehyde, 159

Vanadium pentoxide, occupational asthma from, 183, 186
Vegetable gum-induced occupational asthma, 100–102
Video display terminals, photodermatitis from, 245
Vinyl chloride fumes, 202
Viral infections, and development of occupational asthma, 270–271
Vitallium, pulmonary fibrosis from, 187
VO$_2$MAX, measures of, 30–31
Volatile organic compounds, sick-building syndrome and, 247–248

Waxworms, asthma from, 218, 219
Weeping fig, allergy to, 103
Western red cedar asthma, 48, **87–95**, 276, 296
   chemistry of, 87–88
   clinical features of, 88–92
   diagnosis of, 291
   pathogenesis of, 92–95
Wheat flour, occupational asthma from exposure to, 109–110
Wood dust-induced hypersensitivity pneumonitis, 102
Wood dusts, occupational asthma from exposure to, **87–106**
Wood pulp workers' disease, 102
Wood species, occupational asthma from, 96
Wood trimmers, hypersensitivity pneumonitis in, 102
Wood-burning, residential, emissions from, 155–156
Woodman's disease, 102
Woodstoves, indoor pollution from, 257–258
   formaldehyde and, 155–156
Workers' compensation, and occupational asthma, **9–17**
   history of, 6
   litigious patient and, 262, 264–265
Workers' compensation act, features of, 9
Work place, assessment of, 296–297
Worm infestations, exposure to piperazine in treatment of, 195

Zinc chloride, pulmonary fibrosis from, 187
Zinc exposure, metal fume fever from, 187
Zookeepers, animal facility and, 231

DATE DUE

DEC 0 9 1998			
JA 2 '99			
OCT 0 7 1999 JUL 17 2008			